# Normal and Abnormal Scrotum

Mohamed A. Baky Fahmy
Editor

# Normal and Abnormal Scrotum

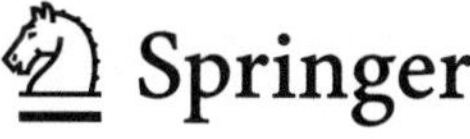 Springer

*Editor*
Mohamed A. Baky Fahmy
Al-Azhar University
Cairo, Egypt

ISBN 978-3-030-83307-7          ISBN 978-3-030-83305-3   (eBook)
https://doi.org/10.1007/978-3-030-83305-3



This Springer imprint is published by the registered company Springer Nature Switzerland AG
The registered company address is: Gewerbestrasse 11, 6330 Cham, Switzerland

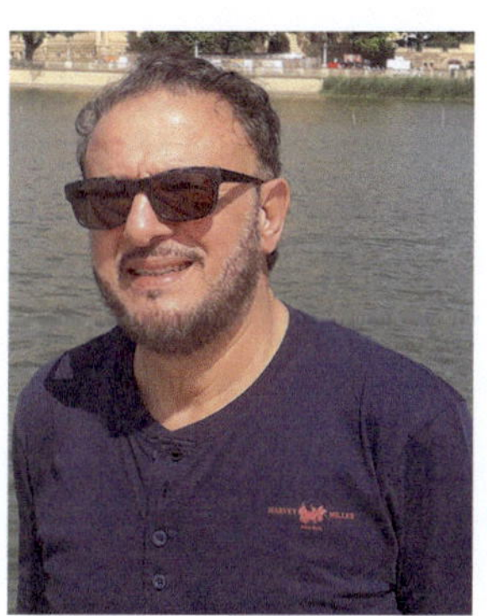

*I wish to dedicate this book with the whole tremendous effort I exerted to bring it to light to my beloved youngest daughter Maha and the soulful youngest son Adam, hoping to trigger both or at least one of them to continue in my hard, long path in pediatric surgery and rare diseases and to join the procession of the strugglers in this field.*

*The Author*

*M A Baky Fahmy*

# Foreword

This book represents a comprehensive review of all aspects of one organ in the human body namely the scrotum and this represents the pursuit of perfection. The editor, doctor Fahmy is to be congratulated on assembling a distinguished group of experts in pediatric surgery and pediatric urology. It is gratifying to see that although some of the surgical techniques which were initiated by plastic surgeons are adopted by pediatric urologists who are now principally concerned with the management of various scrotal surgery. Pediatric urology is one of the most rewarding branches of surgery, it can be exacting and demands meticulous techniques. Being a surgeon who cares for children is a tremendous privilege and we should be grateful for it. As for the scrotal pathology and congenital anomalies, we did not question why these errors of development occur, but arrogantly set out to correct these abnormalities successfully as illustrated in this book.

Moneer K. Hanna, MD, FRCS, FRCS(Ed), FRCS(C)
Clinical Professor of Urology
Institute of Pediatric Urology
Weill-Cornell Medical Center
New York, USA

# Contents

# Contributors

**Gabriela Ambriz-González** Chief of the Department of Pediatric Surgery, Unit of High Specialty, Pediatric Hospital, Medical Center of Western, Mexican Institute of Social Security, Mexico, Mexico

**Mohamed A. Baky Fahmy** Al-Azhar University, Cairo, Egypt

**Lisieux Eyer de Jesus** Fellow Brazilian College of Surgeons, Brazilian Association of Pediatric Surgeons, Pediatric Surgeon Federal Fluminense University and Servidores do Estado Federal Hospital/Ministry of Health, Rio de Janeiro, Brazil

**Francisco Javier León-Frutos** Chief of the Department of Pediatric Surgery, Unit of High Specialty, Pediatric Hospital, Medical Center of Western, Mexican Institute of Social Security, Mexico, Mexico

**Daniel Xavier Lima** Department of Surgery, Faculty of Medicine, Federal University of Minas Gerais, Belo Horizonte, Brazil

**Clécio Piçarro** Department of Surgery, Faculty of Medicine, Hospital das Clínicas, Federal University of Minas Gerais, Belo Horizonte, Brazil;
Division of Pediatric Surgery, Hospital das Clínicas, Federal University of Minas Gerais, Belo Horizonte, Brazil

**Michal Yaela Schechter** Department of Urology, ERN eUROGEN Accredited Centre, Ghent University Hospital, Ghent, Belgium

**Anne-Françoise Spinoit** Department of Urology, ERN eUROGEN Accredited Centre, Ghent University Hospital, Ghent, Belgium

**Alexander Springer** Department of Pediatric Surgery, Medical University Vienna, Vienna, Austria

**Erik Van Laecke** Department of Urology, ERN eUROGEN Accredited Centre, Ghent University Hospital, Ghent, Belgium

# Chapter 1
# Introduction

Mohamed A. Baky Fahmy

One would not guess that the male genitals consisted of anything more than the penis and testicles, as there is a small degree of attention was paid to other part of the male genitals, and bits drawn to scrotum. Scrotum as a structure and its evolution is still inexplicable, attracts and inspired a large and complex literature along the last two decades, but even there is a little progress in providing an adaptive explanation for the scrotal function. Indeed, most workers in the field would still agree with Carrick and Setchell (1977), who lamented that the function of the scrotum "remains something of a mystery" [1]. The conspiracy of silence concerning the role of scrotum in fertility and sexual wellbeing was broken recently by many biologists and psychiatrists, and we will elaborate in this issue in the chapter of scrotal function and the chapter of scrotum in human conscience (Chaps. 3 and 6).

Many textbooks and literature reported testicular anatomy, swellings and other diseases under the title of normal and pathological scrotal issues, but it is very difficult to detect a definitive landmarks between the testicular and scrotal depiction in norm and morbidness, and there is very few bibliographies dedicated exclusively for the scrotum. Despite attention from developmental biologists, reproductive physiologists, and evolutionary biologists, there has been virtually no progress in explaining the wide variability of mammals scrota and little progress achieved in providing an adaptive explanation for the scrotal functions. I think scrotum had both physiological and aesthetic functions, and it may play a pivotal role in sexual conduct not only in human but also in some mammals species, we can recognise the extension of the scrotal development and its essence for masculinity appeal if we can see how much the beauty and fine design of the scrota of some animals like the red-shanked douc and vervet monkeys. (Fig. 1.1).

From the functional point of view; the scrotum's large surface area is the mainstay for the cooling potential provided by this organ, elaborated modifications of local musculature and circulation ensure effective cooling for the testicles. The

M. A. B. Fahmy (✉)
Al-Azhar University, Cairo, Egypt


M. A. B. Fahmy (ed.), *Normal and Abnormal Scrotum*,
https://doi.org/10.1007/978-3-030-83305-3_1

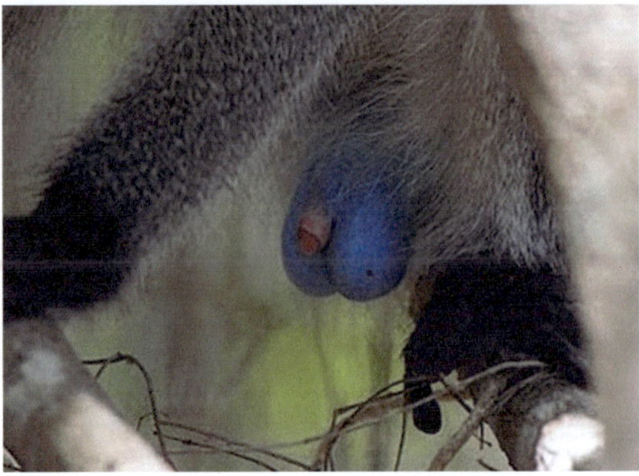

**Fig. 1.1** Vervet monkey Species with blue balls living in Congo. https://upload. wikimedia.org/wikipedia/ commons/a/a8/

3–5 °C temperature differential observed between the scrotum and body core is tightly regulated, chiefly through the action of local scrotal musculature. The tunica dartos and cremaster muscles control the extension of the scrotum in response to temperature; contracting in response to cold and relaxing in response to heat [2].

Scrotal development is fundamentally related to testicular development and its descent; it starts to develop in male fetus from the labioscrotal folds early at the 5th week of intrauterine life after sex differentiation under the influence of the secreted androgen hormone, which produced by fetal Leydig cells (FLC). Normal scrotal development necessities an adequate distribution of androgen receptors and availability of 5-reductase type 2 enzyme [3].

From reviewing the wide spectrum of scrotal anomalies; I could add that the normal scrotal development also necessitates a normally descended testicles, soundly developed abdominal musculature and a well developed caudal area without any intervening embryonic abnormal structure. At delivery of the full term normal male the scrotum is formed of two compartments completely separated by a septum internally and externally at the skin level by a a darker thin line called the median raphe which extend distally from the undersurface of the penis as a penile raphe and caudally as a perineal raphe, the scrotum accommodate a normally descended testicles, with its epididymis. Scrotum is formed of a specially corrugated, well designed thin skin called the scrotal rugosa, which is usually darker than the rest of the body and under this scrotal skin there is a dartos muscle, which is not well studied like other minor body muscles.

Scrotal developmental anomalies are not common and include scrotal hypoplasia, agenesis, ectopic and bifid scrotum; this completely distinguished from other scrotal positional anomalies, which include a wide spectrum of transpositional anomalies, it will be classified and demonstrated distinctly with illustrated cases diagnosed and collected during my practice along the last 40 years. Other rare developmental anomalies which were not reported before will be emphasised in this book; like scrotal dimple, cephalic migration of the scrotum, wide penoscrotal distance and other rarely reported anomalies. I traced all scrotal diseases and anomalies even those reported as a single case report and discussed them all under different headings.

Scrotal reconstruction for congenital abnormalities, trauma, cancer-related extirpation, and aesthetics purpose is a challenging surgery for reconstructive surgeons, at the meantime the scrotal tissues are widely in use to cover penile defects or deformities. Advancements have guided surgical practice while both improved technique and a firm grasp of the reconstructive possibilities have led to fewer complications with improved functional and aesthetic results. So this book will be crucial for demonstrating the proper anatomy and normal anthropometric measures of the scrotal tissues; a separate chapter dedicated solely for the anatomy and anthropometric scrotal dimensions and another for scrotoplasty and its common pitfalls.

As our understanding of genital diseases and anomalies continues to rapidly evolve and advance, this book has been substantially written and incorporates the most current knowledge, understanding, and terminology about the scrotum. This work is designed to provide contemporary, comprehensive, and evidence-based information not only for paediatricians, but also for urologists, pediatric surgeons, plastic surgeons, and other healthcare professionals involved in patient care. In today's era of precision medicine, effective patient care is a collaborative effort requiring medical professionals of various specialties to synthesise new approaches toward pediatric and translational clinical correlations at the patient's bedside.

# References


1. Carrick FN, Setchell BP. The evolution of the scrotum. In: Calaby JH, Tyndale-Biscoe TH, editors. Reproduction and evolution. Canbera: Australian Academy of Science; 1977. p. 165–170.
2. Freeman S. The evolution of the scrotum: a new hypothesis. J Theor Biol 1990; 145:429–445.
3. Hewitt J, Zacharin M. Hormone replacement in disorders of sex development: current thinking. Best Pract Res Clin Endocrinol Metab. 2015; 29:437e447. https://doi.org/10.1016/j.beem.2015.03.002.

# Chapter 2
# Nomenclature and Terminology

**Mohamed A. Baky Fahmy**

**Abbreviations:-**

TV   Tunica Vaginalis
GT   Gubernaculum testis
LC   Lymphangioma circumscriptum

**Accessory scrotum**: Is the rare detection of scrotal skin or scrotal sac outside its normal location, in either the perineum or elsewhere, without an included testicular tissue, in addition to a normally developed scrotum in its normal position,

**Anorchia**: An abnormal physical condition resulting from defective genes or developmental deficiencies characterised by absence of one of both testes, but the term monorchia precisely refer to presence of only one testicle in the scrotum. Anorchidism may have 2 different presentations: true congenital testicular absence, and vanishing of a pre excited testis.

**Beaded Median Raphe "Scrotal pearl"**   Rare cases of brown fine darker nodules replacing the normal smooth line of median raphe, it is rarely reported, and it could be a normal variation.

**Bifid scrotum**: Scrotal midline indentation or cleft with absent scrotal raphe. Bifid scrotum is presented in a wide range of phenotypic forms, and simply classified to partial or complete.

**Buck's fascia**: Deep fascia of the penis, also known as Gallaudet's fascia or fascia of the penis; it is a layer of deep fascia covering the three erectile bodies of the penis and extended to the scrotum. It is a continuation of the deep perineal fascia, but other authors state that it fuses with the tunica albuginea. The name Buck's fascia is named after Gurdon Buck, an American plastic surgeon (1807–1877).

M. A. B. Fahmy (✉)
Al-Azhar University, Cairo, Egypt


M. A. B. Fahmy (ed.), *Normal and Abnormal Scrotum*,
https://doi.org/10.1007/978-3-030-83305-3_2

**Castration:** (Also known as orchiectomy or orchidectomy) is any action, surgical, chemical, or otherwise, by which an individual loses use of the testicles. Surgical castration is bilateral orchiectomy (extirpation of both testicles).

**Cock and ball torture (CBT):** Is a sexual activity involving application of pain or constriction to the penis or the testicles. This may involve directly painful activities, such as genital piercing, wax play, genital spanking, squeezing, ball-busting and other acts.

**Cremaster muscle:** The name of the cremaster muscle is derived from the ancient Greek transitive verb "I hang" (Greek: κρεμάννυμι). It is a thin layer of muscle fibers originating from the internal oblique and transversus abdominis muscles.

**Dartos muscle and fascia:** Sometimes it is also called simply dartos, it is a layer of connective tissue found in the penile shaft, foreskin, and scrotum. The term derived from the Greek δέρνω/derno (beat, flog) and/or δέρμα/derma (skin), meaning "that which is skinned or flayed", possibly due to its appearance.

**Dartos muliebris:** In females, the dartos muscle fibers are less well developed and termed dartos muliebris, it lies beneath the skin of the labia majora, forming a tiny rugae apparent in some females, specially in neonates.

**Ectopic testicles:** A testis is termed ectopic if it lies outside the normal pathway of testicular descent. In contrast to cryptorchidism; ectopic testes have a nearly normal size, the spermatic cord is normal or even longer than normal, and the scrotum may looks well developed.

**Ectopic scrotum:** A rare anomaly characterised by the presence of the normal hemiscrotum away from its normal location; between the penis and the perineum, with deficiency of one hemiscrotum. It is a congenital anomaly in which the scrotum located in a position away from its normal scene.

**Emasculation:** Is the removal of both the penis and the testicles, the external male sex organs, it differs from castration, although the terms are sometimes used interchangeably.

**Fordyce's spots:** A tiny, painless bumps on the scrotum or penile shaft. (also termed Fordyce granules) which are ectopic prominent sebaceous glands, they're totally normal and don't cause any health problems.

**Fournier gangrene:** Is a life-threatening progressive necrotizing fasciitis of the genitalia and perineum, despite the great advances in its treatment, and pathophysiological understanding; it is still carry a great mortality and morbidity rates.

**Gubernaculum:** Gubernaculum testis (GT) is a prenatal cylindrical whitish structure, described for the first time in 1762 by Hunter. Later, it has been described as resembling the Wharton's jelly. The gubernaculum is connected to the caudal part of the male and female mesonephric–gonadal complex during fetal life.

**Haematocele:** Is commonly associated with a history of trauma to the scrotal region, it is a collection of blood inside the potential space between the visceral and parietal tunica vaginalis surrounding the testicle.

**Intertrigo**: Intertrigo is the name given to any dermatosis occurring in skin folds, these sites are especially susceptible to secondary infection, e.g., with *Candida.*

**Kegel exercise**: Kegel exercise known as pelvic-floor exercise, involves repeatedly contracting and relaxing of the muscles that form part of the pelvic floor, sometimes colloquially referred to as the "Kegel muscles", which could be performed multiple times daily.

**Lymphangioma circumscriptum (LC)**: Is a term used for hamartomatous abnormality of the lymphatic channels of the skin, which can be encountered anywhere in the body.

**Lymphangioma scroti**: Large, irregular vascular spaces (similar to cavernous hemangioma and may resembles cysts) lined by one or two layers of flattened, bland epithelial cells with various amounts of fibrous stroma separating the cysts into cavities. Cystic and cavernous lymphangiomas are usually considered the same entity.

**Pampiniform plexus**: (From Latin pampinus, a tendril, and forma, form) is a venous plexus formed of a network of many small veins found in the human male spermatic cord, and the suspensory ligament of the ovary. In male, it is formed by the union of multiple testicular veins from the back of the testis and tributaries from the epididymis. The veins ascend along the spermatic cord in front of the vas deferens. Below the superficial inguinal ring they unite to form three or four veins, which pass along the inguinal canal.

**Penoscrotal fusion**: Is a congenital condition of the male external genitalia, in which the normal insertion of the scrotum at the base of the penis is altered, located higher, along the ventral aspect of the penis, with defective fascial attachment.

**Perineal groove**: Is a sulcus of mucosal tissue with clearly defined margins that can be found in the midline anywhere between the vagina and anus in girls, and rarely reported in boys and if extended anteriorly to involve the scrotum it is considered as a partial bifid scrotum.

**Prepenic muscle**: It is a part of dartos muscle at the root of the penis, the peripenic muscle is composed of unstriped fibers which form an incomplete investment of the penis from its base to the extremity of the prepuce.

**Polyorchia**: Polyorchidism is a rare congenital malformation, characterized by the presence of more than 2 testes in the same individual.

**Pyocele**: Is a purulent collection inside the potential space between the visceral and parietal tunica vaginalis surrounding the testicle and it is often associated with acute epididymoorchitis.

**Raphe**: (/ˈreɪfiː/; from Greek ῥαφή, "seam") plural: raphae or raphes, it has several different meanings in science. In animal anatomy it is used to describe a ridged union of continuous biological tissue. There are several different significant anatomical raphae: like raphe nucleus, buccal raphe, and lingual raphe on the tongue. Raphe means a line of fusion of the two halves of various symmetrical body parts, and in urology the term median raphe refers to the perineal raphe, which is also known as the median raphe of the perineum; and it is divided anatomically to: penile raphe, scrotal and perineal raphae. This line starts just anterior to the anus and extends through the scrotum, continuing on the ventral surface of the penis and prepuce; it is usually darker in colour than the surrounding skin; generally it is deep pink or brown and usually devoid of hair.

**Ruga**: Means a wrinkle, fold, or ridge. Ruga is from the Latin word rūga, it usually used in plural (rugae) . In anatomy, rugae are a series of ridges produced by folding of the wall of an organ. Scrotal rugae is a unique character of the scrotum.

**Scrotum**: In the Middle English the scrotum called "cod". The scrotum or scrotal sac is an anatomical male reproductive structure located caudal to the penis that consists of a suspended dual-chambered sac of skin and smooth muscle. The term is derived from Latin "scrotum", probably transposed from scortum; which means a skin hide.

**Scrotal agenesis**: Congenital scrotal agenesis is the rare scrotal anomaly, and it is characterized by complete absence of scrotal rugae in the perineum between the penis and anus. It is commonly bilateral with an impalpable testicles, but rare cases of unilateral scrotal agenesis are sometimes recognizable.

**Scrotal Asymmetry**: Also known as scrotal ptosis or sagging scrotum. In human male both testicles and the scrotum is clearly asymmetrical in most of the adults, the right scrotum usually being placed higher than its opposite peer.

**Scrotal Calcinosis**: It a skin condition of multiple hard, painless, asymptomatic cutaneous nodules within the scrotal wall and without a detectable abnormalities in the calcium/ phosphorous metabolism.

**Scrotal Dimple**: Is a rare form of minimal partial bifid scrota at the bottom of the scrotum.

**Scrotal Hypoplasia**: Refer to scrotal wall underdevelopment or incompletely developed, the scrotum looks smaller non pendant with a few rugae.

**Scrotal ligaments**: After birth the Gubernaculum testis (GT) is converted to scrotal ligament (SL) , it is located in the posterior lower side of the testis outside of testicular parietal vaginalis.

**Scrotoplasty:** Scrotoplasty, also known as oscheoplasty, is reconstructive surgery to repair or create a new scrotum.

**Scrotal Septum**: Is a vertical layer of fibrous tissue that divides the two compartments of the scrotum. It consists of flexible connective tissue, and its structure extends to the skin surface as the scrotal raphe.

**Scrotal Transposition**: (Shawl scrotum, Prepenile scrotum, doughnut scrotum) In complete penoscrotal transposition (CPST) the base of the penis is entirely covered by the cephalically located scrotum, if only part of the scrotum is located superior to the penis, the term overriding scrotum or partial PST is used instead. In shawl scrotum the superior margins of the scrotum assembled superior to the base of the penis.

**Scrotoschisis:** Is a congenital defect on the scrotal wall through which one or both testes are extruded and become extracorporeal, lying outside the scrotal cavity. The term has been used for testes extruding through scrotum or through an inguinal canal defect, although in this last case; the term **bubonoschisis** would be more appropriate.

**Sebileau's muscle**: Is the deep muscle fibres of the dartos tunica which pass into the scrotal septum. It is named after French anatomist Pierre Sebileau (1860–1953).

**Testicles**: The English words *testis, testiment,* and *testimony* all derive from the Latin root *testari,* meaning to stand and bear witness. Testicle or testis (plural testes) is the male reproductive gland or gonad in all animals, including humans. It is homologous to the female ovary.

**Testicondy**: In biology, testicondy in a species is the condition of having testicles situated within the abdomen as the normal anatomy of that species. Testicondy can be further classified into primary and secondary testicondy.

**Testicular Microlithiasis**: Is a condition involving intratubular calcifications and is typically discovered incidentally on imaging. It is visualized on ultrasound as multiple small echogenic foci disseminated across the testicular parenchyma.

**Transverse Testicular Ectopia** A rare form of ectopic testis, where both testes descend throughout the same inguinal canal and end lodged in the same scrotal pouch.

**Tunica Vaginalis (TV)**: Is the lower end of the peritoneal processus vaginalis. When the fetal testis descends from the abdomen to the scrotum, part of the peritoneum descends with it. This part of peritoneum accompanied with the descending testis is called the peritoneal processus vaginalis.

**Varicocele**: Varicocele is a varicosity of the pampiniform plexus within the upper scrotum. It is very frequent in adults, it affects 15% of the male population.

                                                            

## Further Readings


1. Burdan F, Wojciech Dworzański, Monika Cendrowska-Pinkosz, Maicej Burdan, and A. Dworzańska. Anatomical eponyms unloved names in medical terminology. Folia Morphol. 2016;75(4):413–438.
2. Campbell MF; Wein AJ, Kavoussi LR, McDougal WS, Partin AW, Peters CA, editors. Campbell-Walsh Urology. W.B. Saunders; 2007. p. 65. ISBN 9781416029663.
3. Burdan F, Dworzański W, Cendrowska-Pinkosz M, et al. Anatomical eponyms — unloved names in medical terminology. Folia Morphol. 2016;75(4):413–38. https://doi.org/10.5603/FM.a2016.0012.

# Chapter 3
# Scrotum in Human Conscience

Mohamed A. Baky Fahmy

## 3.1 Scrotum in History

Along the mankind history and throughout different cultures there are a great symbolic value attributed to the male sexual organs, in terms of sexual virility, aggressive threats, procreative power, and moral virtue. Genitalia are a prominent monuments since the Stone Age cave paintings, as it is figured on early Attic vases, the *Herma* columns that decorated ancient Greek houses, and granite phalluses in Medieval churchyards are a good examples. The most prominent feature of these representations is the erect penis; but the testicles are often depicted naturalistically, and are thus accorded their proper place within the male genital system.

From the Neolithic period and the post-glacial period a drawings found in caves in the territory of modern France, where phalluses were depicted, symbolizing the male power and the basis of the genus, these figures are about thirty thousand years old. In Sweden, an images of the Bronze Age were found, in which a hunter with clearly hyperbolic sex organs is clearly visible. It was more recently announced by archeological society that cave art about human-being dated back to 8,000 years ago had been discovered at southern Asia Minor. The primitive human figures involved the phallus pointing the ground almost at the same size with legs [1]. In the Middle Ages, the testicles were often represented by two almonds and the little sac and its contents have played more of a role in human imagination than is reflected in psychoanalytic theory [2]. Herma (Ancient Greek: ἑρμῆς, pl. ἑρμαῖ hermai), commonly called herm in English, is a sculpture with a head and perhaps a torso above a plain, usually squared lower section, on which male genitals may also be carved at the appropriate height, with an obvious well formed scrotum. It is a work by Polyeuktos, at 280 BC.

The Greek classical and pre-classical art, which took great care in its attention to anatomical details, correctly portrayed the right testicle as the higher, but then

M. A. B. Fahmy (✉)
Al-Azhar University, Cairo, Egypt


M. A. B. Fahmy (ed.), *Normal and Abnormal Scrotum*,
https://doi.org/10.1007/978-3-030-83305-3_3

incorrectly portrayed the left testicle as visibly larger. The implication is that the Greeks used a simple mechanical theory, that the left testicle being thought to be lower because it was larger and hence more subject to the pull of gravity [3]. Phidias, the greatest sculptor of antiquity who sculpted divine images of the gods, presented Apollo Parnopios (parnops means locust in ancient Greek) in 450 BCE to thank the god for saving Attica from the locusts that were destroying the crops. The god was presented with an intact penis, scrota and pubic hair. In another bronze status for Apollo at a different period (from 30AC to 313 BC) from the Egyptian museum, one can recognize the intact penis with a precisely designed scrotum (Fig. 3.1a, b).

According to a recent study, an illustrious example of ancient Greek art, is the famous statue the Riace bronzes, also called the Riace Warriors, is a full-size Greek bronzes of naked bearded warrior, casted about 460–450 BC that was found in the sea in 1972 near Riace, Calabria, in Italy, the status was modelled with a reproduction of a left varicocele, which the model was probably suffering from at that time [4]. (Fig. 3.2).

Probably every culture has recognized somehow that the testicles are the essential sine qua non for male gender and masculinity. In the mystery religions of antiquity magical power was attributed to the testicles of rams and bulls to promote male fertility; in certain cannibal tribes of Southeast Africa, male warriors are said to have consumed the testicles of slain enemies to acquire their strength [5]. In the *Zohar* of the Hebrew Kabbala we read that "in the testes are gathered all the oil, the dignity, and the strength of the male from the whole body" [6].

It was suggested that the treatment of the external male genital organs with special care and attention in the mummification process might be derived from the tales of Osiris restored to eternal life when his body was reconstituted by Isis in the Egyptian mythology. That is why a model of the penis and scrotum made of resin

(a)    (b)

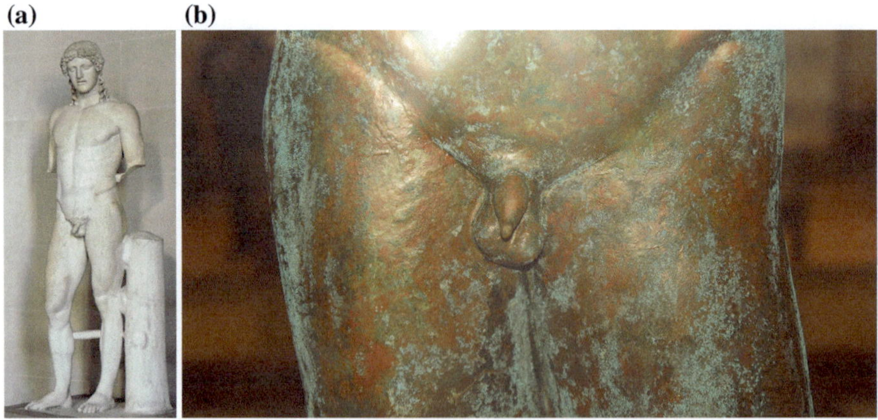

**Fig. 3.1** (**a**) Kassel Apollo, a Roman copy of Apollo Parnopios, second century CE, Louvre, (**b**) Scrotum and the penis of Apollo status in the Egyptian museum, (30 AC–313 BC)

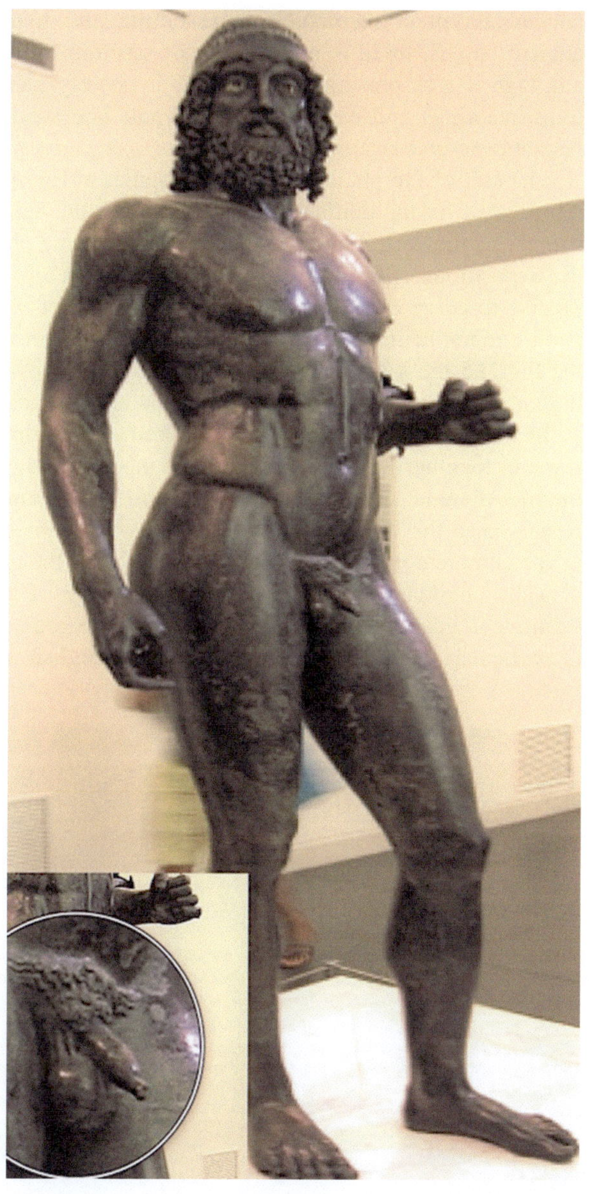

**Fig. 3.2** Riace Warriors status with left varicocele. By Luca Galli - https://www.flickr.com/photos/lucagalli/14936093115/ Bronzo di Riace, CC BY 2.0, https://commons.wikimedia.org/w/index.php?curid=94026571

gilded was laid just below the true external genital organs and kept intact in most adults mummy [7]. (Fig. 3.3) The ancient Egyptians had a rich and varied sexual life, which they found an opportunity to describe in words and pictures. As in the other early primitive civilisations, erotic matters were of prime importance and became an integral part of life. In Pharaonic times, the Egyptians described impotence and recorded several methods to increase the sexual power [8]. In ancient Egyptian medicine, while hernia and hydrocele are well-described in ancient papyri, there is no mention of scrotum and scrotal swellings specifically, although it was presumably detected frequently along other pathologies. Several tomb paintings and reliefs depict servants and workmen with protuberances that resemble scrotal swellings [9].

The cult of the phallus was quite popular in Egyptian ancient mythology and is represented by the deities Ming, Amon Ra, and Asiris. There were legends about the size of the sexual organ of the pharaohs. Some phallic symbols can be found in the expositions of the local history museum in Cairo. In Fig. 3.4 the sculptor is so precise to carve the scrotum of the sandal bearer with a smaller scrota aside the penis and not hanging down as usual, as it may represent a sort of anomalies. But in the Fig. 3.5 the scrota had seen designed precisely with the right side located little higher as a normal finding and the penis is circumcised (Fig. 3.5).

In the Western medical tradition, from Galen through Vesalius, the penis and testicles together were considered to be the standard of perfection against which the internal female genitals were measured and found inferior [10]. During the Renaissance the well-dressed gentleman was adorned with a codpiece emblematic of the complete male genital including not only the erectile power of the penis, but also the abundant seed and nurturant capacity of the testicles. This an obvious example indicating the historical interest of the genitalia in general and the scrotum in particular. The **Codpiece** (from Middle English: cod, meaning "scrotum") is a

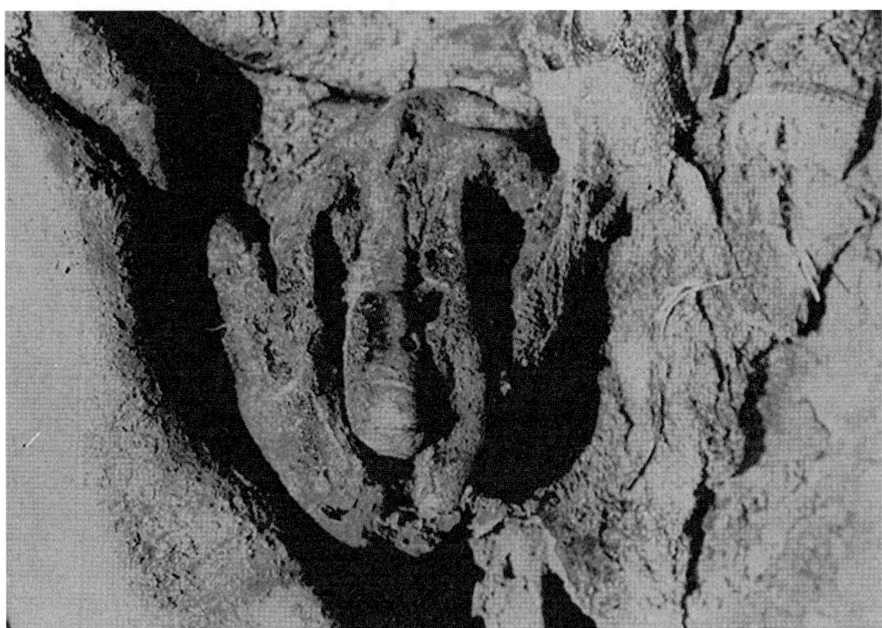

**Fig. 3.3** Anterior view of the mummified external genital organs in the child mummy. The penis and the scrotum including the testes were left intact [7]

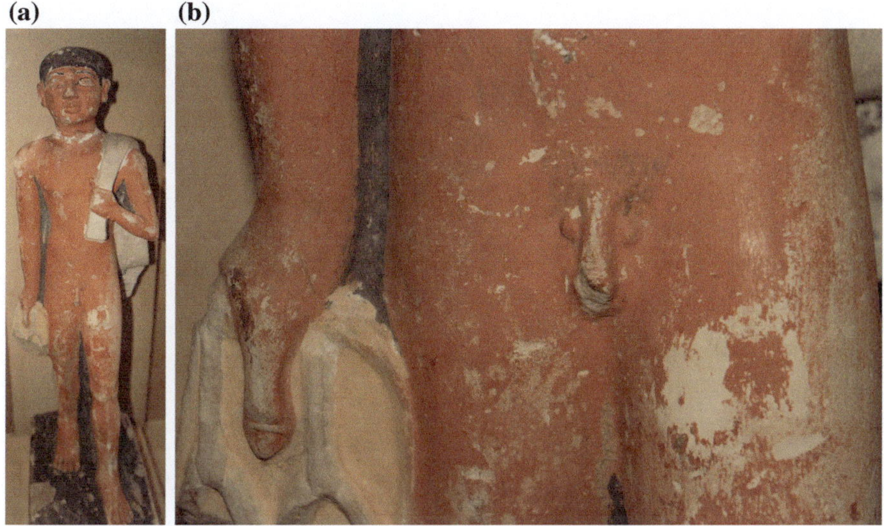

Fig. 3.4  (**a**) Sandal Bearer: Dynasty 5: 2465–2323 BC, Painted limestone, Saqqara Mastaba of Ptahsheps, (**b**) magnification of the genitalia with a small almond like two scrota, located higher at the root of the penis

covering flap or pouch that attaches to the front of the crotch of men's trousers, enclosing the genital area. It may be held closed by string ties, buttons, folds, or other methods. It was an important fashion item of European clothing during the fifteenth and sixteenth centuries, and it reflect the great concern about genitalia [11]. A high spiritual value has also been accorded to the testicles in certain Judea-Christian traditions.

In Biblical times the testicles and scrota had a sacred function; when a man would swear his solemn oath to another, he would first place his hand under the testes. In the Bible the euphemism for testicles is "thigh," so when Abraham exacts a sworn oath from his servant he says, "Put, I pray thee, thy hand under my thigh: And I will make thee swear by the Lord, the God of Heaven" (Genesis 24:1–3). Similarly, the English words *testis, testament,* and *testimony* all derive from the Latin root *testari,* meaning to stand and bear witness. In the Catholic Church the ceremony of enthroning a new pope requires the College cardinals to determine if he has intact genitals: seated on a special marble throne, they must touch his virile parts while pronouncing the formula "Testiculos habet et bene pendentes" (Have testicles and let them hang well) [12].

At 1989, Scott Freeman [13] introduced the adaptive significance of the scrotum after more than 60 years of debate and experimentation, when he published the training hypothesis and suggested that testicular descent and scrotal evolution is a mechanism for improving sperm quality. The hypothesis proposes that: (1) testicular descent decreases blood supply to maturing sperm cells, (2) sperm mitochondria respond to the resulting oxygen stress by enhancing their enzymatic

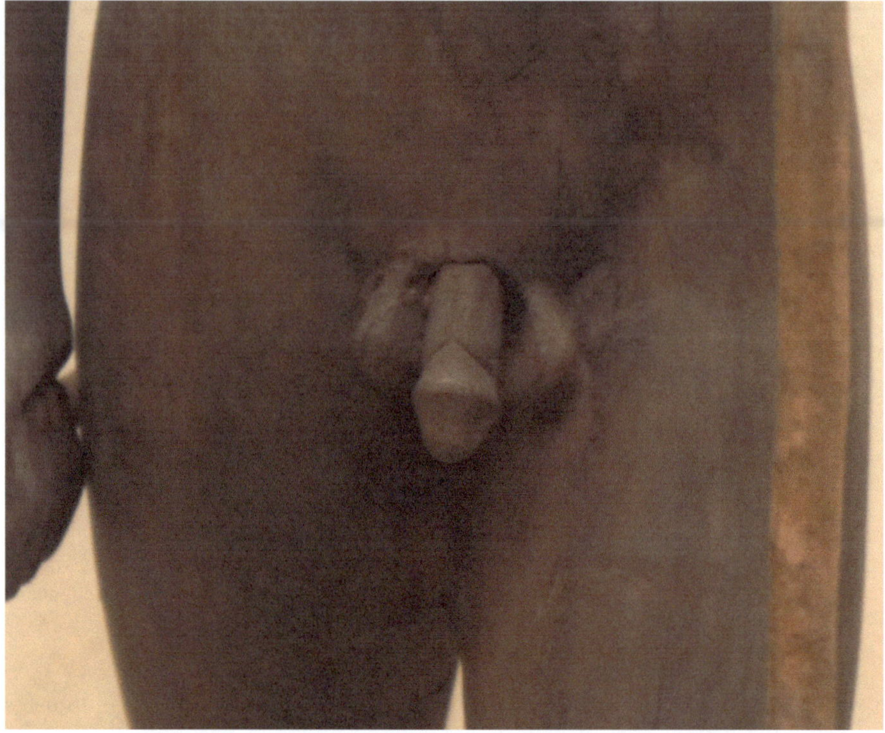

**Fig. 3.5** Statuary present some adult male with a circumcised penis, the right scrotum little bit higher than the left. A few examples of Old Kingdom (2649–2134 B.C.E.). Egyptian museum

machinery for oxidative metabolism, as do oxygen-stressed muscle cell mitochondria, and (3) the resulting increase in aerobic fitness of sperm cells is advantageous in inter-ejaculate competition [13].

## 3.2   Scrotum and Masculine Self-Image

The external position of the testicles in the scrotum is evolved because of their importance in social competition, either as a character in female choice of mates or as a signal of dominance in male-male competition [14]. Pendant scrota containing testes, elongated phallus and rudimentary breasts are the outlines of manliness, and its extension is an avatar of virility. Male body image formation after the phallic stage is a complex emotional and intellectual task involving temporary denial of the inner body and the testicles, it is suggested that a revised account of male sexuality, including both penis and testicles, is a prerequisite for any psychoanalytic theory of gender. Scrotum have an important role in the boys' early feminine identification and bisexuality [15]. Normally, the three factors work together in the same direction to produce an intact core gender identity; the anatomy of the external genitalia, second the infant-parent relationships (the more easily observable components) and the third, which is usually a silent component is a congenitally, inherited biological force [16]. Materials from dreams, folklore, and anthropology all suggest feminine connotations of the testicles and scrotum. Through various symbolic equations the testicles may be paired unconsciously with female breasts, babies, eggs, and uterus. In English, the words balls, nuts, and jewels are used to represent the testicles and scrotum. On the other hand, there is another opinion considering that the symbolism, folklore, and vernacular suggest that the possession of testes and scrotum is a masculine virtue [2]. Probably every culture has recognized somehow that the testicles are essential for male gender and masculinity.

**Testicles as a source of power**: Till 1900 the available scientific data concluded that the ingestion of testicular products could be beneficial as a general bodily tonic and stimulant, "even when all influences of mental suggestion have been excluded. In a remarkable contribution to the history of ideas, Thomas Laqueur at 1990 [17] demonstrated how western thinking has been dominated by the "One Sex Model." According to this viewpoint, the male physical body is assumed to represent the highest level of human development. The female body has exactly the same structure topologically, but is "inside-out" and it is inferior because all the male sexual organs have been retained inside the female body. The vagina is then a kind of unborn penis; the womb is a stunted scrotum; and the ovaries are merely internal testes. In all medical texts until the eighteenth century, the ovaries do not even have a name of their own: their standard designation is "the female testicles."

Romans also mapped male physiology onto female bodies, where the ovaries were women's testicles, the uterus was a deflated scrotum and a weak female 'sperma' was designed to lock in male seed. Adolf Portman (A famous Swiss zoologist) argued that by placing the gonads on the outside, the male was giving a clear indication of his "reproductive pole" a sexual signal important in intergender communication, and his best evidence was a few old world monkeys who have brightly coloured scrota [18]. This theory is not widely accepted because such conspicuous displays are rare (many scrotums are barely visible) and bright coloration seems to have evolved long after the original scrotum. Some have suggested it's not surprising that in its 100 million-year existence, the scrotum has been coopted as a sexual attractant by a handful of groups.


## 3.3  Scrotum and Various Neurotic Symptom

After World War I, Steinach at 1940 [19] pioneered a popular form of vasectomy that was reputed to enhance production of male hormones and thereby ameliorate physical and nervous symptoms.

Male body image formation after the phallic stage is a complex emotional and intellectual task involving temporary denial of the inner body and the testicles.

Finally, it is suggested that a revised account of male sexuality, including both penis and testicles, is a prerequisite for any psychoanalytic theory of gender [19]. Testicular factors may be decisive in various neurotic symptom formations beginning with the early toilet training period. The testicular contribution then takes place along certain preferred pathways of symbolic displacement. Testicular symptoms are observed in many cases of physical and sexual abuse. This finding has application in the treatment of male abuse survivors and to their related sexual dysfunctions.

## 3.4  Scrotum and Castration Psychological Impact

**Castration** (also known as orchiectomy or orchidectomy) is any action, surgical, chemical, or otherwise, by which an individual loses use of the testicles. Surgical castration is bilateral orchiectomy (excision of both testicles). Emasculation is the removal of both the penis and the testicles, the external male sex organs. It differs from castration, although the terms are sometimes used interchangeably. It is not known when castration was first practiced, nor where it was invented, but there are evidences that it was practiced as far back as 4,000 BC based on descriptions in the cult of Ishtar and Uruk (4th millennium BCE). It may have arisen in the Neolithic period in response to animal husbandry, rising populations and population specialisation [20]. Castration was frequently used for religious or social reasons in certain cultures in Europe, South Asia, Africa, and East Asia. At that times after battles, the winners sometimes castrated their captives or the corpses of the defeated to symbolize their victory and seize their power. Over the 13 centuries of the Arab slave trade in Africa, unknown numbers of Africans were enslaved and shipped to the Middle East, most of them were castrated. In 1778, Thomas Jefferson [21] wrote a bill in Virginia reducing the punishment for rape, polygamy or sodomy from death to castration. Over several years the U.S. states have passed laws regarding chemical castration for sex offenders but not one state has mandatory castration.

**Castration anxiety**: Castration anxiety is the fear of emasculation in both the literal and metaphorical sense. In fact, the psychological importance of the scrotum and impaction of its loss along castration has hardly been mentioned. According to Freudian psychoanalysis, castration anxiety can be completely overwhelming to the individual, and can often breach other aspects of their lives. A link has been found between castration anxiety and fear of death. Although differing degrees of anxiety are common, young men who felt the most threatened in their youth tended to show a sort of chronic anxiety, because the consequences are extreme, the fear can evolve from potential disfigurement to life-threatening situations [22].

## 3.5  Scrotum at Early Toilet Training

The earliest situation where testicle problems appear is that of toilet training of boys. Anita Bell at 1964 believed that the common toileting phobias which occur in boy toddlers may be complicated by testicular castration anxieties. She provided three reports of toddlers who suffered toilet phobias along with constipation and nervous anxieties. In each case the symptoms were not fully removed until the parents explained to their boys the nature of testicle retractions and reassured him that his testicles were perfectly safe [23]. It is well-known that for boys at the toddler period there may be a multiple intersection of anxieties connected to toileting, castration, and separation. This is also when toilet training heightens testicular anxiety, and it is natural that the loss and return of the testicles might symbolize the interpersonal back- and-forth of rapprochement, this could be more obvious with children suffering from the physiological retractile testicles.

## 3.6  Scrotum and Cryptorchidism

Surgeons commonly ignoring the scrotal status during their attempts to do orchidopexy or during performing other genital surgery like hypospadias repair, some surgeons may not paying the optimum attention to the scrotal shape and may not considering how the scrotum aesthetically looks after orchidopexy. The pediatric literature recently has recognized the significance of the scrotum, not only medically but also psychologically as well. Research on congenital genitourinary anomalies, DSD and hypogonadism has made its contribution to the understanding of the significance of the scrotum. One often recognizes the importance of an organ only when it is faulty or missing, like the good health. The true nature of the psychologic importance of the testes and the scrotum is illustrated by studying cases which lost that organs either congenitally or post-traumatically. Generally the cryptorchid boys do not tend to be gender-disordered, effeminate, or prehornosexual, but some children who are suffered from congenital genitourinary anomalies, in general and cryptorchidism specifically, may grow up with a social inadequacy and indecision, as noted early by Blos at 1960 [24]. Smith and Lattimer at 1975 [25] found that many emotional problems exist in children lacking one or both testes in the scrotum. But they were impressed with the resolution of these personality deficiencies in children after successful orchiopexy. The best time for surgery for orchidopexy should be performed at or near 1 year of age. Emotional, cognitive, and body image development may be affected profoundly by both the genital deformity and the reconstructive surgery. Psychological factors are of considerable importance, in that a child's reaction to both the surgery and the anaesthetic trauma, which varies dramatically with age. Postoperative behavioral problems such as aggressive or regressive behavior, night terrors, and anxiety may be more common at certain ages, particularly at 1 to 3 years of age [26]. The cosmetic and psychologic sense of genital completeness is so vital that many surgeons may implanted artificial testes when a normal testis was not available at surgery, in both children and adults. Many cases of cryptorchidism are associated with defective or even hypoplastic scrotum, and of less minority; the scrota may be obviously look asymmetrical, all these factors should be considered during orchidopexy, it is the child's rights to have an aesthetic and symmetrically looking scrota. It is not acceptable from any surgeon to leave a child after orchidopexy or hernia repair with a puffy scrotum or to keep the scrotum ended with a bothersome marks or an ugly scar. (Fig. 3.6).

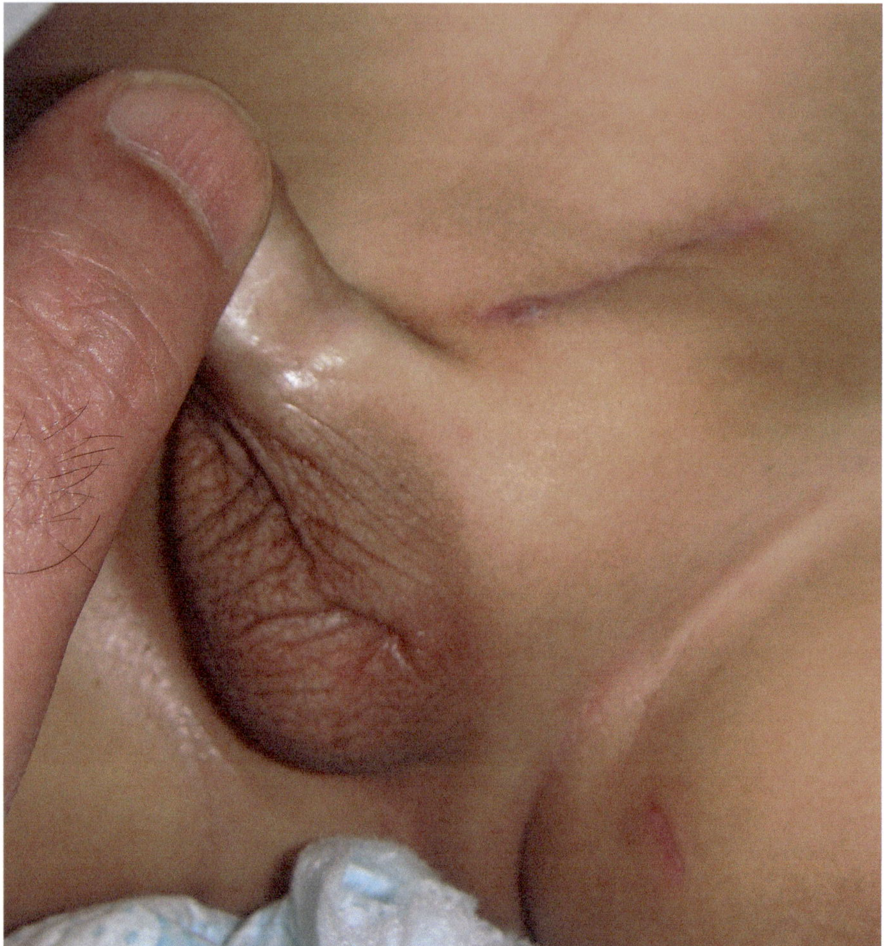

**Fig. 3.6** A 3 years old child with a long left inguinal scar and a scrotal dimple after a non aesthetic orchidopexy

## 3.7  Role of Scrotum in Masturbation and Sexual Activity

Current psychophysiological research rarely studies the role of the scrotal sac and testes in male sexual arousal, in many sexology and andrology literature one may don't find any articles on the psychological role of the testicles in male sexual dysfunction [27]. Masturbation involving the testicles is not infrequent in young boys; the most common practice consists of rubbing and moving the testes inside the inguinal region. Masturbation in latency age boys may include manual manipulation of the scrotum and anus: these sensations, though imbued with an undercurrent of excitation, are primarily experienced as soothing. There is reason to suppose that at least one form of such activity is not uncommon in childhood [28].

**Scrotum and improving sexual arousal**: While some men may be aroused by the feeling of being "owned", the physical feeling of stretching the ligaments suspending the testicles has an effect similar to the more common practice of stretching one's legs and pointing the toes [29]. Preventing the testicles from lifting up so far that they become lodged under the skin immediately adjacent to the base of the penis, is a condition which can be very uncomfortable, especially if the testicle is then squashed by the slap of skin during thrusting in sexual intercourse. Some males may delaying or intensifying ejaculation by preventing the testicles from rising normally to the "point of no return", it is an act to keep reaching an orgasm is harder [15]. Scrotum had a pivotal role in non-penetrative sex; as manual stimulation of a partner's penis, scrotum, clitoris or entire vulva are known as "wanking" in the UK, and "fapping" in modern colloquial terms. Also, the "handjob" is the manual sexual stimulation of the penis or scrotum by a person.

**There are many clinical references to erotic activity involving the testicles and the scrotum:**

**Cock and ball torture (CBT)**, is a sexual activity involving application of pain or constriction to the penis or testicles. This may involve directly painful activities, such as genital piercing, wax play, genital spanking, squeezing, ball-busting, genital flogging, urethral play, tickle torture, erotic electrostimulation, kneeing or kicking. The recipient of such activities may feels a direct physical pleasure via masochism, or emotional pleasure through erotic humiliation. It may be performed using toys and devices to make the penis and testicles more easily accessible for attack, or for foreplay. Many of these practices usually carry a significant health risks [30]. During doggy style, the scrotum sometimes play a role by provides friction to the partner vulva and clitoris, thus possibly producing an orgasm or sexual stimulation [31].

**Ball stretcher:** A metal ball stretcher and cock ring, which forces penis' erection is in use in some countries. A ball stretcher is a sex toy that is used to elongate the scrotum and provide a feeling of weight pulling the testicles away from the body. This can be particularly enjoyable for the wearer as it can make an orgasm more intense, as testicles are prevented from moving up. Intended to make one's testicles permanently hang much lower than before (if used regularly for extended periods of time), this sex toy can be potentially harmful as the circulation of blood can be easily cut off if over-tightened [32]. (Fig. 3.7) While leather stretchers are most common, other models consist of an assortment of steel rings that fastens with screws, causing additional but only mildly uncomfortable weight to the wearer's testicles. The length of the stretcher may vary from 1–4 inches. A more dangerous type of ball stretcher can be home-made simply by wrapping rope or string around one's scrotum until it is eventually stretched to the desired length.

**Ball crusher:** A ball crusher is a device made from either metal or often clear acrylic that squeezes the testicles slowly by turning a nut or screw. The testicle clamped tightly depending on the pain tolerance of the person using it. A ball crusher is often combined with bondage, either with a partner or by oneself.

**Scrotal Parachute:** A parachute is a small collar, usually made from leather, which fastens around the scrotum, and from which weights can be hung. It is conical in shape, with three or four short chains hanging beneath, to which weights can be attached. Parachute used as part of cock and ball torture within a BDSM relationship (Sexual practices or activities involving bondage, discipline, sadism, masochism, or acts of domination and submission), the parachute provides a

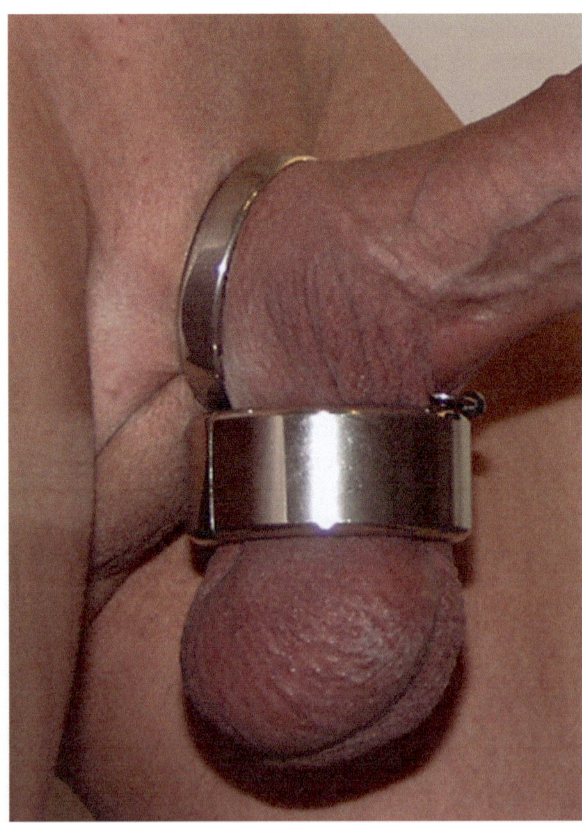

**Fig. 3.7** The penile and scrotal ring, if it is tight enough, strengthens and lengthens the erection, as the veins that supply the penis and the erectile tissue with blood are constricted

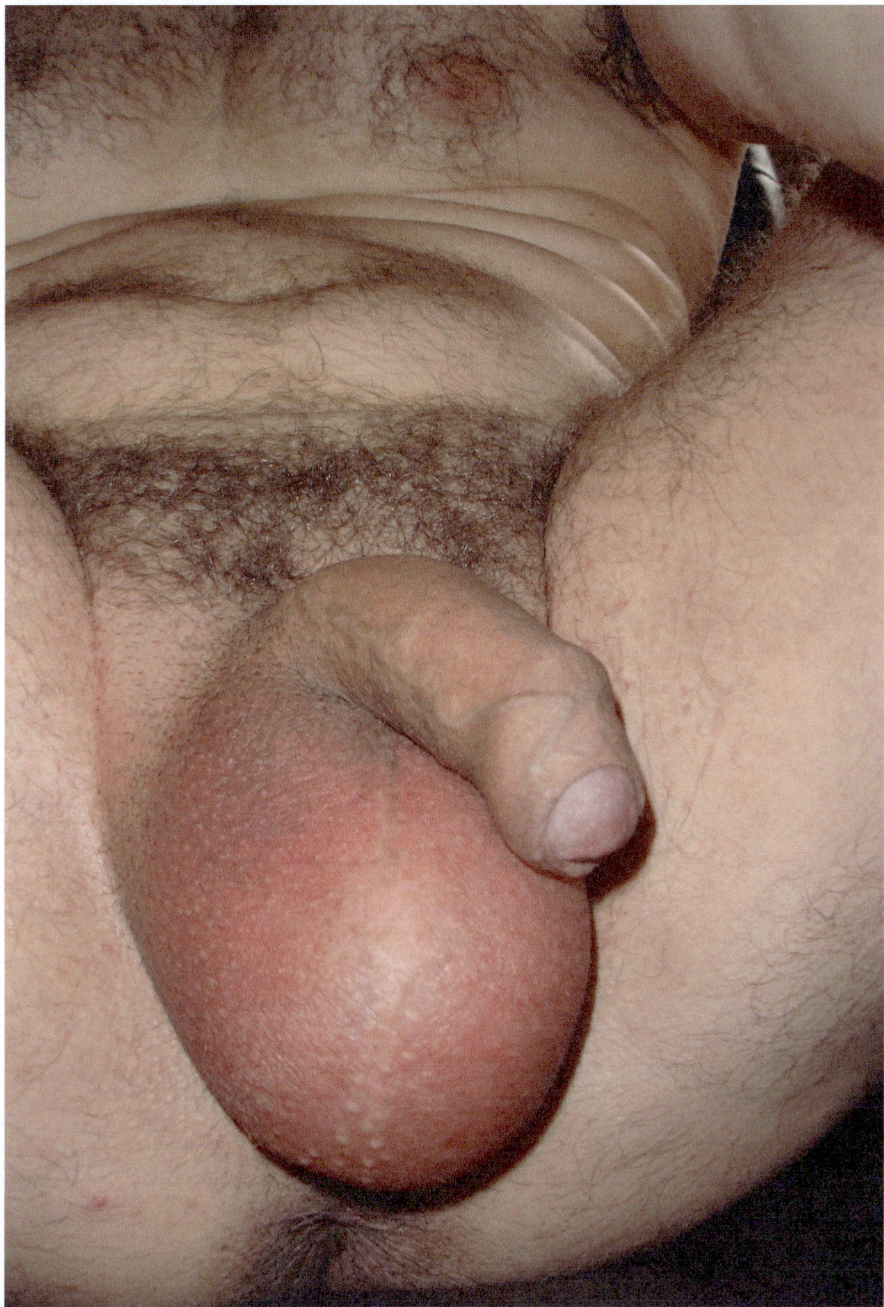

**Fig. 3.8** Scrotal saline infusion

constant drag and a squeezing effect on the testicles. Moderate weights of 3–5 kg can be suspended, especially during bondage. The swinging effect of the weight can restrict sudden movements, as well as providing a visual stimulus for the dominant partner.

**A testicle cuff** is a ring-shaped device around the scrotum between the body and the testicles which when closed does not allow the testicles to slide through it. A common type has two connected cuffs, one around the scrotum and the other around the base of the penis. They are just one of many devices to restrain the male genitalia. A standard padlock, which cannot be removed without its key, may also be locked around the scrotum. Requiring such a man wear testicle cuffs symbolizes that his sexual organs belong to his partner, who may be either male or female. There is a level of humiliation involved, by which they find sexual arousal. The cuffs may even form part of a sexual fetish of the wearer or his partner.

**Scrotal augmentation** By scrotal inflation, or scrotal infusion, it is an unusual sexual practice in which fluid (commonly saline solution, sometimes air or another gas) is injected into the scrotum in order to make it ballooning and increased in size. It carries a number of risks of serious complications, including scrotal cellulitis, subcutaneous emphysema, and possibly fatal complications such as Fournier's gangrene or air embolism [33]. (Fig. 3.8).

# References


1. Verit A. Recent discovery of phallic depictions in prehistoric cave art in Asia Minor. Turk J Urol. 2017;43(4):553–5. https://doi.org/10.5152/tud.2017.52138.
2. MacDougald D. Phallic foods. In: Leach M, editors. Funk and wagnall's standard dictionary of folklore, mythology, and legend. New York: Harper & Row; 1984.
3. McManus IC. Right-left and the scrotum in Greek sculpture. Laterality. 2004 ;9(2):189–99. https://doi.org/10.1080/13576500342000149 PMID: 15382717.
4. Bonafini B, Pozzilli P. Scrotal asymmetry, varicocoele and the Riace Bronzes. Int J Androl. 2012 ;35(2):181–2.
5. Frazer J. The golden bough: a study in magic and religion. 3rd ed. London: Macmillan; 1922. p. 1935.
6. Onians R. 17u Origins of European thought: about the body, the mind, the soul, the world, time, and fate. Cambridge, U.K.: Cambridge Univ. Press; 1954.
7. Morimoto I. External genital organs in male mummies from Qurna, Egypt. J Anthropol Soc Nippon. 1989;97(2):169–87.
8. Shokeir A. Hussein, M: Sexual life in Pharaonic Egypt: towards a urological view. Int J Impot Res. 2004;16:385–8. https://doi.org/10.1038/sj.ijir.3901195.
9. Saber A. Ancient Egyptian surgical heritage. J Invest Surg. 2010 ;23(6):327–34.
10. Arey L. Developmental anatomy: a textbook and laboratory manual ofl embryology, 7th edn. Philadelphia: W.B. Saunders; 1974.
11. Brown JR, Thornton JL. Percival Pott (1714–1788) and chimney sweepers' cancer of the scrotum. Br J Industrial Med. 1957;14:68–71.
12. Derbes VJ. The keepers of the bed: castration and religion. JAMA. 1970;212(1):97–100.
13. Freeman S. The evolution of the scrotum: a new hypothesis. J Theor Biol. 1990;145(4):429–45.

14. Portman A. Animal forms and patterns. New York, NY: Schocken; 1952.
15. Friedman RM. The role of the testicles in male psychological development. J Am Psychoanal Assoc. 1996;44(1):201–53.
16. Stoller RJ. A contribution to the study of gender identity. Int J Psycho-Anal. 1964;45:220–226.
17. Laqueur T. Making sex: body and gender from the Greeks to Freud. Cambridge, MA: Harvard Univ. Press; 1990
18. Ruibal R. The evolution of the scrotum. Evolution 1957; 11(3),376–378. JSTOR, www.jstor.org/stable/2405803.
19. Steinach E. Sex and life: forty years of biological and medical experiments. New York: Viking Press; 1940.
20. Reusch K. That which was missing: the archaeology of castration (PhD). University of Oxford; 2013.
21. Thomas J. A bill for proportioning crimes and punishments 1778 Papers 2:492—504.
22. Sarnoff I, Corwin SM. Castration anxiety and the fear of death. J Pers. 1959;27(3):374.
23. Bell A. Bowel training difficulties in boys. J Amer Acad Child Psychiatry. 1964;3:577–90.
24. Blos P. Comments on the psychological consequences of cryptorchidism. In: The Psychoanalytic Study of the Child, vol 15. New York: International Universities Press; 1960. p. 395–429.
25. Smith A, Lattimer J. Psychosexualimpact of undescended testes and implantation of prostheses. Med Aspects Human Sexuality. 1975;9:62–70.
26. Section on Urology. Timing of elective surgery on the genitalia of male children with particular reference to the risks, benefits, and psychological effects of surgery and anesthesia. Pediatrics. 1996;97(4):590–4.
27. Kaplan . Sexual aversion, sexual phobias, and panic disorder. New York: Brunner/Mazel; 1987.
28. Galatzer-Levy RM. Obscuring desire: A special pattern of male adolescent masturbation, Internet pornography, and the flight from meaning. Psychoanalytic Inquiry. 2012;32(5):480–95.
29. Masters WH, Johnson VE. Human sexual response. Boston: Little, Brown and Company; 1966.
30. Langdridge D; Barker M. Safe, sane, and consensual: contemporary perspectives on sadomasochism. Palgrave Macmillan; 2008. p.174. ISBN 978-0-230-51774-5. Archived from the original on 2013-06-20. Retrieved 2016-10-21.
31. Janssen E, Nicole P, Geer JH. The sexual response. In: Handbook of psychophysiology; 2007. p. 245–266.
32. Hartley N, Levine IS. Nina Hartley's Guide to Total Sex. Avery 2006;136. ISBN 978–1–58333–263–4.
33. Summers J. A complication of an unusual sexual practice. South Med J. 2003;96(7):716–7. https://doi.org/10.1097/01.SMJ.0000078368.00806.A7.

# Chapter 4
# Scrotum Evolution

**Mohamed A. Baky Fahmy**

**Scrotum in phylogeny**: Generally the testes originate in the abdomen in all male creatures, it arrested near the kidneys in birds and some mammals, but it descend to a variable extent to their final mature location in others including man [1]. The scrotum is a curiosity unique to mammals. A recent testicle's-eye view of the mammalian family tree revealed that the monumental descent occurred pretty early in mammalian evolution. And what's more, the scrotum was so important that it evolved twice. The natural selection's tagline reflects the importance of attributes that help to keep creatures alive, which means survival of the fittest, so how scrotality (the scientific term for possessing a scrotum) could fit with this concept with all the obvious handicaps it confers during the journey of testicular exteriorisation? Most investigators have tended to think that the advantages of this curious anatomical arrangement must come in the shape of improved fertility, but this is far from proven [2].

**Variable testicular positions in different species: "Diversity of testes positions in mammals".**

Testes position in mammals ranges through six clearly- definable positions from no descent from the ancestral and embryonic position to permanent descent into a pendant scrotum (Fig. 4.1). Testes in positions 1–4 are within the body cavity, while testes in positions 5–6 are external to the body cavity and held in a different forms of scrota [2].

There are three main categories of mammals recognised according to the testicular location:

1. **Testicondy testes:** mammals in which the testes do not move out of the abdominal cavity and stay close to the kidneys; this group includes the Afrotheria clade of elephants, manatees, duck-billed platypus, male turtles, squamates, birds, crocodiles and other monotremes (Fig. 4.2).

M. A. B. Fahmy (✉)
Al-Azhar University, Cairo, Egypt

     27
M. A. B. Fahmy (ed.), *Normal and Abnormal Scrotum*,
https://doi.org/10.1007/978-3-030-83305-3_4

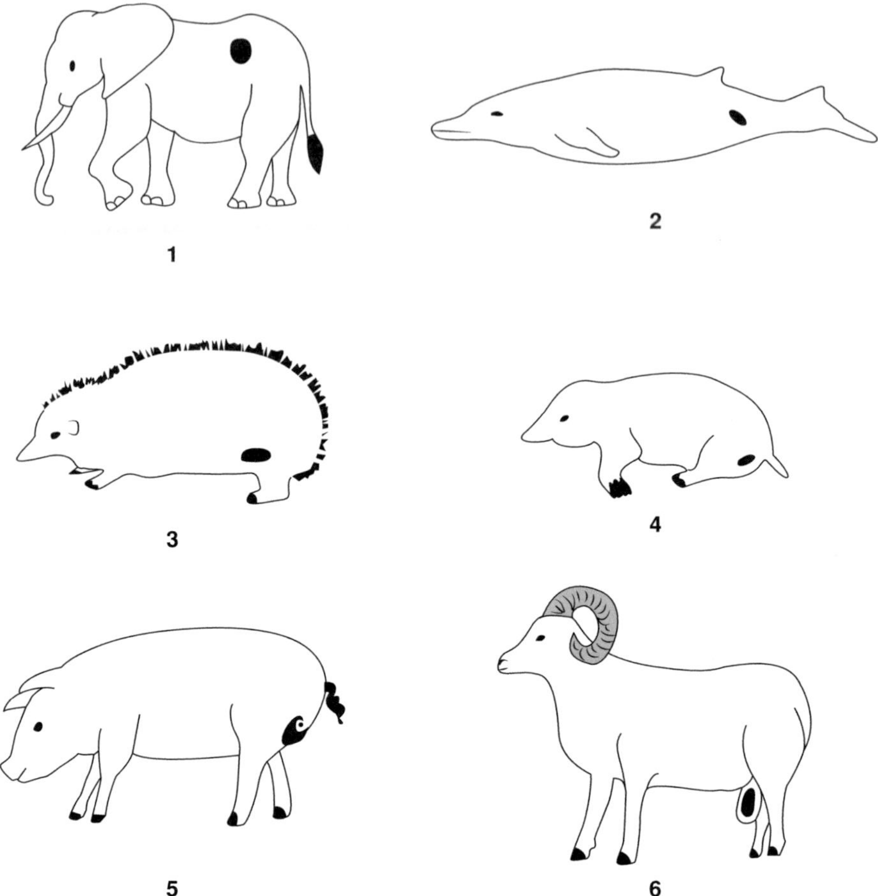

**Fig. 4.1** The six clearly- definable positions of the testicles in mammals, after Carrick and Setchell [2]

2. **Descended ascrotal testes:** mammals with the testes emerges from the abdominal wall, but do not move into a scrotal sac, instead, staying just under the skin, a condition seen in whales, pinnipeds (seals and walruses), sloths, moles, and rhinoceros.
3. **Descended Scrotal:** Although most mammals have descended scrotal testes; mainly the marsupials, bats, rodents, carnivores, and monkeys (Fig. 4.3). Marsupials like kangaroo had a reciprocal relation between scrotum and penis; where the scrotum with an enclosed testicles occupy a cephalic position to the phallus (Fig. 4.4).

In biological evolution the migration of the testes to an external position is a relatively recent mammalian innovation [3]. There are many species of mammal whose testes remain high in the lumbar region near the kidneys, descend only part

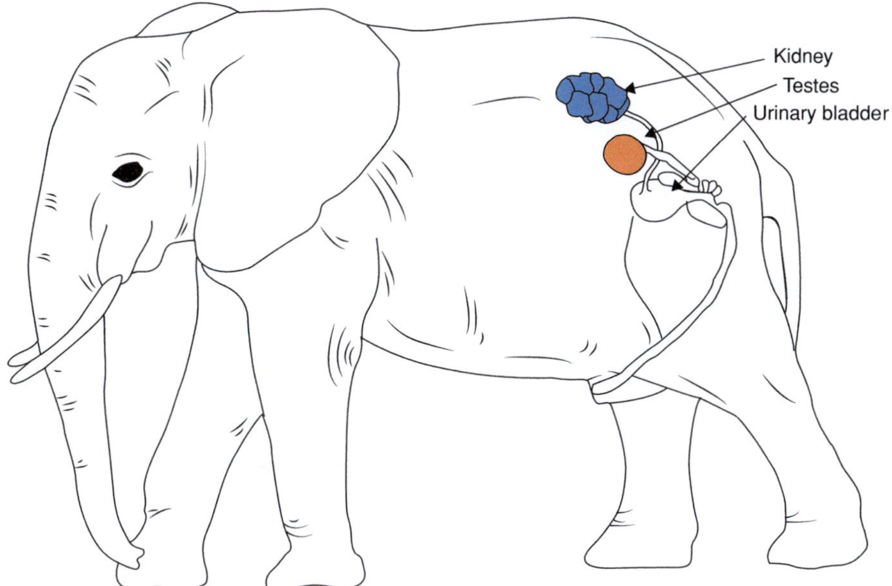


**Fig. 4.2** Testicondy testes in elephant

of the route to the lower abdomen near the bladder, lodge in the inguinal canal, and even retreat back out of the scrotum periodically after the rutting season. While descended scrotal testicles are widespread and represent the prevailing arrangement among mammals, the loss of the scrotum is more common than the loss of testicular descent.

**Theories explaining the variation of testicular location in different species**: Along mankind's history many theories were suggested to explain the goal of testicular descend and subsequently the scrotal development.

**Endothermia theory**: Excessive scrotal heating or cooling may lead to the cessation of spermatogenesis. Data regarding heat exchange rates in scrotal skin can be used to control testicular temperature within the appropriate range. The classical explanation for the evolution of the scrotum is that spermatogenesis can't occur at the high body core temperatures of mammals. In 1926, Moore [4] asserted that the evolution of the scrotum was an evolutionary adaptation to provide an appropriate cool environment of spermatogenesis in response to endothermia. The higher body temperatures hamper sperm production and increase rates of spontaneous mutation. Therefore, a scrotal location would improve sperm production and would also lower the rate of spontaneous mutations. This is of particular importance since the rate of spontaneous mutation rates is higher in the male germ line than the female, particularly affecting the Y chromosome; that's explain normally functioning

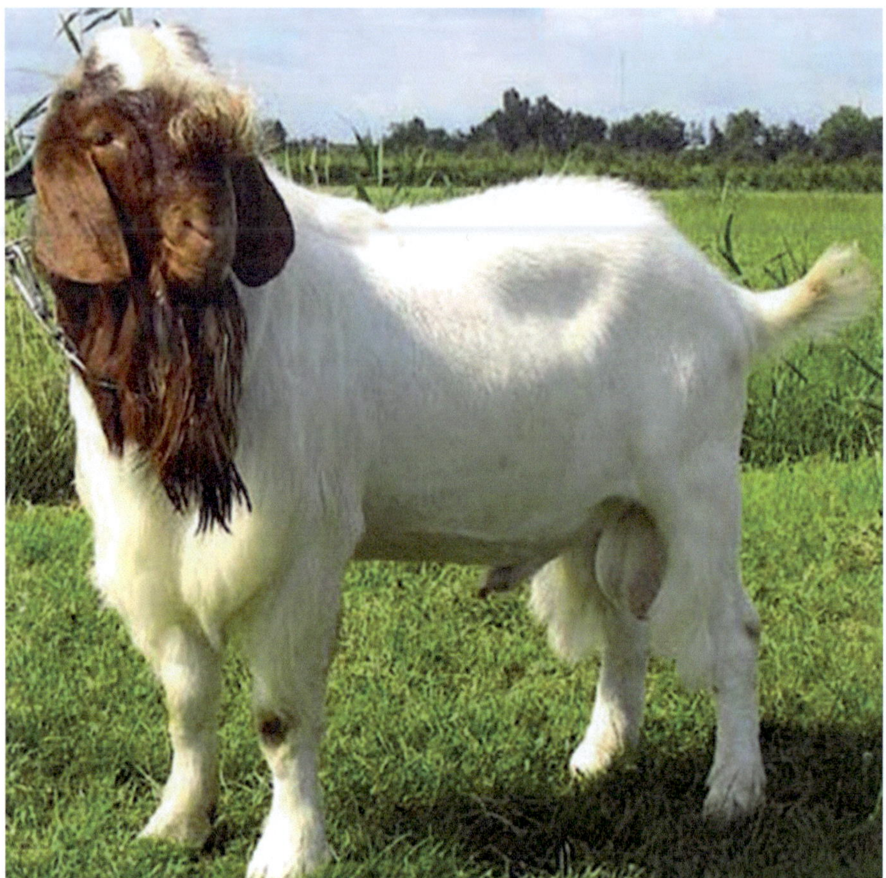

**Fig. 4.3**  Boerbok goat with a markedly pendant scrota

female productive organ without any mutations [5]. This is the most acceptable and also applicable theory for explanting the human testicular descend.

**Activation hypothesis**: descended scrotal testicles might have evolved as a situation-specific mechanism for activating sperm through consistent differences in temperature between the male and female reproductive tracts. A 2–3 centigrade temperature difference links to the activation of sperm in the higher body temperature of the vagina that accompanies insemination. This theory also attempts to explain the cremasteric reflex; as a coital reaction drawing the testicle closer to the abdomen and its higher temperature during sexual arousal to improve sperm motility in preparation for ejaculation [6].

**Training hypothesis**: Testicular descent is a mechanism for improved sperm quality through the imposition of relative hypoxia within the scrotal sac, causing

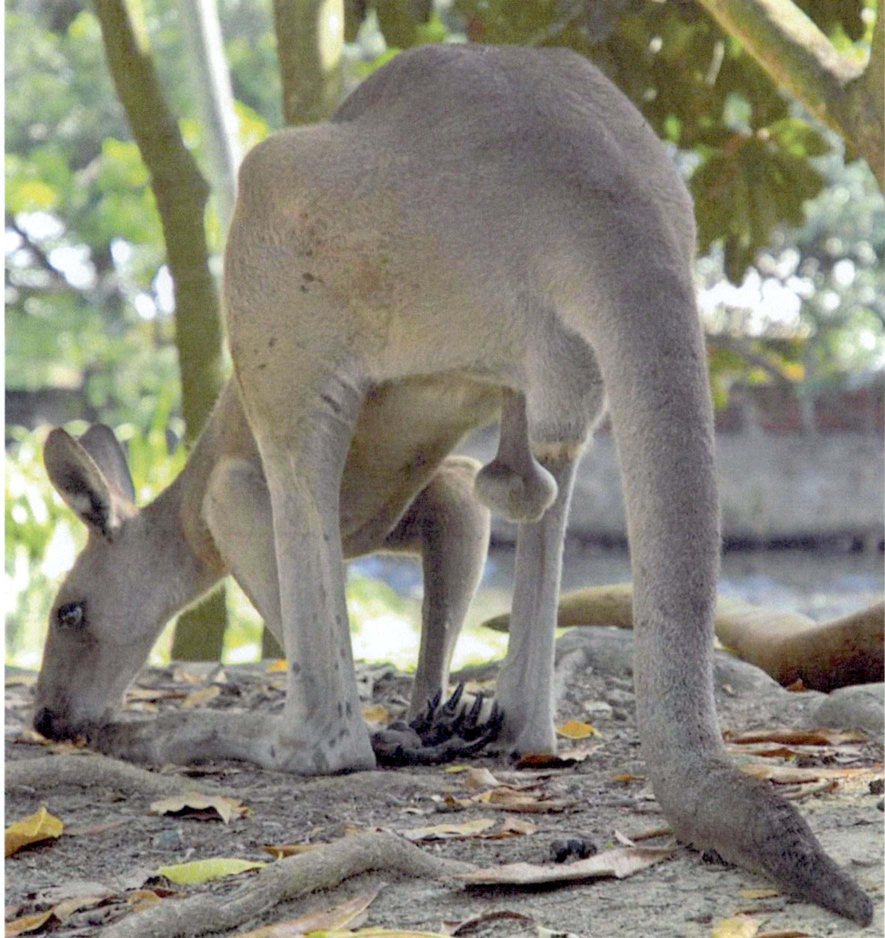

**Fig. 4.4**  Male kangaroo with a scrotum in front of the penis

stress-induced enhanced oxidative metabolism that could result in increased gametic aerobic fitness [7].

**Cool storage hypothesis**: Over a decade ago, Bedford (1977) [8] marked a radical departure from traditional thinking by suggesting that the descent of the epididymis, and not the testis, was the evolutionary "prime mover" in the evolution of the scrotum. In light of these observations Bedford suggested that the primary function of the scrotum was to store sperm in a cool environment, and that testicular descent into a scrotum was a secondary event–merely a mechanism for providing structural support for the epididymides in some species. The cooling requirements of the epididymis were the key issue in testicular descent in support of sperm storage and as a site of gametic optimization in preparation for sperm competition. While these particulars remain theoretical, it is clear that the epididymis is critical for mammalian sperm maturation. It is a highly specific microenvironment for the movement of ions, organic solutes, proteins, and a wide variety of critical hormones such as androgens, estrogens, and retinoids that are necessary for reproduction [8]. Therefore it was the epididymis that was the prime mover for the evolution of the scrotum.

**Sexual display 'handicap hypothesis':** Portman at 1952 [9] suggested that a scrotum and exterior testes were an opportunity for sexual display to attract females, accounting for its ornamentation among some species. In primates the presence of a pigmented scrotum is associated with polygynous and multi-male breeding systems, where male-male competition should be intense and female choice of mates may be important (Fig. 4.5).

This the traditional explanation for the evolution of the scrotum is that the testes descended to an external position because of their importance in social competition, either as a character in female choice of mates or as a signal of dominance in male-male competition. A number of observations are consistent with the social competition hypothesis. There are references to at least 29 genera of mammals with pigmented scrota, either black and furless or colorful. Degree of pigmentation has been shown to be testosterone-dependent in macaques and associated with male

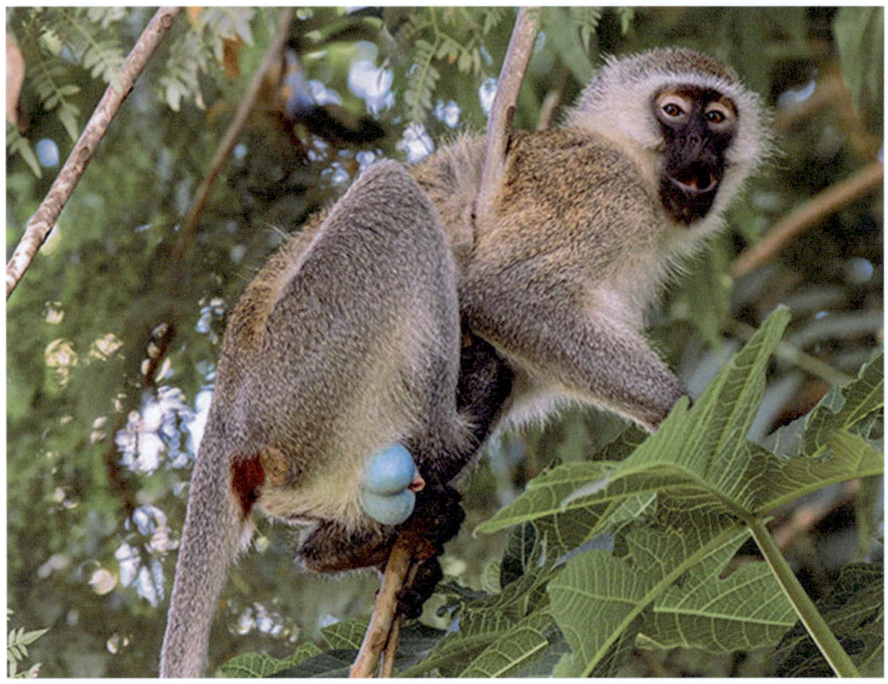

**Fig. 4.5** A vervet monkey displays descended blue balls in a thin, unprotected scrotum

dominance status in macaques and vervet monkeys [10]. Despite observations which support this theoary, the social competition hypothesis begs important questions, for example, if the hypothesis is correct why there are so many nocturnal and fossorial species with scrotal testes? Why is the scrotum so often furred, making it less prominent, and why are pigmented scrota found in such a small percentage of the 698 scrotal genera?. Most importantly, why is testes location variable among taxa that have internal testes? Clearly, neither the temperature-dependent nor the display hypotheses can explain variation in testes position among ascrotal species [6].

Some scientist considering this theory as a 'handicap hypothesis' which postulated the substantive purpose of costly sexual ornamentation was as a representative signal of overall fitness to members of the opposite sex [5]. With the possible exception of coloured scrota among a few species of primates, there is little evidence that this has been the case.

**Galloping hypothesis**: Animals whose mobility is characterized by quick movements or jumping, such as horses, primates, and humans have external testes to avoid concussive hydrostatic rises in intra-abdominal pressure, that is why elephants, whose testicles are internal, do not jump. According to that theory, the testes adjusted to cooler exterior scrotal temperatures as a secondary adaptation [11]. The testes of the males of hippos descend only partially and a scrotum is not present. In addition, the penis retracts into the body when it is not erect. In 1991 Roland Frey [12] reported a number of features of blood vessels of scrotal testes that ensure more constant pressure, possibly to avoid impaired blood drainage during galloping. The specific adaptations are different between marsupials and the rest of us but seem aimed at the same goal. The galloping hypothesis would be a case of evolutionary compromise—the dangers of scrotality being a necessary price for the greater advantages of a new and valuable type of movement [11].

**Gubernaculum Evolution**: John Hunter, for the 1st time, in 1762 described the fetal testis and epididymis in the abdomen, and gave an account of the gubernaculum testis [13]. The gubernaculum appears to be widely distributed across phylogenies. For example, nematodes and almost all mammals have one. Yet, birds do not have a defined gubernacular structure. Their testes originate above their kidneys and stay there. Although bird testes share some commonalities with other mammals, their testes have scattered Leydig cells in the testicular interstitium rather than concentrated around the seminiferous tubules as is the case for mammals [14]. Organisms with a gubernaculum have the capacity to permit testes movement along an anatomical course to reach a consensual location for that cellular ecology and suits homeostatic requirements.

All instances of testicular location can be rationalized by this means. As a particular example, in the elephant, there is no evidence of a gubernaculum, pampaniform plexus, or processsus vaginalis, subsequently there is no scrotum. Other animals have a gubernaculum, but show significant differences in mature location and in the timing of testicular movements. For example, testicular descent in rodents, rabbits, hares, and dogs takes place in the post-natal period. In humans, pigs, cattle and sheep, testis position is settled before birth.

A new study, published in PLOS Biology [15], examined 71 placental mammals for two key genes—RXFP2 and INSL3 that are needed for the development of ligaments gubernaculum. They found that in many Afrotherian mammals without external testes these genes had mutated to the point where they would no longer function. The fact that dysfunctional remnants of the RXFP2 and INSL3 genes are found in mammals without external testicles strongly suggests their ancestors had functioning copies of these genes. Over the course of evolution, when it was no longer an advantage to have external testes for whatever reason, mutations in these genes occurred without reducing the animal's chances of reproduction. These mutated genes were then passed on to the next generation.

Clearly much remains unknown and these ideas need testing.

# References


1. Miller Jr WB, Torday JS. Reappraising the exteriorization of the mammalian testes through evolutionary physiology. Commun Integr Biol . 2019;12(1):38–54. https://doi.org/10.1080/19420889.2019.1586047.
2. Carrick FN, Setchel BP. The evolution of the scrotum. In: Calaby JH, Tyndale-Biscoe TH, editors. Reproduction and evolution; 1977. p. 165–170.
3. Van Tienhoven A. Reproductive physiology of vmebrates. Canbera: Australian Academy of Science, Philadelphia: W.B. Saunders; 1968. Moore CR. The biology of the mammalian testis and scrotum. Quart Rev Biol. 1926;1:4–50. https://doi.org/10.1086/394235
4. Short RV. The testis: the witness of the mating system, the site of mutation and the engine of desire. Acta Paediatr. 1997;86(S422):3–7. https://doi.org/10.1111/j.1651-2227.1997.tb18336.x.
5. Gallup GG Jr, Finn MM, Sammis B. On the origin of descended scrotal testicles: the activation hypothesis. Evol Psych. 2009;7(4):147470490900700400.
6. Freeman S. The evolution of the scrotum: a new hypothesis. J Theoret Biol. 1990;145(4):429–45.
7. Bedford JM. Evolution of the scrotum: the epididymis as the prime mover? In: Calaby JG, Tyndal-Biscoe HD, editors. Reproduction and evolution. Canberra: Australian Academy of Science, 1977. p. 171–182.
8. Jones RC. To store or mature spermatozoa? The primary role of the epididymis. Int J Androl. 2002;22(2):57–66.
9. Portman A. Animal forms and patterns. New York: Schocken; 1952.
10. Dixson AF, Herbert J. The effects of testosterone on the sexual skin and genitalia of the male talapoin monkey. J Repro Fert. 1974;38:217-219.
11. Chance MRA. Reason for externalization of the testis of mammals. J Zool. 1996;239(4):691–5.
12. Frey HL, Peng S, Rajfer J. Synergy of androgens and abdominal pressure in testicular descent. Biol Reprod. 1983;29:1233–9.
13. Beasley SW, Hutson JM. The role of the gubernaculum in testicular descent. J Urol. 1988;140:1191–3.
14. Aire TA. The structure of the interstitial tissue of the active and resting avian testis. Onderstepoort J Vet Res. 1997;64:291–9.
15. Sharma V, Lehmann T, Stuckas H, Funke L, Hiller M. Loss of RXFP2 and INSL3 genes in Afrotheria shows that testicular descent is the ancestral condition in placental mammals. PLoS Biol. 2018;16(6):e2005293. https://doi.org/10.1371/journal.pbio.2005293.

# Chapter 5
# Animals Scrota

Mohamed A. Baky Fahmy

**Abbreviations**

SC  Scrotal circumference
AR  Androgen Receptors

## 5.1  Testicular Position of Animals

Testicondy; means a condition of having testicles situated within the abdomen, it is a feature of Monotremata and most of Atlantogenata, which represent the basal group of all eutherians species. Scrotum is missing in all birds and aquatic animals, but it is present in most mammals, an external scrotum is absent in streamlined marine mammals, such as whales and seals, as well as in some lineages of land mammals, such as the afrotherians, xenarthrans, and numerous families of bats, rodents, and insectivores. Animals that move at a steady pacesuch as elephants, whales, and marsupial moles have an internal testes and had no scrotum. In fact, the degree of testicular descent is highly variable in mammals, and abdominal testes are found in a wide variety and large number of taxa. Testes position in mammals ranges through six clearly- definable positions, and it could be broadly classified to scrotal and ascrotal positions. Furthermore, genera within mammalian families often show variation in testicular position [1] (Chap. 4).

M. A. B. Fahmy (✉)
Al-Azhar University, Cairo, Egypt

© The Author(s), under exclusive license to Springer Nature Switzerland AG 2022
M. A. B. Fahmy (ed.), *Normal and Abnormal Scrotum*,
https://doi.org/10.1007/978-3-030-83305-3_5

## 5.2   Animal Scrotal Pigmentation

At least there are 29 genera of mammals had a pigmented scrota either black and furless or colorful. Degree of pigmentation has been shown to be a testosterone-dependent phenomenon in macaques (The genus Macaca of gregarious old world monkeys of the subfamily Cercopithecinae. The 23 species of macaques inhabit ranges throughout Asia and North Africa) and associated with male dominance status in vervet monkeys [2]. The adult male of each vervet monkey species has a pale blue scrotum and a red penis, and male proboscis monkeys have a red penis with a black scrotum.

Usually in primates the presence of a pigmented scrotum is associated with polygynous and multi-male breeding systems, where male-male competition seems to be intense, and female choice of mates may be an important factor. In pinnipeds the degree of sexual size dimorphism, which is often interpreted as an index of male-male competition, is much greater in genera with external testes than in genera with internally located testes [3].

## 5.3   Variations in Testicular Sizes of Different Animals

According to allometric equation the testes of a 10 g mammal should comprise 1.8% of body mass, whereas testes of a 10,000 kg mammal amount to only 0.04%. Among the smallest mammals, the range of relative testes size is great; the testes of some rodents are as large as 8% of body mass, whereas others are as small as 0.15% [4]. For the testicular size studying, Vahed and his colleagues [5] dissected specimens from 21 bush-cricket species collected around Europe. The testes account for 14% of the body mass of males of this bushcricket species. The previous record holder's testicles—belonging to the fruit fly Drosophila bifurcatipped is about 11% of its body mass. If we have testicles of that size, it would weigh at a staggering 10 kg for a healthy 72 kg man. The testes of a stallion, which are suspended horizontally within the scrotum are ovoids and of about 8 to 12 cm long, and 6 to 7 cm high by 5 cm wide [6]. The male elephant have a most remarkable difference from other mammal species with an intra-abdominal testicles, which can weigh up to 2 kgs each in an adult male. Among mammals in general, we can find no correlation between the size of the testes and their location (abdominal or scrotal), or between the size of testes and the body form and mode of locomotion (terrestrial, aquatic, or aerial). Only there is a functional relationship exists in many mammals between relative size of testes and mating attitude [7]. The evolution of large testes can be attributed to high copulatory frequency and sperm production and the competition among sperm of different males for fertilization of the same female. Size of testes has undoubtedly evolved in each species in response to a variety of other additional factors beyond the first-order influence of body size. The results of Bailey et al. [8] study suggested that prediction of sperm production may be dependent on factors other than scrotal circumference (SC), testicular volume, or weight. Testicular shape may influence sperm output in the mature Holstein bulls.

Also we have to consider that the testis contains both spermatogenic and non-spermatogenic tissue, and the relative proportions of which can vary widely among species. For example, in one survey of 12 mammal species; the percentage of spermatogenic tissue ranged from 32.7% by volume in the woodchuck, and to 92.7% in the degu (Degu is a small hystricomorpha rodent endemic at central Chile) [9]. So it is not necessary for the bulky testes to contain a spermatogenic structure as the nonspermatogenic tissue may share in the semblance of a large mass of some animals testicles. Unlike placental mammals, some male marsupials have a scrotum that is anterior to the penis, which is not homologous to the scrotum of placental mammals, although there are several marsupial species without an external scrotum at all [10] (Chap. 4).

Studies of the testicular size of grazing rams over 3 years showed that testicular volume falls during summer and autumn when forage quality and availability decline and when rams are mating. Loss in testicular size may also occur in summer in the absence of mating activity and at a greater rate than loss in live weight [11] (Fig. 5.1).

## 5.4 Scrotal Swelling in Female Animals (Scrotolisation)

Very rarely the females may carry a vulvar wrinkles resemble the male scrota; Malaivijitnond et al. [12] in an interesting study documented the presence of a sexual skin swelling of adolescent female long-tailed macaques, which is located bilaterally in the inguinal region, it looks globular and phenotypically strongly resembles the male scrotum. Also marsupial reproductive organs differ from the placental mammals, for them, the reproductive tract is doubled. The females have two uteri and two vaginas, and before birth, a birth canal forms between them. The males have a split or double penis lying in front of the scrotum [13]. In spotted hyena; the female possesses no vaginal opening, and the labia are fused to form a pseudo-scrotum.

## 5.5 Scrotal Anomalies in Animals

It may be difficult to assign diseases and anomalies in animals as congenital or acquired; as both categories are interlacing. The environmental pollutants with a hormone-like action might cause several changes in many animals. If we come to the consanguinity as an underlying cause for several congenital diseases in human; it is very common in certain animal species with a special brother-sister matings; as in dogs or pigs, so over several generations it is suspected to find an increases in the incidence of many congenital anomalies. Simply; if consanguinity is considered as

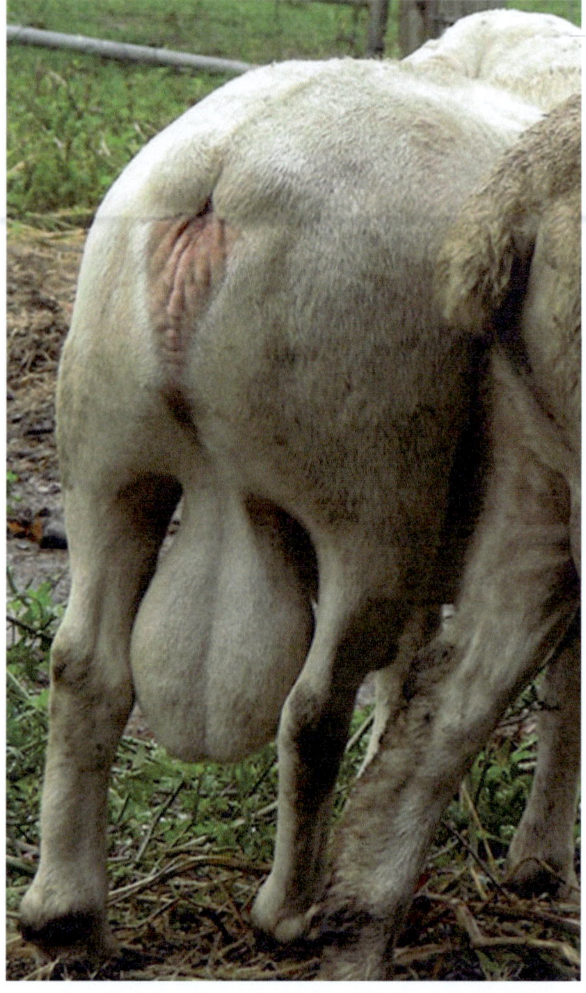

**Fig. 5.1** Ovine (sheep) scrotum, pendulous scrotum characteristic of horned ruminants, with permission from Minnesota Veterinary Anatomy http://vanat.cvm.umn.edu/ungDissect/Lab17/Lab17.html#images

a predisposition for some congenital anomalies in human, such anomalies are expected to be higher in animals, as we can see in cryptorchidism. In some area with a definite pollution, the congenital anomalies may be so high as in male squirrels, where a study documented a 75% of reproductive malformation in Montana [14]. Pesticides like vinclozolin, procymidone, linuron and DDT are AR antagonists. They reduce male rat anogenital distance, and induce a marked areola at relatively low dosages, hypospadias, scrotal tissues agenesis and retained nipples are seen with a middle dosages, while undescended testes and epididymal agenesis are seen at highest doses [15].

**Undescended testicles**: The true incidence of cryptorchidism is very difficult to estimate among taxa, as most discovered cases are typically killed early, as they are deemed unsuitable for breeding and rearing. Probably the incidence of cryptorchidism is higher in dogs, cats and pigs than in cattle or sheep. In dogs and horses, a retained testis most commonly is abdominal. In horses, but not other species, the retention of testes within the inguinal canal is common [16]. Among dogs, the right sided inguinal cryptorchidism was the most common form, followed by right-sided abdominal cryptorchidism. The true incidence of cryptorchidism in a mixed population of cats is estimated to lay between 1 and 1.3%, but it is up to 6.8% in dogs [17].

**Monorchia and Anorchia**: missing one or both testicles with a subsequent scrotal deficiency is not rare in animal kingdom; these anomalies may be congenital or acquired secondary to exposure to the hormonal disruptors. It is not rarely for the Onypterigia tricolor beetle to lacks the left testis. Researchers have found that monorchid beetles are more common than previously thought. In a survey with detailed dissection and study of over 820 species, authors found 174 species, all members of the three lineages, with only one testis. The one-testicle beetles appear and behave in no differently than their two-testicle counterparts, they are mating normally. Authors suggested tentatively that testis loss is driven wholly by an interaction among the internal organs of these beetles, possibly due to selective pressure to maximize the comparatively large accessory glands found in these taxa [18] (Fig. 5.2).

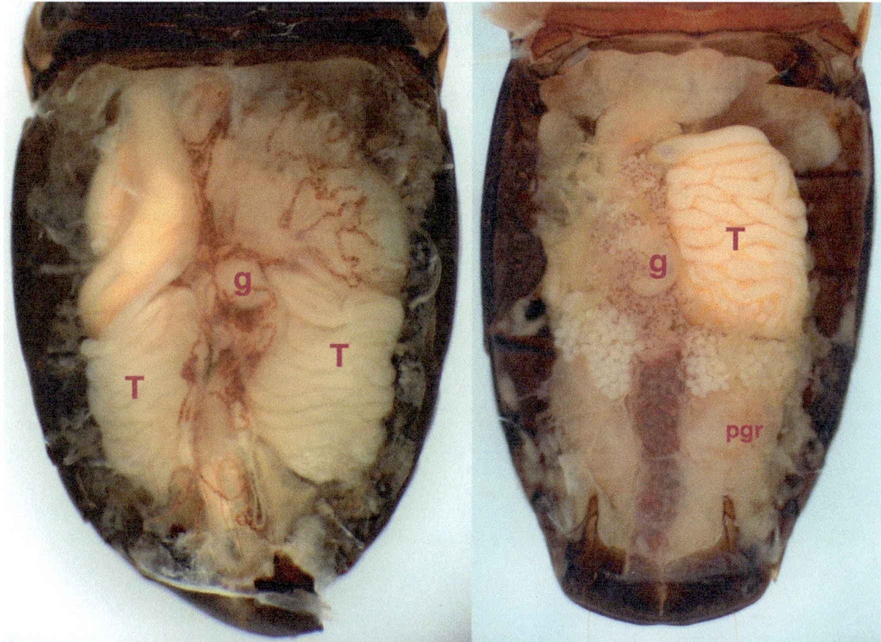


**Fig. 5.2**  Digital images of Amara species from California (Zabrini); with the internal organs of the male carabid beetle abdomen showing size and position of male reproductive organs. T: testis, g: gut, pgr: pygidial gland reservoir. (Ref 4: This photo licensed from the Copyright clearance centre with some modifications)

**Ectopic Testicle**: Judy Hoy [14] have a wide experience in dealing with male reproductive birth defects in Montana animals, and she kindly provided me with a different significant photos for animals; specially the wild fox squirrel, with scrotal anomalies. Exposure to hormone disrupting pesticides during the various stages of embryonic and fetal development of many wild animals can effect the size and placement of each of the reproductive organs, sometimes resulting in quite bizarre looking of the male genitalia.

These are the most common basic birth defects as reported at 2002 in Montana [19]:-

1. Approximately one third of male white-tailed deer have a short scrotum or no scrotum, resulting in both testes being partly or completely ectopic between the external skin and the body wall. There is a very low prevalence of a scrotum comprised of one bursa formed on the external skin, usually the left bursa, with the right testis ectopic in a horizontal position between the external skin and the body wall (Fig. 5.3).
2. There is a high prevalence of misaligned hemiscrota; usually with the left hemiscrota formed directly forward of the right hemiscrota. The prevalence has ranged from 20% to over 80% [19].
   The misaligned hemiscrota malformation is likely because of disrupted gene signaling during early fetal development effecting symmetry. The testes are nearly always descended on Montana ungulates and are either in normal bilateral hemiscrota (30%), in misaligned hemiscrota (60%) or horizontal under the skin with no scrotum formed (10%). Both bilateral scrotums and misaligned

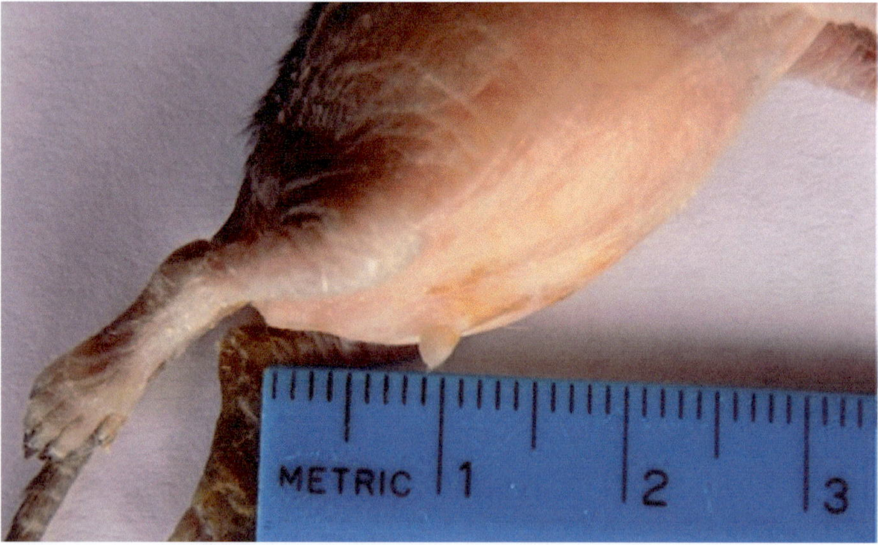


**Fig. 5.3** There is a completely absent scrotum in this chipmunk, which had a penis sheath, but there is no scrotum formed

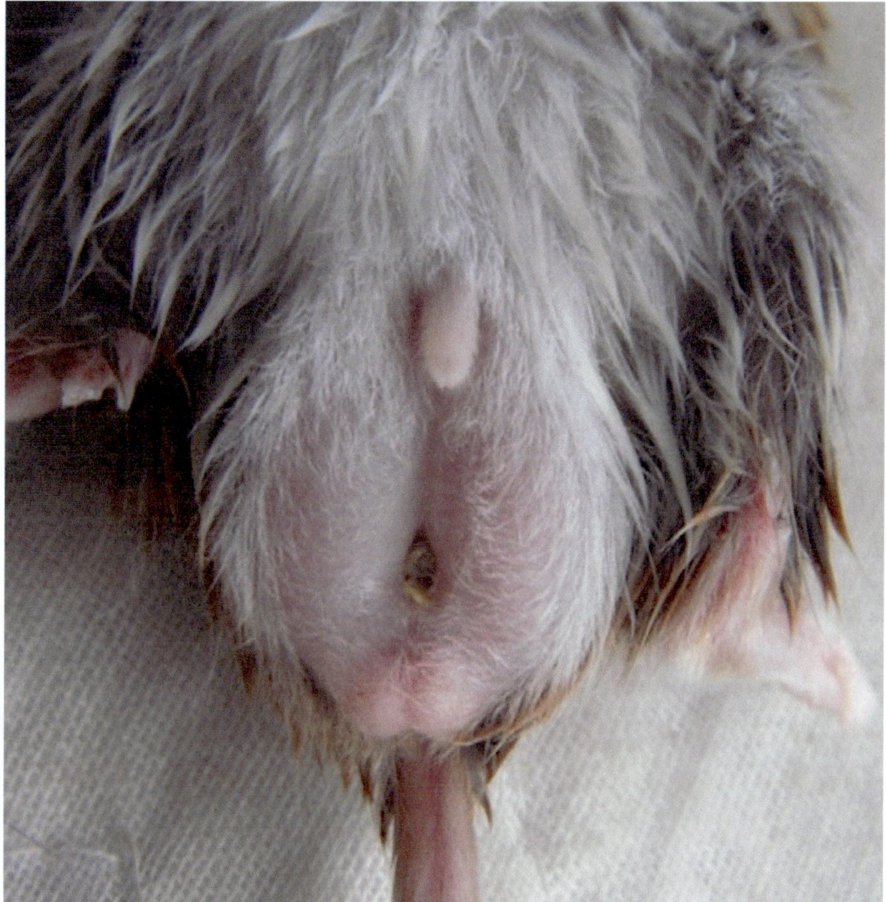

**Fig. 5.4** Ectopic scrotal transposition: This male mouse had a normal length penis sheath, but because the area between the penis sheath and the anus appears to be too short, the left and right hemiscrota were formed caudally on each side of the anus rather than forward of the anus

scrotums are often shorter than the testes they contain, making the testes incompletely ectopic (Fig. 5.4).

3. Some deers, both males and females had their four teats formed forward of normal. This caused the male genitalia to be formed forward on the belly, on some deer the root of the penile sheath lies nearly to the umbilicus. For unknown reasons, in almost all cases it is the left testis that has disappeared.

Biologists have also reported many birth defects on ungulates like misaligned hemiscrota on moose. Male reproductive birth defects on horses, cattle, sheep and goats have been also reported. It is extremely rare to observe a male deer, white-tailed deer or mule deer, with normally placed testes and bursa, normal length

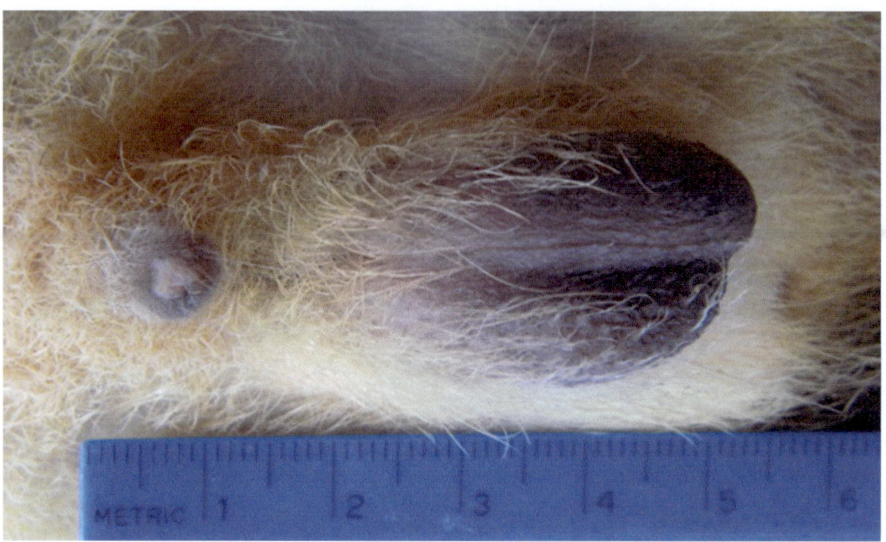


**Fig. 5.5** Normal Fox squirrel scrotum and penis

scrotum and normal penis sheath length [19] (Fig. 5.5). Most are born with at least one of those organs are too short or malformed. The testes have not been observed to be small, too short or in any way abnormal, so the testes themselves do not appear to be affected by the developmental malformations of the scrotum or what is causing them. However, being ectopic results in the sperm being too warm and thus in most cases, damaged and not viable.

The prevalence of ectopic testes with no scrotum or empty misaligned skin flaps where the scrotum should be on wild fox squirrels (*Sciurus niger*) in Ravalli County Montana was extremely high (85%) during a period 2014 when they were collected and examined [19].

**Scrotal dimple and bipartition**: Goats and sheep have morphological characteristics for adaptation to desert and semiarid regions, with the appearance of scrotal division known as scrotum bipartition, which has already been reported in goats. This anatomy increases the surface area of each testicle exposed to environmental temperature, favoring heat dissipation and improving reproductive efficiency. It was concluded that the spermatogenetic line parameters of sheep with scrotal bipartition were different compared to those without scrotal bipartition, with greater efficiencies in spermatogenesis yield and Sertoli cells in the sheep with scrotal bipartition, suggesting that these animals present, as reported in goats, better reproductive indices [20] (Figs. 5.6 and 5.7). Scrotal dimple is very rare in human, and it will be discussed in Chap. 12.

**Wide penoscrotal distance**: Unlike human; many male animals don't have the scrotum surrounding the root of the penis, instead there is a variable gap between the scrotum and the penis. In white-tailed deer male genitalia there is a wide

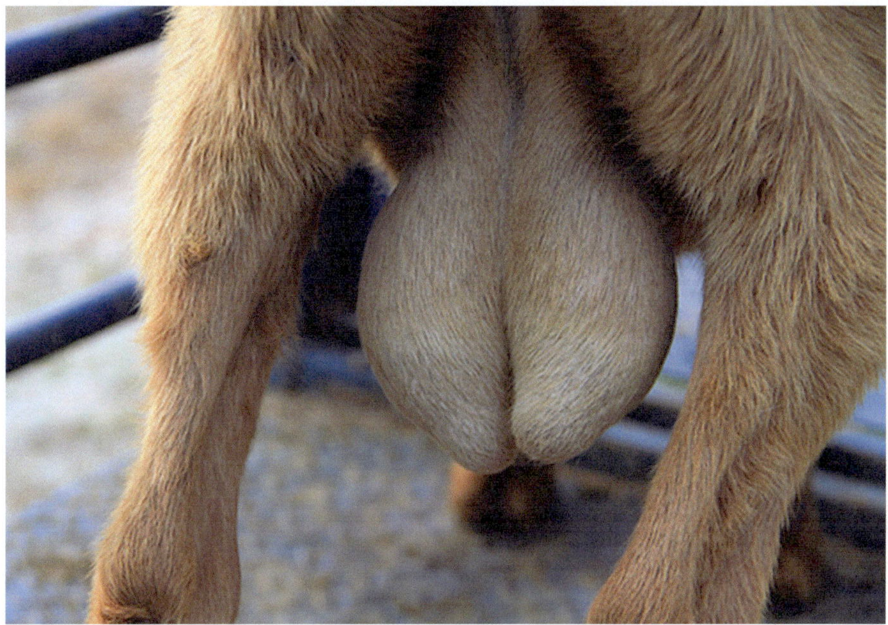

**Fig. 5.6** Two years old ram has a split scrotum and docked tail

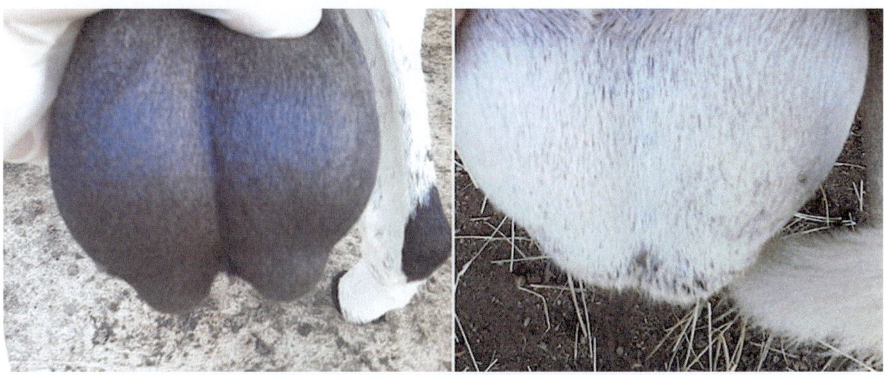

**Fig. 5.7** Scrotum of crossbred rams on left, and sheep with marked scrotal bipartition on the right

distinguishable penoscrotal distance (Fig. 5.8). At the same time this penoscrotal distance is absent in most of the other scrotal animals; where the scrotum lies in the same vicinity around the root of the penis like human (Fig. 5.9). This finding of wide penile separation from the scrotum is rarely seen in human, but we encountered such anomaly either infrequently as an isolated anomaly or in association exstrophy (Chap. 12).

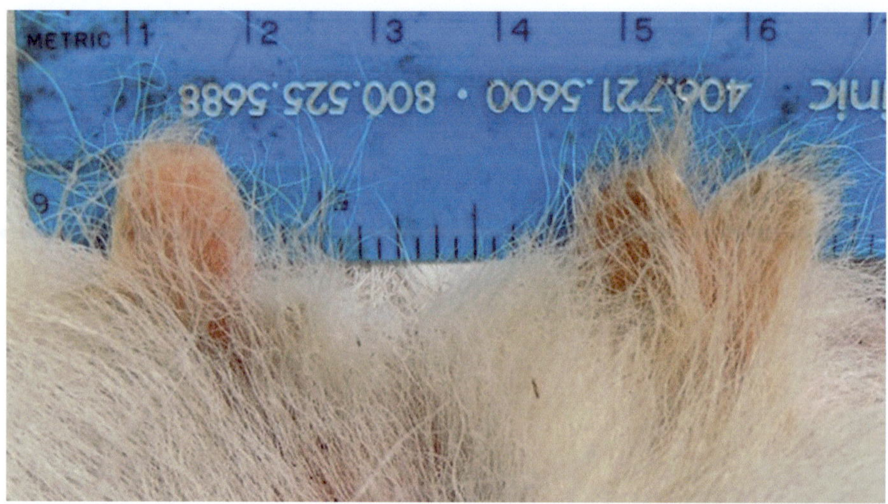

**Fig. 5.8**  A male fox squirrel with a normally wide penoscrotal distance

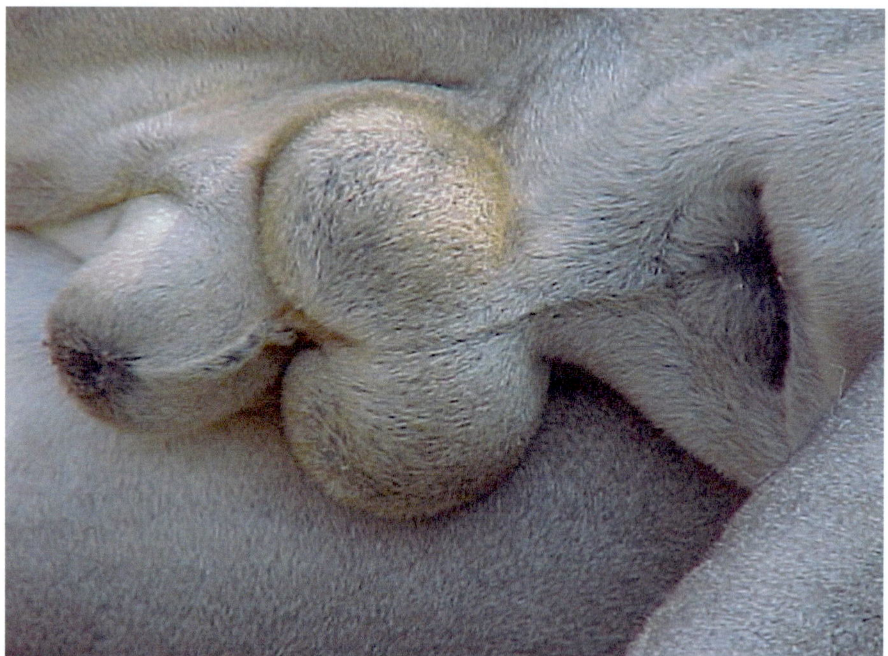

**Fig. 5.9**  A lion genitalia with the scrota sounding the root of penis without any seperation from the root of the penis, with the anus lies just caudally to the scrotum

## 5.6  Interesting Animals Scrota

**Rabbit**: The scrotal sacs lay lateral to the penis and contain epididymal fat pads which protect the testes. The testes of male neonate descend postnatally and are able to retract into the pelvic cavity in order to thermoregulate. The sexually mature male has 2 external testicles that lie on either side of the penis in 2 relatively hairless scrotal sacs. The scrotal skin is thin and the caudal section of the epididymis can be seen through the thin skin of the scrotum at the caudal end of the scrotal sac where the epididymis is attached to the inner layer of the tunica vaginalis. The testicles enlarge with age and sexual maturity (Fig. 5.10). Scrotal and testicular abnormalities, specially cryptorchidism are not rare in rabbits [21].

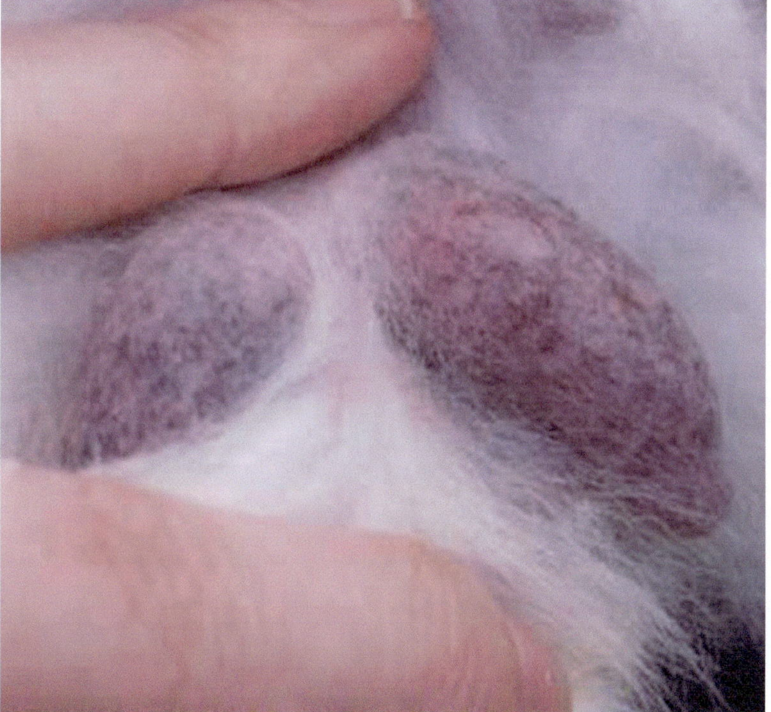

**Fig. 5.10**  A close-up photos of the male rabbit scrota devoid of hair

**Fox squirrel males**: The hemiscrota on this squirrel are bilateral, partially covered by hair and are large enough to contain the normal sized testes. The penis sheath varied widely. Comparison of the normal fox squirrel with the scrotums will help address how severe the reproductive malformations are on squirrels with birth defects (Fig. 5.5).

**Spotted hyena**: The spotted hyena, is a fascinating mammal noted for extreme masculinization of the female external genitalia. The female of spotted hyena is the only extant mammal that mates and gives birth through a pendulous penis-like clitoris. The mating process is complicated, as the male's penis enters and exits the female's reproductive tract through her pseudo-penis rather than directly through the vagina, which is blocked by the false scrotum and testes [22].

**Scrotum Frog**: The Titicaca water frog (Telmatobius culeus), also known as the "scrotum frog" for its loose and baggy skin, which looks like the wrinkled human scrotal skin. In reference to its excessive amounts of skin. This rare frog is characterised by taking its required oxygen from water through its extensive skin folds. This evolutionary adaptation also makes the frog highly sensitive to changes in its habitat, such as environmental contamination [23].

**Male llamas**, had a well defined pyriform scrotal with a distinct penoscrotal distance, it can be vicious and often attempt to injure other males by biting the scrotum. (Fig. 5.11).

**Blue whales** have the largest penises on Earth. An erect blue whale penis is 12 inches (30 cm) in diameter and ten feet in length. It is fibroelastic like those of the blue whale's artiodactyl relatives. The retracted penis curves in an S-shaped loop and stays inside the body. When erect, it peeks out of the genital slit. Cetaceans do not have scrotums like terrestrial mammalian males do. Mammalian scrotums lower ambient temperature to keep sperm viable, so cetaceans had to find a way to compensate [24].

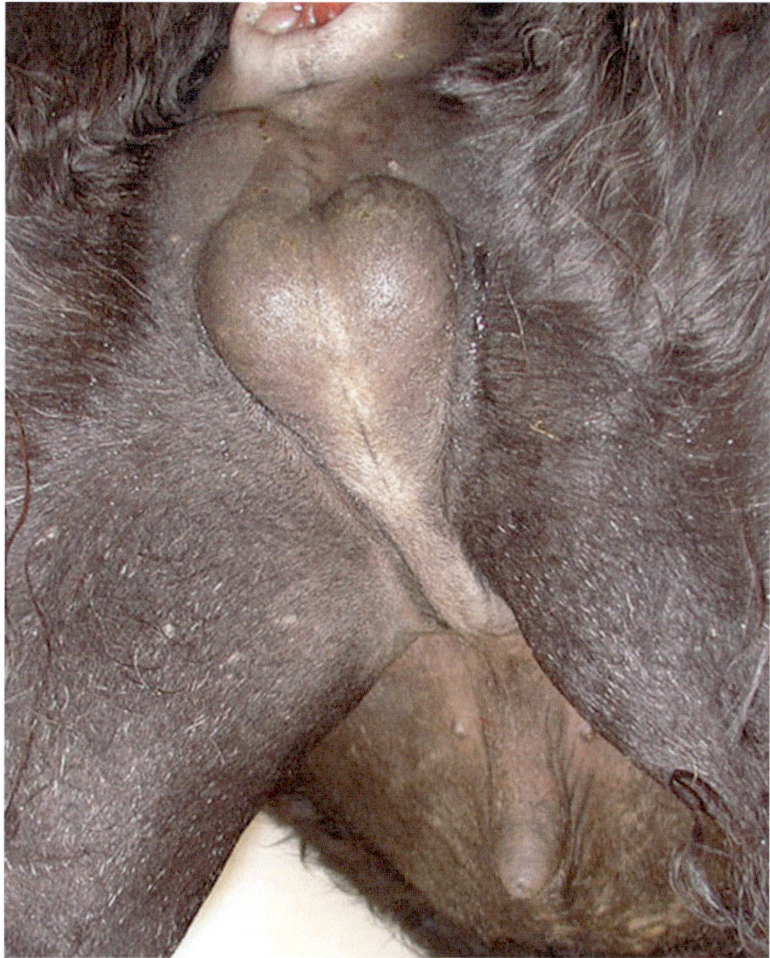

**Fig. 5.11** Male llamas can be vicious and often attempt to injure other males by biting the scrotum, scrotum closeness to the anus is noticeable. This photo reproduced with permission from Minnesota Veterinary Anatomy http://vanat.cvm.umn.edu/ungDissect/Lab17/Lab17.html#images

# References


1. Carrick FN, Setchell BP. The evolution of the scrotum. In: Calaby JH, Tyndale-Biscoe TH, editors. Reproduction and evolution. Canbera: Australian Academy of Science; 1977. p. 165–170.
2. Friderun Ankel-Simons. Primate anatomy: an introduction. Academic Press; 2010. ISBN 978–0–08–046911–9. Archived from the original on 26 March 2014. Retrieved 23 July 2013.
3. Alexander RD. Sexual dimorphism and breeding systems in pinnipeds, ungulates, primates, and humans. In: Chagnon NA, lrons W, Editors. Evolutionary biology and human social behavior, an anthropological perspective. Duxbury Press North Scituate, MA; 1979. p. 402–604.

4. Kenagy GJ, Stephen C. Trombulak, size and function of mammalian testes in relation to body size. J Mammal. 1986;67(1):1–22. https://doi.org/10.2307/1380997.

5. Vahed K, Carron G. Comparison of forced mating behaviour in four taxa of Anonconotus, the Alpine bushcricket. J Zool. 2008;276:313–21. https://doi.org/10.1111/j.1469-7998.2008.00492.x.

6. The Stallion: Breeding Soundness Examination & Reproductive Anatomy. University of Wisconsin-Madison; 2007. Archived from the original on July 16, 2007. Retrieved July 7, 2007.

7. Freeman S. The evolution of the scrotum: a new hypothesis. J Theoret Biol. 1990;145(4): 429–45.

8. Bailey TL, Monke D, Hudson RS, Wolfe DF, Carson RL, Riddell MG. Testicular shape and its relationship to sperm production in mature Holstein bulls. Theriogenology. 1996;46 (5):881–7.

9. Ramm SA, Schärer L. The evolutionary ecology of testicular function: size isn't everything. Biol Rev. 2014;89(4):874–88.

10. Hugh Tyndale-Biscoe C. Life of Marsupials. Csiro Publishing; 2005. ISBN 978-0-643-06257-3.

11. Masters DG, Fels HE. Seasonal changes in the testicular size of grazing rams. Proc Aust Soc Anim Prod. 1984;15:444–447.

12. Malaivijitnond S, Hamada Y, Suryobroto B, Takenaka O. Female long-tailed macaques with scrotum-like structure. Am J Primatol. 2007;69:721–35.

13. Renfree M, Tyndale-Biscoe H. Reproductive physiology of marsupials. ISBN: Cambridge University Press; 1987. p. 9780521337922.

14. Judy H, Swanson N, Seneff S. The high cost of pesticides: human and animal diseases. Poult Fish Wildl Sci. 2015;1–18.

15. Gray Jr LE, Ostby J, Furr J, Wolf CJ, Lambright C, Parks L, Veeramachaneni DN et al. Effects of environmental antiandrogens on reproductive development in experimental animals. Apmis 2001;109(S103):S302-S319.

16. Amann RP, Veeramachaneni DNR. Cryptorchidism and associated problems in animals. Anim Reprod (AR). 2018;3(2):108–20.

17. Yates D, Hayes G, Heffernan M, Beynon R. Incidence of cryptorchidism in dogs and cats. Vet Record. 2003;152(16):502–4.

18. Will KW, Liebherr JK, Maddison DR, Galian J. Absence asymmetry: the evolution of monorchid beetles (Insecta: Coleoptera: Carabidae). J Morphol. 2005;264(1):75–93.

19. Hoy JA, Hoy RD, Seba D, Kerstetter TH. Genital abnormalities in white-tailed deer (*Odocoileus virginianus*) in west-central Montana: Pesticide exposure as a possible cause. J Environ Biol. 2002; 23:189–97. http://www.ncbi.nlm.nih.gov/pubmed/12602857

20. Ramon TGA, Rodrigues et al.: Influence of scrotal bipartition on spermatogenesis yield and sertoli cell efficiency in sheep. Pesq Vet Bras. 2016;36(4):258–262.

21. Harcourt-Brown FM. Disorders of the reproductive tract of rabbits. Vet Clin N Am Exotic Anim Pract . 2017;20(2):555–87. https://doi.org/10.1016/j.cvex.2016.11.010.

22. Szykman M, Van Horn RC, Engh AL, Boydston EE, Holekamp KE. Courtship and mating in free-living spotted hyenas. Behaviour. 2007;144(7):815–46.

23. Gill V. Blobfish wins ugliest animal vote. BBC News. Retrieved 12 September 2013.

24. Mitchinson J, Lloyd J. The book of general ignorance. Random House Digital, Inc; 2007. p. 62. ISBN 9780307394910

# Chapter 6
# Scrotal Functions and Missions

**Mohamed A. Baky Fahmy**

**Abbreviations**

HF     Heat Flux
GDP    Genital Dysmorphophobia
BDD    Body Dysmorphic Disorder
MGIS   Male Genital Image Scale

## 6.1 Physiological Function

**Thermal regulations**: It was found earlier that a normally functioning testis of the adult guinea pig will lose practically all its germinal epithelium when the testis is elevated from the scrotum into the abdomen; the seminiferous tubules show marked degeneration within a week after confinement of the testis in the abdomen, and within 2–3 weeks the tubules are reduced to shrunken, vacuolated, and empty canals except for a single basal row of nuclei. All spermatogenesis ceases, and the testis shows no spermatogenetic activity as long as it remains in the abdomen. If, however, it is replaced in the scrotum after degeneration of the germinal epithelium has occurred, spermatogenesis is re-established and spermatozoa are again produced [1, 2].

It is not only the thin skin and cremasteric muscle of the scrotal sac which promote heat dissipation, but also the arteries that supply blood to the scrotum are positioned adjacent to the veins taking blood away from the scrotum and function as an additional cooling/heat exchange mechanism. As a consequence of these adaptations average scrotal temperatures in humans are typically 2.5 to 3 C lower than body temperature, and spermatogenesis is most efficient at 34 °C [3].

M. A. B. Fahmy (✉)
Al-Azhar University, Cairo, Egypt

It is clear that traditional explanations for the evolution of the scrotum are seriously flawed, according to the alternative hypotheses reviewed, the scrotum mainly evolved to provide a cool environment for sperm storage and testicular descent evolved because it improves sperm quality. These hypotheses offer testable predictions capable of inspiring a new and potentially fruitful round of experimentation on the evolution of a perplexing mammalian character [4].

The scrotum, however, is more than a passive cooling device or cold storage mechanism. There is considerable evidence that the scrotum plays an active thermoregulatory role. When ambient temperature rises not only do testicles descend, but conversely when temperatures fall below a certain point the testicles are drawn up toward the body to conserve heat. The cremasteric muscle, triggered by the cremasteric reflex mediates these moment to moment changes in testicular descent and ascent [5].

Heat flux (HF) in the scrotal skin surface is generated based on the surrounding environment. When a temperature difference exists between an area of the human body and the surrounding environment, (HF) is generated when the scrotal skin surface temperature is different from the ambient temperature [6]. The higher the difference between the scrotum and ambient temperature, the greater the HF generated. If the scrotal temperature is the same as the surrounding temperature, the quantity of heat flow is zero; otherwise, the heat is flowing from the high- to the low-temperature point.

Any account of descended scrotal testicles must also address the enormous potential costs of having the testicles located outside the body cavity where they are left virtually unprotected and especially vulnerable to insult and damage by physical trauma and torsion. Although the testicles actually suffer surprisingly little serious damage they are rather well protected by the tough inner lining of the scrotum; the pain associated with even minor buffeting far surpasses the physical damage. Another advantage is it protects the testes from jolts and compressions associated with an active lifestyle [5]. The cremasteric reflex also appears to function in several other ways to compensate for the vulnerability of descended scrotal testicles and to minimize testicular damage. Fear and the threat of danger have been shown to promote reflexive contractions of the cremasteric muscle and cause the testicles to be drawn up against the body where they are less vulnerable.

## 6.2  Sexual Function

In humans, the scrotum may provide some friction during intercourse, helping to enhance the activity. The rear-entry position of mating may allow the scrotum to stimulate the clitoris and, in this way, may produce an orgasm [7].

Having demonstrated that scrotal stimulation can be pleasurable and used for masturbation and that painful testicular pressure served to evoke masochistic gratification, their is an additional role of attempted mastery of past traumata to the testicles or penis in the testicular masturbation.

It seems that testicles and scrotal sac have the characteristic of an erogenous zone lying between anus and phallus. The CM is solely an involuntary muscle, but it poses some voluntary contraction in adult and its contraction, which occurs during arousal can prevent injury of the testicles during sex, also contraction occurs during ejaculation. The scrotal skin will also contract and thicken when sexual arousal occurs.

**Scrotal Fascism**: Cock and ball torture: is a sexual activity involving application of pain or constriction to the penis or testicles. This may involve directly painful activities, such as genital piercing, wax play, genital spanking, squeezing, ball-busting, genital flogging, urethral play, tickle torture, erotic electrostimulation, kneeing or kicking. The recipient of such activities may receive direct physical pleasure via masochism, or emotional pleasure through erotic humiliation, or knowledge that the play is pleasing to a sadistic dominant [8]. Many of these practices carry significant health risks (Chap. 3) (Fig. 6.1).

## 6.3  Psychological Function

There are few studies presented as evidence of the vital role played by the scrotal sac and testicles in the psychosexual development of the male. Psychophysiological observations demonstrate that in adult subjects under controlled conditions, utilizing structured interviews, the activities of the testes, cremaster muscle, and tunica dartos are very sensitive indicators of changes in psychological mood and are particularly relevant to both consciously and unconsciously perceived anxiety. It is also proved that pronounced scrotal activity occurred with anxiety-provoking discussions [9]. Although the testes are biologically primary, but it have been consigned by analysts to an ancillary role compared to the penis. Freud himself states unequivocally that it is remarkable what a small degree of attention the other part of the male genitals, the little sac with its contents, attracts in children.

Genital dysmorphophobia (GDP) is a condition less frequently diagnosed, which has evolved partly from the contemporary trends, as a sequential part of body dysmorphic disorder (BDD). It is often under-recognized, under-studied, and quite often untreated. Hence, the greater part of recent scientific literature has focused on the advances of cosmetic procedures and/or surgical interventions, without much concern about the role of GDP in the sexual function and self-esteem [10].

Although the sense of masculinity is given not only by the length and shape of the penis but also by an inner sense of belonging to the male sex and gender role, muscularity, breasts, hips, and buttocks, the GDP rather points to the preoccupation and concerns regarding the size, shape, and function of the penis [11].

The genital image is a subset of the overall body image, with an important role in sexual functioning. It is defined by Winter as the degree of feeling satisfaction/ dissatisfaction with various aspects of the genitals. The first measure of male genital image was the Male Genital Image Scale (MGIS) [12]. The MGIS is a 15 item scale, which primarily focuses on penis size, although two items assess pubic hair and two items assess appearance and "hang" of the testicles. Each item is given a satisfaction rating from 1 to 5, with higher scores indicating greater genital satisfaction.

Absent, empty or small scrotum have a great impaction in genital image and management. From the psychophysiological point of view it would seem that the activity of the cremaster and tunica dartos muscles, and testicular retraction constitute very sensitive indicators of changes in psychological mood or functioning [12].

Freud placed major emphasis on areas other than the sac and testes. In his paper on a phobia in a five-year-old boy, he minimized the role of the testes: 'It is remarkable what a small degree of interest the little sac with its contents arouses in the child' [13].

Bell [10] has indicated that the male, during the years two to six, is concretely aware of the uncontrollable retractile movements of his testes during fear, cold, anger, arousal, and defecation. These movements of the testes cause him a great deal of anxiety which he defends against by displacement to the penis. The testes are involved in early fears of object loss and later are a factor in sexual differences in bowel training, usually boys train later.

Niederland (1965) [14] cautions that the presence of an early body defect tends to remain an area of unresolved conflict through its relation to the most primitive body anxieties. Verbal discharge of these anxieties in psycho- analysis is not fully possible because they originate in a preverbal phase of life. The pediatric literature has recognized the significance of the testes and scrotum, not only medically but psychologically as well. Research on congenital urologic anomalies, delayed puberty, and cryptorchidism has made its contribution to the understanding of the significance of the testes and scrotum. One often recognizes the importance of an organ system only when it is faulty or missing, like good health. Richard G. Drus found significant characterologic changes occurring after descent of the testes: disappearance of social inadequacy and lessened chronic indecision, among others. The clarity and stability of the body image exerts an essential influence on the development and structure of the secondary autonomy of the ego [15].

## 6.4   Aesthetic Function

Scrotum had an essential functional and aesthetic roles for the male human being and genital image, and overall men's genital satisfaction and their sexual functioning.

Therefore men with an empty scrotum and subsequently smaller scrota are in need for some sort of testicular prostheses or implants, which have been in use for more than 70 years to guarantee an acceptable scrotal cosmesis in patients who have an empty scrotal sac or an atrophic testis and also when scrotal reconstruction is contemplated. Although various materials have been used in the production of testicular implants, silicone implants still remain the most popular option.

The main indication for implanting a testicular prosthesis is the restoration of the normal scrotal symmetry. The scrotal sac may be empty due to a wide number of causes.

Recently, Wu et al. [16] developed a tissue engineered testicular prosthesis with high-density polyethylene (and polyglycolic acid, after isolating the chondrocytes from swine cartilage, they were seeded onto scaffold and cultured for 2 weeks.

Engineered cartilage testes can be created in bioreactors and implanted in vivo, and can release testosterone for a prolonged period. Furthermore, the levels of testosterone release can be maintained within the physiologic range. This novel technology may be beneficial for patients who require testicular prostheses and chronic hormone supplementation.

In a study carried by Adshead et al. [17] they found that 91% of patients who replied to a questionnaire felt it was extremely important for them to be offered an implant at the time of an orchidectomy. They also demonstrated that 73% of those who had a prosthesis inserted felt that they either had an excellent or good result, but 23% were dissatisfied because of the shape or the position of the prosthesis.

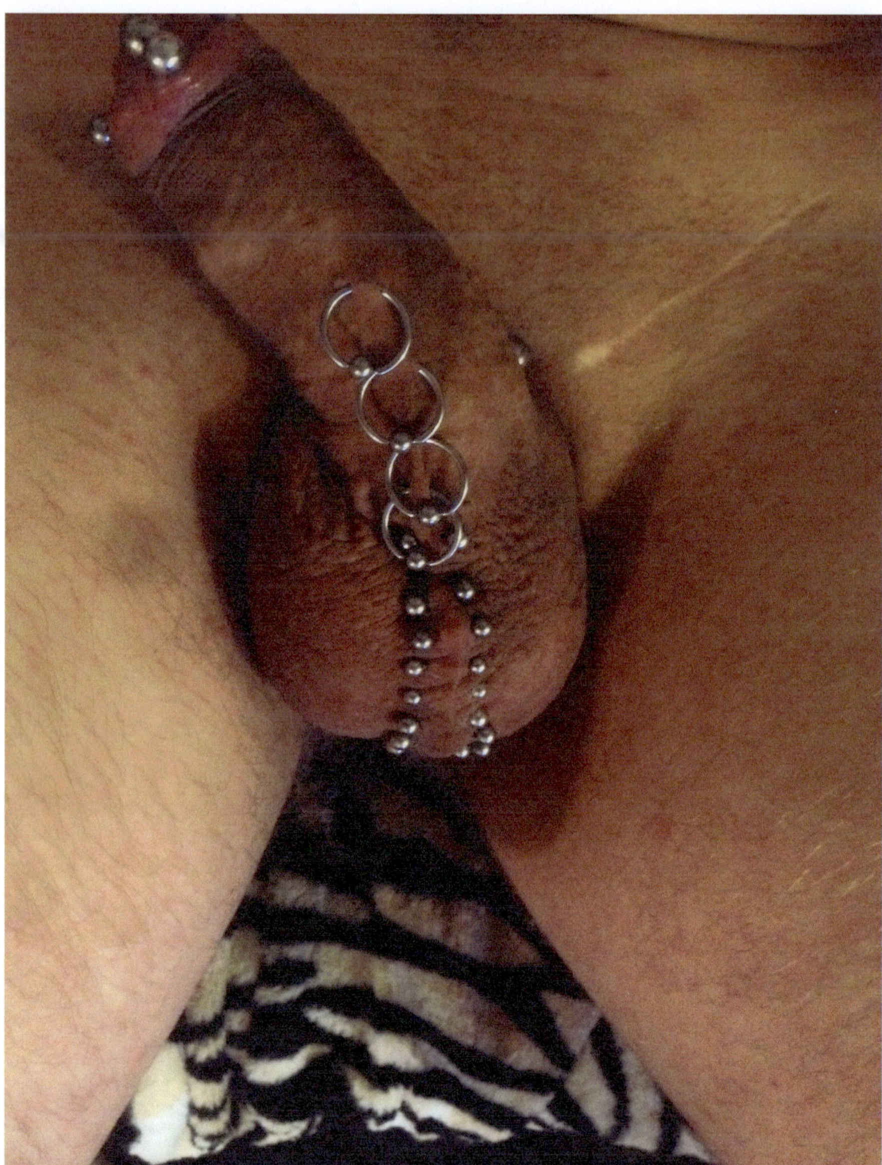

**Fig. 6.1** Scrotal and frenum ladder

# References


1. Moore Carl R, Oslund R. Experiments on the sheep testis- cryptorchidism, vasectomy and scrotal insulation. Amer Jour Physiol. 1924; LXVII:595–607
2. Richard E. Heller: new evidence for the function of the scrotum. Physiol Zool. 1929;2(1):9–17.
3. Valeri A, Mianne D, Merouze F, Bujan L, Altobelli A, Masson J. Etude de la temperature scrotale chez 258 hommes sains, selectionnes par triage au sort dans une population d'hommes de 18 a 23 ans. Analyse statistique, observations epidemiologiques et mesure des diameters testiculaires. Prog Urol. 1993;3:444–52.
4. Freeman S. The evolution of the scrotum: a new hypothesis. J Theor Biol. 1990;145(4):429–45.
5. Gallup GG, Finn MM, Sammis B. On the origin of descended scrotal testicles: the activation hypothesis. Evolution Psychol ISSN. 2009; 7(4): 1474–7049
6. Song GS, Seo JT. Relationship between ambient temperature and heat flux in the scrotal skin. Int J Androl. 2007; 32:288–94. Doi:https://doi.org/10.1111/j.1365-2605.2007.00848.x
7. Richard J. Human reproductive biology. Academic Press; 2013. p. 74. ISBN 9780123821850
8. Langdridge Darren, Barker Meg. Safe, sane, and consensual: contemporary perspectives on sadomasochism. Palgrave Macmillan; 2008. p. 174. ISBN 978-0-230-51774-5
9. Bell A 1. Some observations on the role of the scrotal sac and testicles. J Amer Psa Assn. 1961; IX:261–86
10. Ioana Micluţia. Genital dysmorphophobia in psychiatry and sexual medicine book. Chap 31, pp. 471–80. Springer Nature Switzerland. https://doi.org/10.1007/978-3-030-52298-8
11. Davis SN, Paterson LQ, Binik YM. Male genital image: measurement and implications for medical conditions and surgical practice. Theol Sex. 2011; 21:43–7
12. Winter HC. An examination of the relationships between penis size and body image genital image, and perception of sexual competency in the male. Unpublished doctoral dissertation, New York University; 1989
13. Bell AI, Stroebel CF, Prior DD. Interdisciplinary study: scrotal sac and testes. Psychoanal Q. 1971;40(3):415–34. https://doi.org/10.1080/21674086.1971.11926568.
14. Freud. Analysis of a Phobia in a Five-Year-Old Boy; 1909. Standard Edition X
15. Niederland W. Narcissistic ego impairment in patients with early physical malformation. The Psychoanabtic Study of the Child, 20:518–534. New York: International Universities Press; 1965
16. Druss RG. Cryptorchism and body image: the psychoanalysis of a case. J Am Psychoanal Assoc. 1978;26(1):69–85. https://doi.org/10.1177/000306517802600104.
17. Wu Y. Experimental study on tissue engineered testicular prosthesis with internal support. Zhongguo Xiu Fu Chong Jian Wai Ke Za Zhi. 2007;21(11):1243–6.
18. Adshead J, Khoubehi B, Wood J, Rustin G. Testicular implants and patient satisfaction: a questionnaire based study of men after orchidectomy for testicular cancer. BJU Int. 2001; 88 (6):559–62. 37

# Chapter 7
# Embryology of Scrotum

**Gabriela Ambriz-González and Francisco Javier León-Frutos**

**Nomenclature**

ExG    External genitalia
GT     Genital tubercle
DHT    Dihydrotestosterone
AR     Androgen receptor
CAH    Congenital adrenal hyperplasia
ESR1   Oestrogen receptor 1
ESR2   Oestrogen receptor 2
MIS    Mullerian inhibiting substance

Contemporary understanding of the morphogenetic and molecular mechanisms of sex differentiation of mammalian external genitalia (ExG) is still rudimentary and remains based mainly on principles enunciated by Alfred Jost over half a century ago [1, 2].

The Jost hypothesis states that male sexual differentiation is an active process based on production by the fetal testes of two hormones: testosterone and Mullerian inhibiting substance (MIS). In the presence of androgens, a male phenotype develops, whereas in the absence, the default female pathway occurs. Subsequently dihydrotestosterone (DHT) was shown to be the primary active metabolite responsible for masculinization of external genitalia in mammals. While elicits regression of the Mullerian duct in males. The Jost hypothesis has withstood the test of time and remains a useful model to explain clinical disorders of sex development [1–3].

Over the past decade, we have gather valuable clues regarding how embryonic organ development is organizes by regulatory genes and growth factors in the mechanisms of genital outgrowth and urethral tube closure are beginning to be understood [1, 4, 5].

G. Ambriz-González (✉) · F. J. León-Frutos
Chief of the Department of Pediatric Surgery, Unit of High Specialty, Pediatric Hospital, Medical Center of Western, Mexican Institute of Social Security, Mexico, Mexico


M. A. B. Fahmy (ed.), *Normal and Abnormal Scrotum*,
https://doi.org/10.1007/978-3-030-83305-3_7

Most of the progress in the area of external genital development has come from work on the mouse model; recent comparative studies have shown that early development of external genitalia is evolutionarily conserved across most amniote vertebrates. In mammals, birds, and major reptile clades, external genital development begins with the emergence of one paired genital swelling on either side of the cloacal membrane [4, 6].

At week five of intrauterine life, coelomic epithelium (lining epithelium of primitive peritoneal cavity) covering medial surface of mesonephros proliferates to form a genital ridge. Genitourinary system develops from genital ridge of intermediate mesoderm [3].

The sex of the embryo is determined when fertilization occurs, but the gonads acquire their male or female morphological characters from the 7th week of development [5, 7].

At week four, primordial germ cells migrate to genital ridge along dorsal mesentery. Formation of primitive sex cords: From surface (coelomic) epithelium, numerous cord-like processes develop and enter the genital ridge to form fingerlike cords called primitive sex cords differentiation of primordial germ cells in male is observed for the first time at 21 days [3, 7]

The undifferentiated gonad results from the arrival of the primordial germ cells to the genital crest, this occurs around the 6th week [7].

From this moment on, the coelomic epithelium actively proliferates, originating the primary sex cords that gradually surround the primordial germ cells. The primitive gonad protrudes on the anteromedial side of the intermediate mesoderm, displaying an undifferentiated appearance until the end of the 6th week [3, 7].

At week six of development, male and female embryos have two pairs of genital ducts: (1) the Wolffian ducts, and (2) the Müllerian ducts, which are reformed tubes parallel to the Wolffian also leading to the cloaca [3, 7].

Initially, the Müllerian ducts are separated in the pelvic region by a septum, but later they fuse and form the uterovaginal canal. The distal end of this duct grows caudally until it reaches the posterior wall of the definitive urogenital sinus, between the drainage of the Wolffian ducts. This stage depends on both genetic and hormonal factors [7].

In the male, the gonad undergoes modifications during weeks 6 to 8 of development that can be summarized as follows: The primary sex cords proliferate and form the testicular cords, which in the hilum of the gland originate a network of thin filaments that later derive into the rete testis or Haller's network. At week seven, mesenchymal tissue separates sex cords from coelomic epithelium and form a fibrous layer of tunica albuginea; mediastinal septa and interstitial cells of Leydig. During intrauterine life, these testicular cords are made up of primordial germ cells surrounded by Sertoli cells, remaining solid until puberty [3, 7].

The masculinization of the genital tract occurs during the third-fourth month of development. During the 5th month, the testicular cords transform into seminiferous tubes, inside which the gonocytes transform into spermatogonia [3, 4, 7].

The different seminiferous ducts, once the individual reaches sexual maturity, are channeled and joined to those of the Haller network, which flow into the efferent vessels (which come from the mesonephros), leading to the vas deferens [3, 7].

As for the male genital ducts, when the mesonephros returns, so do the tubules, except for those located in the region of the gonad. These tubules become the efferent vessels of the testis that will join the Haller network. Wolffian ducts persists (except in its cranial portion or appendix of the epididymis) and forms the vas deferens. Immediately below the terminal end of the efferent vessels, it coils itself, forming the epididymis. The portion of the Wolffian duct between the seminal vesicle and its end in the definitive urogenital sinus forms the ejaculatory duct. By the 8th week, Mullerian duct has degenerated in the male, except for its cranial portion, which forms the sessile hydatid. Its caudal end becomes the prostatic utricle located between the ejaculatory ducts [3, 5, 7].

External genitalia (ExG) are the reproductive organs necessary for efficient copulation and internal fertilization in various species. In mammals, male and female external genitalia, the penis and the clitoris, are derived from a common primordium: the genital tubercle (GT). Sexual differentiation of the external genitalia occurs relatively late, after differentiation of the gonads and expression of sex steroid receptors in the genital tubercle [4, 6–8].

The initial development of the ExG is similar in both genders; it is named the undifferentiated or asexual stage. The molecular mechanisms of external genital development are beginning to be identified; however, the origin of cells that give rise to external genitalia is unknown [7, 8].

Distinctive sexual characteristics begin during the ninth week, but the external genitalia are not totally differentiated until the twelfth week. (61 to 83 days of embryonic development). In this undifferentiated period, three progressive formations develop around the orifice of the cloaca in embryos of both genders, corresponding to 1. Cloacal eminence, 2. Cloacal folds and 3. Genital eminences. At this stage, it is impossible to determine the sex of the embryo [3, 7].

At week four, somatopleuric lateral plate mesoderm thickens on the side of cloacal membrane. This thickening produces surface elevation called cloacal folds. The urorectal septum divides the cloacal membrane into ventral urogenital membrane and dorsal anal membrane. The cloacal eminence grows and originates the genital tubercle (GT). The GT is the precursor of the penis and the clitoris, although early development of the tubercle is similar in males and females [3, 4, 6, 7].

Along with the division of cloacal membrane, cloacal fold is also divided into cranial larger urethral folds and caudal anal folds. The cloacal eminence grows and originates the genital tubercle. The GT is the precursor of the penis and the clitoris, although early development of the tubercle is similar in males and females [3, 4, 7].

All three germ layers participate in external genital development; genital mesoderm forms the stromal tissue of the phallus, endoderm derived urethral plate epithelium forms the entire urethral tube, and a tunic of ectodermal epithelium forms the skin and epithelial appendages, such as sweat glands and pilosebaceous units. Although cell lineage analysis of different germ layers within the GT has identified the fates of genital tubercle derivatives, little is known about the embryonic origin of the GT itself [4, 5, 7].

The GT is derived from the latera-most mesoderm. Based on the anteroposterior position of the GT relative to the hind limb buds. Herrera and cols reported that progenitors of the paired genital swellings and the resultant GT could reside in lateral mesoderm at the axial level of the hindlimb buds [3, 4].

The development of the GT requires tight coordination, it has been suggested that several growth factors such as sonic hedgehog, fibroblast growth factors, and bone morphogenetic proteins play orchestrating roles in GT formation before masculinization [8, 9]

The development of the GT can be subdivided into a three-step process: the first phase is characterized for a pre-androgen stage, in which the cloacal membrane forms the lateral genital swellings bilaterally. The second phase is controlled by the presence of masculinizing genetic regulation, and the presence of androgen signaling (DHT) which is secreted by the fetal testes (Leydig cells) [1, 3–5, 8]. However, candidate developmental genes for such processes have been poorly described, Nishada et al., reported three genes detected by real time quantitative PCR analysis (Cyp1b1, Fkbp51 and MafB) with prominently increased expression in male GT. Although expressions of these genes are reported to be correlated with the androgen stimulation in prostate cancer, their functions during GT masculinization processes are unclear [9].

Avendaño and cols, described a syndrome known as 5-alpha-reductase deficiency, results in 46XY males presenting as either feminized males or females at birth due to the inability of testosterone to convert to the more potent androgen, DHT [10].

In other cases, congenital adrenal hyperplasia in 46XX females causes masculinization of the clitoris caused by overproduction of testosterone by the adrenal glands [11, 12]

The third phase of external genitalia development is more genetically complex and relevant in the male than in the female due to the increased distal outgrowth. In this point is taken the tubularization of the urethra throughout the length of the penis. If the male urethra does not tubularize completely, the result is a common congenital defect termed hypospadias [5].

Hypospadias, can be either isolated or present as part of a genetic syndrome and accompanied by other congenital defects. They vary in severity according to how far away the meatus from its intended distal position [13]. Baskin published recently that the male and female developing external genitalia in both the human and mouse express ESR1 and ESR2, along with the androgen receptor (AR). Human clinical data suggests that exogenous estrogens can adversely affect normal penile and urethral development, resulting in hypospadias. Timing of estrogenic exposure, or "window of susceptibility," is an important consideration when examining malformations of the external genitalia in both humans and mice [2, 14].

Around the 10th week in male embryos, the GT lengthens and drags with itself the urethral folds forming the lateral walls of the urethral sulcus of the penis. This groove is delimited by a proliferation of endodermal cells called the urethral plate [3].

At the end of the third month, the two urethral folds close over the urethral lamina and form the penile urethra. This groove runs along the caudal surface of the elongated phallus, but does not reach the most distal portion referred as the glans [1, 2]

In its caudal portion, the penis widens and forms the glans, covered by the foreskin; the most distal portion of the urethra is shaped during the fourth month, when ectodermal cells from the tip of the glans penetrate into the interior and create a short epithelial cord. This cord is then canalized, originating the balanic portion of the penile urethra [2, 8].

Inside phallic mesenchyme, the corpus spongiosum differentiates from the corpora cavernous. A circular epithelial lamina proliferates from the urethral meatus backward allowing the glans to separate from the foreskin shortly before birth. It is the preputial lamina [3].

In the male the labioscrotal swellings migration takes place in the 9th to 11th weeks of gestation and follows in a caudal and medial direction until they fuse at the 12th-week of gestation and form the scrotum, where the testicles will descend (see Fig. 7.1) [15–18].

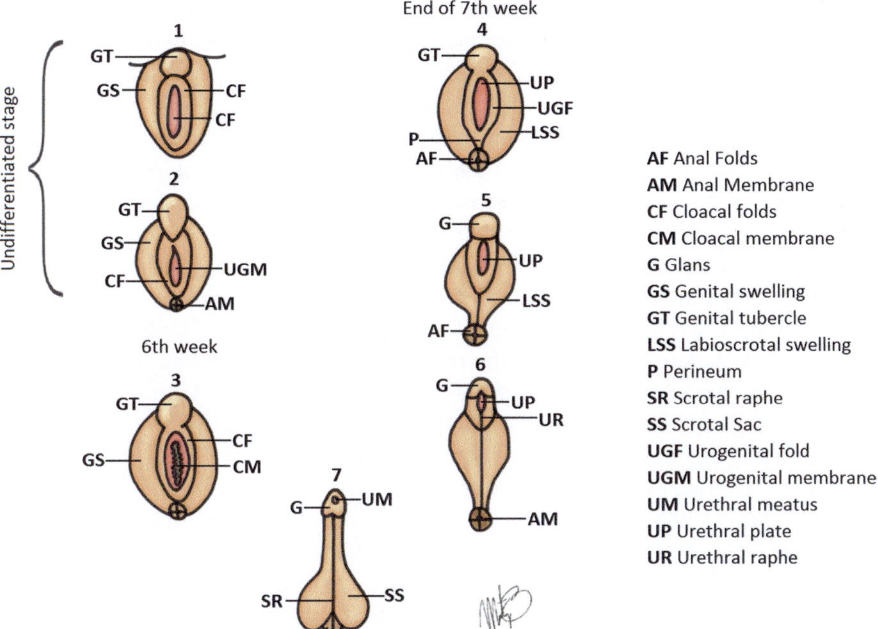


**Fig. 7.1** Embryonic development of male external genitalia

The scrotum may suffer congenital malformations due to abnormal development of the labioscrotal swellings, which occur during intrauterine life. These malformations include accessory scrotum, bifid scrotum, ectopic scrotum, and penoscrotal transposition (PST) [15, 18] (Chap. 12).

Bifid scrotum is a partial or complete separation of normally hemiscrotum in patients, commonly associated with severe hypospadias or chordee. In cases of PST, part or whole of the scrotum is located superior to the penile shaft [17].

PST is defined as the penile malposition of the penis, caudally and posteriorly from the scrotum. Cohen-Addad et al. classified PSTs into three categories: true PST with a normal scrotum, complete PST with bifid scrotum and PST with posterior pelvis deformity. One physiopathological theory is the labioscrotal fold, failure to migrate dorsally, due to absent or insufficient response to androgens in the target tissue. Other theory is the abnormal positioning of the genital tubercle in relation to the scrotal folds [17, 18].

PST also is relationated with genetic factors, familial inheritance can be considered, although most cases are sporadic [18]. Pinke et al. reported 53 cases of incomplete PST and their associated anomalies: genital defects (73.3%), urinary system anomalies (60%), skeletal system anomalies (33.3%), had congenital cardiac defects (20%) facial dysmorphism (13.3%), gastrointestinal tract anomalies (13.3%) and central nervous system anomalies (13.3%). Overall survival was 56.3 and 37.5% neonatal deaths [19].

Ectopic scrotum is positioning in other site of the scrotum which is usually unilateral and suprainguinal, but in some cases infrainguinal (femoral) or on the thigh. The ipsilateral testis is usually present within the ectopic hemiscrotum [17]

There are about 30 cases of accessory scrotum reported in the literature either being solitary or in association with other urogenital or no urogenital abnormalities. This malformation consists in scrotal tissue without testis, which can be present in either the perineum or elsewhere, in addition to a normally developed scrotum. In the absence of a perineal lipoma, accessory perineal scrota are usually associated with other anomalies, including hypospadias, diphallia, defects of scrotal position, anorectal anomalies, and the VACTERL (vertebral, anal, cardiac, tracheoesophageal, renal, and limb anomalies) association [13, 17, 20].

The etiology for an accessory scrotum is not known. Some authors have suggested that the failure migration to the middle of the labioscrotal swelling could be the cause for the occurrence of accessory scrotum [21, 22]. Lamm and Kaplan postulated that one labioscrotal swelling may embryologically divide into two portions with the inferior portion migrating incompletely to form an accessory scrotum [17]. According to Sule et al., the accessory labioscrotal fold usually develops due to intervening mesenchymal tissue disrupting the continuity of developing labioscrotal swelling. Absence of other organ malformations suggests that the causative factor may not have adverse effects on other organ systems undergoing differentiation at the same time, like the musculoskeletal system, spine and central nervous system, even though all these structures get differentiated during the same gestational period [16, 22, 23].

Finally, it is in this pouch where the testicles will settle definitively at the end of a migration that begins during the third month. Testicular migration takes place in two stages: from the 3rd to the 5th month, first because of a phenomenon of relative migration due to the growth of the lumbar region, and later from the 6th to the 8th month, due to an active migration. In the 6th month it is at the level of the pre-peritoneal orifice of the inguinal canal and reaches the final scrotal position in the 8th month [3].

# References


1. Weiss DA, Rodríguez Jr. E, Cunha T, Menshenina J, Barcellos D, Chan LY, et al. Morphology of the external genitalia of the adult male and female mice as an endpoint of sex differentiation. Mol Cell Endocrinol. 2012 May 6; 354(0):94–102. https://doi.org/10.1016/j.mce.2011.08.009
2. Baskin L, Sinclair A, Derpinghaus A, Cao M, Li Y, Overland M, Aksel S, Cunha GR. Estrogens and development of the mouse and human external genitalia. Differentiation. 2021;118:82–106. https://doi.org/10.1016/j.diff.2020.09.004
3. Sontakke Yogesh. Reproductive system male and female reproductive organ. In: Sontakke Yogesh. Texbook of human embriology with clinical cases and 3D clinical illustrations. Published by Satish Kumar Jain and produced by Varum Jain for CBS Publishers & Distributors Pvt. Ltd. 1$^{st}$ edition. 2019, pp. 215–230
4. Herrera AM, Shuster SG, Perriton CL, Cohn MJ. Developmental basis of phallus reduction during bird evolution. Curr Biol. 2012;23:1065–74.
5. Yamada G, Suzuki K, Haraguchi R, Miyagawa S, Satoh Y, Kamimura M, et al. Molecular genetic cascades for external genitalia formation: an emerging organogenesis program. Dev Dyn. 2006;235:1738–52.
6. Herrera AM, Brennan PL, Cohn MJ. Development of avian external genitalia: interspecific differences and sexual differentiation of the male and female phallus. Sex Dev. 2015;9(1): 43–52.
7. Serra RI, Vinaixa F, Serra RJM, Torres B. Estudio embriológico del aparato genital: aspectos clínicos. Acta Pediátric Esp. 1987;45(5):279–86.
8. Perriton CL, Powles N, Chiang C, Maconochie MK, Cohn MJ. Sonic hedgehog signaling from the urethral epithelium controls external genital development. Dev Biol. 2002;247: 26–46.
9. Nishida H, Miyagawa S, Matsumaru D, Wada Y, Satoh Y, Ogino Y, Fukuda S, Iguchi T, Yamada G. Gene expression analyses on embryonic external genitalia: identification of regulatory genes possibly involved in masculinization processes. Congenit Anom (Kyoto). 2008;48(2):63–7. https://doi.org/10.1111/j.1741-4520.2008.00180.x PMID: 18452486.
10. Avendaño A, Paradisi I, Cammarata-Scalisi F, Callea M. 5-α-Reductase type 2 deficiency: is there a genotype-phenotype correlation? A review. Hormones (Athens). 2018;17(2):197–204. https://doi.org/10.1007/s42000-018-0013-9. Epub 2018 Apr 20. PMID: 29858846.
11. Yang JH, Menshenina J, Cunha GR, Place N, Baskin LS. Morphology of mouse external genitalia: implications for a role of estrogen in sexual dimorphism of the mouse genital tubercle. J of Urol. 2010;184:1604–9.
12. El-Maouche D, Arlt W, Merke DP. Congenital adrenal hyperplasia. Lancet 2017;390 (10108):2194–2210. https://doi.org/10.1016/S0140-6736(17)31431-9. Epub 2017 May 30. Erratum in: Lancet. 2017 Nov 11;390 (10108):2142. PMID: 28576284.
13. Baskin L. What is hypospadias? Clin Pediatr (Phila). 2017;56(5):409–18. https://doi.org/10.1177/0009922816684613.

14. Baskin LS. New Insights into Hypospadias: Next-generation Sequencing Reveals Potential Genetic Factors in Male Urethral Development. Eur Urol 2021;79(4):516–518. https://doi.org/10.1016/j.eururo.2021.01.006. Epub 2021 Jan 19. PMID: 33483178.
15. Garcia RA, Sajjad H. Anatomy, Abdomen and Pelvis, Scrotum. 2021 Jul 31. In: StatPearls [Internet]. Treasure Island (FL): StatPearls Publishing; 2021 Jan. PMID: 31751083.
16. Lee JI, Jung HG. Perineal accessory scrotum with a lipomatous hamartoma in an adult male. J Korean Surg Soc. 2013;85(6):305–8.
17. Souvik C, Vishal G, Sasanka N, Dipak G, Sarbani C, Sukanta KD. Perineal accessory scrotum with congenital lipoma: a rare case report. Case Rep Pediatri. 2012;2012:2. https://doi.org/10.1155/2012/757120.
18. Kurt D, Sivrikoz TS, Kalelioğlu Hİ, Has R, Ziylan HO, Yüksel A. Prenatal diagnosis of complete penoscrotal transposition with normal scrotum: Two case reports and review of the literature. J Clin Ultrasound 2020; 48(6):350–356. https://doi.org/10.1002/jcu.22834. Epub 2020 Apr 22. PMID: 32319694.
19. Pinke LA, Rathbun SR, Husmann DA, Kramer SA. Penoscrotal transposition: review of 53 patients. J Urol. 2001;166(5):1865-8. https://doi.org/10.1016/s0022-5347(05)65708–4. PMID: 11586250.
20. Fitouri F, Chebil N, Ben Ammar S, Sahli S, Hamzaoui M. Accessory scrotum. Fetal Pediatr Pathol. 2020;39(1):90–1. https://doi.org/10.1080/15513815.2019.1629133 Epub 2019 Jun 19 PMID: 31215294.
21. Baskin L. What Is Hypospadias? Clin Pediatr (Phila) 2017; 56(5):409–418. https://doi.org/10.1177/0009922816684613. Epub 2017 Jan 12. PMID: 28081624.
22. Yuzo K, Teiichi T. Accessory scrotum: a case report and review of the literature. Br J Plast. 1994;4:579–80.
23. Park KH, Hong JH. Perineal lipoma in association with scrotal anomalies in children. BJU Int. 2006;98(2):409–12.
24. Pananghat AK, Pavai A, Prasanna NK. Accessory scrotum in the perineum. J Indian Assoc Pediatr Surg. 2011;16(4):169–70.

# Chapter 8
# Anatomy of the Scrotum

**Mohamed A. Baky Fahmy**

**Abbreviations**

CM   Cremasteric Muscle
GT   Gubernaculum Testis
SL   Scrotal Ligement
TV   Tunica Vaginalis
BS   Bulbospongiosus

## 8.1   Layers of the Scrotum

The scrotum is developed independently, but anatomically it is considered, to some extant, as an extension of the abdominal wall, thus its layers are similar to it; the comparison between the two walls is shown in Table 8.1. The scrotum is a musculocutaneous pouch, its wall divided into six layers; the skin, superficial (dartos) fascia, external spermatic fascia, cremaster muscle and fascia, internal spermatic fascia, and tunica vaginalis from outside to inside. A poorly defined multilayered appearance can be seen when examining the scrotal wall with sonography (Chap. 27). Actual scrotal wall is formed of skin, dartos muscle and facia, but the other four layers are more or less belonging and surrounding the testicle.

**1. Skin**: Both penile and scrotal skin are thin, elastic and has no adipose fatty layer, and more pigmented than the remainder of the body, irrespective of ethnic background, although this distinct darkness is more obvious in individuals with a black and colored skin. The scrotum is distinguished from the rest of the body by the presence of rugae, which bear thinly scattered, crimped hairs. The scrotal epidermis

M. A. B. Fahmy (✉)
Al-Azhar University, Cairo, Egypt

**Table 8.1** The layer structure relationship between the scrotum and the anterior abdominal wall

| Layer of the scrotum and spermatic cord Layer | Structure of the anterior abdominal wall |
| --- | --- |
| 1. Skin | 1. Skin |
| 2. Superficial (dartos) fascia | 2. Superficial fascia (fatty layer) |
| 3. External spermatic fascia | 3. External oblique aponeurosis |
| 4. Cremaster muscle and fascia | 4. Internal oblique and transversus abdominis muscle |
| 5. Internal spermatic fascia | 5. Transversalis fascia |
| 6. Tunica vaginalis (visceral layer, parietal layer) | 6. Parietal peritoneum |

covers the dermis, which merges with the smooth muscle bundles of the dartos muscle. Scrotal skin has numerous sweat and sebaceous glands whose secretion can react with the local bacteria and produce a special odor characteristic for the inguinal region, specially in adults and adolescent. The external appearance of the scrotum is not constant, it varies according to body temperature; generally it contracts in cold circumstances, but at warm, it stretches and the sweat glands secrete more to keep the local temperature around the testicles lower than the body temperature by 2–3 °C, which benefits the spermatogenesis. The scrotal skin will also contract and thicken when sexual arousal occurs Fig. 8.1.

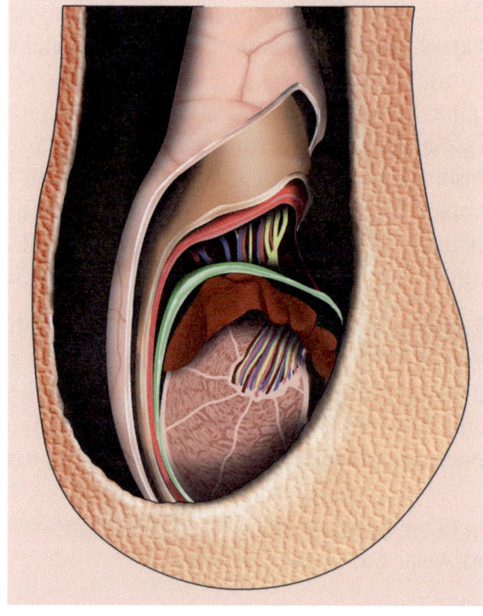

**Fig. 8.1** Six scrotal layers. Photo drawn by Prof Samir A Salam, General surgery Dept, Al azhar University

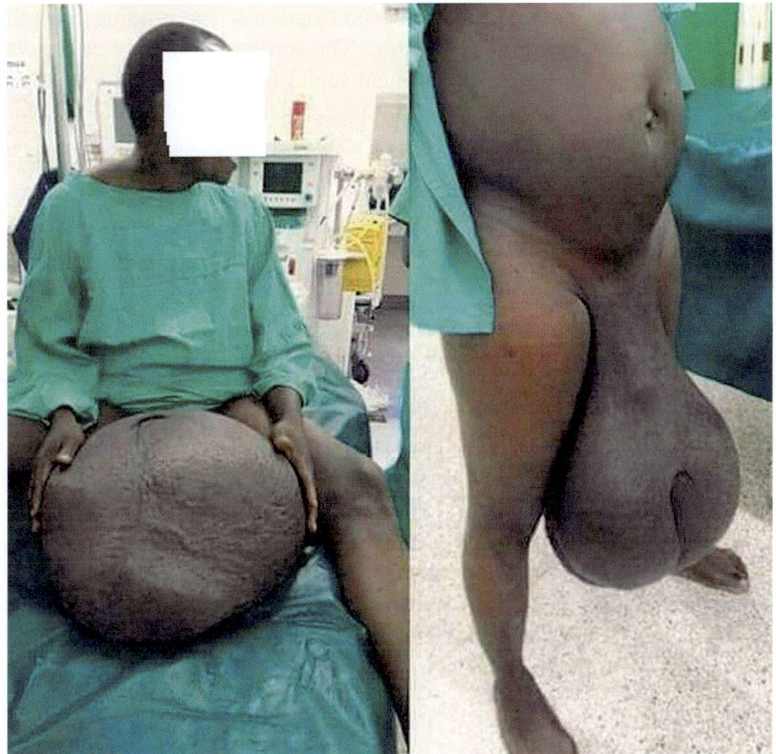

Fig. 8.2 Hugely distended scrotal wall reaching below the knee with a bilateral inguinal herniae

The scrotal skin is highly stretchable and expansile, so in neglected cases of inguinal hernia and hydroceles we may see a hugely expanded scrotal skin reaching down to the level of knees Fig. 8.2.

## 8.2 Scrotal Rugae

In anatomy, rugae are a series of ridges produced by folding of the wall of an organ. Scrotal rugae is a unique character of the scrotum; sometimes the tip of the prepuce poses the same rugae arrangement. These rugae are characteristic by its arrangement and colour, it arranged transversely with a downward inclination in resting position, innumerable minute ridges are superposed upon these. There is no doubt that the purpose of the scrotal muscles is to adapt the skin to the varying volume of the organ, as the changes are greater than could be accommodated by the elasticity of the skin alone, the rugae plays an important role in increasing the scrotal surface area and subsequently adapted the scrotum for a maximum performance in thermal regulation. Scrotal raphe is a slightly elevated ridge of tissue running from the base of the penis to the midline of the perineum. The scrotal raphe is in continuity with the penile raphe superiorly and the perineal raphe inferiorly. Slight hyperpigmentation of the genital raphe is almost invariably present (Fig. 8.3). Surface anatomy and morphology of rugae and raphe are described with details in Chap. 9.

**2. Dartos Muscle and Fascia**: Sometimes it is called simply dartos, or Colles's fascia, it is a layer of connective tissue found in the penile shaft, foreskin, and scrotum. The term "dartos" is derived from the Greek δέρνω/derno (beat, flog) and/ or δέρμα/derma (skin), meaning "that which is skinned or flayed", possibly due to its appearance.

It is a thin layer which contains smooth muscles, dense connective tissues, and elastic fibers forming a well formed fascial sheet. This fascia is 12 mm thick. The penile portion is referred to as the superficial fascia of penis, while the scrotal part is the dartos proper. In addition to being continuous with itself between the scrotum and the penis, it is also continuous with Scarpa's fascia of the anterolateral abdominal wall and with Colles's fascia of the perineum. The dartos fascia is closely attached to the skin for the lack of adipose tissues, and this attachment is responsible for the designated scrotal rugae, which are specially obvious when the dartos muscle fibers are in a tonic contracture, but once these contraction is lost the scrotum will looks smooth and lax. The skin and dartos fascia is just superficial to the external spermatic fascia in the scrotum and to Buck's fascia in the penile shaft.

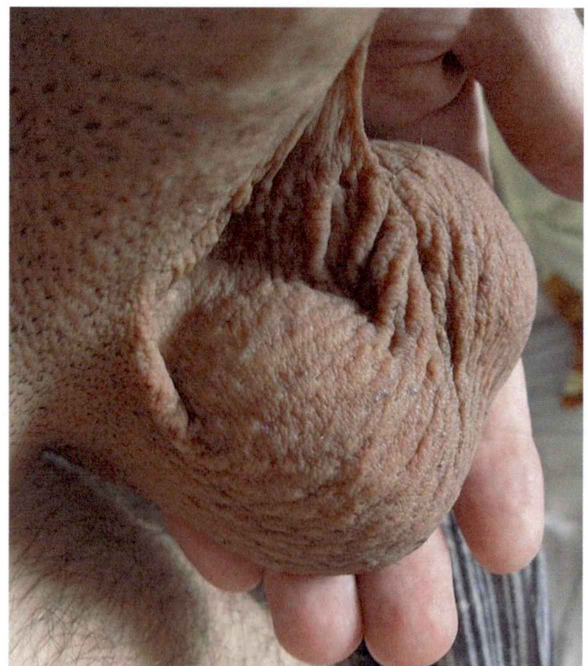

**Fig. 8.3** Typical configuration of the scrotum in adult with a minimal extension of the scrotal skin to the root of the penis

Weicker [1] postulated a rhythmic contraction pattern of the tunica dartos which was influenced by changes in temperature, weight, psychological factors, and by drugs, fatigue, and sleep. The dartos fascia extends into the scrotal septum, which connects the raphe to the inferior surface of the penile radix and divides the scrotum into the left and right chambers. The two compartments hold the testis, epididymis, and part of the spermatic cord separately. The smooth muscle of the dartos fascia stretches or contracts depending on the variations of temperature in the environment to regulate the temperature within the scrotum. Contraction reduces the surface area available for heat loss, thus reducing heat loss and warming the testicles. Conversely, expansion increases the surface area, promoting more heat loss and thus cooling the testicles. The dartos muscle works in conjunction with the cremaster muscle to elevate the testis but this should not be confused with the cremasteric reflex [2].

In females, the same muscle fibers are less well developed and termed dartos muliebris, lying beneath the skin of the labia majora, it forms a tiny rugae, apparent in some females, specially in neonates. Dartos facia and muscles receive innervation from postganglionic sympathetic nerve fibers arriving via the ilioinguinal nerve and the posterior scrotal nerve [3].

The origin of the dartos muscle and facia as well the bilateral dorsolateral perineal complex is derived from the dermatomes of the same somites that provide the tissue for the striated muscles of the perineum. Dartos is a double-layered construction, this construction is shown to be the result of an early division into two components, superficial and deep. The latter participates in the strong proliferation of the stroma dorsal to the urethral orifice, thereby forming a continuous layer of parallel bundles of smooth muscle cells extending from the external anal sphincter to the free margin of the prepuce. Meanwhile, the superficial component keeps its distinct structure and remains restricted to the skin of the scrotum. Together, the two components provide the dartos fascia of the scrotum with its remarkably intricate bilaminate histologic structure, which clearly recognized in adult. The dartos stroma, which originally formed the main constituent of both scrotal swellings, keeps also its bilaminate structure. The deep lamina, with its characteristic ventralward orientation, differentiates into relatively large ventralward oriented and isolated bundles of smooth muscle cells embedded in a finely fibrillar connective tissue rich in blood vessels. The bundles begin at the ventral extremity of the external anal sphincter, fan out into the scrotal halves, converge toward the shaft of the penis where the pattern becomes predominantly oblique-transverse because the bundles maintain their ventralward direction around a penis, which stands almost perpendicular to the scrotum, and end at the free margin of the prepuce. The configuration of the stromal elements does not change during the shift of the urethral orifice to the tip of the penis during early development of the male urogenital area [4] (Fig. 8.4).

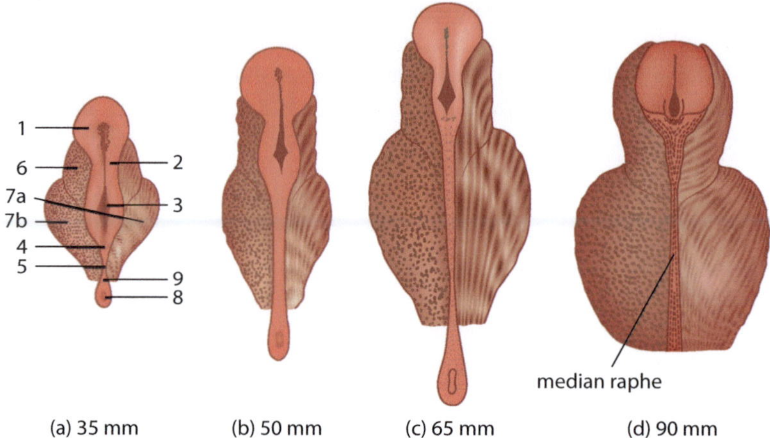



**Fig. 8.4** Schematic drawings of the external perineum of male fetuses of 35 to 90 mm, dartos layers consisting of a deep lamina passing into a superficial lamina (7b) confined to the scrotum (shown at the right side only). 8, Anal orifice; 9, Perineal raphe. ( modified from Ref 4)

**Peripenic muscle**: The peripenic muscle have been described for the first time by Sappey in 1860, but it is passed over with the briefest mention by the majority of anatomical textbooks [4]. It is not generally realised that the dartos muscle of the scrotum is continued forward beneath the skin of the penis to from the peripenic muscles, this muscle sheet has a certain practical importance (Fig. 8.5).

It has been thought that the dartos muscle extends into the penis only for a short distance on its underside, in the so-called area scroti of Klatsch. These are two areas, one on either side of the root of the penis on its under surface, and presented externally by a skin corrugation differing from the rest of the penile skin in presenting a darker, rougher appearance, in being very rich in sebaceous glands, and plentifully provided with hairs. This is too conservative an estimate of the extent of the dense muscle tissue (Fig. 8.6). But Delbert [5] and others reported that this muscle extends over the whole length of the penis. Many authors indicated that the peripenic muscle is composed of unstriped fibers which form an incomplete investment of the penis from its base to the extremity of the prepuce [4–6]. The muscle is situated 1 or 2 mm beneath the skin, from which it is quite separate except inferiorly in the region of the median raphe. The muscle bundles are very slender and are made up of a few muscle-cells only, but they run in every direction transversely, longitudinally, and obliquely. The development and strength of the whole dartos sheet varies greatly in different individuals, and the peripenic muscle is not always well formed. It is particularly weak in persons with dependent, lax, and smooth scrotums.

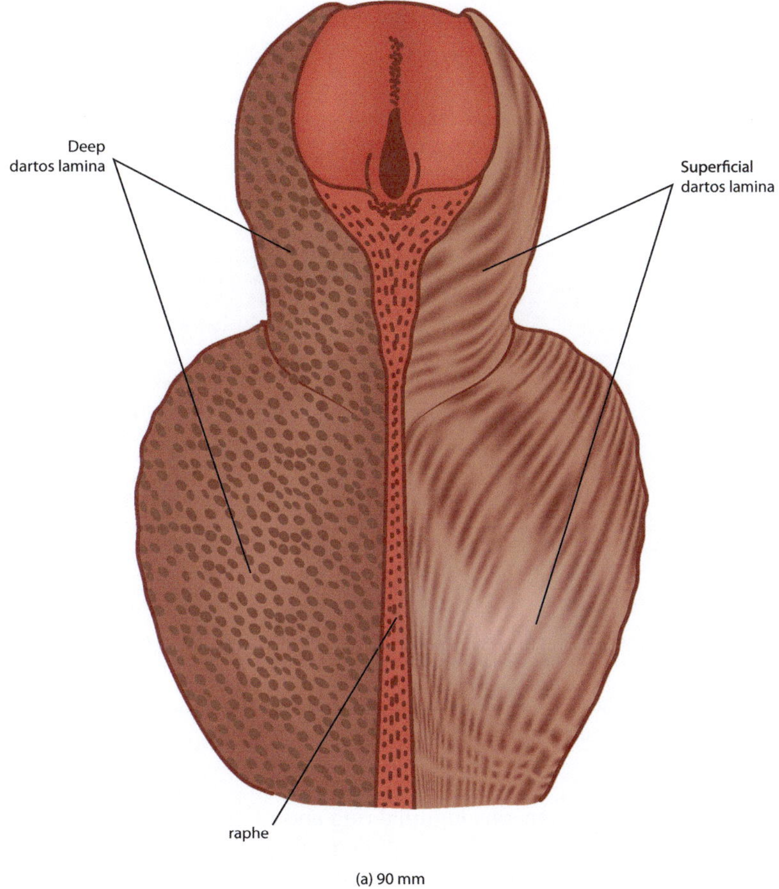


**Fig. 8.5** Extension of dartos lamina to the shaft of the penis during penile development

I think peripenic muscle fibers are of paramount importance to preserve a normal penoscrotal angle, and to keep scrotal contents (testicles) away from the root of the penis, as it act as a diaphragm separated scrotal contents from the penis, this will be discussed in the chapter of scrotal anomalies (Chaps. 11 and 13).

Distorted or dysgenetic abnormal prepenic muscle is responsible for penile chordee, which may associates some cases of hypospadias and really this chordee standing alone as an isolated anomaly, also distorted dartos or its component "prepenic muscles" may be the underlying pathology for different cases of webbed penis and penoscrotal fusion (Fig. 8.7).

Defective dartos muscle and facia and its clinical impaction will be discussed in details with scrotal congenital anomalies (Chap. 13).

**3. External Spermatic Fascia**: It is a thin membrane of connective tissue which contains collagen fibers and connects to the dartos fascia loosely. It is originates

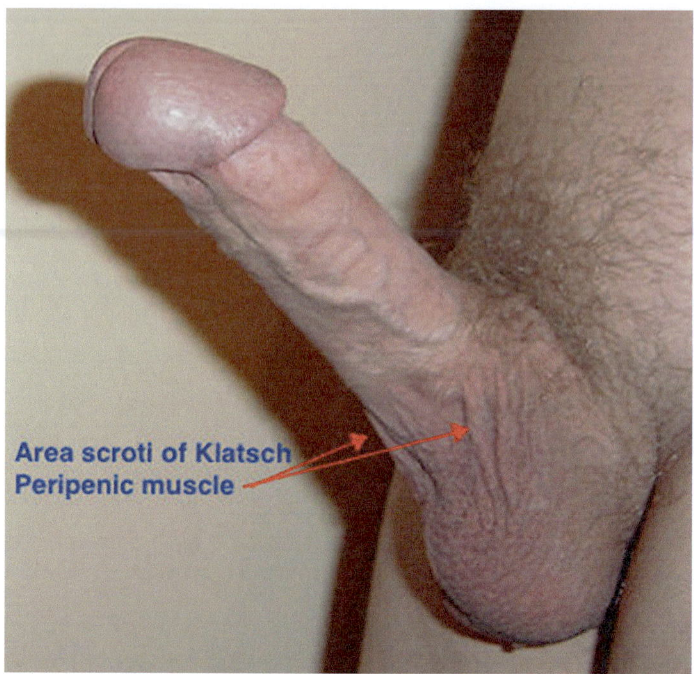


**Fig. 8.6** Erected penis showing the extension of prepenic muscles manifested as a scrotal lateral extension to both sided of the root of the penis

from the edge of the subcutaneous inguinal ring and extends to the deep layer of the abdominal superficial fascia and the abdominal external oblique aponeurosis. Around the spermatic cord this layer is well formed, and should be dissected carefully during varicocelectomy and herniotomy.

**4. Cremaster Muscle (CM):** The name of the cremaster muscle is derived from the ancient Greek transitive verb "I hang" (Greek: κρεμάννυμι). It is a thin layer of muscle fibers originating from the internal oblique and transversus abdominis muscles. The cremaster muscle and spermatic cord enter the scrotum through the superficial inguinal ring and surround the testis and epididymis. When the skin of lower abdomen or upper thigh is stimulated, the cremaster muscle will contracts, which results in ascending of the testis and scrotum, that is known as the cremasteric reflex. The CM maintains the testis in a suspended position. The cremaster muscle is a paired structure, there being one on each side of the body (Fig. 8.8).

The CM develops to its full extent only in males; in females it is represented by only a few muscle loops and is found on the round ligament. In rats, it has been shown that cremaster muscles developed from the gubernacular bulb, also in human embryo the bottom of the CM is attached to the dome of gubernaculum. Anatomically, the lateral cremaster muscle originates from the internal oblique muscle, just superior to the inguinal canal, and the middle of the inguinal ligament.

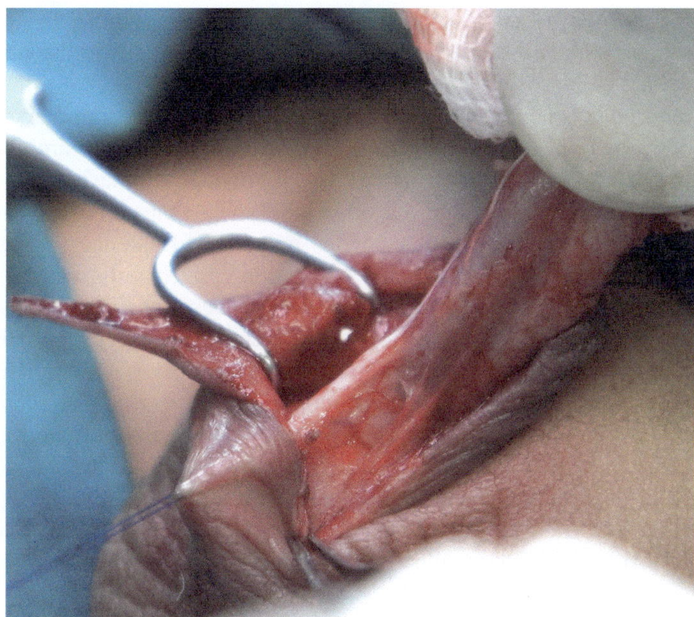

**Fig. 8.7** Dissection of the distorted dartos anchoring the penis to the scrotum and manifested as a penile webbing

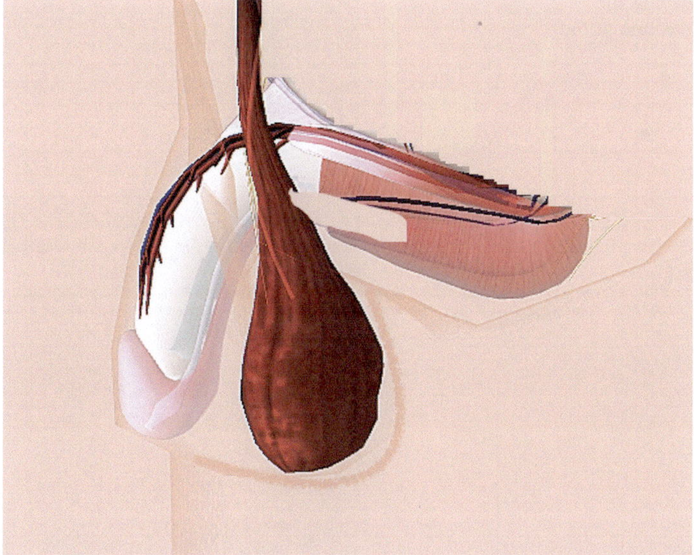

**Fig. 8.8** Diagrammatic presentation of CM, with its fibers sloping over itself, and hanging the testicle

The medial cremaster muscle, which sometimes is absent, originates from the pubic tubercle and sometimes the lateral pubic crest. Both inserted into the tunica vaginalis underneath the testis [7].

CM is an "embryogenic" striated muscle contains a large number of smooth muscle fibers, and the excessive electromyographic discharges are due to the presence of multifocal motor end-plates, it had a polyneural innervation both at the muscle fibre and/or at the spinal cord level in adult males, thus it has a weak cortical control but mostly excited by the cutaneous inputs [8]. Evidence suggests differences in contractility in CM associated with undescended testis caused by alterations of autonomic innervation. These differences may contribute to the pathophysiology of undescended testis [9]. The cremaster muscle is supplied by the cremasteric artery which is a branch of inferior epigastric artery, and it is innervated from the genital branch of the genitofemoral nerve. So it receives distinctly different innervation and vascular supply in comparison to the internal oblique muscle.

The cremaster muscle's function is to raise and lower the testes in order to regulate scrotal temperature for optimal spermatogenesis and survival of the produced spermatozoa. It does this by increasing or decreasing the exposed surface area of the surrounding tissue, allowing faster or slower dissipation of body heat (Fig. 8.9).

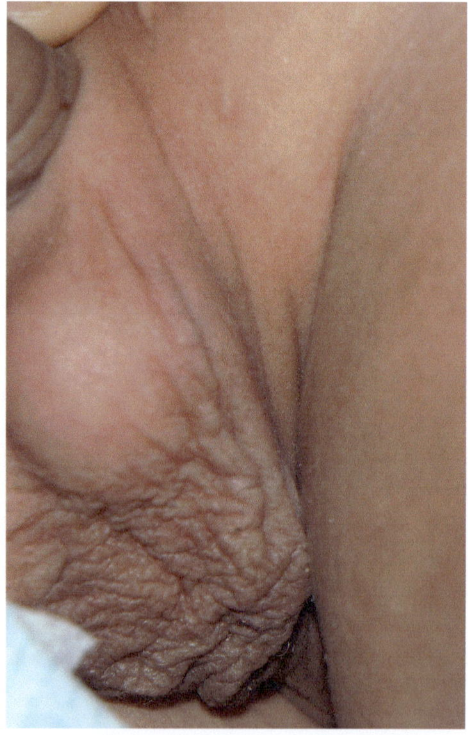

**Fig. 8.9** Obvious cremasteric contraction pulling up the testes and leaving the corrugated scrotum at the bottom

The CM is solely an involuntary muscle, but it poses some voluntary contraction in adult and its contraction, which occurs during arousal, can prevent injury of the testicles during sex, also contraction occurs during ejaculation. Cremasteric contraction can also occurs during moments of extreme fear, possibly help to avoid injuring the testes while dealing with a fighting situation. Kegel exercise which is known as pelvic-floor exercise, involves repeatedly contracting and relaxing the muscles that form part of the pelvic floor, sometimes colloquially referred to as the "Kegel muscles", which could be performed multiple times each day, for several minutes at a time, but takes one to three months to begin to have an effect. CM can also be contracted voluntarily, by performing Kegels (which somehow contracts the cremaster), or by flexing and tightening the abdominal muscles [10]. Clinically, a reflex arc termed the cremasteric reflex can be demonstrated by lightly stroking the skin of the inner thigh downwards from the hip towards the knee. This stimulates the sensory fibers of the ilioinguinal nerve, which enters the spinal cord at L1. The sensory fibers stimulate the motor fibers of the genital branch of the genitofemoral nerve (also at spinal level L1), which provides innervation to the cremaster muscles causing the contraction of the muscle and elevation of the testes.

**Clinical significance**: The cremaster muscle occasionally experiences painful spasms or cramps in adult males which may be chronic and debilitating. Treatment for these spasms ranges from minor surgery to injection with botulinum toxin to the regular application of heat to relax the muscle. Surgery, including the excision of the cremaster muscle, which has apparently been able to provide complete relief from this condition without a significant side effects [11].

The genitofemoral nerve, which supplying the CM, or the muscle itself may be compressed or injured during hernia repair or orchidopexy operations, this is mostly transient in nature and rarely causes persistent symptoms, but in some cases the CM reflex is either absent on the operated side or the CM reflex response to the physical or electrical stimulation on the operated side is weak in comparison to the normal side. Weak or absent ipsilateral CM reflex on the affected side may result in a descended testis; in contrast, the contralateral intact CM becomes more excitable and the testis ascends, which may results in a testicular positional distortion [12].

**5. Internal Spermatic Fascia**: It lies beneath the cremaster muscle, it is extremely thin and connects with the transversalis fascia. There are a few smooth muscle fibers within it.

**6. Tunica Vaginalis**: The tunica vaginalis (TV) is the lower end of the peritoneal processus vaginalis. When the fetal testis descends from the abdomen to the scrotum, part of the peritoneum descends with it. This part of peritoneum accompanied with the descending testis is called the peritoneal processus vaginalis. After birth, the proximal part of the peritoneal processus vaginalis contracts and is commonly obliterated, forming the ligamentous remnant of the processus vaginal and leaving a closed distal sac which the testis is invaginated into; otherwise a congenital inguinal hernia and communicating hydrocele could occur (Fig. 8.10). The tunica is reflected from the testis onto the internal surface of the scrotum, forming the visceral and parietal layers of the tunica. The visceral layer covers the sides and anterior aspects of the tunica albuginea and lower part of the spermatic cord. The cavity between the visceral and parietal layer is called the tunica vaginalis cavity "mesorchium", which accommodate a little fluid in the cavity between the two layers helping with the movement of the testis in the scrotum, and act as a cushion protecting the testis from minor trauma. When there are pathological changes of the tunica vaginalis, testis, or epididymis, the secretion or absorption of the fluid may also change. Thus the balance breaks and hydrocele, pyocele or haematocele could occur. The relationship between the testis and the TV gradually changed with age, so that the mesorchium was obliterated by secondary adhesion between the mesothelium of the TV and the posterior half of the testis, so that by middle age and the elderly male the TV lumen had shrunk to the point that it appeared to be only in front, of the testis, rather than completely encasing it [13].

## 8.3    The Septum of the Scrotum

**The septum of the scrotum** is a vertical layer of fibrous tissue that divides the two compartments of the scrotum. It consists of flexible connective tissue, and its structure extends to the skin surface as the scrotal raphe. It is an incomplete wall of connective tissue and nonstriated dartos muscle fibers dividing the scrotum into two sacs, each containing a testis [14] (Fig. 8.11). Scrotal compartments are an internal

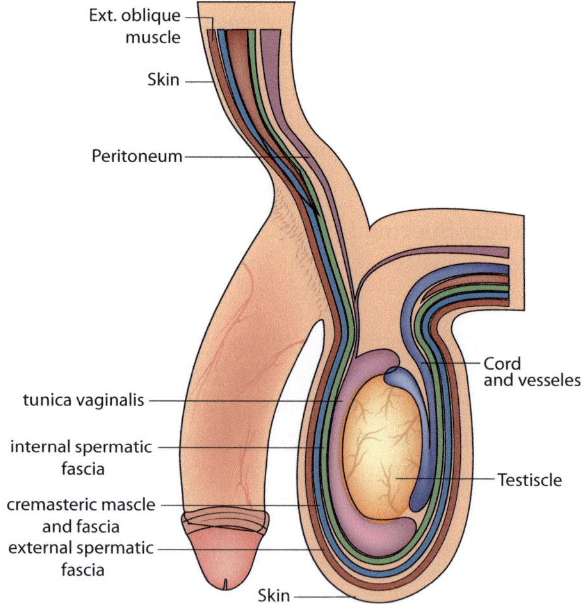



**Fig. 8.10** Scrotal layers with both layers of tunica vaginalis forming a potential cavity in front of the testicle

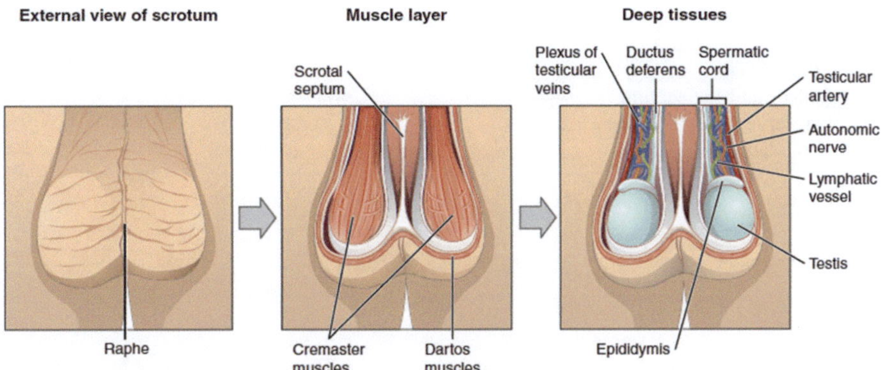


**Fig. 8.11** Scrotal septum with external, and deeper configurations. 3D anatomy of the layers surrounding the testis. This file is licensed under the Creative Commons Attribution-Share Alike 4.0 International license. Illustration from Anatomy & Physiology, Connexions http://cnx.org/content/col11496/1.6/, Jun 19, 2013

structures; which means that the person himself or the examining clinician could not appreciate a two distinct chambers, as the scrotal septum is cross-wall and it is not so dense or hard to be, be palpable, but it is formed of dense collagen fibres which usually extend out into the softer adjacent tissues. Externally both scrota commonly semblances as a one unit, with the median raphe slightly separating the two scrota with either a shallow depression or a slight prominence, in a very rare occasions the two scrotal compartments looks bipartition at the distal end which give raise to a **Scrotal dimple** (discussed in Chap. 14). Scrotal septum will be obviously distinguishable if there is a pathological condition confined to one scrotal compartment; so in cases of huge testicular swellings like hernia or hydrocele it will result in an over stretching of the affected side only with sparing the contralateral one by the well formed septum (Fig. 8.12). The same is applicable in acute testicular pathology; like cases of acute idiopathic scrotal oedema, pyocele and haematocele, where the scrotal septum clearly protect the counter side from the spreading of the pathology from one side to the other (Fig. 8.13). In cases of blunt perineal trauma or penile fracture; in which Buck's fascia remains intact, extravasated blood or urine is confined to the penile shaft. The limitation of ecchymosis and edema leads to the commonly described eggplant deformity. Traumatic disruption of Buck's fascia, however, leads to a different pattern; because dartos fascia will contain extravasations in the superficial perineal pouch, which manifests as a perineal hematoma in a butterfly distribution. Finally, disruption of dartos fascia allows for spread of hematoma, urine, or even infection to the abdominal wall and scrotum [15] .

This original superficial scrotal septal element becomes less distinct later with aging, when it develops into a thinning central core flanked by broader zones of homogenous collagen, lateralward-spreading connective tissue, smooth muscle tissue of the dartos fascia, and numerous blood vessels and nerves. These blood

                                                                      

**Fig. 8.12** Left sided haematocele confined to one side of the scrotal compartment and the septum clearly preserve the other side, which looks normal

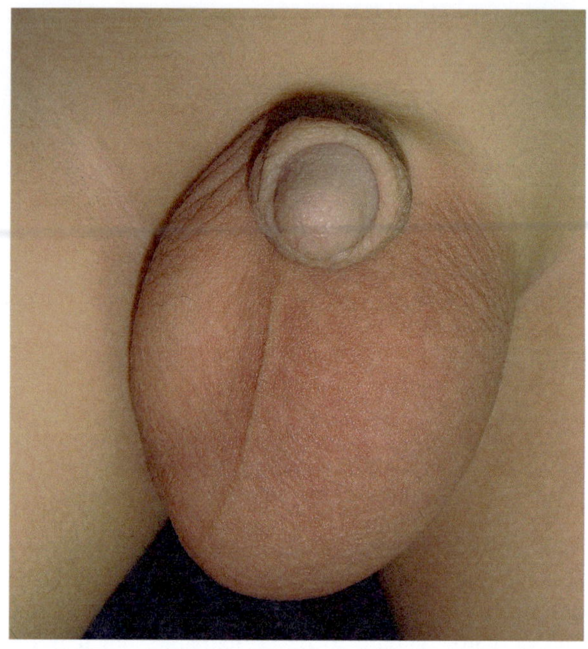

**Fig. 8.13** Acute scrotal oedema with early signs of inflammation confined only to one side (left)

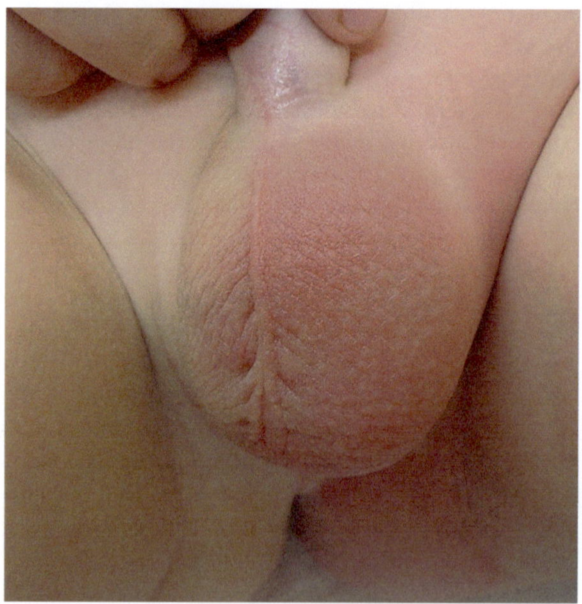

vessels and nerves run in a distinct and contrasting ventralcaudalward direction, which had their original direction toward the urogenital scrotal swellings. All elements together form the definitive (anatomical) septum. This structure of the raphe and superficial septum is far less distinct in the penis than in the scrotum. The perineal body and adjacent deep scrotal septum develop from that portion of the deep dorsal urogenital stroma, initially positioned dorsal to the urogenital sinus. Originally there is a distinction between a dense peripheral zone that extends into the adjacent medial sides of the puborectal and bulbospongiosus and the caudal extremity of the external urethral sphincter muscles. As a result, all neighbouring bilateral structures positioned laterally, i.e., the bulbourethral glands, and puborectal, internal and external urethral sphincters, bulbospongiosus, transversus perinei superficialis [4].

Histological septa are seen throughout most tissues of the body, particularly where they are needed to stiffen soft cellular tissue, and they also provide planes of ingress for small blood vessels [16].

**Sebileau's muscle** is the deep muscle fibres of the dartos tunica which pass into the scrotal septum. It is named after French anatomist Pierre Sebileau (1860–1953) [17].

## 8.4  Raphe of Scrotum

Is also called Vesling line, sometimes a term "perineal raphe" is applied to a raphe behind the root of penis (Fig. 8.14). The ventral perineal raphe originates from the fibrovascular tissue of the urethral folds just dorsal to the urogenital orifice, where for a short time the cloacal groove existed as a remnant of the original communication between the urogenital and anal compartments of the cloaca, from a short V-shape it lengthens into the narrow median raphe. The raphe is characterized by dense fibrovascular tissue with a conspicuous parallel and longitudinal orientation. It may for some time reveal a groove in the midline in which some pseudostratified columnar epithelium may extend from the dorsal margin of the urethra [18] (Chap. 17).

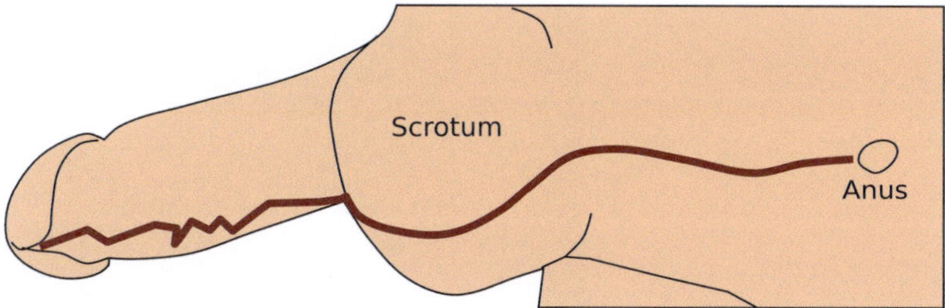


**Fig. 8.14** Extension of the median raphe from the frenulum down to the perineum; forming penile, scrotal and perineal raphae

A variably narrow median zone of the raphe is permanently devoid of hair follicles and glands. This long ventral raphe is complemented dorsally by a similar extension in the perineum, i.e., dorsal perineal raphe. So raphe is an epithelial-mesenchymal interaction (subcutaneous fibrous plate), it has been hypothesized that raphe formed by the delayed fusion under control of androgen hormone, extending from the penile frenulum, along the penile shaft and scrotum and toward the anus. According to van der Putte [4], the human raphe appears at 9th week of gestation and becomes thicker and continuous with the anus at 12–13 weeks, he did not consider the raphe as a remnant of fusion of the bilateral genital folds but a secondary structure formed after disappearance of the genital folds. One of the mainstay gender difference in topographical anatomy is the fusion of scrotal raphe in male and its dehiscence in the female, this embryological difference is secondary to fusion or separation of bilateral bulbospongiosus muscle (BS), which make the midline reinforced intermuscular septum internally and scrotal raphe superficially in male, but in female fetuses, the bilateral BS are widely separated to keep the vestibule opening [19].

Normally the median scrotal raphe is little bit darker and raised in comparison to the adjacent scrotal skin, normal variations include absent or non distinguishable raphe, and the other extreme of normal variation is to have an expansively raised or darker raphe (Fig. 8.15). In adults and children, the penile and scrotal raphe vary in shape and thickness between individuals [20]. Raphe anomalies include pearly

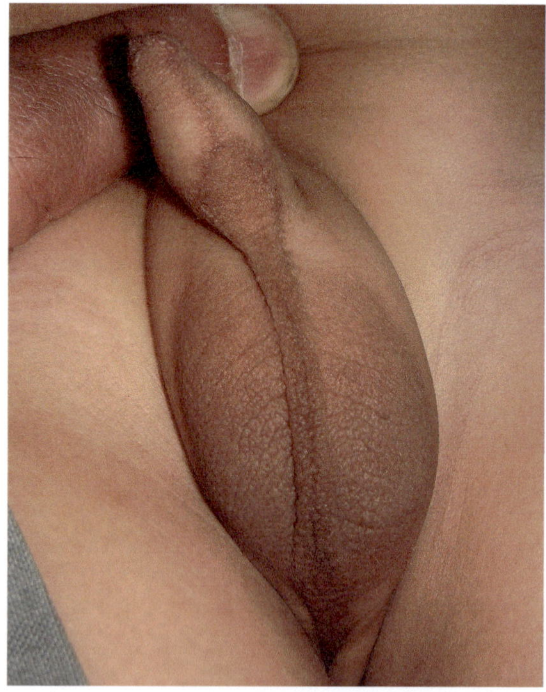

**Fig. 8.15** Scrotal raphe raised and wider than normal, distal penile raphe also widened and looks as diamond shape

pigmented, prominent, or wide raphe. Abnormal scrotal raphe will be described in details with the scrotal congenital anomalies (Chap. 17).

## 8.5  Scrotal Ligament (SL)

Gubernaculum testis (GT) is a prenatal cylindrical whitish structure, described for the first time in 1762 by Hunter. Later, it has been described as resembling the Wharton's jelly. The gubernaculum is connected to the caudal part of the male and female mesonephric–gonadal complex during fetal life. It is noteworthy that after birth the GT is converted to scrotal ligament (SL) [21]. The description of this ligament and its attachments after birth is important, because of two main pathologies; cryptorchidism and spermatic cord torsion. The SL is located in the posterior lower side of the testis outside of testicular parietal vaginalis. Macroscopically the GT is covered by the tunica vaginalis on all its sides except the posterior wall and is surrounded by the vaginal process. The growth of the vaginal process divides GT into three parts.

1. The bulb corresponds to the caudal region, which has not been invaded by the vaginal process.
2. The cord attaches the testis and the epididymis to the bulb. The cord is covered by the visceral layer of the vaginal process.
3. The vaginal gubernaculum corresponds to the portion which externally surrounds the parietal portion of the vaginal process.

Histologically the GT consists of undifferentiated spindle-shaped cells. It presents as a dense organization of longitudinally oriented collagenous fibers and predominance of fibroblasts. The fibroblasts number increases till 28 weeks of gestation before decreasing after this. Also a fibrofatty tissue containing some vessels and striated muscles cells are recognizable at its scrotal end in postnatal age [22]. The GT involved during testicular descent; firstly, during the trans-abdominal step, an enlargement of GT occurs with regression of the cranial suspensory ligament. This step is called the "swelling reaction" with the gubernaculum bulging out of the external ring [23].

During inguinoscrotal testicular descend, GT could be anchored to the scrotum according to various authors, but this attachment is challenged by others. Some of them described many forms of attachments, whereas other identify no distal attachment between the gubernacular bulb and the scrotal wall. Different studies have shown that the proximal extremity of the gubernaculum fixes the lower pole of the testis and the tail of epididymis with two bundles. The description of scrotal ligament as a firm attachment from the lower pole of testes to the scrotum is controversial. Furthermore, its role in prevention of testicular torsion is also questionable. While the anatomy of the GT and the testicular descent in the human fetus is often discussed, but postnatal anatomy of the GT or SL is rarely described

[24]. Some authors such as Dajusta et al. [25] and Favorito et al. [26] stated that firm scrotal attachment to testis could prevent spermatic cord torsion especially in cases of intra-vaginal testicle. The frequency of spermatic cord torsion remains higher in adults than in young children, which may be attributed to the demolition of SL. So it seems that the SL disappears with age.

The absence of SL is not enough to induce a spermatic cord torsion, because there are many other spermatic cord torsion predisposing factors. However, others such as Heyns [27] denied any scrotal attachments after the inguinal passage of the testicles.

The typical SL is described as a "Y-shape" ligament with the testis and epididymis as proximal insertions and the scrotum as distal attachment, sometimes, two bundles are identified: one bundle is attached from the tail of epididymis to the scrotum and the other one is attached from the lower pole of the testis to the scrotum, giving the SL its "Y form" [23].

Cadaveric examination of 25 testicular samples (Sixteen old aged cadaveric testicular specimens and fourteen fetal testicular specimens), where the lack of proximal and distal attachment was found in the majority of cases (56%). However, the main proximal attachment found in the SL; is the epididymal attachment (28.0% of cases), whereas no cases of testicular attachment was found. Distally, there were more variations with a scrotal attachment, a cremaster attachment (12% of cases) and multiple adherences in 16% of cases [24].

Histological examination showed the presence of patchy areas of dense collagen fibres of variable density amidst loose areolar connective tissue. In contrast, fetal specimens showed the presence of a definitive gubernaculum testes and revealed the presence of mesenchymal tissue, collagen, elastic fibres, and myocytes which varied according to gestational age of fetuses. Structure of scrotal ligament and gubernaculum testes is highly variable. In adults, the lower pole of testes is attached to the scrotum by connective tissue. After birth, gubernaculum testes gradually involutes and is present as scattered patches of dense regular connective tissue of different densities. It merges with the testicular coverings probably helping in the fixation of tunica vaginalis. Such arrangement indicates that gubernaculum blends with the fascia covering the testes and involutes gradually after birth [28].

There is no available studies about the global prevalence of SL or GT persistence at different age groups, but from my experience with inguinoscrotal surgeries for a considerable number of children; I appreciated different forms and dimensions of GT attached to the lower pole of the testicle and forming either an orthotopic or ectopic pathway to the bottom of the scrotum. These infrequently seen with cases of cryptorchidism and in the rare cases of ectopic testicles Figs. 8.16, 8.17.

Even in some cases of inguinal hernia repair, specially at younger ages, a well formed scrotal attachment between the lower pole of testes and the internal scrotal wall could be seen. In Fig. 8.18 one can see a well formed GT along the round ligament and its distal end is anchored to the labia majora in a 2 years girl with a left sided inguinal hernia.

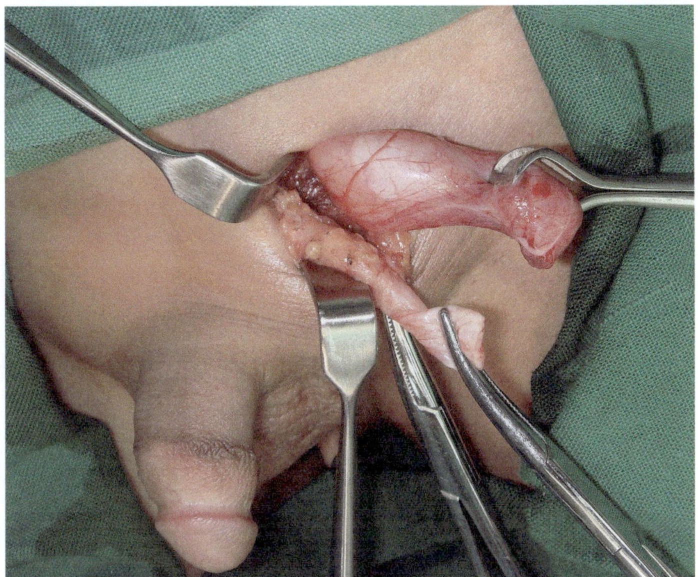

**Fig. 8.16** A well formed gubernaculum (scrotal ligament), during dissection for a left undescended testicle (2 years old child)

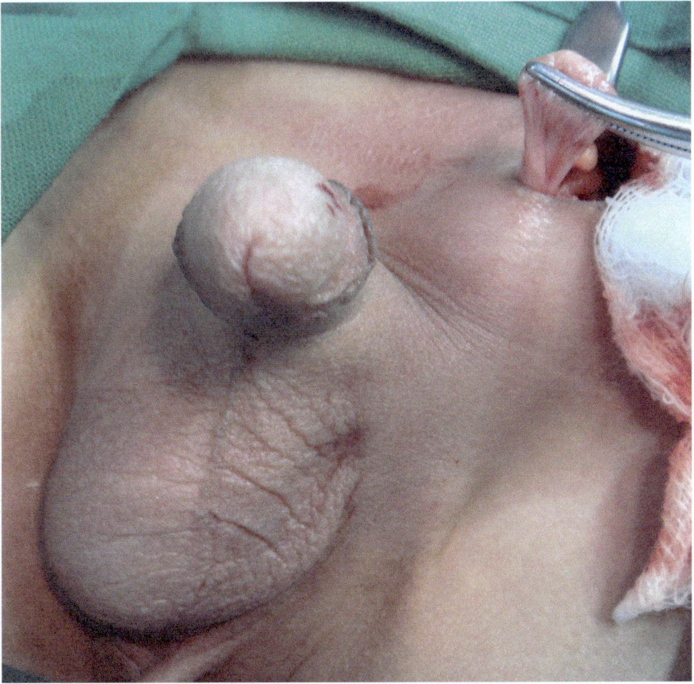

**Fig. 8.17** A case of cryptorchidism and a well formed gubernaculum with its distal end inserted ectopically in the uppermost medial aspect of the thigh

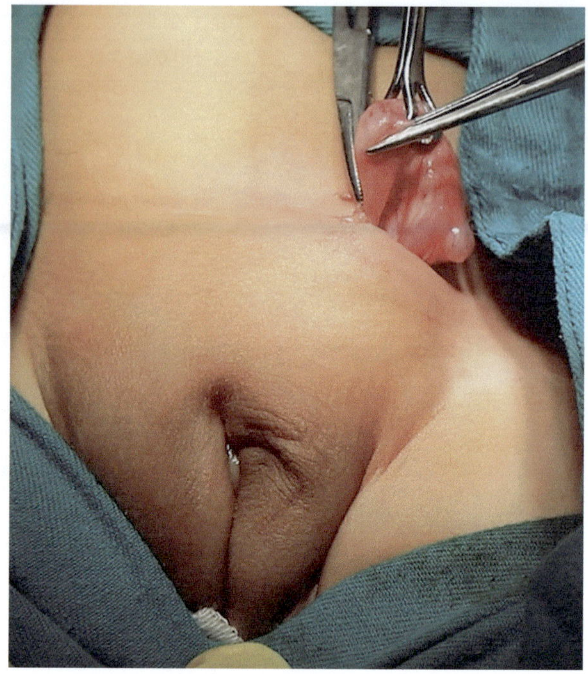

**Fig. 8.18** A well formed GT along the round ligament, with its distal end anchored to the labia majora in a 2 years girl with a left sided inguinal hernia

## 8.6  Blood Supply of Scrotum: Arterial Blood Supply: (Fig. 8.19)

The scrotal and perineal skin has a uniquely rich blood supply. The prominent vascularity of this region is advantageous for reconstruction as it allows for the design of various local flaps to cover perineal and penile skin defects. Scrotal flaps necrosis is extremely rare and so, even if a larger artery is transected [29]. It is noticeable that generous scrotal blood supply is in counter to the restricted testicular blood supply as suggested by Scott Freeman [30], he hypothesized that the poor testicular blood supply keeps the testicles in an oxygen-starved environment and so toughens up the sperm. Deprived of oxygen, the sperm might react like "muscle cells reaction to aerobic training"; increasing the number and size of mitochondria they contain and therefore becoming better prepared for the herculean task of ascending a cervix, uterus, and fallopian tube.

Scrotal skin is well vascularized due to the confluence of two main arterial systems; femoral artery via the external pudendal arteries and the internal iliac artery via the internal pudendal artery. The anterior scrotum is nourished by the anterior scrotal arteries, branches of the superficial and deep external pudendal arteries. These arteries are variable in course. Within the scrotum, near the peno-scrotal junction, superficial branches supply a subdermal plexus that travel toward apex of the scrotum to anastomose with the posterior circulation. These arteries are

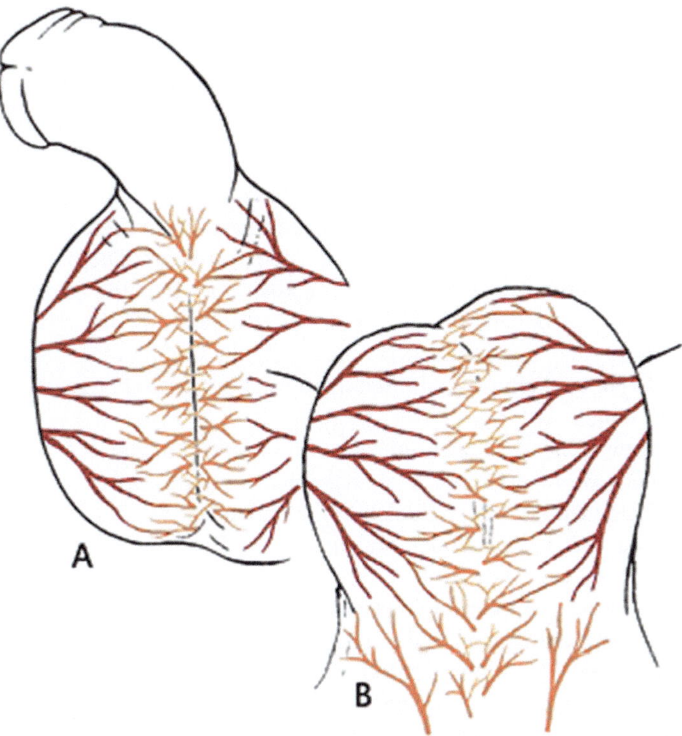


**Fig. 8.19** Vascular scrotal territories. Branches from inferior external pudendal artery (in red) and branches from septal arteries (in orange). A, Anterior face of scrotum. B, Posterior face of scrotum

distributed in three cutaneous territories, two lateral and one central, which are widely inter-anastomosed. Each lateral territory receives an inferior external pudendal artery which accesses at the midpoint of the scrotal root and fans out to cover the entire corresponding hemiscrotum. The central cutaneous territory is vascularized through the branches of two main scrotal arteries which are a continuation of the perineal arteries and which access via the posterior face, running deeply on both sides of the septum. In the perineum, the internal iliac artery continues as the internal pudendal artery. After emerging from Alcock's canal, it travels through the perineal membrane to continue as the perineal artery. The course of this artery is between ischiocavernosus and bulbospongiosus muscles, in the membranous layer of the superficial perineal fascia. From there, posterior scrotal arteries are given off in a variable pattern and travel toward apex of the scrotum. Interconnections are made with the anterior circulation, as well as across the central septum combining left and right-sided circulations. In addition, it has been shown that the scrotal raphe receives branches through a separate branch of the perineal artery [31].

Knowledge of this perineal vascular anatomy facilitates designing of different local pedicled flaps, specially for reconstruction of perineogenital defects as well as in male-to-female sex reassignment surgeries. As scrotal-perineal flaps based on the internal pudendal arteries have come into increased use, vaginoplasty has evolved from the strict use of split-thickness skin grafts and abdominally based penile flaps [32].

**Venous Drainage**: The anterior scrotum is drained by veins in the subdermal plexus and then come together at the base of scrotum. From there they travel to the external pudendal veins and ultimately to the femoral veins. The posterior scrotum is emptied by coalescence of subdermal plexus veins into the perineal vein and finally the internal pudendal vein, mirroring course of the arterial system. Generally, there are no connections between the subdermal plexus and the Dartos-based venous drainage, although there is an occasional large communication in some individuals.

**Nerve supply**: Classical anatomical studies revealed that the scrotum has a complex pattern of innervation. The main nerve supply arises from the scrotal branches of the perineal nerve, a branch of the pudendal nerve. A small contribution arises from the inferior pudendal branch of the femoral cutaneous nerve. The anterior and lateral aspects of the scrotum receive contributions mainly from the genital branch of the genitofemoral nerve and the anterior cutaneous branches of the iliohypogastric and the ilioinguinal nerves; which are called 'border nerves' [33].

The nerves innervating the ventral side of the proximal penis and scrotum originated mainly from the perineal nerves arising from pudendal nerves. The nerves travelling along the ventral side of penis coalesced at the penoscrotal area to be directed into the scrotal septum. At the penoscrotal junction, nerves on both sides of the ventral penis shifted to the interscrotal septum in a triangular fashion. The interscrotal septum was densely occupied by nerve fibres. Nerves were distributed horizontally to both hemiscrotal walls through this interscrotal septum. Both hemiscrota seem primarily to be innervated separately [34].

The interscrotal septum has a dense innervation. Both hemiscrota were innervated mainly by horizontally distributed nerve fibres arising from the interscrotal septum. Any procedure violating the penoscrotal and interscrotal septal area may jeopardize scrotal innervation (Fig. 8.20). Spinal anaesthesia covering only the level of the sacral nerves is frequently found to be satisfactory for scrotal surgery based on dermatome charts. The spinal or epidural anaesthesia affecting only the perineal nerves originating from S2, 3 and 4 is generally considered to be adequate for scrotal skin procedures [35]. The interscrotal septum has a pivotal role in scrotal sensation, as it carries a high density of scrotal nerves. In many scrotal surgical techniques the interscrotal septum is violated. After scrotal surgery, de novo scrotal pain and abnormalities of sensation are not uncommon. In the light of these anatomical findings, a probable explanation may be the disturbance of the nerves travelling in the septum. Horizontal incisions on each hemiscrotum and preservation of the interscrotal septum are critical, so as not to harm the neural structure of the scrotum. In some of the orchidopexy techniques for undescended testis and testicular torsion, the midline approach to the scrotum has been encouraged,

**Fig. 8.20** A median raphe incision, which may jeopardize the scrotal innervation

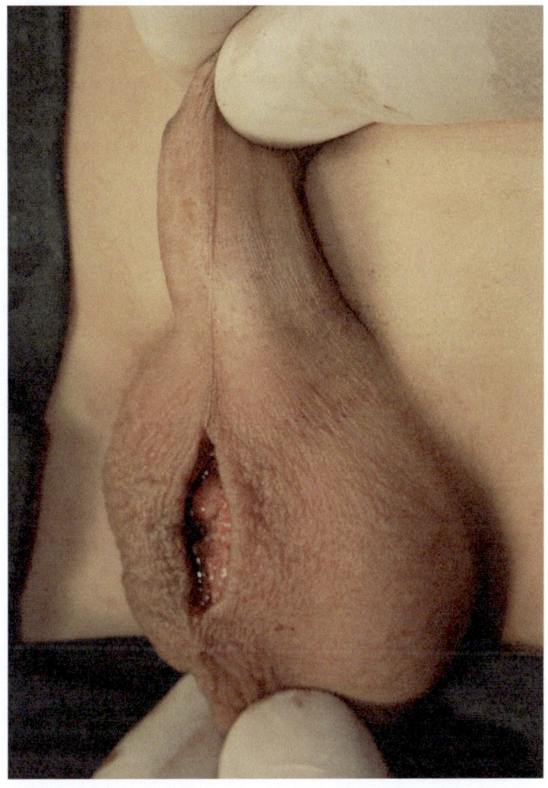

claiming a lower risk of retorsion or ascent of the testis. Although transeptal approaches have also been described. The advantages of this approach have also not been documented, compared with the original dartos pouch technique, and it may lead to neuronal injury. The classic dartos pouch technique (without harming the interscrotal septum) is still the reference standard for treating an undescended testes. Yucel S and Baskin [34] in their study showed that any fixative surgery disturbing the interscrotal septum is not anatomically appropriate as there is a high risk of nerve injury. We usually advocate surgical manipulation of both hemiscrota through two different horizontal incisions that do not destroy the scrotal innervation (Fig. 8.20).

## 8.7   Lymphatic Drainage of the Scrotum

Lymphatic drainage of the penile skin, is to the superficial inguinal as well as the subinguinal lymph nodes. The lymph of the scrotum drains into the superficial inguinal lymph nodes and femoral lymph nodes. There are many communicating branches between the lymphatic vessels of the scrotum and the penis, but there is no communication between the lymph of the scrotum and the lymphatic drainage of the testis. Also there is no connection between the lymph of the scrotum and the lymph of each layer of the tunica vaginalis of the spermatic cord either. Thus, the scrotal lymph does not go along with the pudendal blood vessel. As a result, the range of lymph dissection in scrotal surgery is the same as in penile cancer surgery which includes the inguinal lymph nodes and parailiac artery lymph nodes. The lymphatic vessels of the testis are abundant, which can be divided into superficial and deep plexus. The superficial plexus is located at the inner surface of the visceral layer of the tunica vaginalis. The deep plexus is situated in the parenchyma of the testis and converges into 4–6 lymphatic vessels, and then ascend with vessels in the spermatic cord and enter the retroperitoneal space through the inguinal canal and drain into the lumbar lymph nodes. These lymph nodes distribute from the aortic bifurcation to the celiac artery which is nearby the renal hilum [36].

# References


1. Weicker B.: Ober rhythmische kontraktionen der tunica dartos und ihre beinflussung durch mechanische, physikalische, Psychische und Pharma kologische Mittel, durch Schlaf und Infektiose Erkrankungen. Ztschr. f. die Gesamte Experimentelle Medizin, LIV; 1927
2. Heyns CF, Theron PD. Fournier's gangrene. In: Hohenfellner M, Santucci RA, editors. Emergencies in urology. New York, NY: Springer-Verlag; 2007. p. 50–3.
3. Campbell. In: Alan J. Wein, editor. Campbell-Walsh Urology. Philadelphia: Elsevier Saunders; ISBN 978–1–4160–6911–9
4. van der Putte. The Devlopment of the Perineum in the Human, Vol. 177. Advances in Anatomy Embryology and Cell Biology, pp. 1001–109. ISBN 3–540–21039–3 Springer Berlin Heidelberg New York
5. Delbert Paul. Section "Verge" Traite d'anat. humaine, Poirier and Charpy, 2d edit. 1907, vol. v, part I
6. Jefersson G Victoria. The Peripenic muscle; some observations on the anatomy of phimosis. Surg Gynecol Obstet (Chicago). 1916; 2(23):177–81
7. Hrabovszky Z, Pilla ND, Yap T, Farmer PJ, Hutson JM, Carlin JB. Role of the gubernacular bulb in cremaster muscle development of the rat. Anat Rec. 2002;267(2):159–65. https://doi.org/10.1002/ar.10092.PMID11997885.
8. Özdemirkirana T, Ertekinb C. Cremaster muscle motor unit action potentials. Clin Neurophysiol. 2011;122(8):1679–85.
9. Tanyel FC, Ertunç M, Büyükpamukçu N, Onur R. Mechanisms involved in contractile differences among cremaster muscles according to localization of testis. J Pediatr Surg. 2001;36(10):1551–60.
10. Shafik A, et al. J Sexual Medicine. 2007;4:1022–7.
11. Baty, John A. Cremasteric cramp with testicular retraction. British Med J. 5 May 1956; 1 (4974):1014–1015. doi:https://doi.org/10.1136/bmj.1.4974.1014. ISSN 0959-8138. PMC 1979762
12. Zempoalteca R, Martínez-Gómez M, Hudson R, Cruz Y, Lucio RA. An anatomical and electrophysiological study of the genitofemoral nerve and some of its targets in the male rat. J Anat. 2002;201:493–505.

13. Lopez-Marambio AF, Hutson JM. The relationship between the testis and tunica vaginalis changes with age. J Pediatr Surg. 2015;50:2075–7. https://doi.org/10.1016/j.jpedsurg.2015.08.032.
14. Berkow, MD, editor, Robert. The Merck manual of medical information; home edition. Whitehouse Station, New Jersey: Merck Research Laboratories; 1977. ISBN 0911910875
15. Rosenstein DI, Morrey AF, McAninch JW, et al. Penile trauma. In: Graham SD, Keane TE, Glenn JF, et al., editors. Glenn's urology. Philadelphia, PA: Lippincott Williams & Wilkins; 2010. p. 514–6.
16. Male Sexual Dysfunction: Pathophysiology and Treatment, edited by Fouad R. Kandeel, ISBN 978–0824724399 ISBN 0824724399 Edition: 1st, 2007. New York. p. 502
17. Sebileau Pierre. Coverings of testicles: purses, cremaster, vagina, descent of a testicle. Imprimerie des Arts et Manufactures & Dubuisson; 1897
18. Baskin LS, Erol A, Jegatheesan P, Li Y, Liu W, Cunha GR. Urethral seam formation and hypospadias. Cell Tissue Res. 2001;305:379–87.
19. Zhe Wu Jin, Jin Y, Wu Li X, Murakami G, et al. Perineal raphe with special reference to its extension to the anus: a histological study using human fetuses. Anat Cell Biol. 2016; 49:116–124. http://dx.doi.org/https://doi.org/10.5115/acb.2016.49.2.116
20. Baky Fahmy MA. The spectrum of genital median raphe anomalies among infants undergoing ritual circumcision. J Pediatr Urol. 2013; 9(6 Pt A):872–7
21. Costa WS, Sampaio FJB, Favorito LA, Cardoso LEM. Testicular migration: remodeling of connective tissue and muscle cells in human gubernaculum testis. J Urol. 2002;167:2171–6.
22. Favorito LA, Costa SF, Julio-Junior HR, Sampaio FJB. The importance of the gubernaculum in testicular migration during the human fetal period. Int Braz J Urol Off J Braz Soc Urol. 2014;40:722–9.
23. Hutson JM, Nation T, Balic A, Southwell BR. The role of the gubernaculum in the descent and undescent of the testis. Ther Adv Urol. 2009;1:115–21.
24. Cavalie G, Bellier A, Marnas G et al. Anatomy and histology of the scrotal ligament in adults: inconsistency and variability of the gubernaculum testis. Surg Radiol Anat. DOI https://doi.org/10.1007/s00276-017-1904-1
25. Da Justa DG, Granberg CF, Villanueva C, Baker LA. Contemporary review of spermatic cord torsion: new concepts, emerging technologies and potential therapeutics. J Pediatr Urol. 2013;9:723–30.
26. Favorito LA, Cavalcante AG, Costa WS. Anatomic aspects of epididymis and tunica vaginalis in patients with spermatic cord torsion. Int Braz J Urol. 2004;30:420–4.
27. Heyns CF. The gubernaculum during testicular descent in the human fetus. J Anat. 1987;153:93–112.
28. Ganapathy A, Pushpaja JJ, Kapoor K et al. Structural and functional significance of scrotal ligament: a comparative histological study. Anatom Sci Int. https://doi.org/10.1007/s12565-020-00566-8
29. Isken T, Onyedi M, Sen C, Izmirli H, Yucel E. A novel application for repair of skin defects of the penis: anterior scrotal artery flap. Plast Reconstr Surg. 2009;124(1):181e–2e.
30. Freeman S. The evolution of the scrotum: a new hypothesis. J Theoret Biol. 1990;145(4):429–45.
31. Carrera A, Gil-Vernet A, Forcada P, et al. Arteries of the scrotum: a microvascular study and its application to urethral reconstruction with scrotal aps. BJU Int. 2008;103:820–4.
32. Gil-Vernet A, A, Forcada P, Morro R, Llusa M, Arango O. Arteries of the scrotum: a microvascular study and its application to urethral reconstruction with scrotal flaps. BJU Int. 103:820–4. doi:https://doi.org/10.1111/j.1464-410X.2008.08167.x
33. Elhilali MM, Winfield HN. Genitourinary pain. In: Wall PD, Mclazck R, editors. Textbook of pain. Edinburgh: Churchill Livingstone; 1989. p. 500–1.
34. Yucel S, Baskin, LS. The neuroanatomy of the human scrotum: surgical ramifications. 2003 BJU Int. 2003; 91:393–397. doi:https://doi.org/10.1046/j.1464-4096.2003.04087.x

35. Sprung J, Wilt S, Bourke DL, Thomas P. Is it time to correct the dermatome chart of the anterior scrotal region. Anesthesiology. 1993;79:381–3.
36. Longfei Liu. Applied anatomy of the scrotum and its contents. Chapter 1 in Scrotoscope. DOI: https://doi.org/10.1016/B978-0-12-815008-5.00001-7

# Chapter 9
# Morphology and Anthropometric Measurements of Scrotum

**Mohamed A. Baky Fahmy and Alexander Springer**

**Abbreviation**

MSH   Melanin Stimulating Hormone
AGD   Anogenital distance
LSF   Labioscrotal Fold

## 9.1   Surface Anatomy

The mainstay morphological difference between male and female is the large phallus over a pendant scrota and exteriorised reproductive organ. The scrotum suspends below the pubic symphysis and between the anteromedial sides of both thighs and separated from the anus by the perineum. There is a longitudinal line in the middle of the scrotum called the scrotal raphe externally and a scrotal septum internally; which gives rise to a two completely separated compartments, the left side usually lies lower than the right one, with a minor variabilities. Both scrota commonly semblances as a one unit, with the median raphe slightly separating the two scrota with either a shallow depression or a slight prominence, but in a very rare occasions the two scrotal compartments looks bipartite at the distal end which give raise to the **scrotal dimple** (discussed in Chap. 12). Generally, the scrotum is in a contracted state with a lot of corrugations on its surface, which known as the scrotal rugae, but these rugae are hardly visible if the scrotum is in a relaxed status or stretched; so rugae are prominent in winter and cold environments but flatten in warm circumstances. In infants and children the rugae are more prominent, but at old age and due to generalised hypotonia and musculature laxity these rugae are flat with more or less smooth scrotal skin (Fig. 9.1).

M. A. B. Fahmy (✉)
Al-Azhar University, Cairo, Egypt

A. Springer
Department of Pediatric Surgery, Medical University Vienna, Vienna, Austria

          91
M. A. B. Fahmy (ed.), *Normal and Abnormal Scrotum*,
https://doi.org/10.1007/978-3-030-83305-3_9

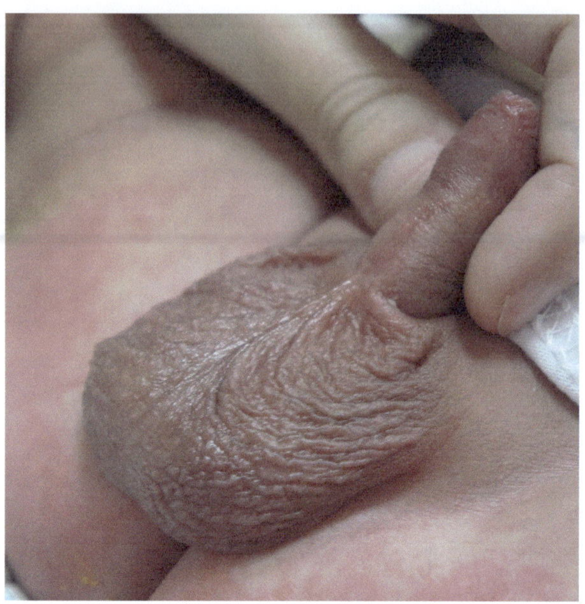

**Fig. 9.1** Normal scrotum of a newborn

The scrotum naturally designed to accommodates the testicles outside the body without interfering with the penile erection, and not to be irritated with urine drippling by keeping an appropriate penoscrotal distance and a normal penoscrotal angles, also without intervene with walking and movements of the thighs. As well the scrotum positioned with a considerable anoscrotal distance away from the anus, so not to be soiled with faces in early neonatal life.

## 9.2 Scrotal Shape

Normal scrotum is oval shaped, that's why the testis is known among children and in different vernacular languages as "eggs" or balls. Anatomically the scrotum is either conical or pyramidal, with its dome at the root of the penis and a free base united with its peer of the of the other side through the raphe. Sometimes the scrotum of both sides is more or less rounded looks like ball with a difficulty to distinguish both sided (Fig. 9.2).

Scrotums are usually, but not always, a little darker than the rest of body skin, and are usually wrinkly and covered with sparse hair. Many people have a lots of tiny, painless bumps on their scrotum or penile shaft. These are called Fordyce's spots (also termed Fordyce granules) which are ectopic prominent sebaceous glands, they're totally normal and don't cause any health problems (Fig. 9.3).

**Scrotal boundaries:** Normally a characteristic scrotal skin is extended to the root of penis at the midline, with a minimal extension to the ventral penile surface,

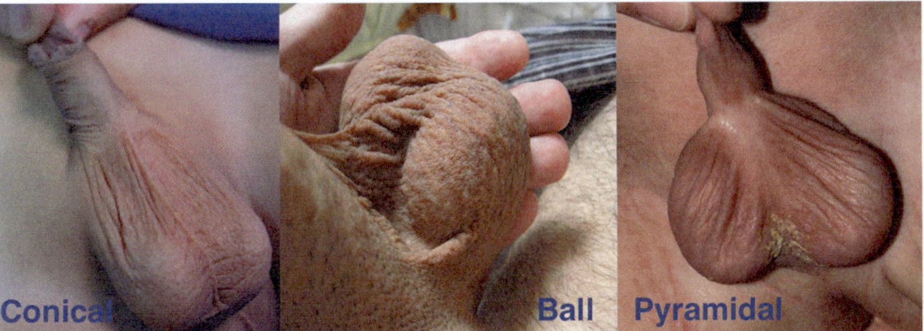



**Fig. 9.2**  Different shapes of scrotum

**Fig. 9.3**  Prominent Fordyce spots obviously seen in the penile skin with minimal spots in the scrotum

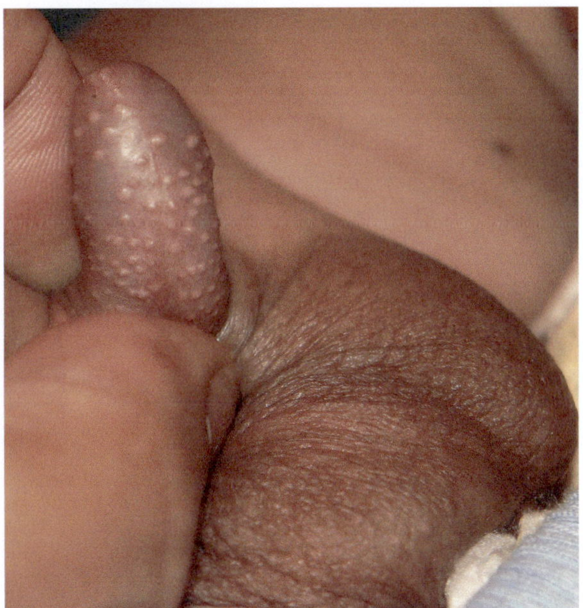

but preserving a distinguished penoscrotal angle, which separate penile skin from the scrotum and this gives a chance for penis to extend freely during erection (Fig. 9.4). We will see in chapter of scrotal anomalies that abnormal high insertion of scrotal skin may end with a form of webbed penis, and in other rare occasions there is complete fusion between both scrotal and penile skin, but minimal degree of encroachment of the scrotal skin to the base of the penis is acceptable and will not affect the functional penile length (Figs. 9.5, 9.6).

Lateral to the root of the penis the scrotum end up at both sides, where the scrotal skin forming a triangular extension which vanish in the normal inguinal skin, usually forming an acute angle, and normally it stop at both sides of the penis, and

                                                          M. A. B. Fahmy and A. Springer

**Fig. 9.4** Normal penoscrotal junction with a scrotal skin not encroaching over the ventral penile skin

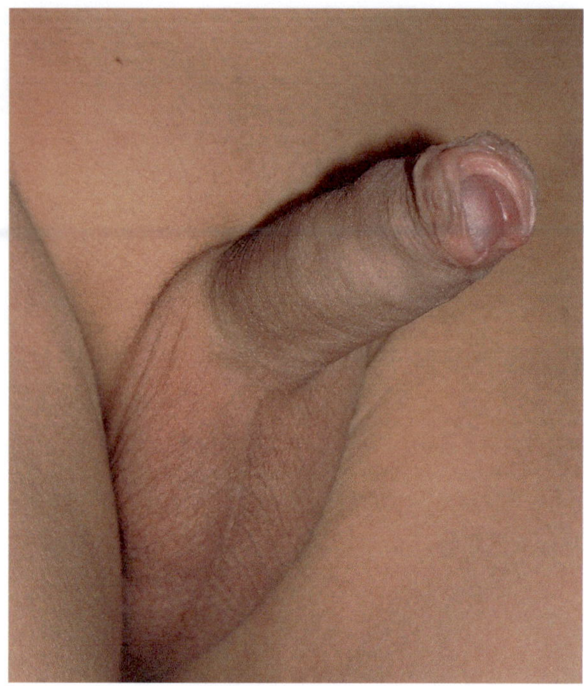

**Fig. 9.5** Minimal extension of the middle scrotal skin to the ventral penile skin

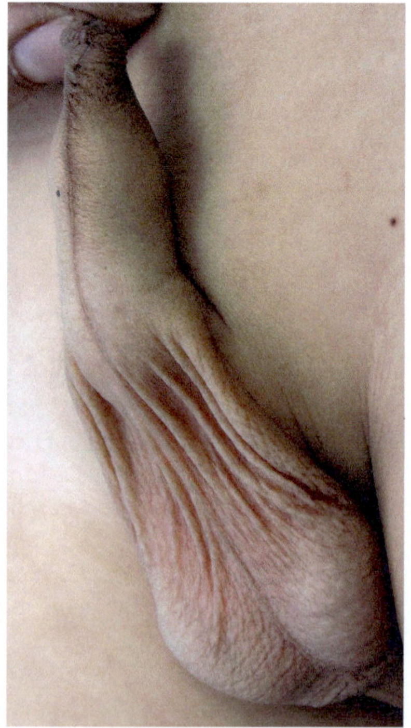

**Fig. 9.6** Significant midline creeping of the scrotal skin over the root of the penis

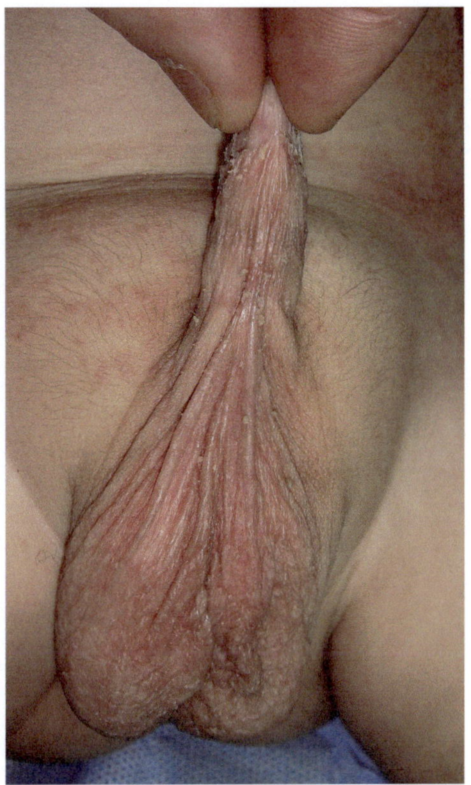

each side didn't met the corresponding other side (Fig. 9.7). It has been thought that the dartos muscle extends into the penis only for a short distance on its underside, in the so-called area scroti of Klatsch. A minimal degree of creeping of the upper lateral scrotal angles is acceptable and may not affect neither the normal penile length nor the penile movement during erection (Fig. 9.8), but if the upper lateral scrotal skin extend above the penis; to encircle its root completely, we will end with some sort of shawl scrotum (a variant of scrotal transposition), which will be discussed with scrotal anomalies (Chap. 12) (Fig. 9.9).

In a rare occasions the lateral upper scrotal skin is inserted higher at both sides penile shaft, and in such cases the abnormally attached scrotal skin will results in hindering the proper erection and it may deserves surgical correction (Fig. 9.10). In some cases of proximal hypospadias the upper angles of the scrotum are inserted higher in the penile shaft at both sides of the unfolded urethral plate; such cases also deserve proper scrotal repositioning before or at the time of hypospadias repair (Fig. 9.11).

**Laterally deficient scrotum:** Normally the lateral scrotal skin furl and wind around itself to form a pear shaped scrotal sac, to envelopes the whole normally suspended testicle, (Fig. 9.1) and the entire conical scrotum formed of the special

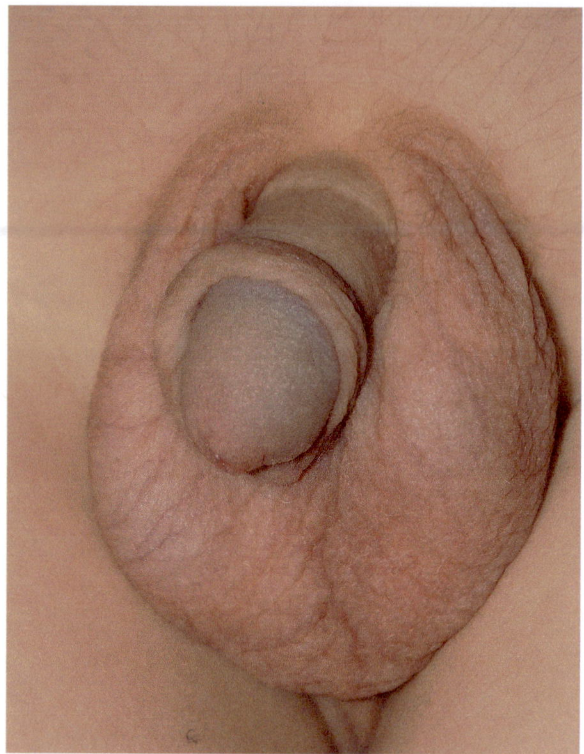

**Fig. 9.7** An acceptable degree of minimal extension of the lateral scrotal angles towards the midline

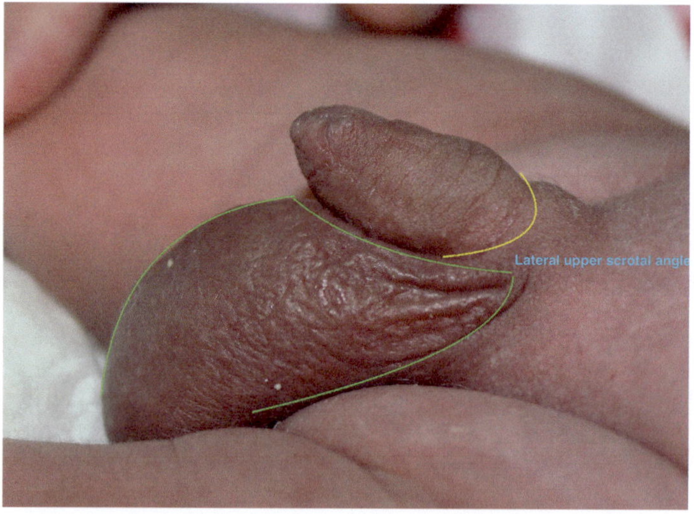


**Fig. 9.8** Triangular upper scrotal extension at both sides of the penis

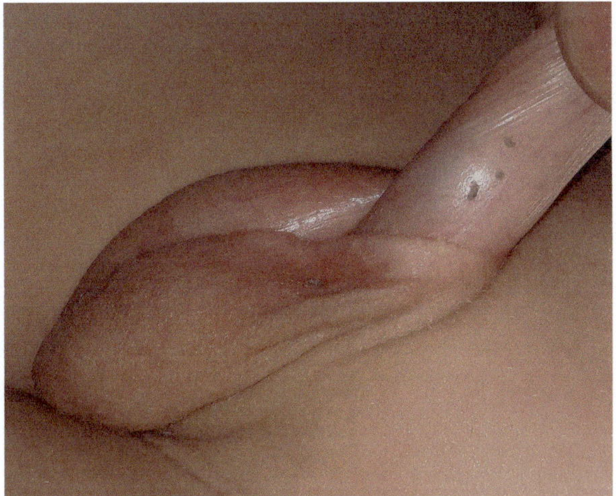

**Fig. 9.9** Lateral upper scrotal angles inserted higher at the both sides of the penis

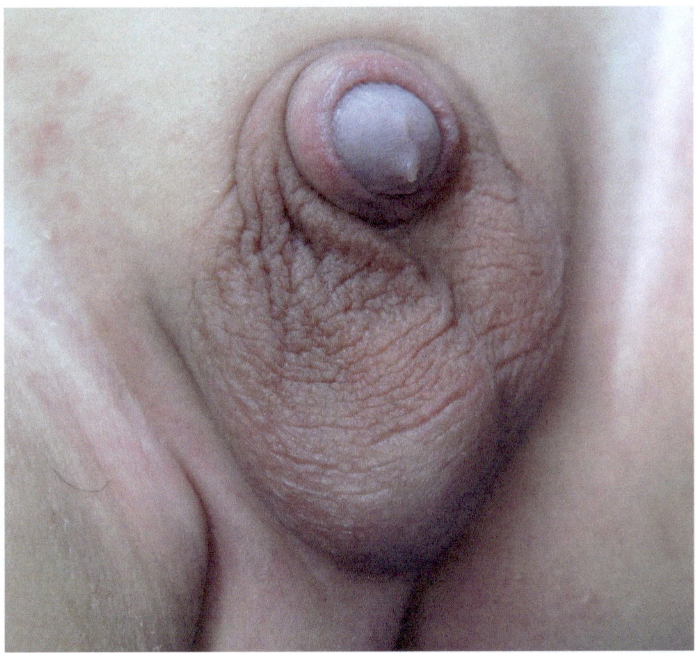

**Fig. 9.10** Obvious scrotal tissues overriding the root of the penis forming a minimal degree of shawl scrotum

**Fig. 9.11** Upper lateral scrotal angles inserted higher at both sided of urethral plate in a case of penoscrotal hypospadias

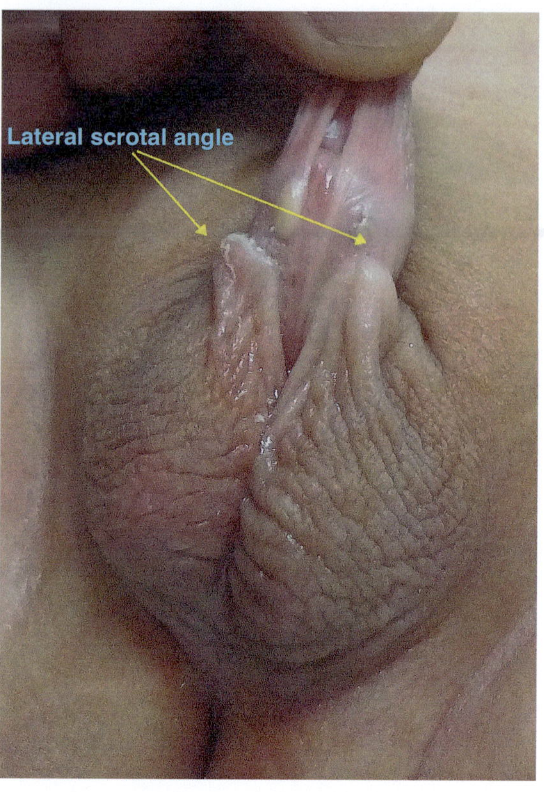


scrotal skin, but very rarely the lateral scrotum may be deficient of rugae for a variable extents and replaced by a normal skin identical to the inguinal skin (Fig. 9.12). Such cases of lateral scanty or deficient scrotal skin are usually an isolated cases without any associated genital anomalies, these cases may be considered as a minimal degree of scrotal hypoplasia (Chap. 11) The skin denuded of rugae may be extended above the root of the penis with a marked accumulation of subcutaneous fat recognisable beneath this skin (A normal scrotum, doesn't include any subcutaneous fat) (Fig. 9.13) Current evidence suggests that androgen inactivation might be a predominant in adipose tissue, particularly in subcutaneous depots. Therefore, androgen inactivation could retain the subcutaneous fat in the scrotal skin; this might have prevented transmission of the dartos fascia and muscle contraction directly to the epidermis, which then failed to form the rugae scrotal skin [1].

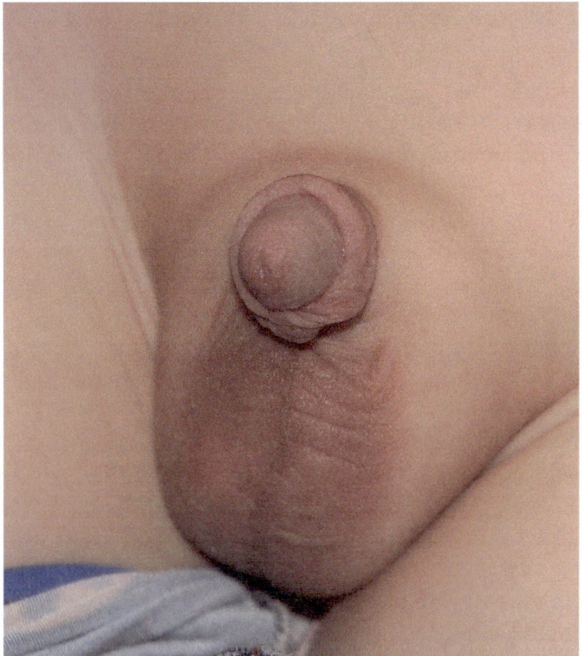

**Fig. 9.12** Laterally symmetrical deficient scrotal skin which minimize the scrotal surface area

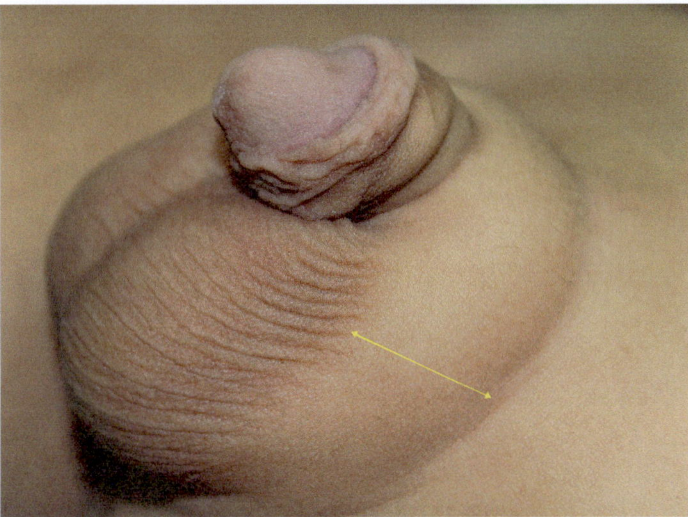

**Fig. 9.13** Excessive fat deposition in the scrotal skin which is devoted of rugae, this abnormal skin is going above the penis encircling its root

## 9.3 Scrotal Rugae

Ruga mean a wrinkle, fold, or ridge. Ruga is from the Latin word rūga, it usually used in plural (rugae). Normally the scrotal rugae are a transverse ridges, extended from the scrotal raphe medially, and attached laterally to the lower end of the inguinal region proximally and wind dorsally to attach again in the dorsal scrotal raphe distally to form the round base of the conical scrotum. Rugae poses a slight downward inclining if the penis is in a flaccid status, these folds will be raised and arranged obliquely merging from the midline and directed downwards at the periphery, if the penis stretched or erected (Fig. 9.14).

Rugae are a raised skin folds formed by the fine attachment of dartos muscle to the scrotal skin. Between every two rugae there is a minute depression, and its number is variable; we found that the main rugae are between 12 to 25 normally, there are innumerable minute less prominent superposed rugae between the main one. Rugae should not be confused with the normal scrotal skin folds, which are commonly seen during upward penile movements and during erection (Fig. 9.15). The wrinkled scrotal skin with the rugae give this organ a large surface area, which acts as a cooling chamber, scrotal skin requires adequate testosterone stimulation and a normally functioning androgen receptors for its normal development to gives raise of these unique semblance [2].

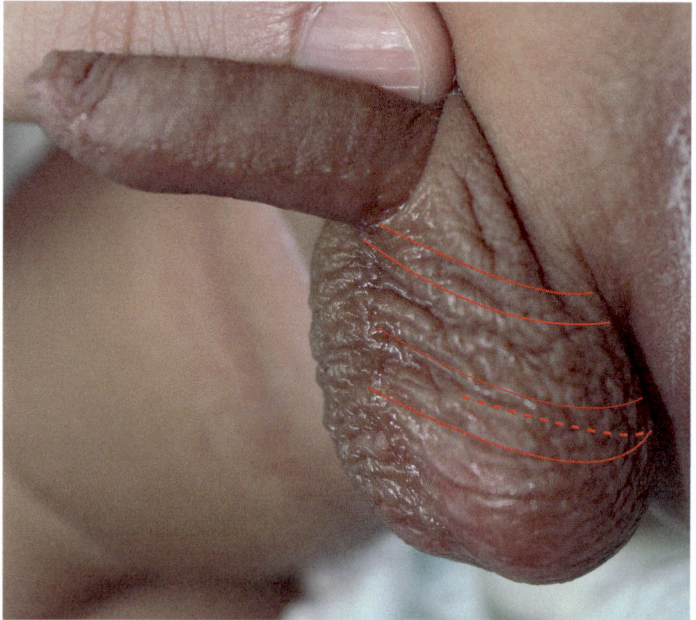

**Fig. 9.14** Scrotal rugae extend to inguinal skin proximally, but wind around to insert posteriorly to form a ring distally

**Fig. 9.15** Rugae and skin folds

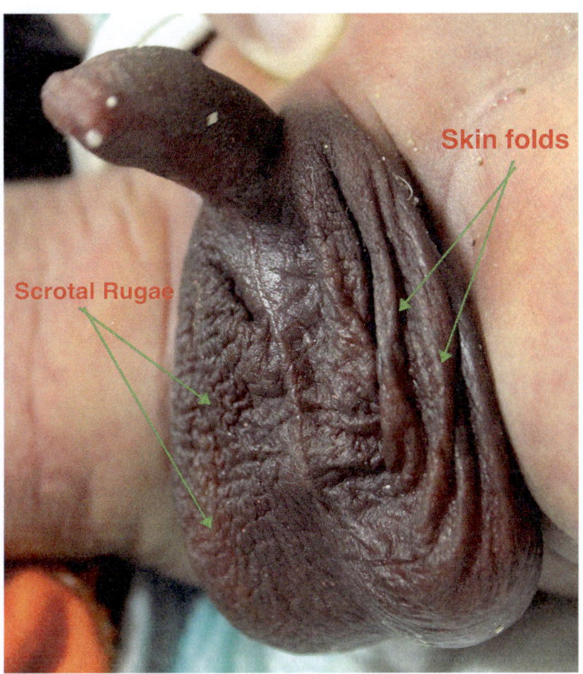


Low expression of androgen receptor, steroid-5-alpha-reductase, and alpha polypeptide 2 in the affected side of the scrotum are likely resulted in absence of the characteristic scrotal rugae, and pigmentation on histological and biological analyses. So the entire scrotum or its rugae may be absent or scanty in cases of androgen insensitivity syndrome due to localized partial androgen insensitivity and 5α-Reductase type 2 deficiency, with enough dihydrotestosterone production to prevent labia formation, but not enough to stimulate scrotal development, as evidenced by the presence of the midline raphe. This condition may be unilateral, but commonly it is bilateral [3].

In neonates, and due to wetness of the inguinal region by urine and frequent washing; we may see a prominent oedematous scrotal rugae, of course this condition may end with some sorts of contact or nonspecific dermatitis (Fig. 9.16). Scrotal dermatitis will be discussed in Chap. 26.

**Testicular appearance inside the scrotum:** In normal males the midpoint of the testis is at or below the level of mid-scrotum. Normally and due to thickening and wrinkling of the scrotal wall the testicle is non-discernible from the scrotal skin in majority of men, but in some children the testicle is obviously well seen and distinct with its boundaries, this is also may be seen in adults with a relaxed thin scrota. This could be attributed to the normal variation of the thickness and development of the cremasteric muscle and dartos fascia (Fig. 9.17).

**Fig. 9.16** Scrotal rugae oedema and prominence in neonate

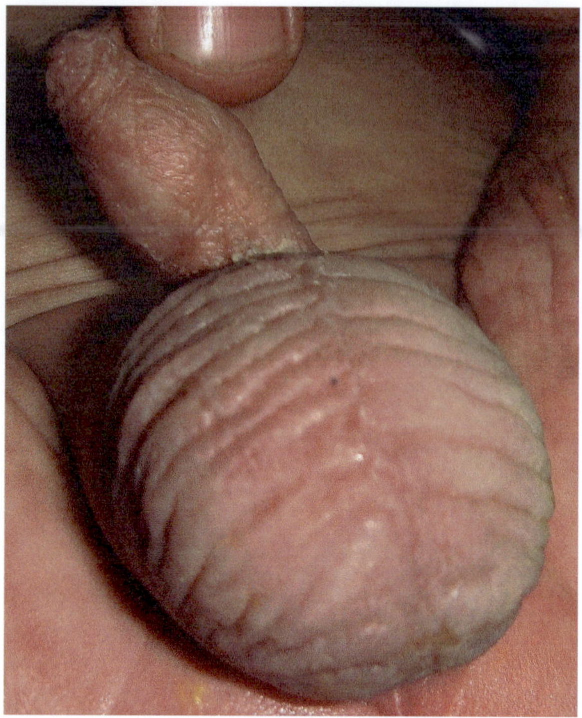

**Fig. 9.17** Bilaterally distinct testicles in a child with thin scrotal wall

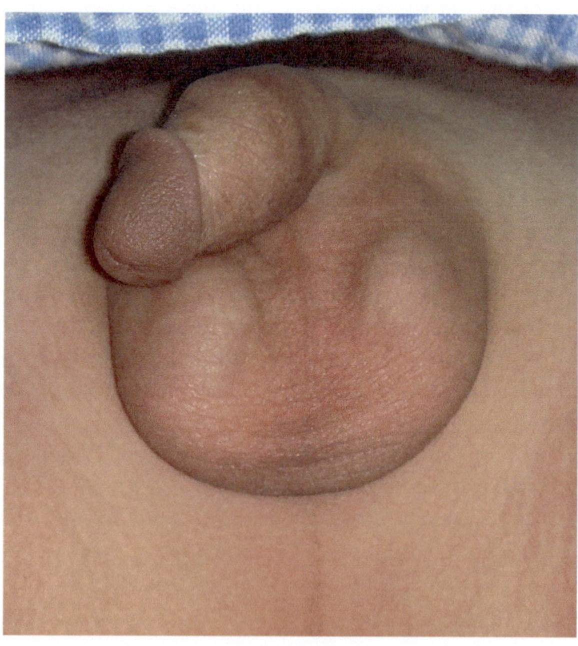

## 9.4  Scrotal Colour

Pigmentation of the genital area is probably influenced by sex hormone impregnation prior to birth, which results in normal darkness of the scrotum and median raphe, but later on the friction or chronic irritation may partly explain an acquired scrotal hyperpigmentation, which may be manifested after puberty. Human genital melanocytes are target cells for androgen, which stimulates tyrosinase activity; androgens modulate tyrosinase activity through regulation of cyclic adenosine monophosphate, which is a key regulator of skin pigmentation [4]. Therefore, androgen inactivation might also have result in the absence of pigmentation during the fetal period.

**Hyperpigmented scrotum:** It is more common in black skinned infants (Fig. 9.18), but it is detectable in 20% of Mongolian and in 5% of Caucasian infants [5]. The hyperpigmentation is believed to be due to a Melanin Stimulating Hormone (MSH) stimulation in the uterus, but the precise mechanism is not clear. The physiological hyperpigmentation of the scrotum must be differentiated from the rare hyperpigmentation due to a congenital adrenal hyperplasia. Where the accumulation of 17-hydroxyprogesterone leads, after its transformation in the liver, to an increased concentration of testosterone and therefore leads to the hyperpigmentation of the genitalia, which in male is associated with an increased volume of the penis, and the clitoris in female.

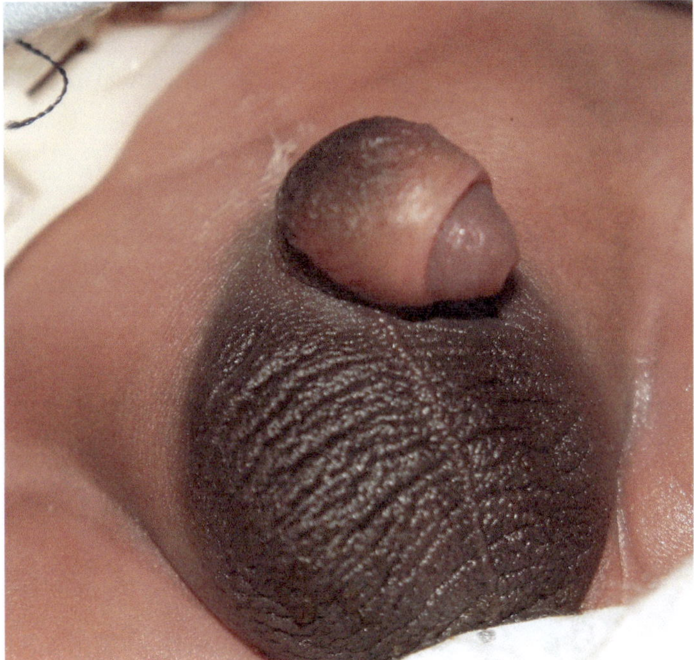

**Fig. 9.18** A darker scrotum in a normal hispanic child, a congenitally small prepuce is obvious (Hyposthia)

## 9.5 Scrotal Surface Area

Some people's scrota are longer and hang lower, others sit up a little higher. Most of studies are concerned mainly with the size of the testicles at different ages, without any concern for the scrotal surface ares. Testicular size could be measured and assisted roughly by palpation and comparison with a Prader's orchidometer (Fig. 9.19) and precisely by ultrasound; which measures the testicular volume. In the Handbook of Normal Physical Measurements [Hall et al., 2007] [6] there is a detailed descriptions of measurement techniques and growth standards, with abundant data on penile growth in individuals of different ethnic backgrounds, but there is no data about the surface anatomy of the scrotum.

The average size of a man testicle is about 4 × 3 × 2 cm in size and it is oval in shape. The mean actual testicular volume was 10.6 ± 3.5 ml. In both adults and foetuses it is clear that the right testicle is both the heavier and also the greater in volume. The scrotal boundaries determined by the posterior margin of the four-chette or first fold of the scrotum (the line from the beginning of the transverse rugae; scrotalperineal junction), to the root of the penis and the lateral normal skin. The clinical assessment of the scrotal skin surface area could be detected through multiplying the scrotal length (from the root of the penis to the perineal limit of the scrotum) with the scrotal width, which could be measured precisely by an electronic digital caliper (0–6/0–150 mm; Resolution of 0.01/0.1 mm; Accuracy: 0.01/± 0.2 mm) (Figs. 9.20 and 9.21).

Also the number of scrotal rugae can gives a rough idea about the scrotal surface area; the number of main rugae is normally variable widely between individuals (normally from 12 to 25), an ill developed or scanty scrotal rugae should be

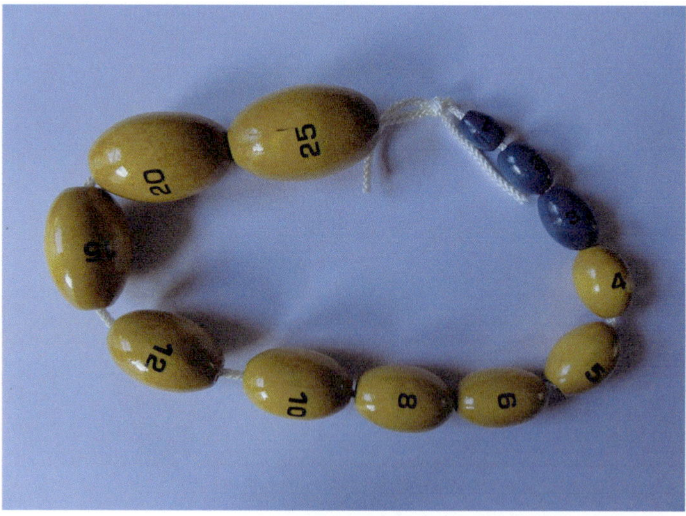

**Fig. 9.19** Prader's orchidometer

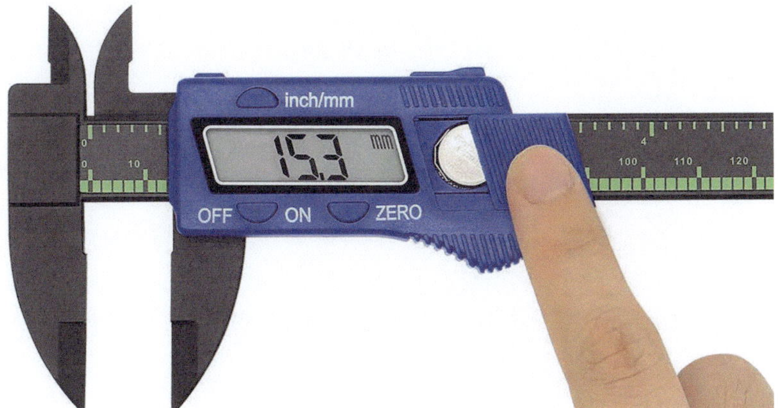

**Fig. 9.20**  Electronic digital caliper

**Fig. 9.21**  Measurement of scrotal surface area by multiplying the scrotal length with the scrotal width

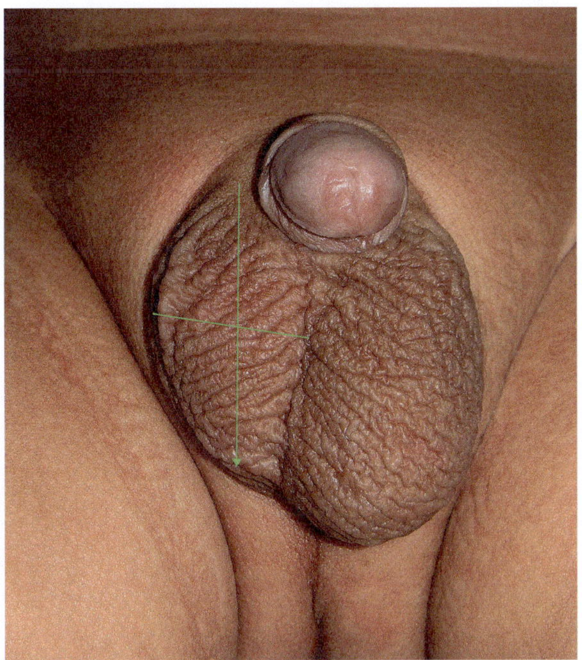

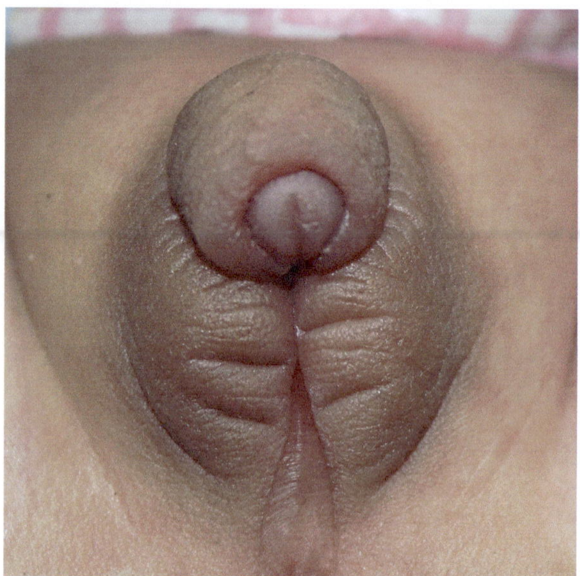

**Fig. 9.22** Scanty rugae with wide raphe and a deficient prepuce

considered as a scrotal hypoplasia, and in scrotal agenesis there is no detectable rugae. (Fig. 9.22) (Chap. 11).

I think detection of scrotal surface area is crucial for evaluation of the genital growth and may be helpful in diagnosis of hypogonadism, also the scrotal size increment could be an indicator for the treatment progress of the cases of hypogonadism and scrotal hypoplasia (Fig. 9.23).

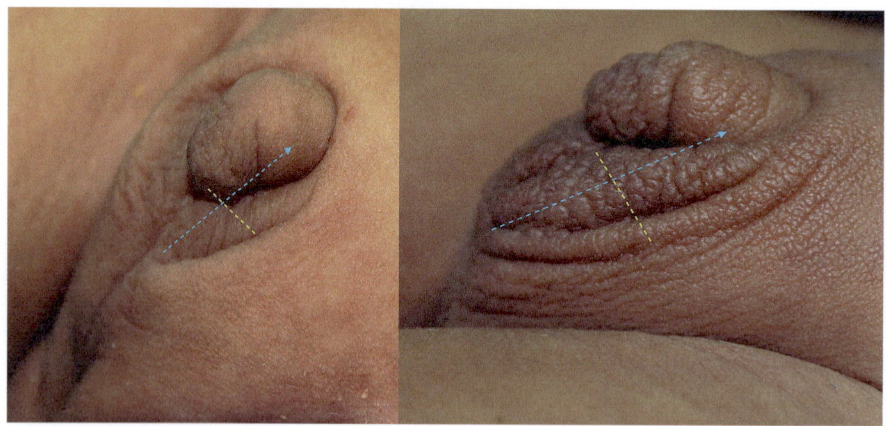

**Fig. 9.23** Scrotal surface area increment after local testosterone treatment for a case of scrotal hypoplasia

Abnormal small scrotum may be attributed to hypogonadism or scrotal hypoplasia, but on the other hand the extensively long scrotum without any intrascrotal swelling is known as a pendant scrotum.

## 9.6  Position of the Scrotum

The penis and scrotum as a one unit had a fixed location, with very minimal normal variations and rarely subjected to congenital anatomical positional anomalies. Scrotal position is limited cephalically by the penis and its attachment to the symphysis pubis, and caudally by the anal position, from which it is separated by the anogenital raphe. This position is determined embryologically by the degree of infromedial migration of the labioscrotal folds. Normally the scrotum lies immediately posterior (caudal), to the penis, separated from it by the penoscrotal angle and junction, with a commonly shared wall (skin and dartos). Also the scrotum is cephalic or anterior to the anus, separated from it by the perineal body, and communicated to the lips of the anus by the perineal raphe. The anoscrotal distance is more or less fixed, with a minimal variations. Caudal migration of the penis and scrotum is seen in some cases of bladder exstrophy; as the eviscerated bladder wall pushes the genitalia downward. In rare cases of caudal regression syndrome and secondary to the disturbed pelvic bone architecture the penis and the scrotum may be positioned ectopically caudal (Chap. 12).

**Factors determine scrotal position:**

**Symphysis pubis**: The penis is supported in the prepubic position in its flaccid and erect states by a support system called the penile suspensory ligamentous system. The superior margin of this ligament corresponded to the upper border of the pubic symphysis and its posterior margin attached to its anteroinferior surface, and it is attached the tunica albuginea of the corpora cavernosa inferiorly [7]. So the lower border of symphysis pubis limits the upper border of the penis, by the suspensory ligament attachment, and this also limits any cephalic migration of the scrotum.

**Genetic and Hormonal**: Dihydrotestosterone induces virilization, which includes vertical lengthening of the perineum; fusion of the urogenital folds to form the penile shaft, glans and urethra; and fusion of the LSF to form the scrotum [8]. Some authors suggested a genetic basis for normal penoscrotal relationship, but the embryological sequence responsible for this relation defect remains unclear [9].

One of the main features determining the sex difference between male and female is the difference of the positions of scrotum or its analogue labia majora, so abnormal scrotal positioning may be a sort of sex indifference or masculinity (Fig. 9.24).

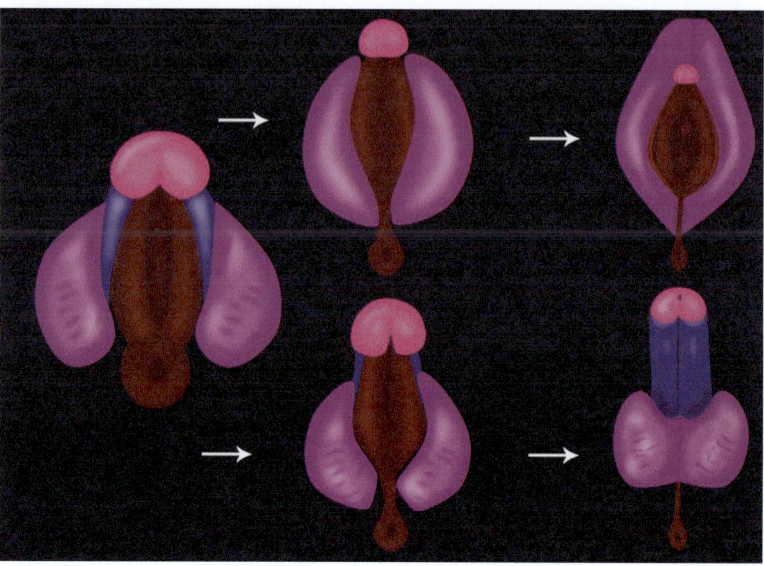

**Fig. 9.24** Labioscrotal folds migration and sex difference

Abnormal positioning of the genital tubercle in relation to the scrotal swellings during the critical fourth to fifth week of gestation may affect the inferomedial migration and fusion of the scrotal swellings. The penis and scrotum achieve their usual arrangement when, under the influence of androgens, the genital tubercle elongates to become the penis, while migration of LSF brings scrotum downwards. Lamm and Kaplan suggested that scrotal anomalies result from early division and/or abnormal migration of the labioscrotal swelling [10]. Congenital perineal lipoma have been described as an associated condition of abnormal scrotal position; however, they are very commonly associated with accessory scrotum in up to 83% of cases. Sule et al. [11] hypothesized that the accessory LSF develops because a perineal lipoma in the perineum, which disrupts the continuity of the developing caudal labioscrotal swelling, and this support the view of field defect which interfere and hinder proper penoscrotal configuration.

## 9.7 Anoscrotal Distance (Anogenital Distance)

Understanding the anogenital anatomy is critical for any medical practitioner. It is, therefore, important for health care providers to know the proper techniques for anogenital examinations, normal anatomy, and to know when findings are forensically relevant, warrant treatment, or require referral to a sub-specialist for further evaluation and management [12].

By the end of the sixth week, a down-growth of splanchnic mesoderm called the urogenital septum reaches the cloacal membrane, dividing it into the urogenital and anal membranes. The site of fusion between the urogenital septum and the cloacal membrane is the future perineal body. As the cloacal membrane becomes divided into the urogenital and anal membranes, these swellings become the urogenital swellings anteriorly and the anal folds dorsally, with the perineal body developing between the two swellings. Lateral to the urogenital swellings, a pair of elevations develop, called the genital swellings. During the eighth week of gestation, the urogenital and anal membranes rupture, so that the urogenital sinus and anal canal communicate freely with the amniotic cavity [13]. Failure of midline fusion may be manifested as a different grades of bilateral scrotal compartments separation" Bifid Scrotum". Anogenital distance (AGD) has been suggested to represent a phenotypic signature reflecting in utero androgen action, and throughout life. AGD is longer in males than in females in both rodents and humans, and it has been associated with other reproductive end points in humans. Boys born with cryptorchidism or hypospadias have shorter AGD, and cross-sectional studies have found an associations between shorter AGD and lower testosterone levels, poorer semen quality, and infertility in adult men [14]. So normal scrotum had a fixed position confined by the penis and perineal body, and it is very rarely seen ectopic cephalically or caudally. But we may have a wide AGD (wider separation of the scrotum from the anus) normally in few cases, which will gave a false impression of more cephalically positioned scrotum (Fig. 9.25) and this may be attributed to a posteriorly

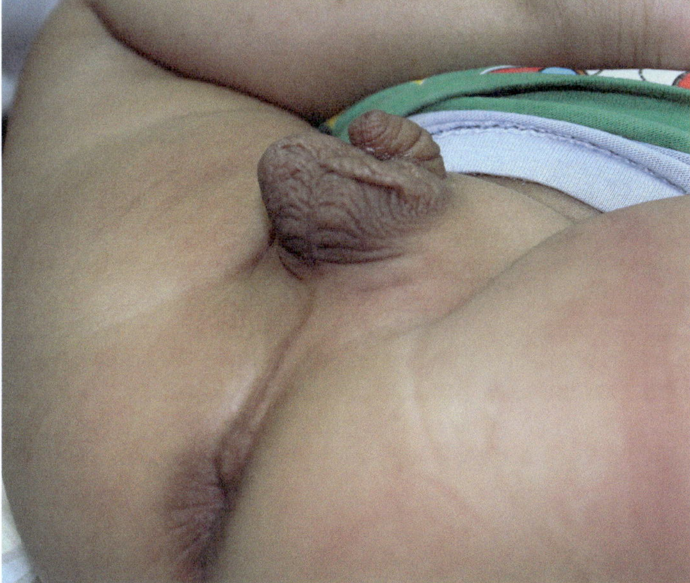

**Fig. 9.25** Wide distance between scrotum and anus in a normal child

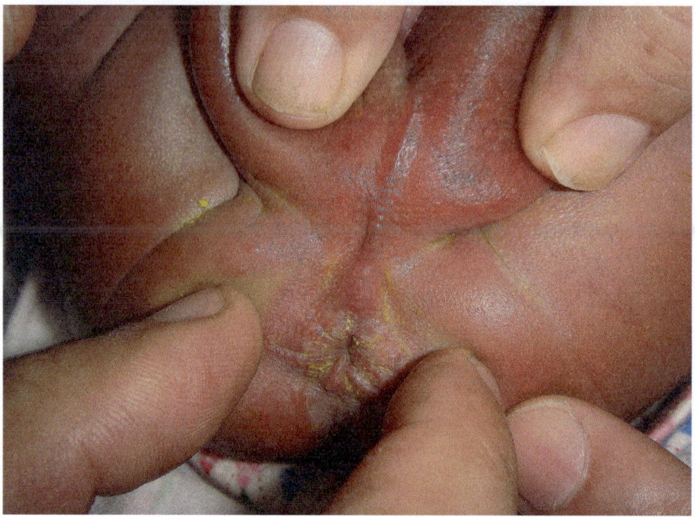

**Fig. 9.26** Short anoscrotal distance in a normal neonate

positioned anus. In the other way around this AGD distance may be normally shorter, with the lower limit of scrotum approaching the anal verge (Fig. 9.26).

## 9.8   Penoscrotal Angle

Normally the penis and scrotum is in intimacy relation, but not in a common vicinity, and as mentioned before, normally the scrotal skin may creep over the penile median raphe at the root of the penis, and the lateral upper scrotal angles are normally incorporated with the penile skin at both sides. At puberty the penis maintained at a right or slightly obtuse angle with main scrotal axis (Fig. 9.27). In early fetal development the rotation of the penis ventralward, as illustrated by the changing angle between the axis of the corpora cavernosa and the ventral side of the pubic symphysis from 160 degrees (fetus of 35 mm) to 90 degrees (fetus 90 mm) is secondary to the lengthening of the penis that actually moves ventralward between the two scrotal swellings [15]. In any age group there is considerable variation in the angle at which the erect penis is carried on the standing male. The average position, calculated from all ages, is slightly above the horizontal, but there are approximately 15 to 20 percent of the cases where the angle is about 45 above the

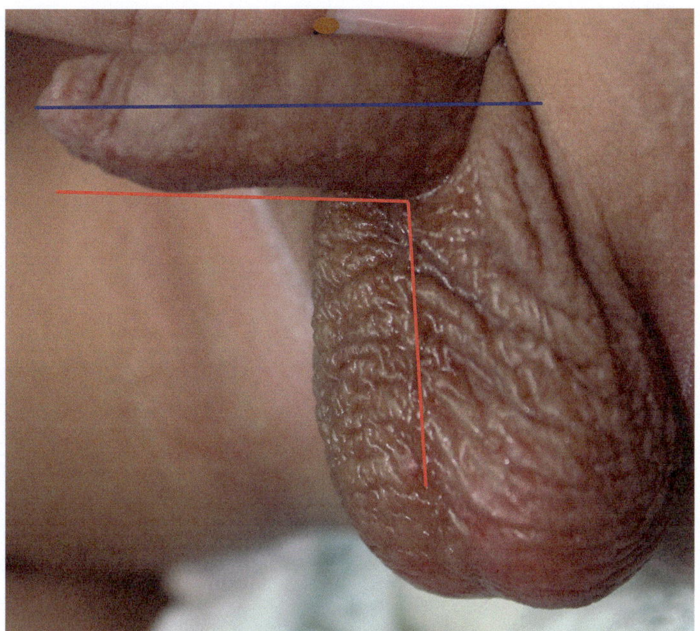

**Fig. 9.27** Penoscrotal angle

horizontal, and 8 to 10 percent of the males who carry the erect penis nearly vertically, more or less tightly against the belly. The angle of erection is, in general, higher in the early twenties, and lower in more advanced ages [16] (Fig. 9.28). Abnormal penoscrotal relation may ends with inability to perform vaginal intromission, painful coitus for the partner or embarrassment leading to psychic problems.

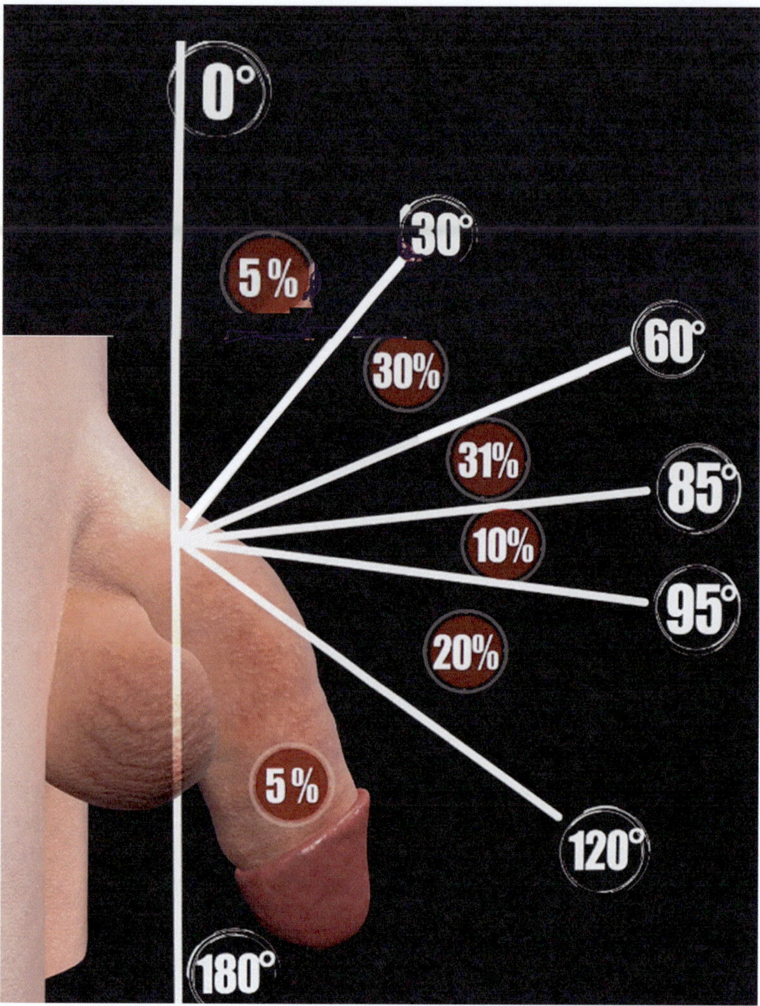


**Fig. 9.28** Different penoscrotal angeles of erection [20]

## 9.9 Penoscrotal Distance

The anatomically correct location of the penis in adults is typically 1 to 1.5 cm superior to the upper margin of the scrotum, with a defined penoscrotal angle along with the skin. It is not rare to have a normal variation of the penoscrotal junction; wheres the most common one is obscuring of the normal junction with a scrotal creeping over the ventral penile surface. Over liaison results in abnormally concealed or webbed penis, and in very rare cases a complete penoscrotal fusion may be seen. In cases of webbed penis; ventrally, at the base of the penis, the dartos

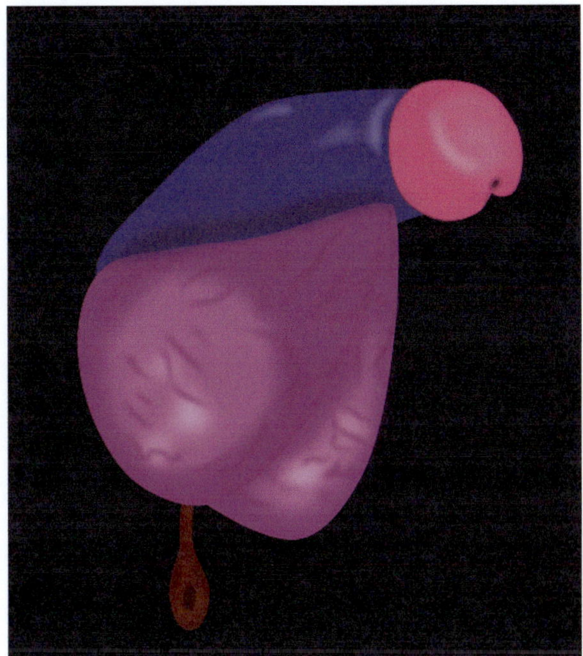

**Fig. 9.29** Diagram showing the scrotal tissue creeping over the penile ventral surface; obscuring the normal penoscrotal angle

fascia combines with more smooth muscle fibres and closely adheres to the skin of the scrotal wall, making the penis look diminutive (Fig. 9.29).

Inadequate fixation of penile skin and poor basal attachment of the shaft result in a pile of narrowed skin on the ventral surface of the penis, whereas the scrotal skin ascends to the middle shaft, thereby compensating for the paucity of cutaneous coverage [17]. The reciprocal of penoscrotal fusion is a very rare anomaly of wide penoscrotal distance; where the penis is widely separated by a normal skin from the upper scrotal edges, this is seen either sporadically or with cases of bladder exstrophy [18] (Fig. 9.30) (Chap. 12).

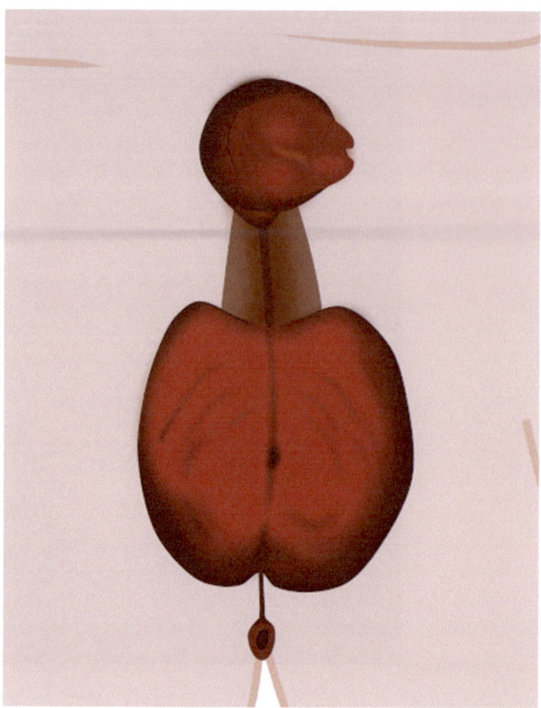

**Fig. 9.30** A diagram showing a wide penoscrotal distance

## 9.10 Normal Scrotal Asymmetry

In humans, the asymmetry is much more subtle and usually invisible. Genital asymmetry seems to occur in human males, also it has been found to occur in many species of the animal kingdom. Scrotum normally not fully symmetrical, with the left side usually hanging lower than the right, which may be due to a greater length of the spermatic cord (Fig. 9.31).

Physiologically, one testis is typically lower than the other to avoid compression in the event of impact. An alternative view is that testis descent asymmetry evolved to enable a wider surface area for both scrota and subsequently a more effective cooling of the testicles. In both adults and foetuses it is clear that the right testicle is both the heavier and also the greater in volume; but the larger and heavier is also the higher in position. Testicular asymmetry has been attributed to more well-developed and greater flexion of the muscles on one side of the lower abdomen relative to the other side [19] and/or the different length, angle and source of the blood vessels supplying the two testicles [19] (Chap. 18).

Scrotal and testicular asymmetry is not a constant phenomena; as we may have many cases in health and diseases where both sides are identically symmetrical without any obvious changes between both side, in Fig. 9.32 a 2 years child who had an idiopathic small phallus, but both scrota are a little bit enlarged but still symmetrical in shape and size.

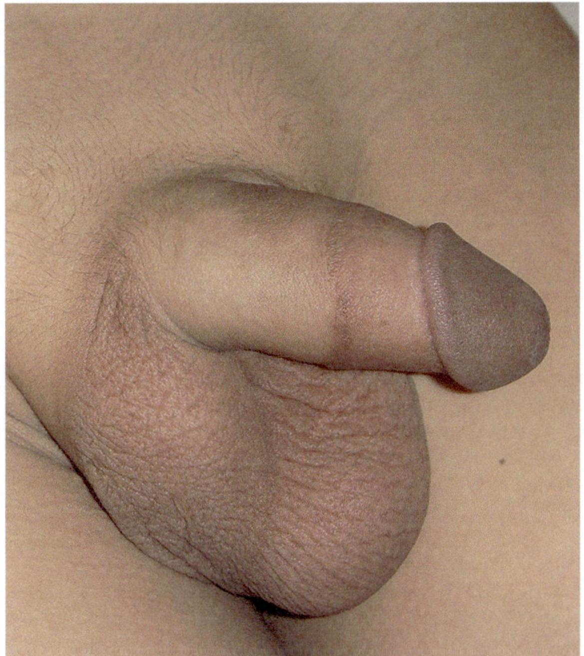

**Fig. 9.31** Normal scrotal asymmetry with a lower seated left side

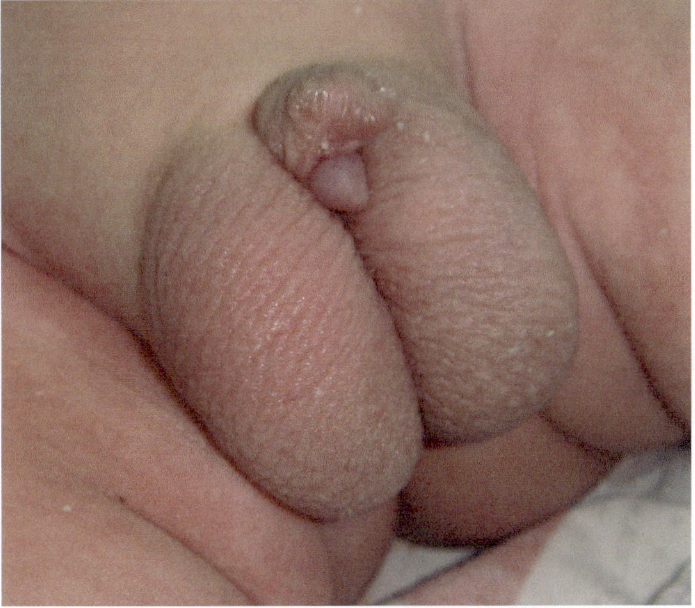

**Fig. 9.32** A child with microphallus, but had a symmetrical and identical bilateral scrota

# References

1. Blouin K, Richard C, Brochu G, et al. Androgen inactivation and steroid-converting enzyme expression in abdominal adipose tissue in men. J Endocrinol. 2006;191:637–49.
2. Wright JE. Congenital absence of the scrotum: case report and description of an original technique of construction of a scrotum. J Pediatr Surg. 1993;28:264–6.
3. Nishio H, Mizuno M, Moritoki Y, et al. Hemiscrotal agenesis: pathogenesis and management strategies. Int J Urol. 2016;23:523–6.
4. Tadokoro T, Rouzaud F, Itami S, Hearing VJ, Yoshikawa K. The inhibitory effect of androgen and sex-hormone-binding globulin on the intracellular cAMP level and tyrosinase activity of normal human melanocytes. Pigment Cell Res. 2003;16:190–7.
5. Rivers JK, Frederiksen PC. Dibdin C: a prevalence survey of dermatoses in the Australian neonate. J Am Acad Dermatol. 1990;23:77–81.
6. Hall JG, Allanson JA, Gripp K, Slavotinek A. Handbook of normal physical measurements. 2nd ed. New York: Oxford University Press; 2007.
7. Chen X, et al. Visualization of the penile suspensory ligamentous system. Med Sci Monit. 2017;23:2436–44. https://doi.org/10.12659/MSM.901926.
8. Flum AS, Chaviano AH, Kaplan WE. Hemiscrotal agenesis: new variation in a rare anomaly. Urology. 2012;79:210–1.
9. Pinke LA, Rathbun SR, Husmann DA, Kramer SA. Penoscrotal transposition: review of 53 patients. J Urol. 2001;166:1865–8.
10. Lamm DL, Kaplan GW. Accessory and ectopic scrota. Urology. 1977;9:149–53.
11. Sule JD, Skoog SJ, Tank ES. Perineal lipoma and the accessory labioscrotal fold: an etiological relationship. J Urol. 1994;151:475–7.
12. Deye KP, Jackson AM. Children: normal anogenital anatomy and variants. Encycl Foren Legal Med. 2016, 1. Elsevier Ltd. doi:https://doi.org/10.1016/B978-0-12-800034-2.00073-2
13. Schoenwolf GC, Bieyl SB, Brauer PR, Francis-West P. Larsen's human embryology. 4th ed. Philadelphia, PA: Churchill Livingstone; 2008.
14. Eisenberg ML, Jensen TK, Walters RC, Skakkebaek NE, Lipshultz LI. The relationship between anogenital distance and reproductive hormone levels in adult men. J Urol. 2012;187:594–8.
15. van der Putte. The development of the perineum in the human, vol. 177. Advances in anatomy embryology and cell biology. pp. 1001–109. ISBN 3–540–21039–3 Springer Berlin Heidelberg New York
16. Kolligian ME, Franco I, Reda EF. Correction Of Penoscrotal Transposition: A Novel Approach The Journal Of Urology. 0022–5347/00/1643–0994/0
17. Liu X, He DW, Hua Y, Zhang DY, Wei GH. Congenital completely buried penis in boys: anatomical basis and surgical technique. BJU Int. 2013;112:271–5.
18. Fahmy MAB, El Shennawy AA, Edress AM. Spectrum of penoscrotal positional anomalies in children. Int J Surg. September 2014; 12(9):983–988. https://doi.org/10.1016/j.ijsu.2014.08.001
19. Chang RH, Hsu FK, Chan ST, et al. Scrotal asymmetry and handedness. J Anat. 1960;94:543–8.
20. Sparling J. Penile erections: shape, angle, and length. J Sex Marital Ther. 1997;23(3):195–207. https://doi.org/10.1080/00926239708403924.

# Chapter 10
# Congenital Scrotal Anomalies

Mohamed A. Baky Fahmy

## 10.1 Introduction

The scrotum is relatively resistant to embryological misadventure. Congenital malformations of the scrotum are rare, but it may significantly affecting the scrotal aesthetic appeal, and hindering adult sexual performance. Many authors classified scrotal anomalies into four main categories; bifid scrotum, accessory scrotum, scrotal transposition and ectopic scrotum, but scrotal hypoplasia, agenesis and penoscrotal fusion are not included in such simple classification. The congenital anomalies of scrotum are commonly associated with hypospadias, testicular maldescend, and intersex. Congenital scrotal anomalies are included in various syndromic features including gross psychomotor delay, facial dysmorphism, ophthalmological abnormalities, skeletal deformities, cerebellar malformations, or gastrointestinal defects; which are included in a known syndromes like; Cutis marmorata telangiectasia congenital, Prader–Willi syndrome, PHACE syndrome, Popliteal pterygium syndrome [1]. Theoretically it was believed that scrotal development is closely related to penile development, but observationally this is not true; as many cases had a normally developed phallus. At the fourth week of gestation, the phallus developed from the genital tubercle to form the penis, while at the same time, genital swellings appear at both sides of the inguinal region from the labioscrotal folds and gradually move to the posterior site and form the labioscrotal swellings at 10–12 weeks of gestation. In male this swelling migrates further to the caudal area of the penile site and forms the right and left parts of the scrotum. Although the etiology of scrotal anomalies remains unclear, the most accepted etiopathogenetic hypothesis for these conditions is an abnormal migration of labioscrotal swelling mainly due to distention of an associated perineal swelling or compression by the fetus heel in utero [2].

M. A. B. Fahmy (✉)
Al-Azhar University, Cairo, Egypt

## 10.2 Spectrum and Classifications of Scrotal Congenital Anomalies

In the following chapters we will assess the extent of the biased representation of those cases, classifying these anomalies into main categories and subtypes, and discussing the different modalities of diagnosis and managements. Further research is needed along with greater clinical experience in the treatment of those patients to better define their management options and refine the aesthetic scrotoplasty techniques.

Herein scrotal anomalies are classified into main groups and subgroups:

1 Scrotal Maldevelopment Anomalies:

    A Scrotal Agenesis

      Unilateral
      Bilateral

    B Scrotal Hypoplasia

      Unilateral
      Bilateral
      Focal

2 Positional Anomalies of the Scrotum "Scrotal Transposition"
3 Penoscrotal Fusion
4 Bifid Scrotum
5 Ectopic Scrotum
6 Accessory Scrotum
7 Scrotal Median Raphe Anomalies
8 Scrotal Asymmetry
9 Scrotoscchiasis
10 Congenital Scrotal Calcinosis
11 Scrotal Vascular Anomalies

# References


1. Kendirci M, Horasanlı K, Miroğlu C. Accessory scrotum with multiple skeletal abnormalities. Int J Urol. 2006;13:648–50.
2. Sule JD, Skoog SJ, Tank ES. Perineal lipoma and accessory labioscrotal fold: An etiological relationship. J Urol. 1994;151:475–7.

# Chapter 11
# Scrotal Maldevelopment Anomalies

Mohamed A. Baky Fahmy

**Abbreviations**

CSA   Congenital scrotal agenesis
SH    Scrotal hypoplasia
AR    Androgen receptor
DSD   Disorders of sex development
AMH   Anti Mullerian hormone
HCG   Human chorionic gonadotrophin

**Scrotal Maldevelopment Anomalies**
**Scrotal Agenesis**
    Unilateral
    Bilateral
**Scrotal Hypoplasia**
    Bilateral
    Unilateral
    Focal

## 11.1   Scrotal Agenesis

**Definition**: Congenital scrotal agenesis (CSA) is a rare scrotal anomaly, and it is characterized by complete absence of scrotal rugae in the perineum between the penis and anus [1] (Fig. 11.1).

CSA is commonly bilateral with an impalpable testicles, but rare cases of unilateral scrotal agenesis are sometimes recognizable (Fig. 11.2).

M. A. B. Fahmy (✉)
Al-Azhar University, Cairo, Egypt

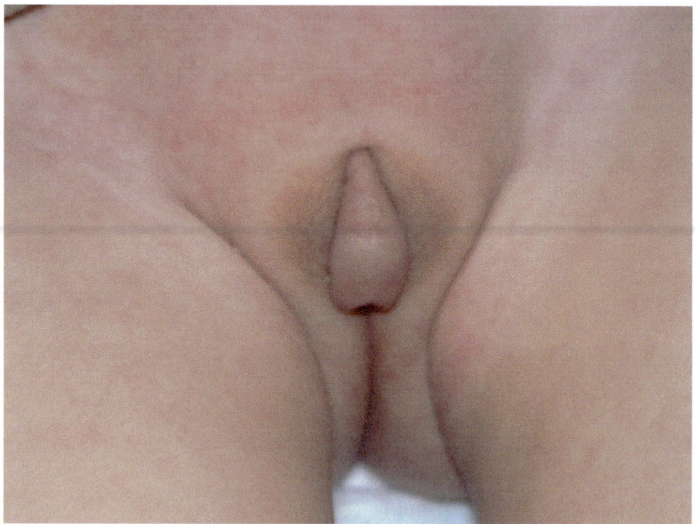

**Fig. 11.1** Case of bilateral scrotal agenesis with a well developed penis

**Incidence**: Preventing and treating non reported rare or mismatch diseases will require both expanding the studies design to sample diverse populations and contexts, and fully incorporating evolutionary perspectives. Literature review identified few cases reported with congenital scrotal agenesis, mainly in surgical reconstructive journals, other cases are reported briefly along other chromosomal and endocrinal syndromes. As many cases escape reporting and publication; either due to early pass away of the baby or non recognizability, so it is extremely difficult to plot out an exact figure about the incidence of CSA or hypoplasia among population.

**Etiology**: The etiology of CSA could be either chromosomal, or a local field defect during early fetal development with or without androgen receptors defectiveness. Several hypotheses were postulated in literature to explain scrotal agenesis; including a dermatological anomaly or the presence of amniotic bands that may cause loss of scrotal skin. However, these hypotheses seem unlikely because of the presence of a normal median raphe in some reported cases. The association of scrotal agenesis with dihydrotestosterone was hypothesized also, but hormonal assays performed in several cases were normal. However, functional work on MAB21L1 gene function may evidence its role in steroid biogenesis, and its deficiency could explain scrotal underdevelopment [2].

Nishio et al. [3] carried out at 2016, for the first time, an evaluation of the normal and abnormal scrotal skin in hemiscrotal agenesis in a boy with non-syndromic CSA using histological and biological analyses to assess the AR in agenetic scrotum. They carried out biopsies of both edges of the rugae and non-rugae scrotal skin, histologically they found more subcutaneous adipose tissue and less melanin in the non-rugae than in the rugae scrotal skin. Conspicuously, expressions of androgen receptor and SRD5A2 were significantly lower in the non-rugae scrotum

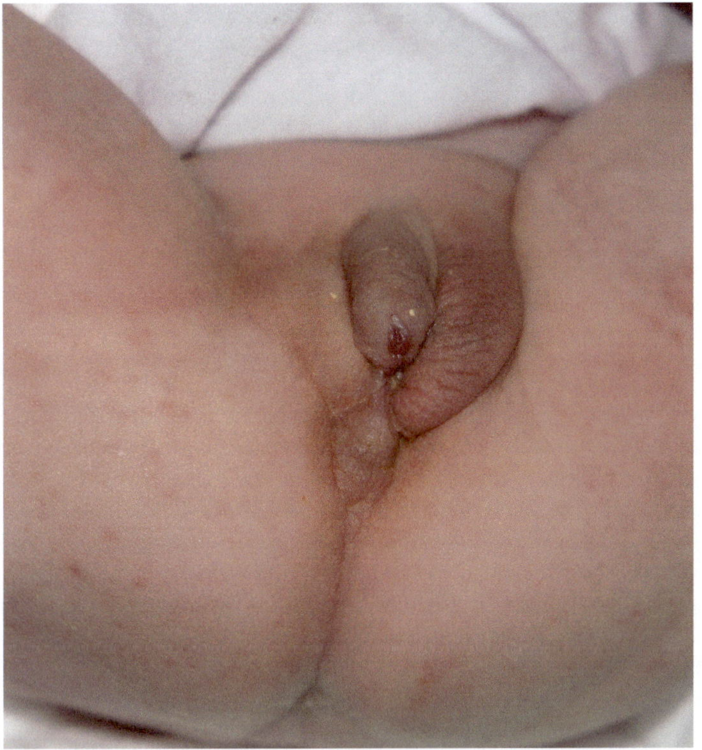

**Fig. 11.2** Rare case of unilateral right scrotal agenesis with imperforate anus

skin, which was shown by quantitative reverse transcription polymerase chain reaction analysis. These new findings showed that scrotal skin with absent rugae and pigmentation has low activity against androgen owing to the low expression of androgen receptor and SRD5A2. The abundance of subcutaneous adipose tissue and pigmentation deficiency in the non-rugae scrotal skin were also attributed to androgen inactivation in the affected skin. Thus, inadequate function of both androgen receptor and SRD5A2 in the pathogenesis of HSA was well documented in this study [3]. Although the cause of androgen inactivation remains unknown and in consequence, exclusion of alternative etiologies requires additional investigation using genetic technologies, such as exome sequencing, together with ascertainment of further patients. Mohan et al. [4] reported the treatment of 2 cases of scrotal agenesis with topical testosterone with a subsequent development of scrotal skin with normal rugosity, which was used to construct a new scrotum. This would suggest that the labioscrotal folds were present but did not properly develop into a scrotum, they contended that this might be due to a localized partial 5a-reductase, with enough dihydrotestosterone produced to prevent labia formation but not enough to stimulate scrotal development. In 1 of the 2 reported cases, scrotal rugae developed over an ectopic testis in the medial thigh, which might suggest some role for abnormal migration of the labioscrotal folds.

**Clinically**: Most of the affected boys with bilateral agenesis of scrotum presented a normal median raphe, flat, non pigmented and non rugose skin between the base of the penis and anus. They had a maldescended testes; either cryptorchid or ectopic.

We classified CSA into:

- Unilateral CSA
- Bilateral CSA
- Syndromic scrotal agenesis
- Isolated CSA

Unilateral agenesis, also known as hemiscrotal agenesis, it is more rare than the bilateral cases, and usually presented as an isolated anomaly, without any recognizable syndrome (non syndromic) with a well developed penis (Fig. 11.3). Many cases of unilateral CSA are associating a different forms of anorectal malformations (Fig. 11.4) A broad spectrum of clinical features were associating CSA; including ophthalmologic abnormalities, low-set ears, micrognathia, short neck, clubfoot, coarse facial dysmorphism, hypothyroidism, gross psychomotor delay, and intellectual disability. Atrial and ventricular septum defects are also a common associates [5].

Bilateral CSA are commonly one of the manifestation of other chromosomal syndromes, but sporadic isolated cases are rare and associated with bilateral cryptorchidism, ectopic testicles or anorchia (Figs. 11.5 and 11.6). Common syndromes associated with CSA are Prader–Willi syndrome, genitopatellar syndrome,

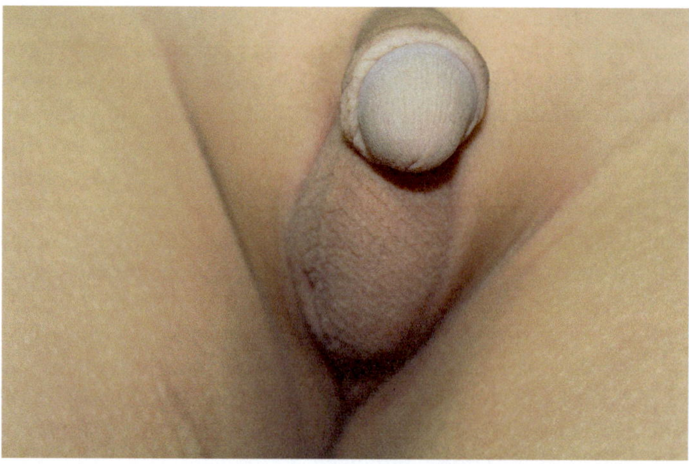

**Fig. 11.3** Isolated unilateral left CSA without any other detectable anomaly except an ipsilateral cryptorchidism

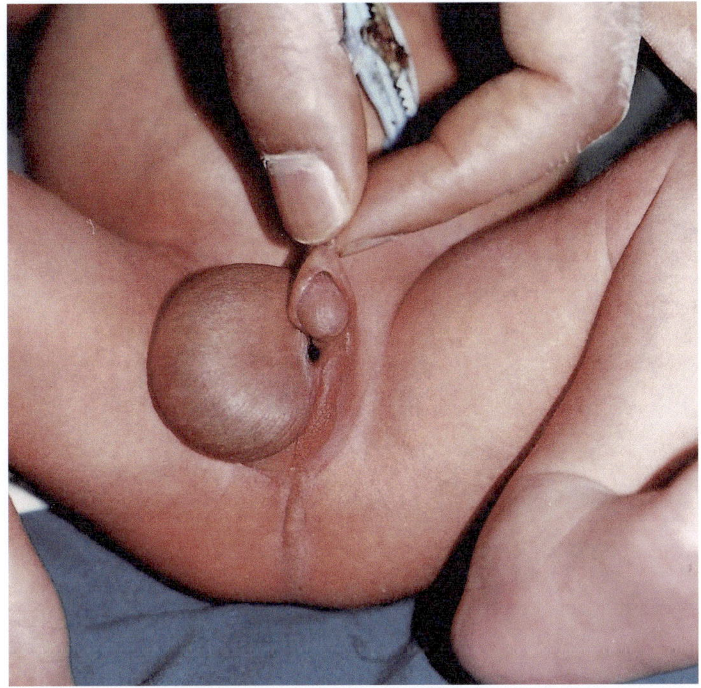

**Fig. 11.4** Right sided CSA with imperforate anus and rectourethral fistula, the right side shows a compensatory hypertrophy

Cutis marmorata telangiectasia congenital, and popliteal pterygium syndrome. This supporting the existence of genetic heterogeneity in this anomaly [6, 7]. Popliteal pterygium syndrome is a rare congenital condition involving craniofacial and genitourinary anomalies as well as malformation of the extremities, and the striking characteristic of this syndrome is a popliteal pterygium, which consists of a net of connective tissue spreading from the ischial tuberosity to the calcaneus.

We diagnosed three cases of scrotal agenesis with caudal regression syndrome (Fig. 11.7), two of them had of different forms of aphallia (Fig. 11.8), and most cases of sirenomelia had aphallia and bilateral CSA (Fig. 11.9). Caudal Regression Syndrome is a spectrum of congenital malformations, which consist of anomalies of the rectum, the urinary and genital systems, the lumbosacral spine, and the lower limbs. Though exact cause that leads to caudal regression syndrome is still unknown but it is believed that genetic influence as well as maternal pathologic factor related to carbohydrate metabolism play an important roles [8]. Anorectal malformations, specially higher anomalies may be associated with CSA; either bilateral or unilateral (Figs. 11.2 and 11.4) Also hypospadias is not a rare associate (Fig. 11.10) There are few differential diagnoses that can be mentioned, but in few cases with absent scrotal sac, but only had a traces of scrotal rugae, a confusion between agenesis and hypoplasia may be raised, but without any impaction in the

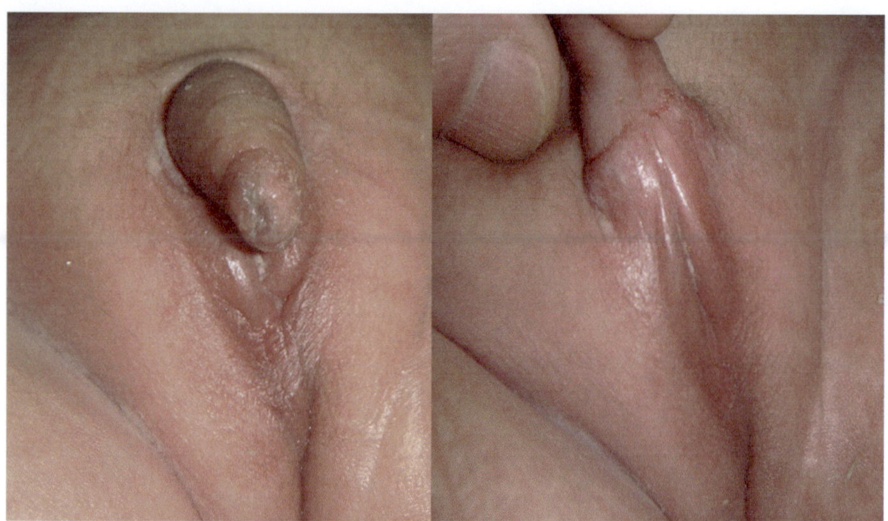

**Fig. 11.5** A case of bilateral CSA with a normal phallus and bilateral impalpable testicles

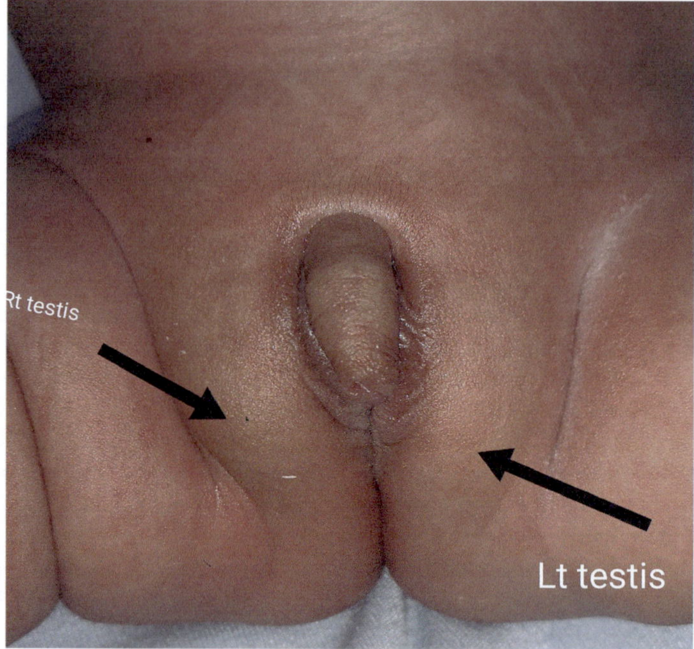


**Fig. 11.6** Bilateral scrotal agenesis with a bilateral ectopic testicles

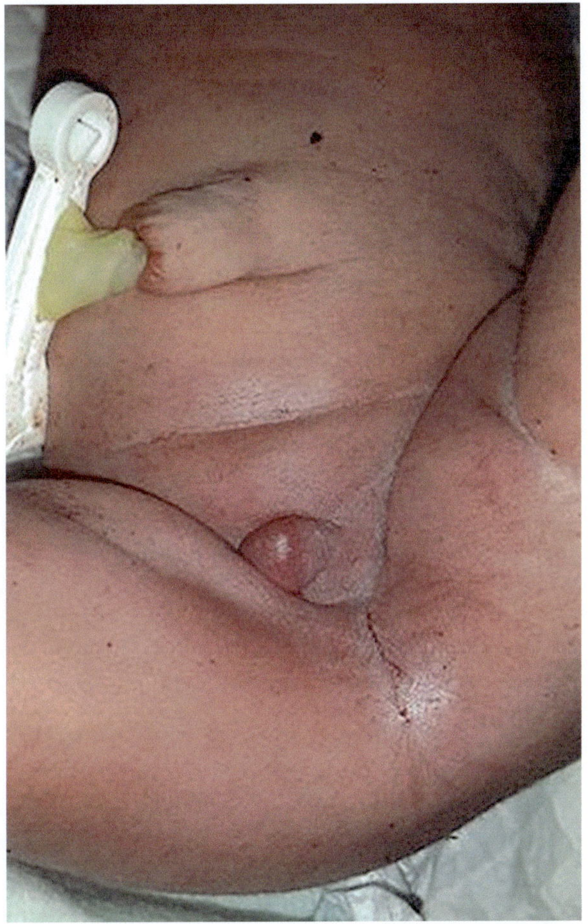

**Fig. 11.7** Neonate with caudal regression syndrome, aphallia and CSA

management and prognosis. In such cases a skin biopsy from the intended area of scrotum before commencement of treatment will differentiate between agenesis and hypoplasia, also a quantitative androgen receptor assessment is helpful to evaluate such cases (Fig. 11.10).

Usually the skin between the penis and the perineum is flat and smooth, as in Fig. 11.5, where a two longitudinal skin ridges are replacing the deficient scrotum. Sometimes an accumulated subcutaneous fat is replacing the deficient scrotum. It is documented that normally the testosterone activity (systemically available hormone and normal local androgen receptors) minimize fat deposition in the genital area [9]. Karyotypic is mandatory to rule out cases of DSD from an isolated cases of CSA; as many cases may be thought, at the first impression, as a case of intersex [10]. Specific cytogenetic studies, if available, are essential to detect any abnormal genetic disorders.

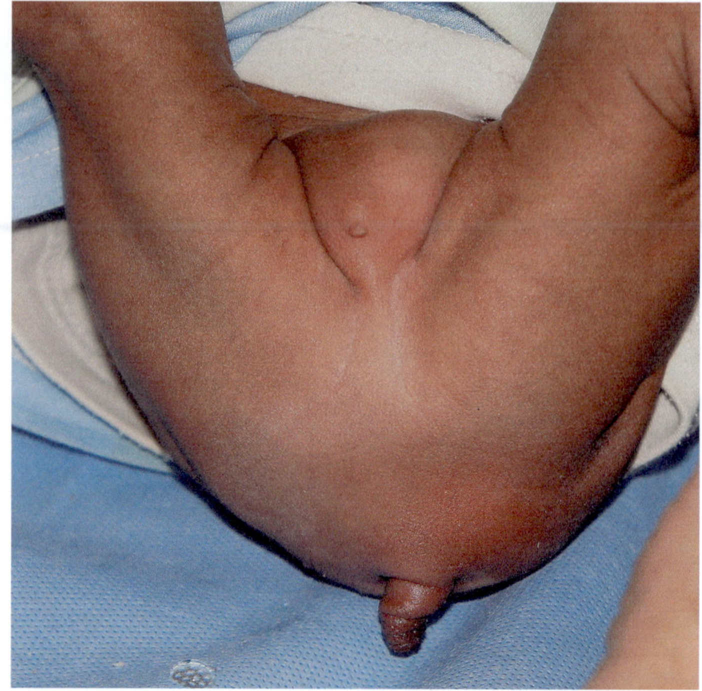

**Fig. 11.8** CSA in a cases of severe caudal regression with a sacral ectopic phallus

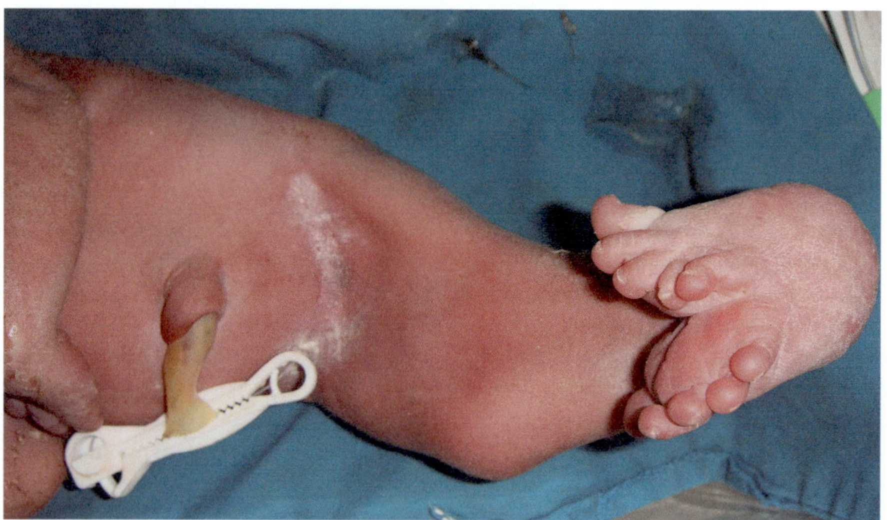

**Fig. 11.9** Aphallia and CSA in a case of Sirenomelia

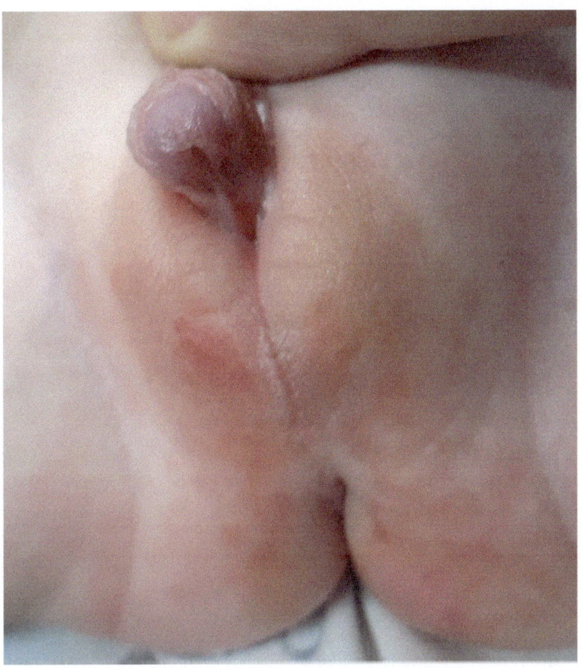

**Fig. 11.10** Case of absent scrotum with a hypospadia, which may raise a confusion between scrotal agenesis and hypoplasia, but absent rugae and pigmentation is obvious

Endocrinology tests usually revealing a normal levels of LH, FSH and testosterone, supposing that both testicles are palpable, but syndromic cases and cases associated with anorchia will have a disturbed hormonal profile, with a low testosterone. We found that AMH is significantly low with different grades of CSA, specially the bilateral one.

**Relations to the testicles**: Most cases of CSA had a bilateral maldescended testicles; either in the form of undescended but palpable testicles, or an ectopic testicles. (Figs. 11.1 and 11.6) Some cases may have the testes descended, specially with cases of hemiscrotal agenesis, which suggests that scrotal agenesis might not be closely related to testicular descent. Many cases of syndromic bilateral CSA; specially cases of aphallia and caudal regression syndrome will had no testicles at all (anorchia). Location of the gonads was determined by palpation, and assessed by ultrasound, but MRI may be indicated in some cases.

**Managements of CSA**: Scrotal sac is basically crucial to accommodates testicles, and it also posses an essential role in psychic make up and genital images. It is impossible to bring down a maldescended testicles in a hypoplastic or absent scrota. So management of CSA should start earlier to any attempts of orchidopexy, such attempts to manipulate testicles before solving the problem of CSA will be disastrous (Fig. 11.11). Priority should be given to management of general, or systemic anomalies; for example the cardiac defect. Once the general condition of the baby is

**Fig. 11.11** A child with
bilateral CSA and
microphallus after an attempt
to fix an atrophic testicles

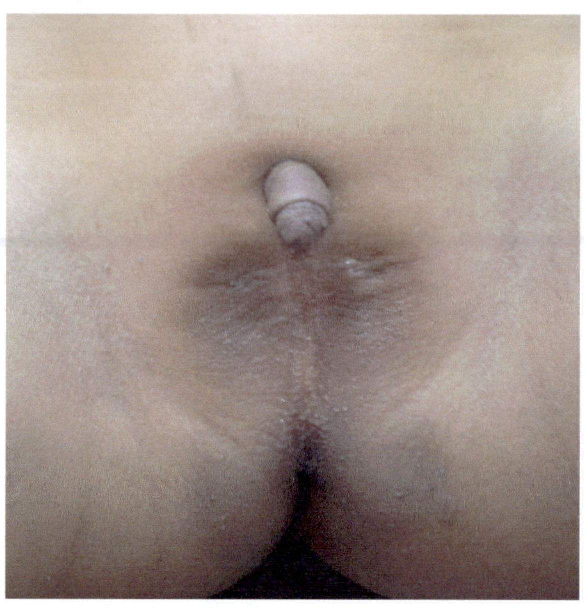

stabilised; attention to manage CSA should start after proper investigations. There are a different modalities for treatment of each group.

**Medical treatment**: Mohan et al. [4] reported the treatment of 2 cases of scrotal agenesis with topical testosterone with a subsequent development of scrotal skin with normal rugosity, which was used to construct a new scrotum.

Testosterone is a medication and naturally occurring steroid hormone. It is used to treat male hypogonadism. Common side effects include acne, swelling, and breast enlargement. Serious side effects may include liver toxicity, heart disease, and behavioral changes. Children may develop an early masculinization. Testosterone was first isolated in 1935, and approved for medical use in 1939 [11]. Rates of use had have increased three times in the United States between 2001 and 2011. It is on the World Health Organization's List of Essential Medicines, the safest and most effective medicines needed in a health system and it is available as a generic medication [12].

We advocate the use of local testosterone early at the age around 2 years for 1–2 months, either alone or in combination with Human Chorionic Gonadotrophin (HCG) injection. If there is facility to assess AR; both quantitively and qualitatively before commencement of treatment, it will give an impression about the possible response to testosterone therapy. Considering the complexity of the procedures for scrotal reconstruction, the relatively harmless intervention with topical testosterone before undertaking any surgical procedures for scrotal agenesis is recommended (Fig. 11.12).

The only side effect we encountered with topical testosterone therapy is redness and darkness of the genital skin, which is reversible after cession of the treatment.

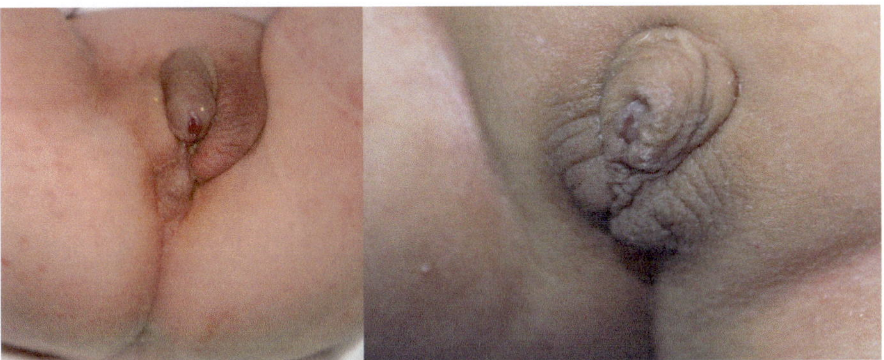

**Fig. 11.12** Case of unilateral CSA before and 6 weeks after topical testosterone treatment

Partial response to medical treatment could facilitate and precede the further surgical reconstruction, but if there is no response to hormonal therapy, this is an indication of complete deficiency of AR and mandates scrotoplasty.

**Surgical reconstruction**: Different surgical techniques have been used to create a functional and aesthetic appearing neo-scrotum. Silay et al. [13] used tissue expanders in the perineum to create a scrotal space and later performed a staged bilateral orchidopexy. A small tissue expander could be inserted into a skin pouch created caudal to the root of penis, this may be effective in unilateral cases of CSA, definitely it is also beneficial in cases of hypoplasia (Fig. 11.13). Theoretically this modality could be applied for bilateral cases, either concomitantly or at alternative sessions. The self-inflating tissue expander is preferable in such cases. Wright and Verga [14] used the Beck-Ombrédanne technique to raise a preputial flap, which was then buttonholed over the glans penis and secured to the ventral surface of the base of the penis as a neoscrotum. In general, even a small appearing scrotum is able to accommodate the testicles. More recently a well-vascularized preputial skin flap rotated to the perineum based on its ventral dartos pedicle provided an excellent source of tissue for creation of a neoscrotum [15]. Myocutaneous flaps; including anterolateral thigh fasciocutaneous islands, perineal, adductor longus, gracilis and rectus abdominis muscles, have been used in adult patients. The results from a cosmetic standpoint may be suboptimal because of the obvious unmatched look of the neoscrotum [16] (Chap. 28).

## 11.2 Scrotal Hypoplasia (SH)

Scrotal hypoplasia is a minor degree of scrotal tissue maldevelopment; it could be unilateral, bilateral or focal and commonly it is an isolated anomaly without any systemic or syndromic malformation, but few cases were rarely reported with

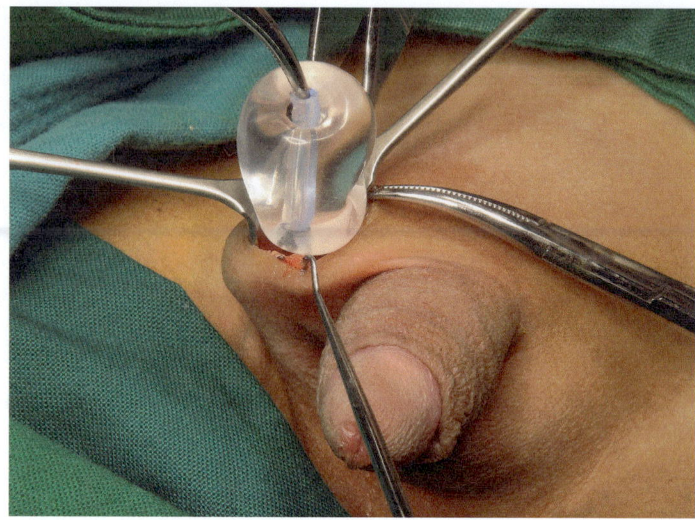

**Fig. 11.13** Insertion of tissue expander in case of unilateral CSA

different syndromes. Unilateral cases are more common and usually associated with undescended testicle and hypospadias.

**Definition**: There is no uniform definition of SH, as the term "hypoplasia" itself is not always used precisely, it properly refers to an inadequate or below-normal number of cells. SH refer to scrotal wall underdevelopment or incompletely developed scrotum, which looks smaller non pendant with a few rugae.

We classified cases of scrotal hypoplasia into three subtypes:

Bilateral
Unilateral
Focal

**Clinically**: Scrotal hypoplasia, occurs most commonly in boys with an undescended testis and in infants with genital ambiguity. There is no specific investigations to diagnose such cases, which usually recognized clinically; in bilateral cases the scrotum looks small hanging up under the phallus, which may be normally developed, the location of deficient scrotum is occupied by a normal skin, sometimes give a false impression of a wide anoscrotal distance (Fig. 11.14). We adopted measurement of scrotal surface area (Length of scrotum multiplied by its width) and the number of rugae (normally 12–25) to detect cases of SH, specially in unilateral cases when compared to the ipsilateral normal side. Median scrotal raphe is usually preserved (Fig. 11.15).

Focal scrotal hypoplasia is an entity which was not described before; and it includes a partial deficient scrotum, which is not involving the entire hemiscrotum (Fig. 11.16).

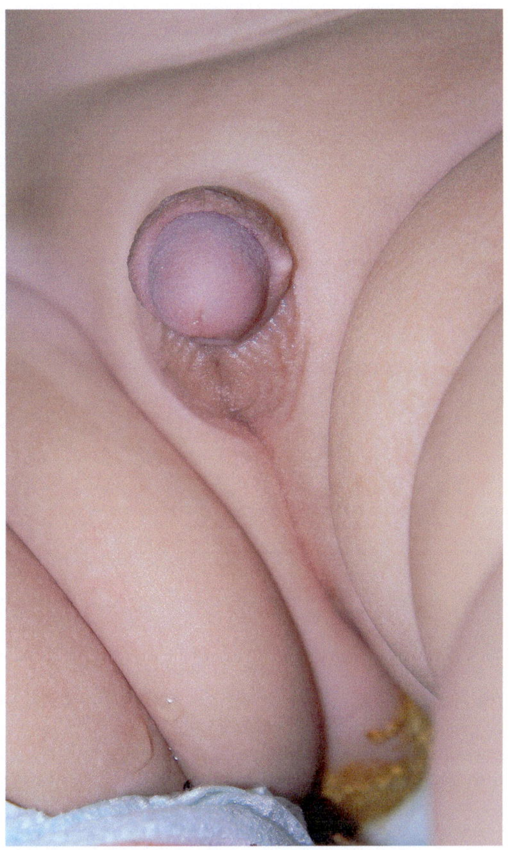

**Fig. 11.14** Bilateral scrotal hypoplasia with a normally developed penis and wide anoscrotal distance

Scrotal rugae may be only deficient laterally leaving only a central patch of rugae around the raphe; so this considered as a focal SH (Fig. 11.17). Some cases of bifid scrotum may had a midline deficient scrotum (Fig. 11.18), also cases of ectopic scrotum may exhibit a deficient scrotum and hypoplasia at the native scrotum. (Fig. 11.19).

SH may be associated with undescended testicle (Fig. 11.20), or ectopic testicles (Fig. 11.21), very rarely a hypoplastic scrotum may envelope a normally descended testicles [17] (Fig. 11.22). Many cases of either uni or bilateral SH are associating different grades of hypospadias, and few cases are reported with anorchia. Investigations could be required to locate the impalpable testicle, to assist the hormonal profile; to diagnoses cases of hypogonadism and to rule out any other associated anomalies.

**Etiology**: It seems likely that this anomaly is multifactorial in origin, with localized androgen insensitivity, localized 5α-reductase deficiency, and failure of formation of the labioscrotal fold; all possibly playing some role. Scrotum in cases of

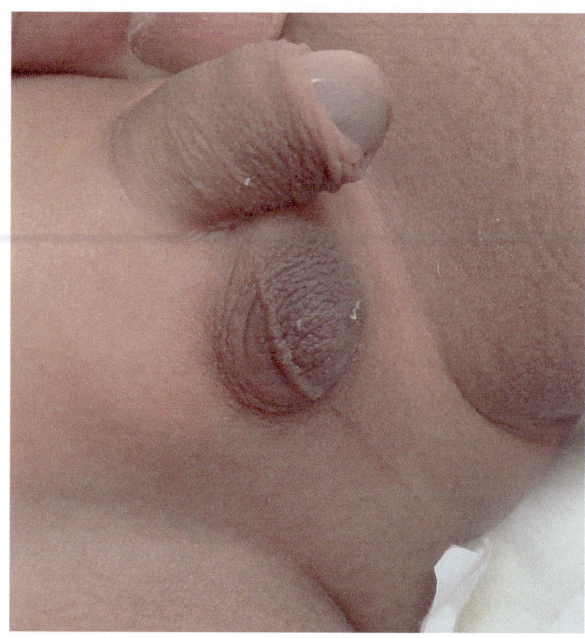

**Fig. 11.15** A case of right side SH with a traces of scrotal rugae and preserved raphe

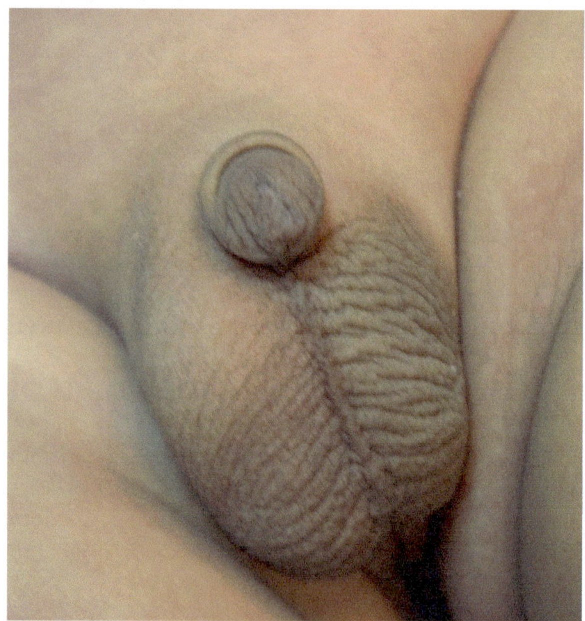

**Fig. 11.16** Child with a focal hypoplasia of the uppermost part of right scrotum, testicles are descended

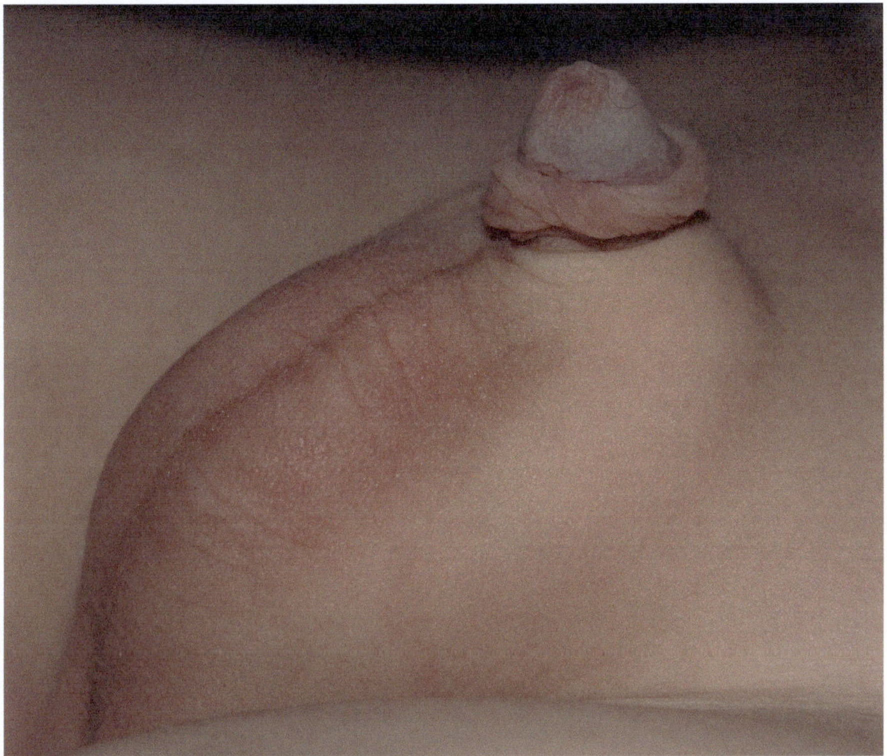

**Fig. 11.17** Laterally deficient scrotal rugae replaced by normal skin and subcutaneous fat

complete Androgen Insensitivity Syndrome (AIS) is usually hypoplastic either bilaterally (Fig. 11.23), unilateral or even with focal hypoplasia.

- We reported one case of focal scrotal hypoplasia as a part of generalised hypogonadism in a 4 years old boy with chromosomal translocation between chromosomes 4 and 7. (Fig. 11.24)

**Many explanations were suggested to explain the pathogenesis and etiology of SH:**

- This deformity may result from lack of gubernacular swelling of the labioscrotal folds. Scrotal hypoplasia may indicate a congenital hypogonadotropic hypogonadism [18].
- In congenital bilateral anorchidism the patients have male external genitalia, but the internal genitalia consists only of normal Wolffian derivatives without Müllerian derivatives, patients have male external genitalia with hypoplasia of both the scrotum and penis. The disorder may be associated with other malformations, such as anal atresia, rectourethral and rectovaginal fistula, and bladder exstrophy [19].

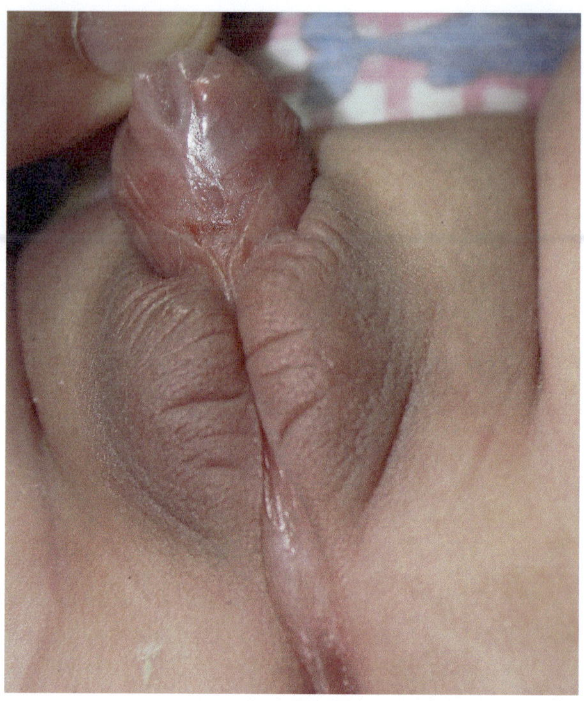

**Fig. 11.18** Bifid scrotum with a centrally deficient scrotal tissue and scanty rugae

- Baraitser–Winter syndrome (BRWS) is a rare but well-defined developmental disorder recognized by the combination of congenital ptosis, high-arched eyebrows, hypertelorism, ocular coloboma and a brain malformation, and it is commonly associated with bilateral scrotal hypoplasia [20].
- Genitopatellar syndrome is caused by mutations in the *KAT6B* gene, and SH is usually manifested with other genital anomalies [21].
- In patients with 47,XXX they have mental retardation, gynecomastia, normal stature, scrotal hypoplasia, well-formed small penis, small testes, and scant pubic hair. Serum testosterone level is markedly decreased [22].
- Patients with Down syndrome usually have cryptorchidism, small testes, hypoplasia of the penis and scrotum, and hypospadias [23].

**Management**: Many cases of minimal degree of SH, specially if it is an isolated anomaly, could be followed up till the time of puberty, as some cases may improve with the normal hormonal serge. Bilateral SH with a diminutive scrotal sac and accompanied with undescended testicles should be managed before any attempt to bring a normal sized testis in a hypoplastic scrotum (Fig. 11.25).

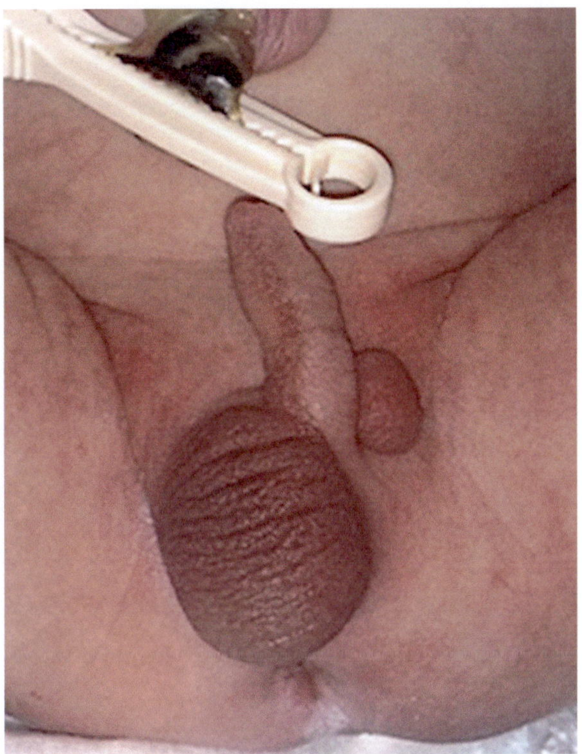

**Fig. 11.19** Left side accessory scrotum with an ipsilateral scrotal hypoplasia

Hormonal therapy proved to be effective in improving many cases of SH [4, 24]. We used topical testosterone for six weeks in all diagnosed cases of SH before any attempts to do orchidopexy or hypospadias repair, with a strict follow up. A promising results and minimal side effects were encountered. Scrotal surface area increments is appreciated in 80% of the cases [25] (Fig. 11.26).

Few cases which showed no response to hormonal therapy, or had a scared or defective skin at the scrotal location, may need a sort of scrotoplasty, which described earlier with cases of scrotal agenesis. Unilateral cases could be managed by either a preputial flap or a mobilized flap from the ipsilateral normal side. As scrotal maldevelopment is not so common and doesn't attract more recent advances for its managements; there is no reported researches about the use of tissue engineering for scrotal replacement. Recently, the scrotoplasty has received more attention than before. Scrotoplasty has the goal of creating an aesthetically pleasing and accurate scrotum from other tissues of the patient (Chap. 28).

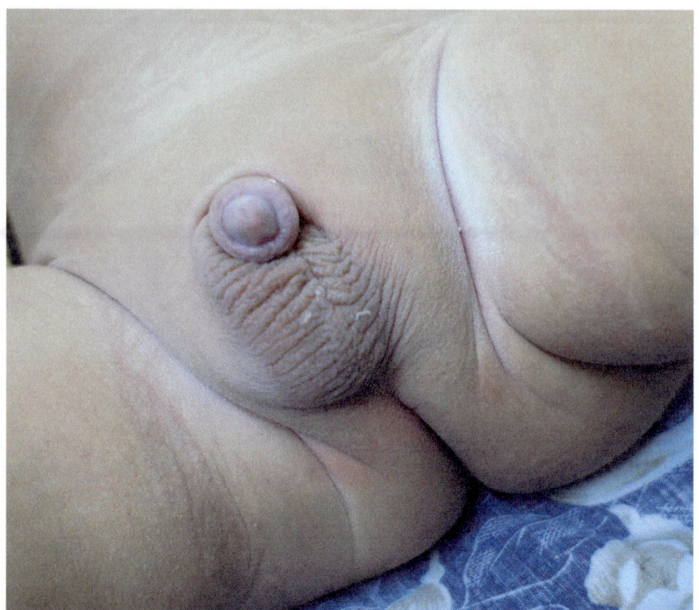

**Fig. 11.20** Left scrotal hypoplasia with undescended testicle

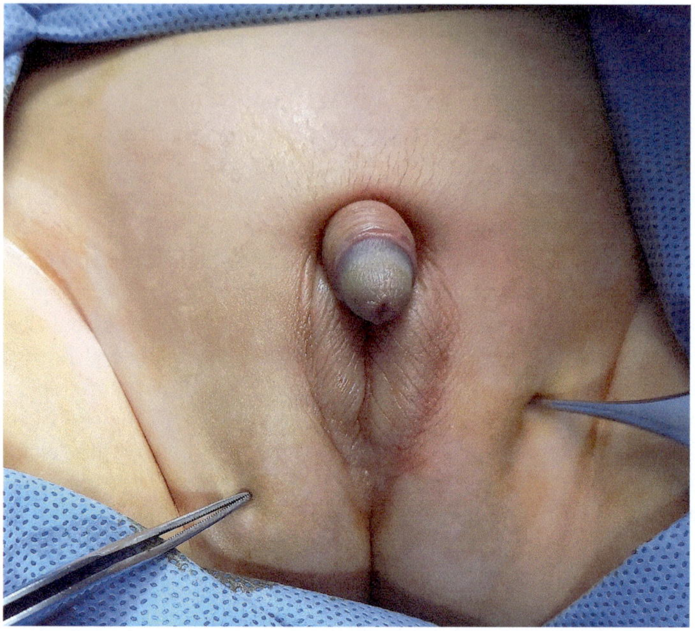

**Fig. 11.21** Bilateral SH with an ectopic testicles

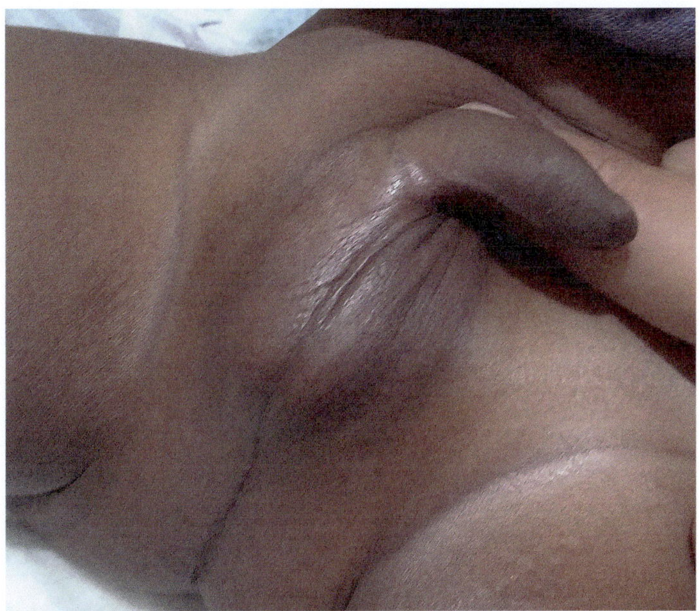

**Fig. 11.22** Bilateral SH with well formed scrotal sac but absent rogue and a normally descended testicles

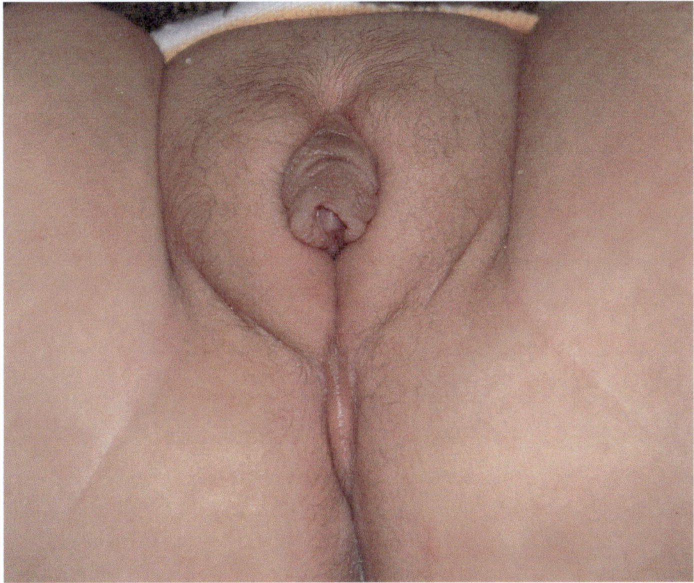

**Fig. 11.23** A case of Complete AIS with bilateral scrotal hypoplasia, the scrotal sac replaced by an accumulated subcutaneous fat

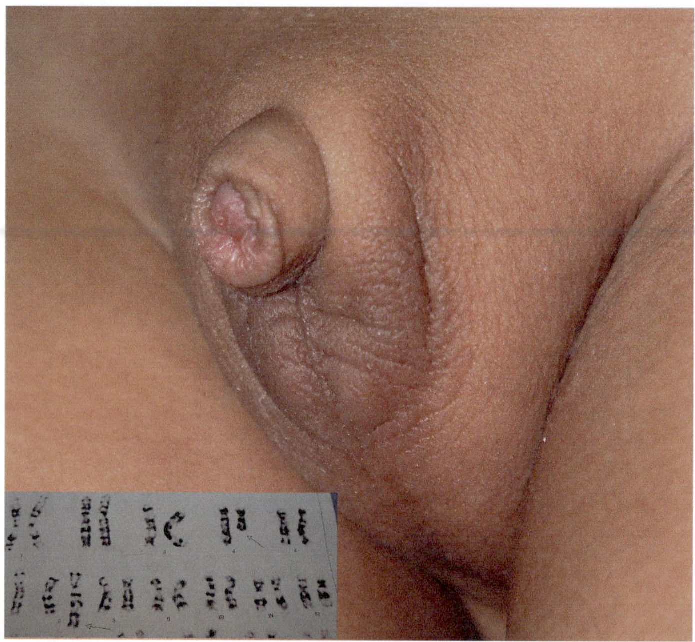

**Fig. 11.24** A 4 years old child with chromosomal 4& 7 translocation, hypogonadism and focal scrotal hypoplasia

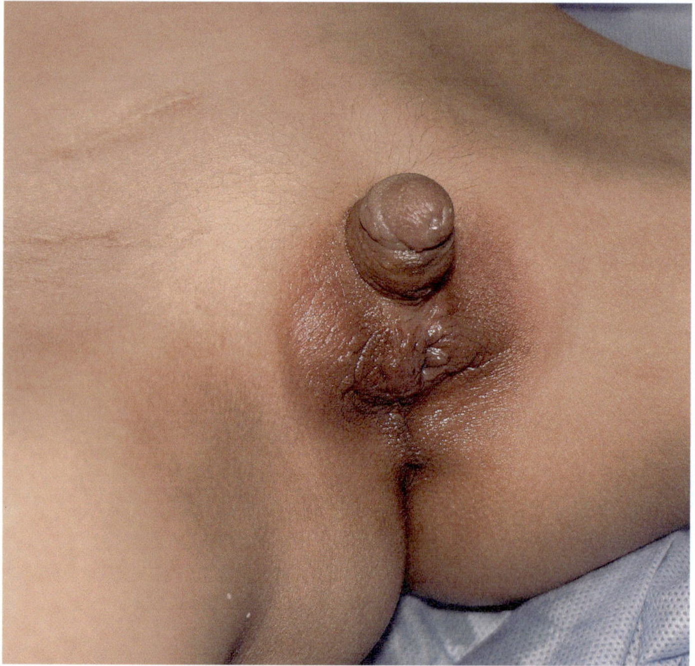

**Fig. 11.25** A case of bilateral SH and hypospadias with both testicles brought down in a hypoplastic scrotum

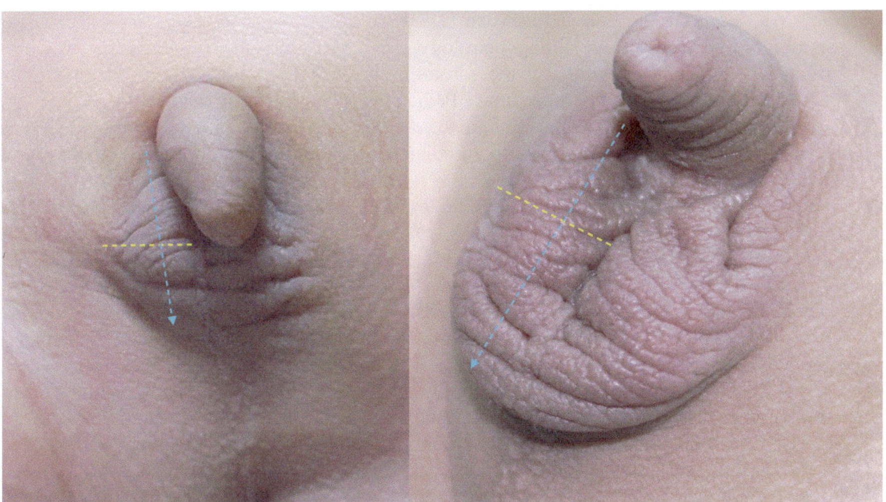

**Fig. 11.26** Improved scrotal skin quality, 6 weeks after application of testosterone in a a child with bilateral SH

# References


1. Yilmaz E, Afsarlar CE, Karaman I, Ozguner IF, Karaman A, Hızlı F. Congenital hemiscrotal agenesis: report of a rare entity. J Pediatr Urol. 2013;9:e76–7.
2. Bruel, et al. Autosomal recessive truncating *MAB21L1* mutation associated with a syndromic scrotal agenesis. Clin Genet. 2017;91:333–8.
3. Nishio H, Mizuno K, Moritoki Y, Kamisawa H, Naiki T, Kurokawa S, Nakane A, Okada A, Yasui T, Hayashi Y. Hemiscrotal agenesis: Pathogenesis and management strategies. Int J Urol. 2016;23:523–6. https://doi.org/10.1111/iju.13079.
4. Mohan PP, Woodward MN, Chandran H, Parashar K. Topical testosterone in scrotal agenesis. Pediatr Surg Int. 2006;22:565–6.
5. Flum AS, Chaviano AH, Kaplan WE. Hemiscrotal agenesis: new variation in a rare anomaly. Urology. 2012;79(1):210–1.
6. Janoff DM, Skoog SJ. Congenital scrotal agenesis: description of a rare anomaly and management strategies. J Urol. 2005;173(2):589–91.
7. Corona-Rivera JR, Acosta-León J, León-Hernández MÁ, Martínez- Macías FJ, Bobadilla-Morales L, Corona-Rivera A: Co-occurrence of hemiscrotal agenesis with cutis marmorata telangiectatica congenita and hydronephrosis affecting the same side of the body. Am J Med Genet A. 2014;164A(1):199– 203.
8. Semba K. Etiology of caudal Regression Syndrome. Hum genet Embryol. 2013;03(02).
9. Blouin K, Richard C, Brochu G, et al. Androgen inactivation and steroid-converting enzyme expression in abdominal adipose tissue in men. J Endocrinol. 2006;191:637–49.
10. Ogilvy-Stuart AL, Brain CE. Early assessment of ambiguous genitalia. Arch Dis Child. 2004;89(5):401–7.
11. Taylor WN. Anabolic Steroids and the Athlete (2 ed.). McFarland; 2002. p. 180. ISBN 978-0-7864-1128-3. Archived from the original on September 14, 2016.
12. Hamilton R. Tarascon Pocket Pharmacopoeia 2015 Deluxe Lab-Coat Edition. Jones & Bartlett Learning. 2015. p. 197. ISBN 978-1-284-05756-0.

13. Silay MS, Yesil G, Yildiz K, Kilincaslan H, Ozgen IT, Armagan A. Congenital agenesis of scrotum and labia majora in siblings. Urology. 2013;81(2):421–3.

14. Wright JE. Congenital absence of the scrotum: case report and description of an original technique of construction of a scrotum. J Pediatr Surg. 1993;28(2):264–6.

15. Benson M, Hanna MK. A novel technique to construct a neo-scrotum out of preputial skin for agenesis and underdeveloped scrotum. J Pediatr Urol. 2018. https://doi.org/10.1016/j.jpurol.2018.03.022.

16. Datubo-Brown D D: Alternative techniques for scrotal recon- struction. Br J Urol. 1990;65:115.

17. Jafarov V. Perineal ectopic testis with unilateral scrotal hypoplasia. J Pediatr Surg Case Rep. 2019;51:101298.

18. Hoar RM, Calvano CJ, Reddy PP, Bauer SB, Mandell J. Unilateral suprainguinal ectopic scrotum: the role of the gubernaculum in the formation of an ectopic scrotum. Teratology. 1998;57:64–9.

19. Bernasconi S, Ghizzoni L, Panza C, Volta C, Caselli G. Congenital anorchia: natural history and treatment. Horm Res. 1992;37(Suppl 3) 50–4.

20. Shawky RM, et al. Baraitser-Winter syndrome: An additional Egyptian patient with skeletal anomalies, bilateral iris and choroid colobomas, retinal hypoplasia and hypoplastic scrotum. Egypt J Med Hum Genet. 2016;17:119–23. https://doi.org/10.1016/j.ejmhg.2015.04.004.

21. Cormier-Daire V, Chauvet ML, Lyonnet S, et al. Genitopatellar syndrome: a new condition comprising absent patellae, scrotal hypoplasia, renal anomalies, facial dysmorphism, and mental retardation. J Med Genet. 2000;37:520–4.

22. Karaer K, Ergun MA, Weise A, et al. The case of an infertile male with an uncommon reciprocal X-autosomal translocation: how does this affect male fertility? Genet Couns. 2010;21:397–404.

23. Mercer ES, Broecker B, Smith EA, Kirsch AJ, Scherz HC, A Massad C. Urological manifestations of Down syndrome. J Urol. 2004;171:1250–3.

24. Corona G, Rastrelli G, Forti G, Maggi M. Update in testosterone therapy for men. J Sexual Med. 2011;8:639–54.

25. Al Samahy O, Doa O, Dalia G, Fahmy MAB. Efficacy of topical testosterone in management of scrotal hypoplasia and agenesis. J Pediatr Urol. 2021. https://doi.org/10.1016/j.jpurol.2021.02.014

# Chapter 12
# Positional Anomalies of the Scrotum "Scrotal Transposition"

Mohamed A. Baky Fahmy

**Abbreviations**

PST    Penoscrotal Transposition
PSD    Penoscrotal Distance
CPST   Complete Penoscrotal Transposition
AIS    Androgen Insensitivity Syndromes
DSD    Disorders of Sex Development
ARM    Anorectal Anomalies

## 12.1  Introduction

Our understanding of sexual differentiation has recently improved dramatically, but one aspect of sexual differentiation that is still poorly understood is the mechanism controlling the position of genitalia, which represents one of the most substantial differences between the sexes [1]. The embryological origins of the penis and scrotum are the genital tubercle and labioscrotal folds, respectively. At the end of the fourth week of development, males and females have indistinguishable external genitalia. The penis and scrotum achieve their usual arrangement when, under the influence of androgens, the genital tubercle elongates to become the penis, and at a caudal position to it the labioscrotal folds develop, which migrate inferomedially and fuse in the midline to form the scrotum. Abnormal location of the genital tubercle or abnormal migration of the labioscrotal folds may be the origin of penoscrotal transposition [2]. The scrotum is a unique anatomical feature of human males and most terrestrial land-dwelling male mammals. The scrotum is continuous with the skin of the lower abdomen and is located directly behind the penis in front

**Electronic supplementary material** The online version of this chapter (https://doi.org/10.1007/978-3-030-83305-3_12) contains supplementary material, which is available to authorized users.

M. A. B. Fahmy (✉)
Al-Azhar University, Cairo, Egypt

of the anus. It is a dual-chambered suspended sack, and its wall is formed by a thin layer of skin lined with delicate smooth muscle tissue (dartos fascia and muscle). Some mammals, such as lagomorphs and kangaroos, have scrota located in front of their penis. Although the testes and scrotum formed early in embryonic life, sexual maturation begins upon entry into puberty, when the increased secretion of testosterone causes a darkening of the skin and the development of sparse hair on the scrotum.

Complete penoscrotal transposition (CPST) is a rare and unusual malformation in which the scrotum is located cephalic to the penis. This condition was described in detail by Appleby in 1923 [3]. Factors determining the normal scrotal position and their alterations may result in different forms of PST being divergent and include genetic, hormonal and local anatomic alterations. We adopted a newer classification that considered other unreported minor subtypes and contemplated the two directions of scrotal transposition: either cephalic or caudal. Caudal migration of the scrotal sacs away from the penis is a positional anomaly that will leave the genitalia with an abnormal semblance. PST is rarely reported as an isolated anomaly in a normal male, and the most common association is hypospadias. Over the last 60 years, a very wide spectrum of urogenital and systemic anomalies have been reported with PST. Some of these associating anomalies are correctable, such as hypospadias and chordee, but others may be a life-threatening malformations and may even be incompatible with life. These associated anomalies may be in the form of specific well-known syndromes or just as single or multisystemic malformations. Surgical correction of uncomplicated transposition is relatively simple through a one-stage procedure: by bisecting the scrotum and suturing the 2 halves around the base of the penis or by repositioning the penis through a subcutaneous tunnel dissected beneath the anterior scrotal wall. However, when transposition is accompanied by severe hypospadias, additional factors demand consideration. The Glenn-Anderson technique is still the most successful method for transposition repair. Pinke et al. [4] managed this anomaly with a single-stage Thiersch-Duplay urethroplasty with bladder or buccal mucosa or a staged procedure in complicated cases. Other similar procedures are also described.

## 12.2 Synonyms

Scrotal transposition is the commonly used scientific term; other names are less frequently used, such as shawl scrotum, prepenile scrotum, scrotum dislocation, scrotopenile inversion and doughnut scrotum.

## 12.3  Definition

Penoscrotal transposition may be defined simply as a congenital abnormal positioning of the scrotum superior to the penis, but this definition does not cover the whole spectrum of these malformations. In complete penoscrotal transposition (CPST), the base of the penis is entirely covered by the cephalically located scrotum; if only part of the scrotum is located superior to the penis, the term overriding scrotum or partial PST is used instead.

In shawl scrotum, only the superior margins of the scrotum assemble superiorly to the base of the penis. Partial or complete positional exchange between the penis and the scrotum is a divergent rare anomaly that may manifest in different phenotypes.

We simply define PST as an abnormal positioning or extension of the scrotum above the base of the penis, but a detailed description will be given for each type and subtype with our advocated new classification. The International Classification of Diseases classified this anomaly with ID number 752.81; and the full ID is retrievable from: http://purl.bioontology.org/ontology/ICD-9/752.81.

**Incidence**: PST is a rare congenital anomaly, and some authors reported its prevalence at the birth to be less than 1/10,000 newborns [5]. Pinke et al. [4] in 2001 reported a large, single-institution series of 53 patients aged from 1 day to 30 years old with PST, and Sunay M et al. in 2007 [6] revised the results of the reconstruction of the largest reported series of 64 cases.

**Historical Background**: Complete transposition of the penis and scrotum was first reported by Bergman in 1911 [7]. Appleby in 1923 [3] reported a case of complete PST, and he claimed that this was the 1st reported case. McIlvoy and Harris in 1955 [8] reported the first surgery to move the penis into a more cranial position through a subcutaneous tunnel beneath the prepenile scrotum. Forshall and Rickham in 1956 [9] reported the ninth case in the literature, the second to be operated upon and the first where an associated hypospadias was also repaired. Sakamoto et al. in 1978 [10] and Paramo et al. [11] in 1981 used the term "doughnut scrotum" to describe a configuration in which the penis is centrally placed and surrounded by a scrotum that is continuous both anterosuperiorly and posteroinferiorly. In 1985, Cohen-Addad et al. [12] distinguished between complete PST with a prepenile scrotum of normal appearance and PST with a bifid scrotum.

## 12.4  Factors Determining Scrotal Position

The factors that determine the normal scrotal position and their alterations that may result in different forms of PST are divergent and include the following:

1. **Genetic control and scrotal evolution:**

The scrotum is structure unique to mammals. A recent testicular view of the mammalian family tree revealed that monumental descent occurred early in mammalian evolution. Humans and all other brethren primates have scrotums that bounce between the limbs, dangling behind the penis. Differences between animals and humans can reveal important insights into human biology. In the male marsupial foetus, the scrotum initially develops independently of androgens in the same location as the mammary buds in females (in the groin, cranial to the pubis). Testicular descent occurs in two stages, which is similar to rodents and humans, but as the scrotum in marsupials is located over the external inguinal ring (cranial to the penis), the inguinoscrotal phase is much simpler than in humans, which is why cryptorchidism is rare [13].

Some authors have suggested a genetic basis of the normal penoscrotal relationship, but the complete embryological sequence responsible for this defect remains unclear [4]. In studies on the Tammar wallaby (a small macropod native to South and Western Australia) and other marsupials, it has been proven that scrotal development is not under hormonal control, and the development of the marsupial scrotum, gubernaculum and processus vaginalis are under direct genetic control [14]. However, in humans, all secondary sexual differentiation, including that of the scrotum, is assumed to be under hormonal control rather than direct genetic control. The occasional apparent "reversion" in humans to the metatherian state of scrotal transposition (humans are more closely related to marsupials than to placentals) suggests the possibility of a potentially functional copy of the primitive genetic control mechanism, which is normally active in metatherians and certain lower primates and may exist in the human genome. At least some forms of prepenile scrotal development are under the control of specific genes [15]. Gualtieri and Segal [16] suggested that a prepenile scrotum occurred through genetic mutation, which may be spontaneous in nature or induced by radiation. In pigs, an abnormal location of the gubernaculum appears to be genetically controlled, and in rats, a suprainguinal ectopic scrotum with the contained descended testis appears to be influenced by multiple genes and alleles. Ikadai et al. [17] developed an inbred stain of rats in which a suprainguinal ectopic scrotum occurs in 70% of males, suggesting a genetic aetiology. Datta et al. [18] suggested a 'spontaneous alteration' in the genetic configuration as an explanation for the transposition of the penis and scrotum. The detection of PST in humans as a major finding in many syndromes with specific gene alterations points to possible genetic implications in its aetiological pathogenesis. Many reported cases of PST have been sporadic, a fact that might suggest that the condition is not inherited; however, familial occurrence has been frequently reported. The patient reported by Cohen-Addad et al. [12] in 1985 had trisomy 18 mosaicism, with 8% of the studied cells being trisomic. Pinke et al. [4], in their series of 53 cases, identified one family in whom inheritance occurred in an X-linked recessive manner. Chromosomal studies were performed in 7 cases of partial PST, with a normal male karyotype being reported in 6 of them; in the remaining case, mosaicism was found in skin fibroblasts (16 of 24 cells being 46,XY and 8 cells being 46,XX) [10]. Cases of PST associated with androgen insensitivity syndrome (AIS) indicate both genetic and hormonal control of scrotal position.

2. **Hormonal Control:**

Sixty years ago, the famous French biologist Alfred Jost [19] showed that sexual development is regulated mostly by androgens from the foetal testis. Androgen deficiency leads to 46,XY DSD, with severe phallic hypoplasia and penoscrotal or perineal hypospadias. The primary role of androgens in the masculinization of the embryonic genital tubercle into a penis is well accepted. On the other hand, it has been proven in the human foetus that dihydrotestosterone induces virilization, which includes vertical lengthening of the perineum; the fusion of the urogenital folds to form the penile shaft, glans and urethra; and the fusion of the LSF to form the scrotum [20]. There is evidence that 5-alpha-reductase type 2 deficiency may be involved in PST. 5-Alpha reductase type 2 deficiency is an autosomal-recessive sex limited condition that prevents the conversion of testosterone to dihydrotestosterone [21].

One of the main features determining the sex difference between males and females is the difference in the positions of the scrotum or its analogue labia majora; therefore, abnormal scrotal positioning may be a sort of sex indifference or masculinity (Video animation).

Abnormal positioning of the genital tubercle in relation to scrotal swellings during the critical period extending from the fourth to fifth weeks of gestation may affect the inferomedial migration and fusion of scrotal swellings [22]. The penis and scrotum achieve their usual arrangement when, under the influence of androgens, the genital tubercle elongates to become the penis, while the migration of the labioscrotal folds brings the scrotal sacks opposite each other and caudally to the penis. Lamm and Kaplan [23] suggested that scrotal anomalies result from early division and/or abnormal migration of labioscrotal swelling. Penoscrotal transposition may be the result of a failure of the labioscrotal folds to move caudally either through migration or differential growth followed by subsequent merging of the cranial extent of the scrotal folds. This growth and merging together with the retardation of the development of the genital tubercle places the scrotum cranial to the base of the penis, a position normally seen in marsupials and some lower primate species (*Tupaia* and tarsier) [1]. In cases of a unilateral suprainguinal ectopic scrotum, there is a normal penis, and the contralateral scrotum and testis are normally positioned; therefore, it would seem that the defect must be in movement either through migration or through differential growth of the labioscrotal fold itself [24]. A teratogenic aetiology has also been postulated; some authors have reported that the administration of hormonal treatments in the first weeks of pregnancy can cause this type of malformation [25].

3. **Androgen receptors**

   Different forms of PST are diagnosed with AIS, and it is believed that PST defects are related to a poor response of the target organs to androgens due to a mutation in the gene for androgen receptors and that it is transmitted with a recessive inheritance linked to the X chromosome. Bals-Pratsch et al. [26] were the first authors to describe this association when they presented three siblings with penoscrotal transposition in whom androgen receptor alterations were detected. Additionally, one family in the Pinke et al. [4] series had X-linked recessive inheritance of PST. This finding led those authors to suggest an androgen receptor disorder, which would also be inherited in this manner, as the main aetiology of PST.

4. **Abnormal local anatomical factors**

   Local anatomical defects may act alone or in combination with other previously mentioned factors that induce PST:-

1. **Perineal lipomas:** Congenital perineal lipoma has been described as an associated condition of abnormal scrotal position; however, it is very commonly associated with accessory scrotum in up to 83% of cases. Sule et al. [27] hypothesized that the accessory labioscrotal fold develops secondary to perineal lipoma in the perineum, which disrupts the continuity of the developing caudal labioscrotal swelling. Perineal lipoma might be closely related to abnormal development of the labioscrotal swelling, which supports the view of field defects that interfere with and hinder proper penoscrotal configuration [28]. Additionally, sacrococcygeal teratomas have been reported with PST [29].

   Stephens [30] proposed that pressure from the contralateral heel causing compression during intrauterine life could give rise to abnormal scrotum formation. This could also explain perineal abnormalities associated with PST, such as anorectal malformations [30]. In addition to pregnancy-related complications such as oligohydramnios and breech presentation, the abnormally flexed limb in early foetal life could also be responsible for the reduction deformity of the contralateral limb with resultant PST [30]. The association of PST with different forms of congenital skeletal deformities, such as popliteal pterygium syndrome, indicates the possibility of local mechanical factors as embryological mesenchymal disorders in the aetiology of this anomaly.

2. **Symphysis pubis:** The penis is supported in the prepubic position in its flaccid and erect states through the support of the penile suspensory ligamentous system [31]. The superior margin of this ligament corresponds to the upper border of the pubic symphysis, its posterior margin is attached to the anteroinferior surface of the pubic symphysis, and it is attached the tunica albuginea of the corpora cavernosa inferiorly. Therefore, the lower border of the pubic symphysis limits the upper border of the penis by suspensory ligament attachment and subsequently limits any cephalic migration of the scrotum. Congenital deficiency of the suspensory ligament may be associated with bilateral creeping of the lateral scrotal edges and result in partial PST (Fig. 12.1).

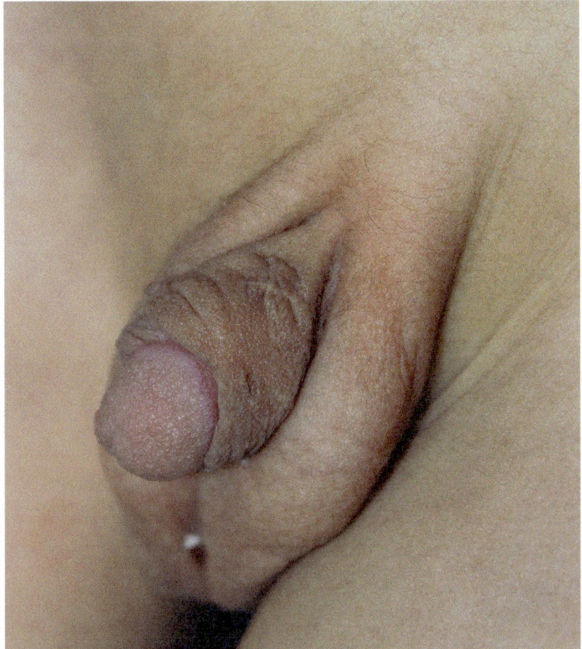

**Fig. 12.1** Congenital deficiency of the suspensory ligament with an incomplete PST

Additionally, the scrotum is normally located anterior to the anus, separated from it by the perineal body, and is connected to the lips of the anus by the perineal raphe. The anoscrotal distance is more or less fixed, with a minimal variation [32] (Chap. 9).

Therefore, disturbed anal anatomy, as in cases of ARM, is commonly associated with PST. Additionally, abnormal pelvic bone configurations in the form of dysplasia or caudal regression syndrome may result in ectopic genitalia [33] (Fig. 12.2).

## 12.5 Classifications of Penoscrotal Transposition

Penoscrotal transposition is a heterogeneous anomaly in which the scrotum is positioned abnormally, superior to the penis or away from it. The penis lies entirely behind the scrotum in the complete types. In less severe forms, the penis may appear to arise from the centre of the scrotum or to be enveloped by the scrotum; by contrast, the distance between the scrotum and the penile shaft may be so wide in isolated cases or in association with other anomalies.

Many authors classified PST into only complete and partial forms [4, 34]. Glenn and Anderson at 1973 [31] incorporated other unrelated anomalies, and broadly,

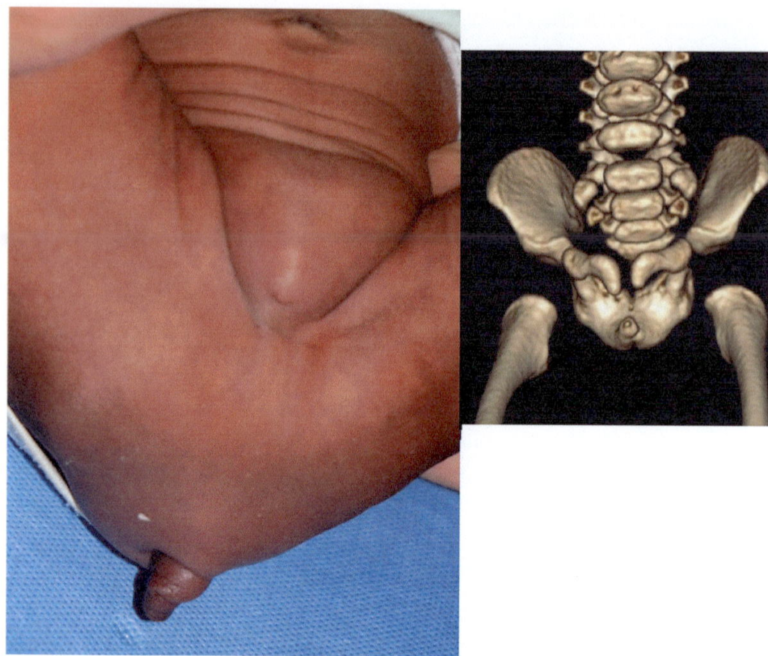

**Fig. 12.2** A very rare case of caudal migration of the phallus to the anal position, complete scrotal agenesis. CT scan showed crowded and fused pelvic bones with deficient ischial bones; these anatomical pelvic anomalies may explain the caudal migration of the genitalia

they classified penoscrotal abnormalities into the following categories according to severity:

- Bifid scrotum
- Incomplete or partial penoscrotal transpositions

- Complete penoscrotal transposition or prepenile scrotum
- Ectopic scrotum

Bifid and ectopic scrotum are different entities unrelated phenotypically to PST, the pathogenesis and aetiology are different in those divergent anomalies. (Chaps. 14 and 15).

We adopted a newer classification that considered other unreported minor subtypes and contemplated the two directions of scrotal transposition: either cephalic or caudal [35]. After diagnosing more variant cases (a total of 65 cases), we revised and simplified our previously published classification into the following categories and subcategories:

- **Cephalic scrotal transposition**

  - Major "complete"
  - Minor "partial": which is sub classified to:-

    Unilateral (asymmetrical)
    Bilateral (symmetrical)
    Central median penile scrotalization

- **Caudal scrotal regression**
- **Iatrogenic penoscrotal transposition**

In major scrotal transposition, the two scrotal sacs are completely cephalic to the penis, which points downward and caudally (Fig. 12.3).

Minor transposition is a more common congenital anomaly; in such cases, the penis lies in the middle of the scrotum, or the penis is engulfed in the middle of the scrotum. Incomplete PST could be a severe form where most of the scrotal sac lies above the penis, but part of the scrotum still lies caudal to the penis. This type of PST may hide an associated severe proximal hypospadias with penile chordee (Fig. 12.4).

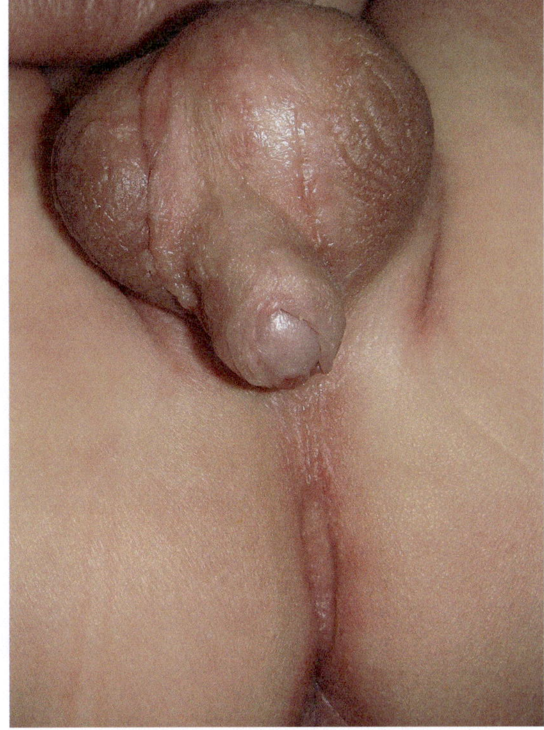

**Fig. 12.3** Complete PST: The normal-sized penis with a normal urethra and meatus directed downward under the cephalically transposed scrotum

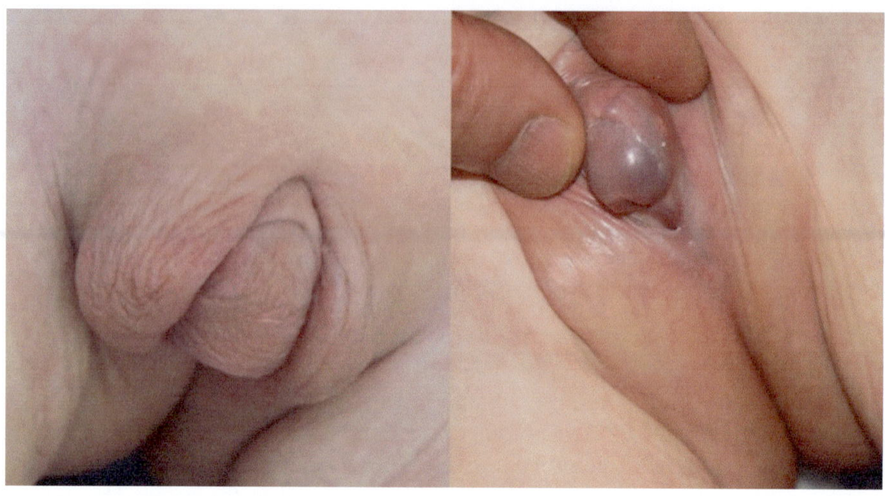

**Fig. 12.4** Incomplete major PST; the scrotum was not completely transposed cephalically, with proximal hypospadias

A minor degree of PST could be a unilateral transposition, which is less frequent than bilateral transposition. (Fig. 12.5) Most cases of unilateral PST we encountered are left sided without any clear explanation [36] (Fig. 12.6).

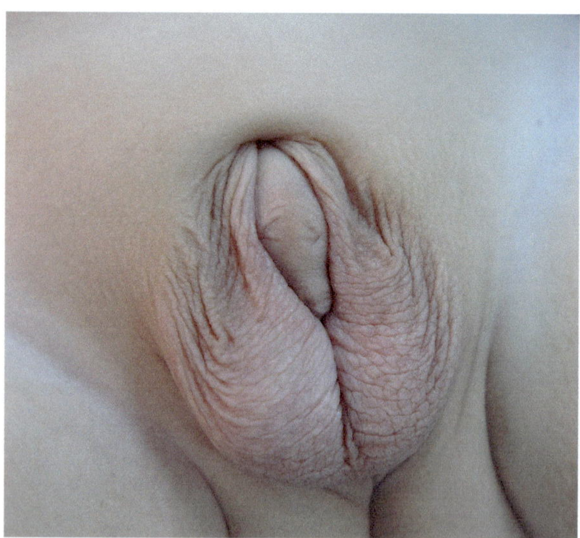

**Fig. 12.5** Incomplete bilateral PST, with obvious prepenile depression secondary to a deficient suspensory ligament

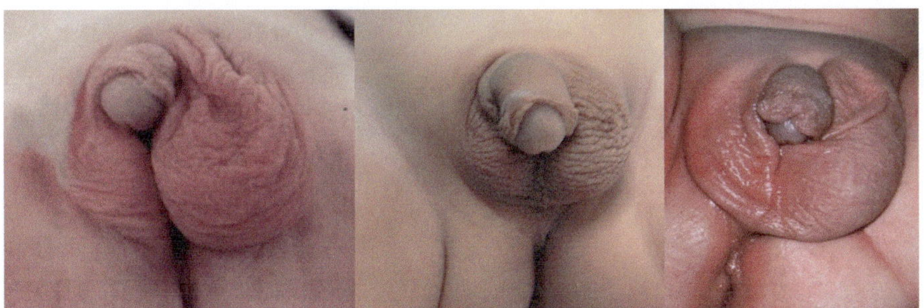

**Fig. 12.6**  Different forms of unilateral partial PST, all are left sided

Central cephalic migration of the scrotum to the ventral penile skin was described in the literature as a webbed penis or penoscrotal fusion, but this is not accurate, as a minimal degree of scrotalization of the penile skin at the base of the penis may be seen as a normal variant (Fig. 12.7). Scrotal skin may extensively enclose the penis, and the characteristic hairless smooth penile skin is replaced by wrinkled darker scrotal skin. In the rare case presented in Fig. 12.8, the scrotal skin extends distally down to the prepuce. Extensive scrotalization of the ventral penile surface will affect the functional length of the penis during erection and may require correction to restore the normal penoscrotal junction with a right angle between the penis and a caudally advanced scrotum (Fig. 12.9).

Caudal scrotal regression is an unreported anomaly in which the scrotum migrates more caudally, leaving a wide distance between the fixed penis and the scrotal sac. A wide distance between the base of the penis and the scrotum is a normal finding in some animals, with a wide variation between different species (Figs. 12.10 and 12.11). However, in the normal human penoscrotal configuration, the scrotum is in a sort of continuity with the penis through the dartos muscle and fascia, but the scrotal skin is distinctive from the penile skin, with a more or less acute penoscrotal angle. Caudal migration of the scrotal sacs away from the penis is a positional anomaly that will leave the genitalia with an abnormal semblance. Some cases were recognized along with other associated anomalies, such as penile rotation, hypospadias and chordee (Figs. 12.12 and 12.13).

It is interesting to recognize that most boys with a bladder exstrophy had a definite wide penoscrotal angle, with an explicit  caudal migration of the scrotum, which is commonly of normal size, and in some cases, the scrotal sacs are divergent laterally from the midline (Fig. 12.14).

Iatrogenic scrotal transposition complicating improper scrotal reconstruction during hypospadias repair has been recently recognized as a deformity, and cursory scrotoplasty by incompetent surgeons for cases of posttrumatic penile or scrotal skin loss may end with an iatrogenic forms of scrotal transposition or malposition (Fig. 12.15).

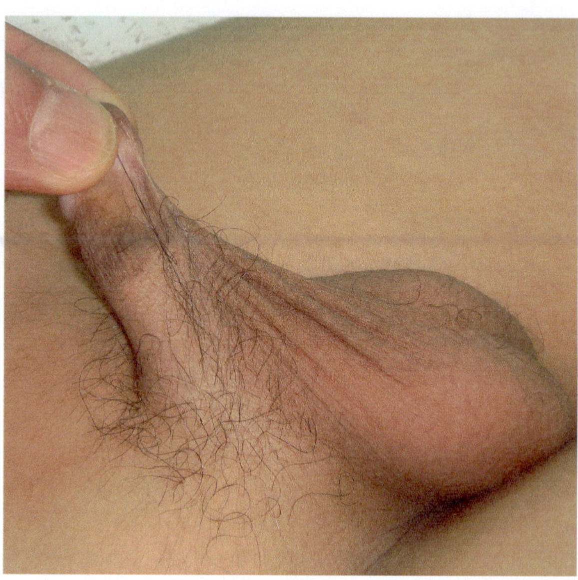

**Fig. 12.7** Central scrotalization of the ventral penile skin

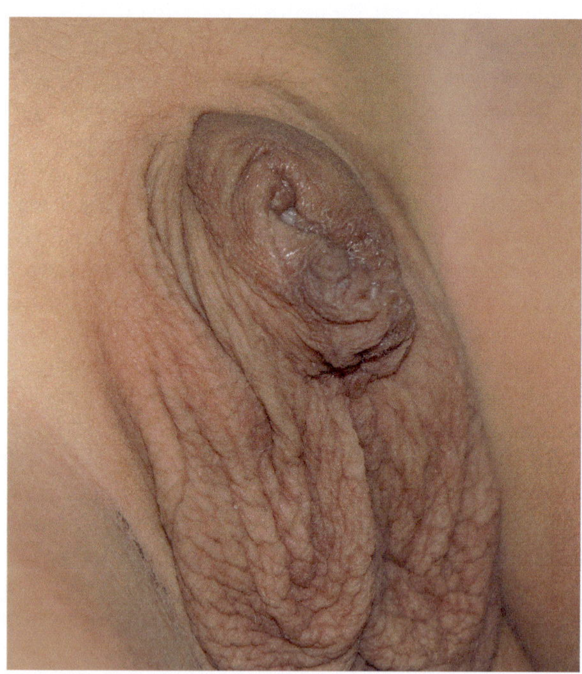

**Fig. 12.8** Rare case of extensive scrotalization of the penile skin distal to the prepuce

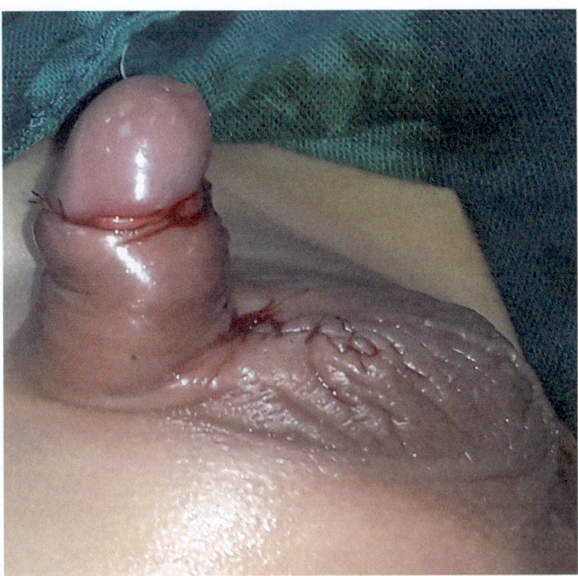

**Fig. 12.9**  Reconstruction of the central scrotum to restore the normal penoscrotal angle

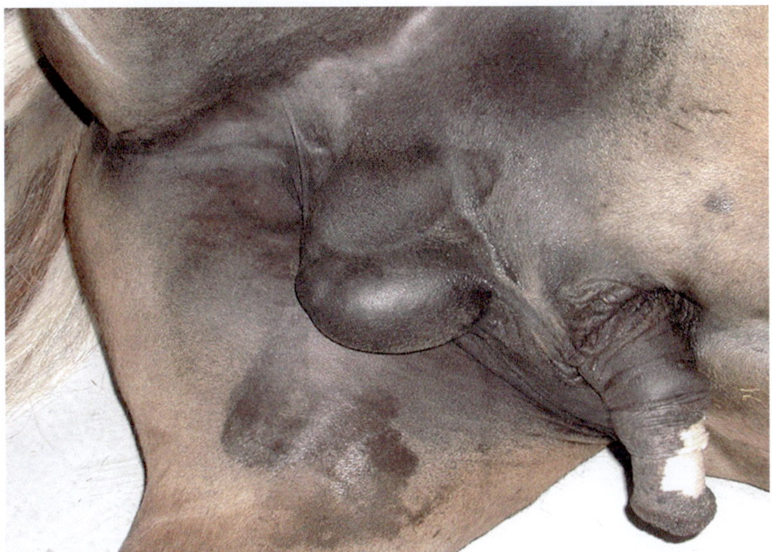

**Fig. 12.10**  Normal equine scrotum and penis, with testes covered by scrotal skin; external layer of prepuce; and preputial ring retracted with an evident space between the scrotum and the root of the penis. From the Minnesota Veterinary Anatomy website, http://vanat.cvm.umn.edu/ungDissect/Lab17/Lab17.html#images with permission

                                                                        M. A. B. Fahmy

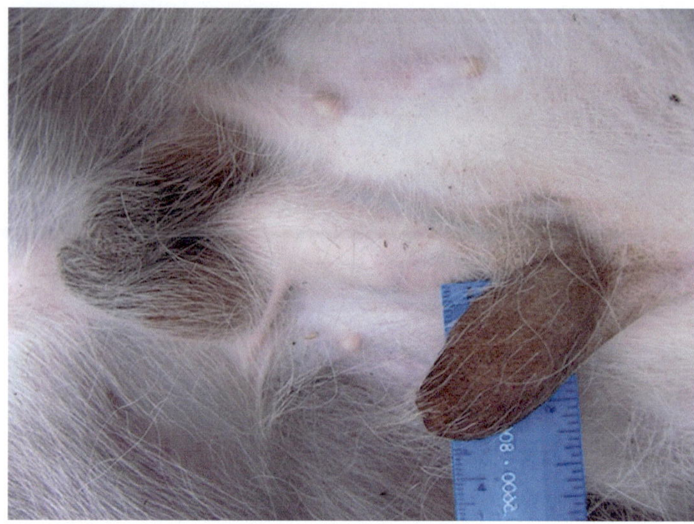

**Fig. 12.11** Genitalia of a 2 1/2-year-old white-tailed deer. The penis sheath is normal in length (6 cm), and the scrotum is normal in length with bilateral hemiscrota and an abnormally wide penoscrotal distance. (This photo was provided by Judith Hoy)

**Fig. 12.12** A wide penoscrotal distance in a child with otherwise normal genitalia

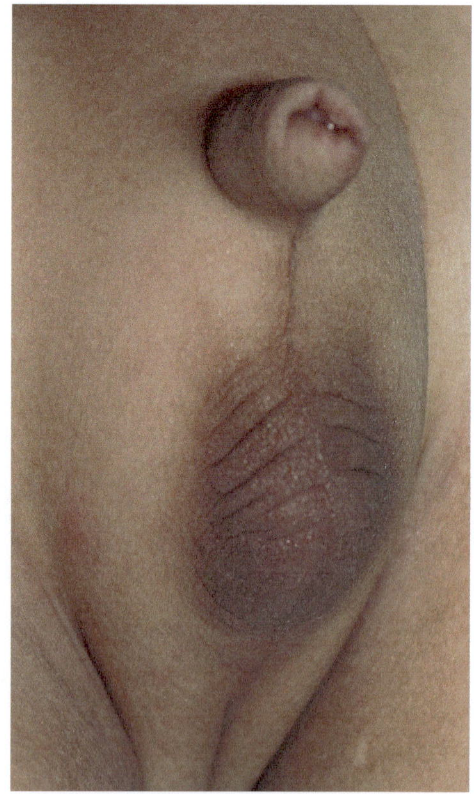

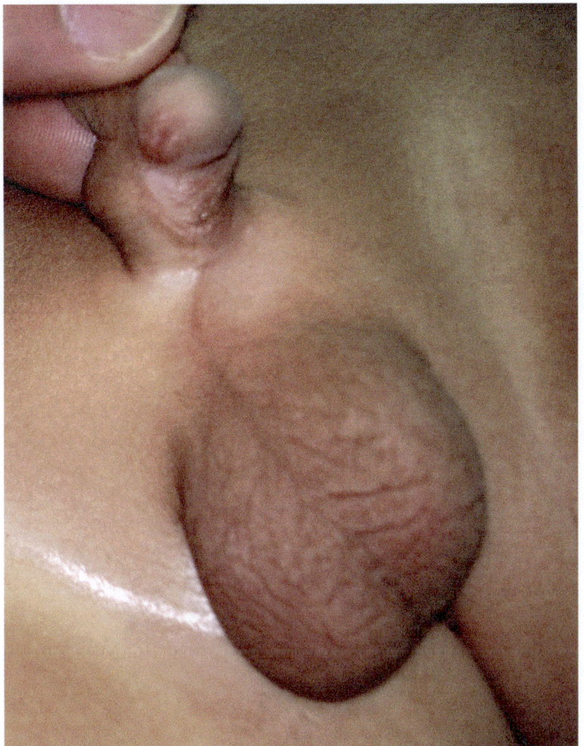

**Fig. 12.13** A case of right-sided penile rotation, ventral deficiency of the prepuce, chordee without hypospadias and a wide penoscrotal distance

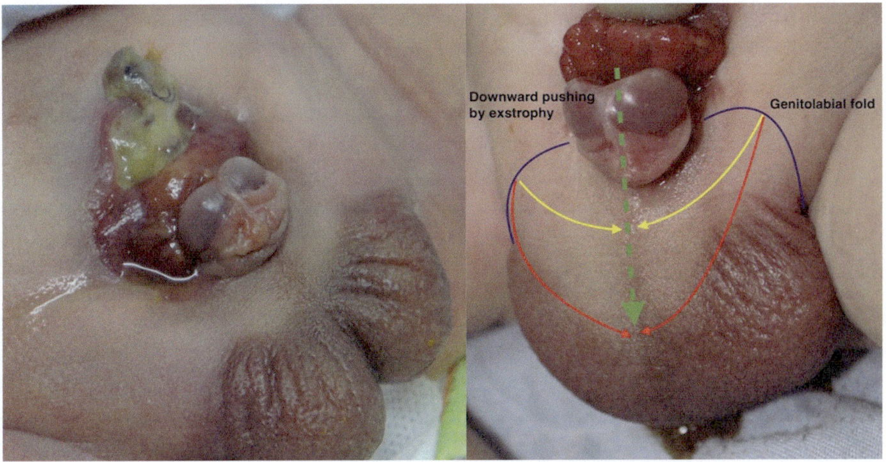


**Fig. 12.14** Neonate with bladder exstrophy and a wide penoscrotal distance and a laterally divergent scrota

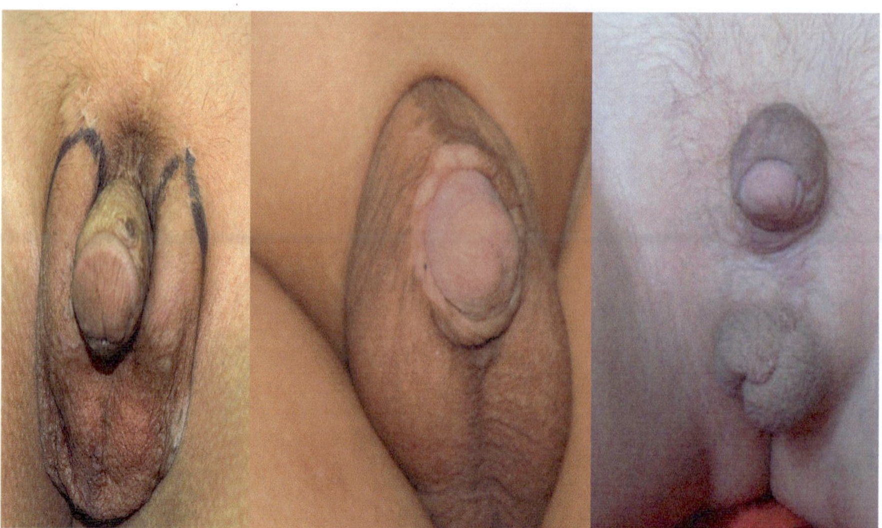

**Fig. 12.15** Different forms of iatrogenic scrotal transposition secondary to improper scrotal reconstruction

## 12.6   Associated Anomalies

PST is scarcely reported as an isolated anomaly in a healthy male, and the most common associations are hypospadias, penile chordee and rotation. Over the last 60 years, a very wide spectrum of urogenital and systemic anomalies have been reported with PST. Some of these associated anomalies are correctable and can be reconstructed during PST repair, such as hypospadias and chordee, but other anomalies may be life-threatening malformations and may even incompatible with life, such as urinary tract agenesis or major cardiovascular anomalies. These associated anomalies may be in the form of specific well-known syndromes or just as single or multisystemic malformations. Parida et al. [34] noted a 90% incidence of major renal anomalies associated with CPST. The most common non-urogenital abnormalities associated with PST were mental retardation (60%), anorectal malformations (33%), central nervous system anomalies (29%), vertebral defects (29%), preaxial limb defects including radial dysgenesis (24%), and congenital heart disease (19%) [35].

**Urinary anomalies**: Urinary tract agenesis or only renal agenesis, horse-shoe kidney, ectopic and dysplastic kidney, obstructive uropathy and hydronephrosis were reported with CPST [36]. Presumably, renal agenesis results from a failure in the formation of the ureteric bud, precluding its inductive effect on metanephrogenic tissue. Perhaps the same defect that interferes with scrotal migration interferes with ureteral development, which occurs in the fourth week of gestation [37]. Different forms and variable sizes of prostatic diverticulum are reported with both

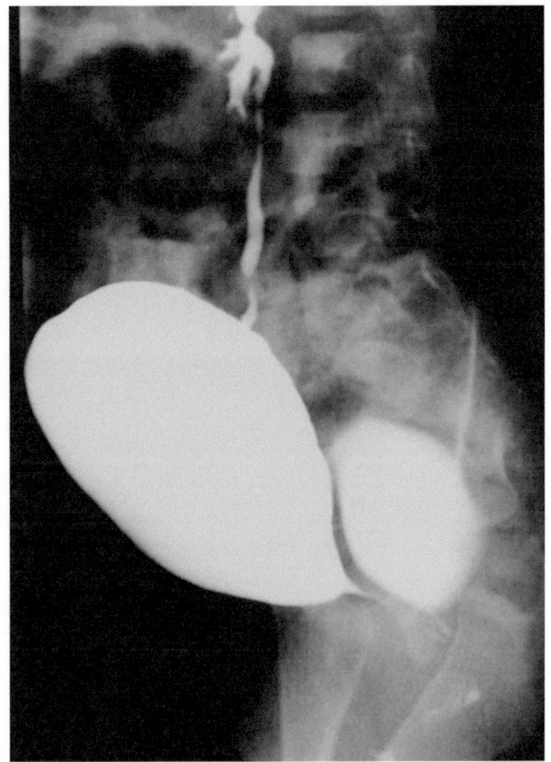

**Fig. 12.16** Large prostatic utricle in a 2-year-old boy with complete PST. Right-sided vesicoureteral reflux was also remarkable

partial and complete PST [8, 34]. (Fig. 12.16) Congenital inguinal hernia, either unilateral or bilateral, is frequently associated with PST but has not been previously reported, some cases presented to us with a huge inguinal hernia (Fig. 12.17).

**Penile Anomalies**: Penile anomalies such as hypospadias are frequently associated with partial or complete PST; hypospadias is reported in 79% in some series and 90% in others, and minor forms of scrotal transposition are sometimes overlooked in patients with proximal hypospadias [37, 38]. Penile rotation secondary to ipsilateral failure of the migration of the urethral fold, resulting in the rotation of the penile raphe to the side of the defect, has been reported [38] (Fig. 12.13). Chordees with or without hypospadias are not rare (81% of the cases) [3].

Pinke et al. [4] reported 26% of either unilateral or bilateral undescended testes in their series. Median raphe anomalies such as wide, deviated, rotated or bifid raphae were also reported [39]. A deficiency of the suspensory ligament, which results in prepenile depression, may be associated with PST (Figs. 12.1 and 12.5).

Epispadias has also been described in a few cases, especially with incomplete PST [40]. We diagnosed 2 cases of minor PST with epispadias, and one of them had an intact prepuce (Fig 12.18).

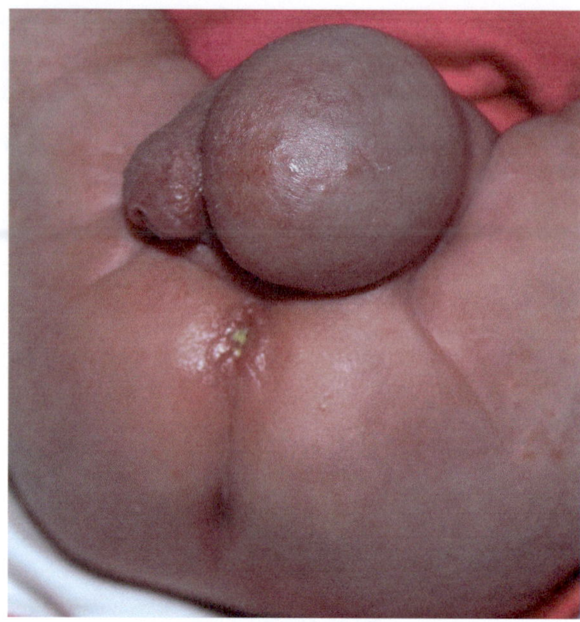

**Fig. 12.17** A neonate with complete PST and a large left-sided inguinal hernia

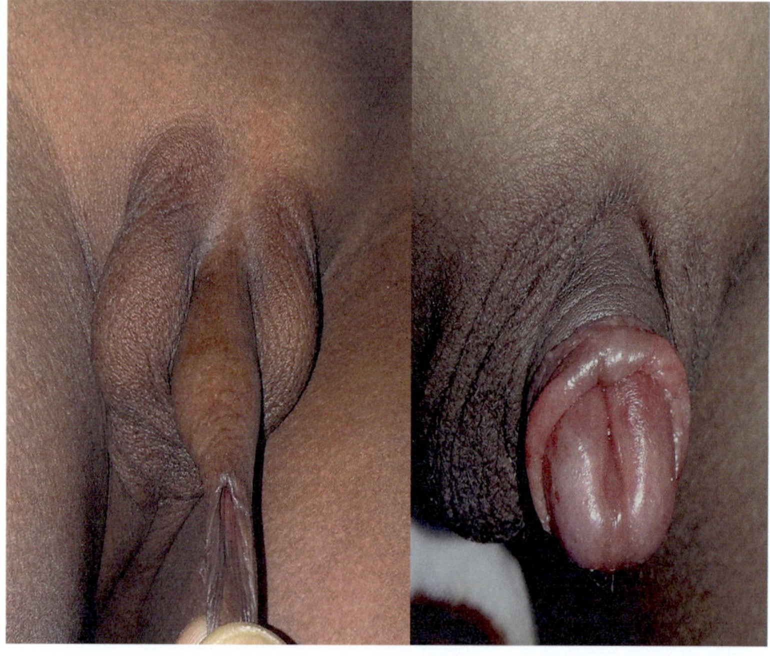

**Fig. 12.18** A patient with an intact prepuce, bilateral incomplete PST and isolated epispadias

**Skeletal Anomalies**: Skeletal and vertebral anomalies are frequently reported with PST, either in the form of single-bone dysplasia or multiple skeletal anomalies as specific well-known syndromes or as an isolated single anomaly [39]. Interestingly, Chappel in 1958 [40] reported a case of PST in a patient with Fanconi syndrome, with other anomalies; including a shortened and defective upper limb and an absence of the right forearm. In addition, the patient with PST reported by Burkitt in 1961 [41] also had left radial aplasia with a rudimentary thumb and absent first metacarpal bone.

**Popliteal pterygium syndrome**: This syndrome, as described by Gorlin and Pindborg [33], manifested with various genitourinary anomalies, including abnormal positioning of the penis; hypospadias; cryptorchidism; and absent, bifid, or ectopic scrota. PST associated with this syndrome may be secondary to local limb deformities; which could hinder the normal scrotal configuration of the foetus (Fig. 12.19).

**Caudal Regression syndrome**: In 1982, Johnslon [42] reviewed cases of PST, and he documented sixty patients with PST, of whom 23 had associated caudal regression syndrome (9 of them had complete PST and 14 cases had incomplete PST). This syndrome represents a wide variety of pelvic, spinal and limb anomalies, and PST may be secondary to the whole pelvic anatomical disturbance [43, 44]. Both the penis and scrotum could be displaced caudally as a part of the whole pelvic displacement (Fig. 12.2).

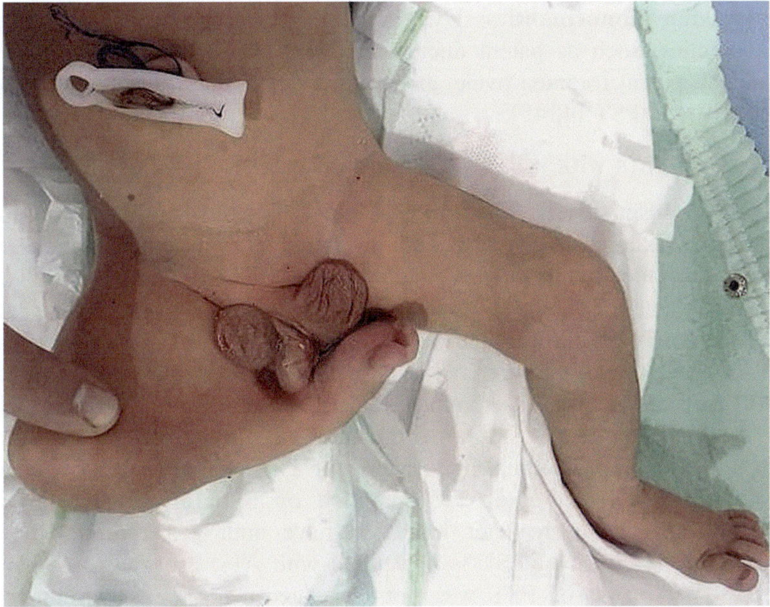

**Fig. 12.19** A case of a neonate with PST and popliteal pterygium syndrome

**Fig. 12.20** PST with incomplete AIS

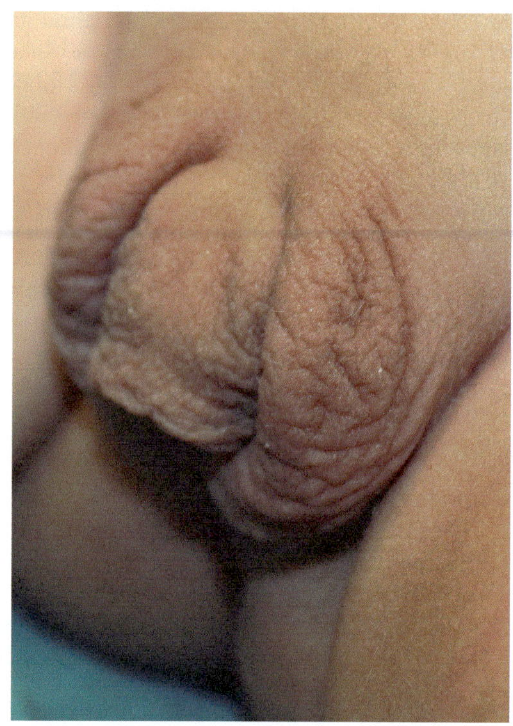

**Cardiovascular abnormalities**: Hypertrophic, obstructive cardiomyopathy and other anomalies, such as patent ductus arteriosus, Fallot's tetralogy, ventricular septal defect, patent foramen ovale, atrial septal defect, and mitral valve prolapse, are reported with PST [4, 45].

**Specific syndromes with a PST as a main criteria**:

- **Androgen Insensitivity Syndrome (AIS):** This syndrome is diagnosed with various grades and is caused by mutation in the androgen receptor gene, which is located on the X chromosome, and its mutation is transmitted in an X-linked recessive manner [15]. In complete androgen insensitivity syndrome (CAIS), there are no visible clinical signs of androgen action, and patients are born with normal female external genitalia. Partial androgen insensitivity syndrome (PAIS) includes a broad spectrum of male undermasculinization. The genitalia may be morphologically similar to those of a healthy male, though small, or there may be simple coronal hypospadias or a prominent midline raphe of the scrotum. Bals-Pratsch et al. [26] reported on 3 brothers with penoscrotal transposition who were later found to have androgen receptor disorders. A different spectrum of PST is detectable with AIS, especially the complete forms. The degree of PST was not correlated with the spectrum of AIS. Complete AIS may be present with incomplete PST; on the other hand, partial AIS may be present with complete PST (Fig. 12.20). Patients with congenital

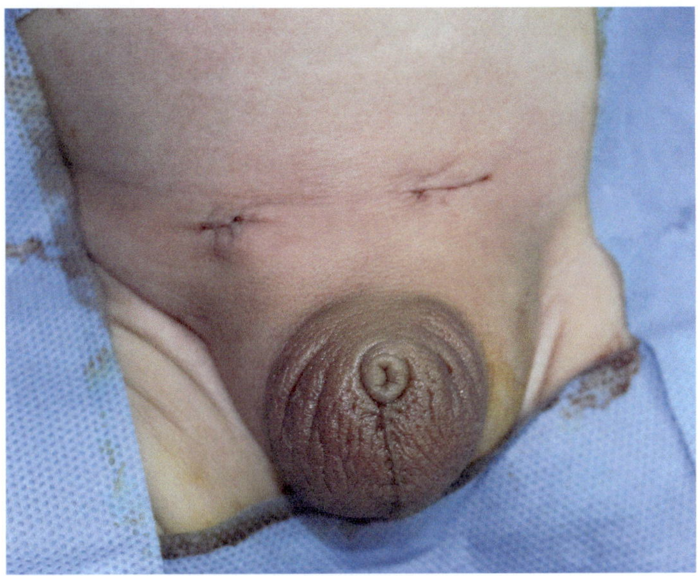

**Fig. 12.21** An infant with trisomy 13 and bilateral inguinal hernias, microphallus and a partial scrotal transposition

adrenal hyperplasia (CAH), either female or male, commonly have different forms of PST.

We diagnosed and treated a non-reported case of complete PST in a baby with congenital hypothyroidism (Cretinism).

- **Chromosomal Anomalies:** PST malformation has been described as part of genetic syndromes in 6% of cases. Both autosomal and X chromosomal anomalies have been reported with PST [2]. Reports of alterations in chromosome 13 include ring chromosome 13, deletions located in the distal region of chromosome 13q and translocations, the inversion of chromosome 4, mosaicism (45,XO and 46,XY) and Klinefelter syndrome (47,XXY) [46].

We diagnosed a neonate who had trisomy 13 and incomplete PST with a bilateral inguinal hernia (Fig. 12.21). Cohen-Addad et al. [12] reported a case of trisomy 18 mosaicism with PST.

Turner's syndrome is a relatively common type of human X chromosome monosomy that occurs in females and is characterized by partial or complete loss of an X chromosome [47]. Herein, we present an interesting case of a neonate girl with a scrotal-like labia, which poses as complete PST, and large hernia on the left side; an ovotestes was detected in the hernial sac (Fig. 12.22).

Aarskog-Scott syndrome (faciodigitogenital syndrome): It is an X-linked recessive syndrome characterized by short stature, facial abnormalities, low-set

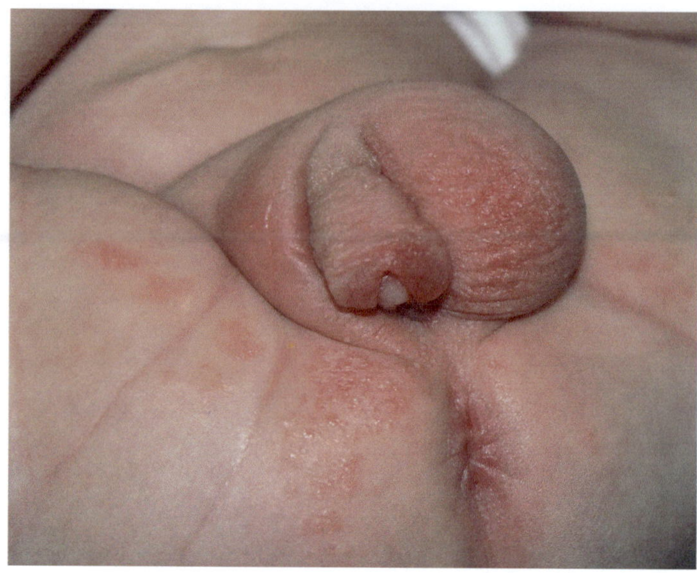

**Fig. 12.22** A case of Turner's syndrome with labial scrotalization with transposition and a left-sided inguinal hernia

drooping ears, down-slanted palpebral fissures, ophthalmoplegia, hyperopic astigmatism, and cleft lip/palate, PST was reported with this syndrome [48].

Many less common syndromes had different forms of PTS as a minor component of their presentation [4]:

- Rubenstein-Taybi syndrome
- Craniofrontonasal dysplasia
- Hunter Carpenter McDonald syndrome
- Naguib syndrome
- Saito Kuba Tsuruta syndrome
- Ieshima Koeda Inagaki syndrome
- Cystic fibrosis gastritis megaloblastic anaemia
- Willems de Vries syndrome
- Schinzel syndrome and Seaver Cassidy syndrome
- Duhamel's syndrome [49].
- Simpson-Golabi-Behmel syndrome [50, 51].
- We recognized a case of prune belly syndrome with minimal bilateral scrotal transposition, such association was not yet reported. (Fig. 12.23).

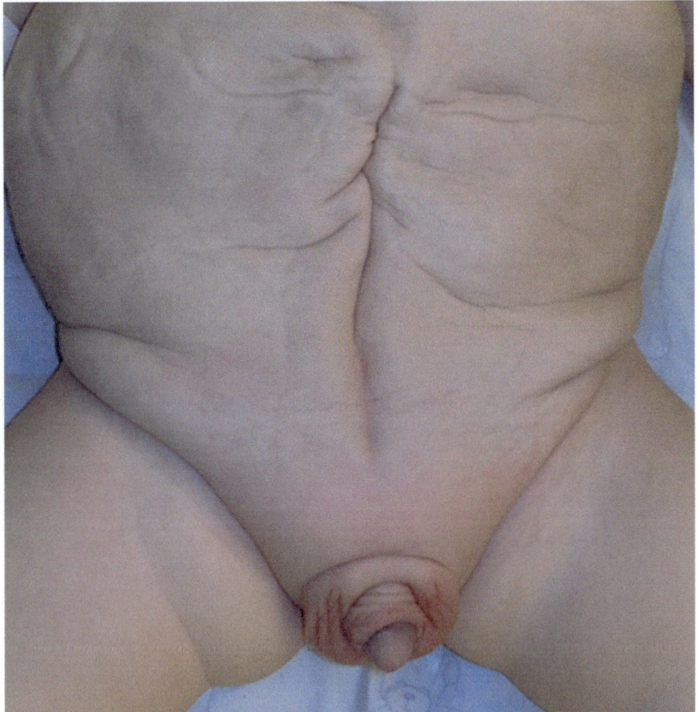

**Fig. 12.23**   An infant with prune belly syndrome and minor PST

## 12.7   Presentation and the Impact of PST on Health

Recently, and especially in developed countries, most penoscrotal anomalies have been recognizable immediately in the delivery rooms. We diagnosed most cases of partial PST and other variants during the evaluation of babies with complex or advanced forms of hypospadias or DSD, but a considerable number of cases had either complete or partial PST with a normal-sized penis, normal urethra and an orthotopic urinary meatus (Fig. 12.3).

We diagnosed 2 cases of CPST and 5 cases of partial PST in infants and children referred with an inguinal hernia (Figs. 12.17, 12.21 and 12.22).

Adults with such anomalies have been reported before, and they may still be diagnosed in developing countries. Morton et al. [52] in 1965 reported a 28-year-old patient with scrotal transposition who had been married for 2 years and was apparently well adjusted to his abnormality with intromission and ejaculation into the vagina by lifting the scrotum away from the penis; the angulation of the erect penis, caused by chordee, effectively aided intromission, and he voided in a standing position by a similar manoeuvre of manually elevating the scrotum [52]. Although the diagnosis of most reported cases of PST is sporadic, many families

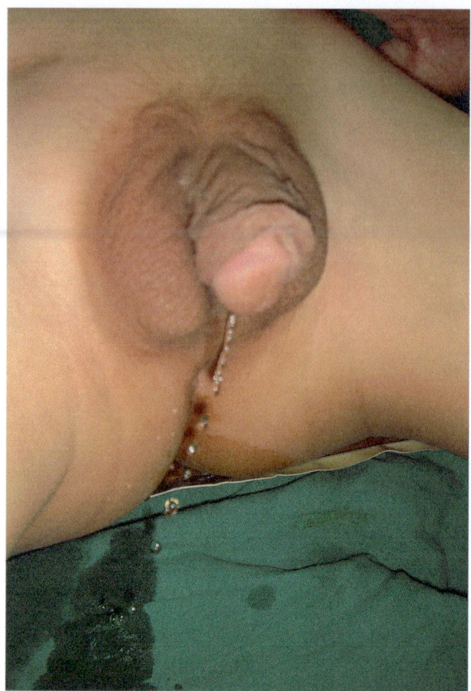

**Fig. 12.24** Downward and backward urine stream in a child with incomplete PST

with affected siblings have been reported in the literature, where parental consanguinity was not specified. However, consanguinity is reported in some other cases [53]. In the Pinke et al. [4] series, 13% of the patients had a family history of PST.

PST may create hygienic and mechanical difficulty with voiding, difficulty in putting on a condom and sexual activity, and psychological problems affecting the adult patients and the parents of children with PST. The inability of the child or adolescent to void in a standing position is a substantial psychological problem, and later on  the cosmetic deformity can lead to demands for surgery (Fig. 12.24).

The presence of any form of PST will definitely affect the functional length of the penis, as the normal-sized penis will be functionally shortened due to engulfment by the transposed scrota. It is not true that penoscrotal transposition is an asymptomatic deformity. Most cases we diagnosed with different forms of PST exhibit severe and resistant dermatitis secondary to an abnormally directed urine stream (Fig. 12.25).

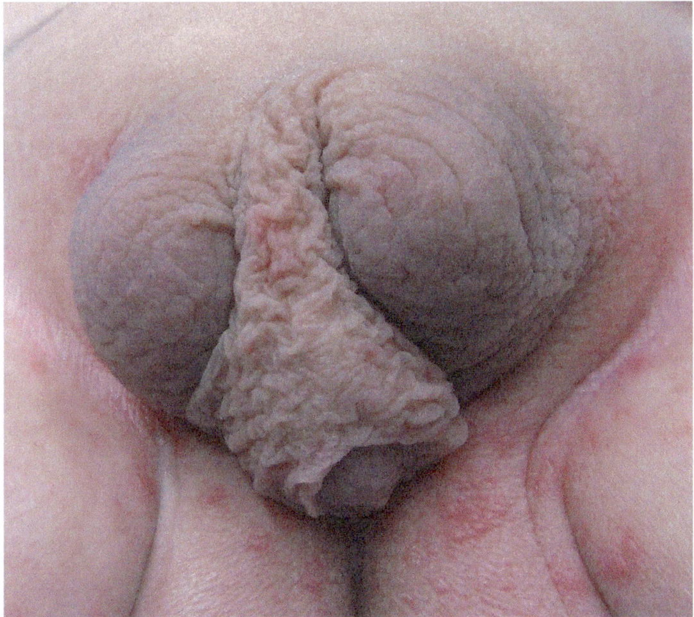

**Fig. 12.25** Severe dermatitis secondary to abnormal urine stream in a case of partial PST

## 12.8   Diagnosis

The diagnosis is mainly clinical and usually obvious in complete cases, but the clinician should be aware of incomplete, unilateral and minor cases. General awareness about the normal scrotal surface anatomy and normal penoscrotal angles is mandatory to diagnose minor cases. Many cases are usually recognizable during precise evaluation of cases of DSD. Cases of wide penoscrotal distance and caudal scrotal migration are diagnosed during the management of patients with bladder exstrophy, either before reconstruction or after failed repair. Iatrogenic cases are usually recognizable during the follow-up after unsatisfactory penile or scrotal reconstructions. Investigations are mainly required for the early detection of any associated local or systemic anomalies.

## 12.9   Prenatal Diagnosis

The first published case of prenatal ultrasound diagnosis of PST dated from 1995, when Mandell [54] published a series of a total of 17 foetuses sonographically diagnosed with genital malformations, of which 2 were PSTs. Later, in 2002, another case was published, with an ultrasound image of the scrotum in a prepenile position, which appeared between the penis and the insertion of the umbilical cord.

Colour Doppler was presented as a useful tool for confirmation of the diagnosis and imaging of the urinary tract [55].

Differential Diagnosis: PST should be differentiated from conditions such as penoscrotal fusion, webbed and concealed penis, penoscrotal hypospadias, pseudohermaphroditism, micropenis, intrauterine penile amputation, and especially penile agenesis with a midline skin tag anterior to the anus [56]. Most important is to differentiate cases of incomplete PST from cases of ectopic and accessory scrotum.

## 12.10  Treatment

Surgical correction of uncomplicated transposition is relatively simple through a one-stage procedure. Campbell et al. [57] restored the normal anatomical relations by bisecting the scrotum and suturing the 2 halves around the base of the penis. Mcllvoy and Harris [58] achieved the same result by repositioning the penis through a subcutaneous tunnel dissected beneath the anterior scrotal wall. However, when transposition is accompanied by severe hypospadias, additional factors demand consideration. The Glenn-Anderson [31] technique is the most successful method for transposition repair, and most patients require complex urethroplasty for hypospadias and release of chordee. Pinke et al. [4] managed this anomaly in a single stage by Thiersch-Duplay urethroplasty in 6 patients and complex repair with bladder or buccal mucosa or a staged procedure in 34 cases. Surgery is performed usually between 12 and 18 months. Forshall and Rickham [9] used a different technique where cranially located scrotal flaps were elevated, rotated medially and caudally and sutured beneath the penis. This technique was also used by Glenn and Anderson [31]. M-plasty was claimed to be an excellent technique for the correction of penoscrotal transposition, with a low incidence of penile lymphedema, which could be attributed to the preservation of the dorsal penile skin. This procedure may provide an excellent cosmetic appearance and allows early correction of hypospadias [59]. Pinke et al. [4] reported a 70% incidence of complications when performing urethral plastic surgery and penile scrotal displacement correction

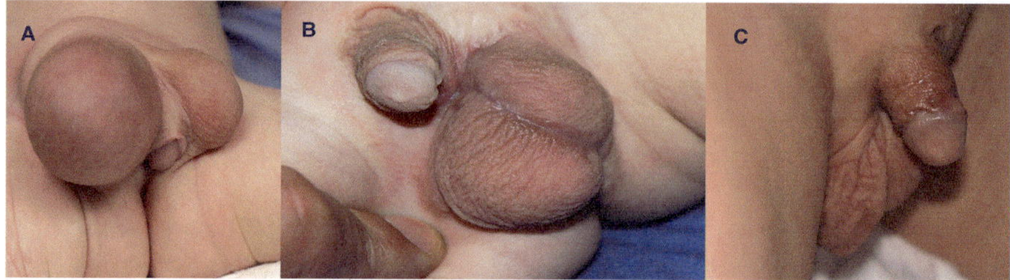

**Fig. 12.26** Staged repair of penoscrotal transposition; A: 1st presentation at neonatal period with a huge Rt inguinal hernia, penoscrotal hypospadias and CPST, B: Staged repair anterior view and C: Lateral view

simultaneously. It is generally not advisable to perform both urethral plastic surgery and scrotoplasty in one setting. Kim K S [60] thought that transposition surgery is mainly useful as a secondary surgery after hypospadias correction.

For repair of CPST, we used a circumferential incision at the base of the penis. This incision was then extended vertically at 12 o'clock in the midline between the fused scrotal folds. The vertical incision was stopped at a point where the penis had to be transposed, and a racket-shaped incision was made laterally, on either side from the 12 o'clock position, to outline the scrotal folds. Multiple stages are frequently required (Fig. 12.26).

Caudal scrotal regression could be repaired at the end of bladder exstrophy reconstruction through a vertical midline incision in the normal skin between the root of the penis and scrotal raphe with the advancement of the scrotal sacs. However, in some cases, scrotal repair could be achieved during subsequent surgeries after primary reconstruction for correction of other penile anomalies, i.e., during the correction of epispadias or penile lengthening.

# References


1. Sugita TC, Hutson JM. Genital anomalies in human and animal models reveal the mechanisms and hormones governing testicular descent. British J Urolo. 1997;78:99–112.
2. Moore KL, Persaud TV. The developing human: clinically oriented embryology. Philadelphia: WB Saunders; 2003.
3. Appleby LH. An unusual arrangement of the external genitalia. Can Med Ass J. 1923;13:514–6.
4. Pinke LA, Rathbun SR, Husmann DA, Kramer SA. Penoscrotal transposition: review of 53 patients. J Urol. 2001;166:1865–8.
5. Burgos J, et al. Transposicio´n pene-escrotal completa: diagno´stico prenatal. Prog Obstet Ginecol. 2012. https://doi.org/10.1016/j.pog.2011.09.012.
6. Sunay M, Emir L, Karabulut A, Erol D. Thiersch-duplay technique following correction of penoscrotal transposition. Urol Int. 2009;82:28–31.
7. Bergmann JF. Normale und abnormale Entwicklung des Menschen. Wiesbaden; 1911.
8. Mcllvoy DB, Harris HS. Transposition of the penis and scrotum: Case report. J Urol. 1955;73:540–3.
9. Forshall I, Rickham PP. Transposition of the penis and scrotum. Brit J Urol. 1956;28:250.
10. Sakamoto K, Kuroki Y, Fujisawa Y, Yoshimine K, Morital KM. XX/XY chromosomal mosaicism presenting a chordee without hypospadas associated with scrotal transposition. J Urol. 1978;119:841–3.
11. Paramo PG, Hinderer U, San Antonio J, Paramo Jr PS, Silmi A, Rabada M. Prepenile scrotum. Eur Urol. 1981;7246–51.
12. Cohen-Addad N, Zarafu IW, Hanna MK. Complete penoscrotal transposition. Urology. 1985;26:149–52.
13. Coveney D, Shaw G, Hutson JM, Renfree MB. Effect of an antiandrogen on testicular descent and inguinal closure in a marsupial, the tammar wallaby (Macropus eugenii). Reproduction. 2002;124:865–74 PubMed: 12530924.
14. Renfree MB. The role of genes and hormones in marsupial sexual differentiation. J Zool Lond. 1992;226:165–73.
15. MacKenzie J, Chitayat D, McLorie J, Balfe J, Pandit PB, Blecher SR. Penoscrotal transposition: a case report and review. Am J Med Genet. 1994;49:103–7.

16. Gualtieri T, and A.D. Segal () Prepenile scrotum in a double monster: Teratological considerations. The hazards of radiation. J. Urol. 1954;71:488–96.
17. Kadai, H., C. Ajisawa, K. Taya, and T. Imamichi (1988) Suprainguinal ectopic scrota of TS inbred rats. J. Reprod. Fertil., *84:*701–707
18. Datta NS, Singh SM, Reddy AVS, Chakravarty AK. Transposition of penis and scrotum in two brothers. J Urol. 1971;105:739–42.
19. Jost A. Problems of fetal endocrinology: the gonadal and hypophyseal hormones. Rec Prog Horm Res. 1953;8:379–418.
20. Flum AS, Chaviano AH, Kaplan WE. Hemiscrotal agenesis: new variation in a rare anomaly. Urology. 2012;79:210–1.
21. Blaschko SD, Mahawong P, Ferretti M, et al. Analysis of the effect of estrogen/androgen perturbation on penile development in transgenic and diethylstilbestrol-treated mice. Anat Rec (Hoboken). 2012;296:1127–41.
22. Patten BM. Human embryology. New York: McGraw-Hill Book Co.; 1968, pp. 449–94.
23. Lamm DL, Kaplan GW. Accessory and ectopic scrota. Urology. 1977;9:149–53.
24. Flanagan MI, McDonald JH, Kiefer JH. Unilateral transposition of the scrotum. J Urol. 1961;86:273–5.
25. Meguid NA, Temtamy SA, Mazen I. Transposition of external genitalia and associated malformations. Clin Dysmorphol. 2003;12:59–62.
26. Bals-Pratsch M, Schweikert HU, Nieschlag E. Androgen receptor disorder in three brothers with bifid prepenile scrotum and hypospadias. Acta Endocrinol (Copen). 1990;123:271–6.
27. Sule JD, Skoog SJ, Tank ES. Perineal lipoma and the accessory labioscrotal fold: an etiological relationship. J Urol. 1994;151:475–7.
28. Park KH, Hong JH. Perineal lipoma in association with scrotal anomalies in children. BJU Int. 2006;98:409–12.
29. Bhat NA, Mathur M, Bhatnagar V. Sacrococcygeal teratoma with anorectal malformation. Indian J Gastroenterol. 2003;22:27.
30. Stephens FD. Embryology of the cloaca and embryogenesis of anorectal malformations. Birth Defects Orig Artic Ser. 1988;24:177–209.
31. Glenn JF, Anderson EE. Surgical correction of incomplete penoscrotal transposition. J Urol. 1973;110:603–5.
32. Fahmy MAB, Alaa Aldin A, Alshennawy AA, Edress AM. Spectrum of penoscrotal positional anomalies in children. Int J Surg. 2014;12(9):983–8. http://www.sciencedirect.com/science/article/pii/S1743919114004853.
33. Gorlin RJ, Pindborg JJ. Syndromes of the head and neck. New York: McGraw-Hill Book Co.; 1964. pp. 122–5.
34. Parida SK, Hall BD, Barton L, Fujimoto A. Penoscrotal transposition and associated anomalies: report of five new cases and review of the literature. Am J Med Genet. 1995;59:68–75.
35. Fahmy M. Penoscrotal Positional (PSP) Anomalies. In: Congenital Anomalies of the Penis. Cham: Springer; 2017. https://doi.org/10.1007/978-3-319-43310-3_15.
36. Eisenberg ML, Jensen TK, Walters RC, Skakkebaek NE, Lipshultz LI. The relationship between anogenital distance and reproductive hormone levels in adult men. J Urol. 2012;187:594–8.
37. Morton C. Wilson, Carl l. Wilson and Jack N. Thicksten: transposition of the external genitalia. J Urol. 1965; 94. Patten BM. Human embryology. New York: McGraw-Hill Book Co.; 1968. pp. 449–94.
38. Wilson MC, Wilson CL, Thicksten JN. Transposition of the external genitalia. J Urol. 1965;94:600.
39. Remzi D. Transposition of penis and scrotum. J Urol. 1966;96:555.
40. Chappel BS. Transposition of external genitalia in a case with Fanconi type deformity. J Urol. 1958;79:115–8.
41. Burkitt D. Transposition of the scrotum and penis. Brit J Surg. 1961;48:460.

42. Johnslon JH. Abnormalities of the scrotum and the testes. In: Williams DI, Johnslon JH, editors. Ped-Urology. 2nd ed. London: Butterworth Scientific; 1982. p. 451–66.
43. Al-Zaiem MM. Caudal regression syndrome and peno-scrotal transposition. Saudi Med J. 2001;22(6):545–6.
44. Lage JM, Driscoll SG, Bieber FR. Transposition of the external genitalia associated with caudal regression. J Urol. 1987;138:387–9.
45. Anlar B, Ayabakan S. Transposition of the external genitalia: a case with cardiovascular malformations and polycystic kidneys. Eur J Pediatr. 1986;145:161.
46. Gershoni-Baruch R, Zekaria D. Deletion (13) (q22) with multiple congenital anomalies, hydranencephaly and penoscrotal transposition. Clin Dysmorphol. 1996;5:289.
47. Cui X, Cui Y, Shi L et al. A basic understanding of turner syndrome: incidence, complications, diagnosis, and treatment. Intractable Rare Dis. Res. 2018;7(4):223–8.
48. Shinkawa T, Yamauchi Y, Osada Y, Ishisawa N. Aarskog syndrome Jour Urolog. 1983;22(6): P624-626. https://doi.org/10.1016/0090-4295(83)90311-4.
49. Miller SF. Transposition of the Genitalia and Duhamel's Syndrome of Caudal Regression. J Pediatr Surg. 1972;7(4).
50. Griffith CB, Probert RC, Vance GH. Genital anomalies in three male siblings with Simpson-Golabi-Behmel syndrome. Am J Med Genet A. 2009;149A:2484–8.
51. Villarreal DD, Villarreal H, Paez AM, Peppas D, Lynch J, Roeder E, Powers GC. A Patient With a unique frameshift mutation in GPC3, causing Simpson–Golabi–Behmel Syndrome, presenting with craniosynostosis, penoscrotal hypospadias, and a large prostatic utricle. Am J Med Genet Part A. 2013;161A:3121–5.
52. Morton C. Wilson, Carl l. Wilson and Jack N. Thicksten: transposition of the external genitalia. J Urol. 1965;94.
53. Meguid et al: Transposition of external genitalia and associated malformations. Clinical Dysmorphology 2003, Vol 12 No 1. DOI: https://doi.org/10.1097/01.mcd.0000046502.50562.82
54. Mandell J, Bromley B, Peters CA, Benacerraf BR. Prenatal sono- graphic detection of genital malformations. J Urol. 1995;153:1994–6.
55. Vijayaraghavan SB, Muruganand SK, Ravikumar VR, Marimuthu K. Prenatal sonographic features of penoscrotal transposition. J Ultrasound Med. 2002;21:1427–30.
56. Kendirci M, Horasanlı K, Miroğlu C. Accessory scrotum with multiple skeletal abnormalities. Int J Urol. 2006;13:648–50.
57. Campbell MF, Harrison JH. Urology. Philadelphia: W. B. Saunders Co. 1970. pp. 1576–7.
58. McIlvoy DB, Harris HS. Transposition of the penis and scrotum. Case report J Urol. 1955;73:540.
59. Mylarappa P, Puvvada S, Nayak KA. Evaluation and outcome of M plasty for the management of doughnut scrotum. J Clin Urol. 2017;10(4):364–7. https://doi.org/10.1177/2051415816686762
60. Kim KS. The individualized surgical approach of penoscrotal transposition according to the anatomical position of the penis. Korean J Urol. 2006;47:287–92. https://doi.org/10.4111/kju.2006.47.3.287.

# Chapter 13
# Penoscrotal Fusion

Mohamed A. Baky Fahmy

**Abbreviations**

PSF   Penoscrotal Fusion
PP    Palmate Penis
AGD   Anogenital distance
DF    Dartos fascia
WP    Webbed Penis
AR    Androgen Receptor

**Synonyms**: Webbed penis, palmate penis, penis palmatus, inconspicuous penis

**Definition**: Penoscrotal fusion is a congenital condition of the male external genitalia, in which the normal insertion of the scrotum at the base of the penis is altered, located higher, along the ventral aspect of the penis, with defective fascial attachment. Thus, a normal penoscrotal angle evanescences. There are different forms and degrees of PSF, more or less pronounced, according to the height where the scrotum is inserted into the penis and the degree of penile concealment. In isolated cases of PSF the penis is tethered to the scrotum in the midline, so the penoscrotal angle is obscured. The tethered scrotal skin will then be pulled distally with the penile skin during erection, creating the impression of a "sail of skin" tethered to the ventral penile shaft (Fig. 13.1).

PSF is a broad term includes the webbed, concealed and inconspicuous buried penis (Fig. 13.2).

PSF may be referred as webbed penis, which is also known as penis palmatus. It is not necessary for all cases of PSF to be webbed, webbing will be seen if the penoscrotal fusion is not only at skin level but extended deeply to include dartos fascia and muscle. If PSF extended allover the penile shaft; the term concealed or

M. A. B. Fahmy (✉)
Al-Azhar University, Cairo, Egypt

     173
M. A. B. Fahmy (ed.), *Normal and Abnormal Scrotum*,
https://doi.org/10.1007/978-3-030-83305-3_13

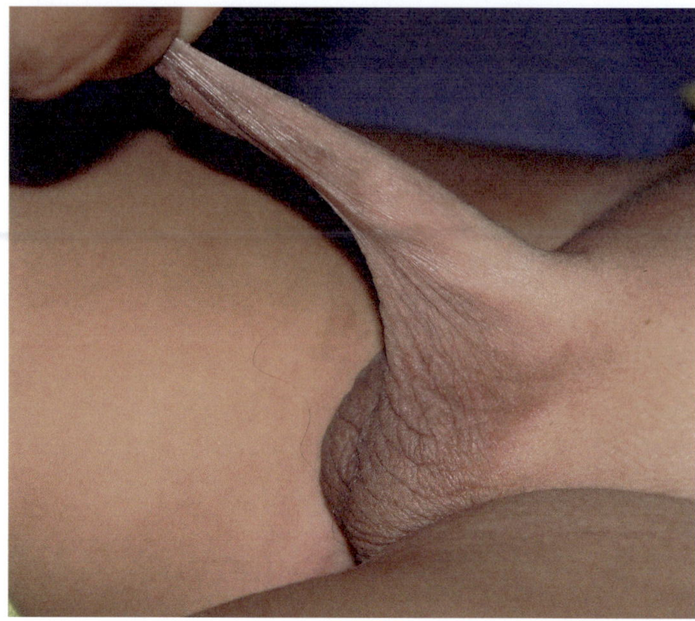

**Fig. 13.1** PSF with an apparent scrotal skin attached to the middle of the stretched penile skin, this type of fusion doesn't affect the penile length

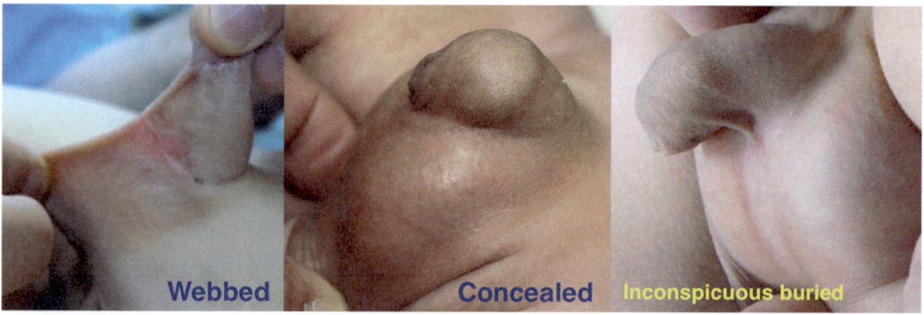


**Fig. 13.2** Webbed, concealed and inconspicuous buried penises

inconspicuous will be more appropriate. Penile scrotolisation is the condition of just creeping of the scrotal skin over the ventral penile surface without fusion between the scrotum and penis (Fig. 13.3). Concealed penis is appropriately applied for a normally developed penis which is hidden in the mons pubis [1]. The terms of buried and concealed penises are neither precise nor scientific.

**Incidence**: PSF is more frequent than thought, the only thing missing to detect it is performing a thorough physical examination of the patients. Matsuo et al. [2] reported a prevalence of 3.7% in Japanese newborn infants.

**Fig. 13.3** A case of scrotolisation of the proximal penile shaft; the scrotum creeped all around the base of the penis

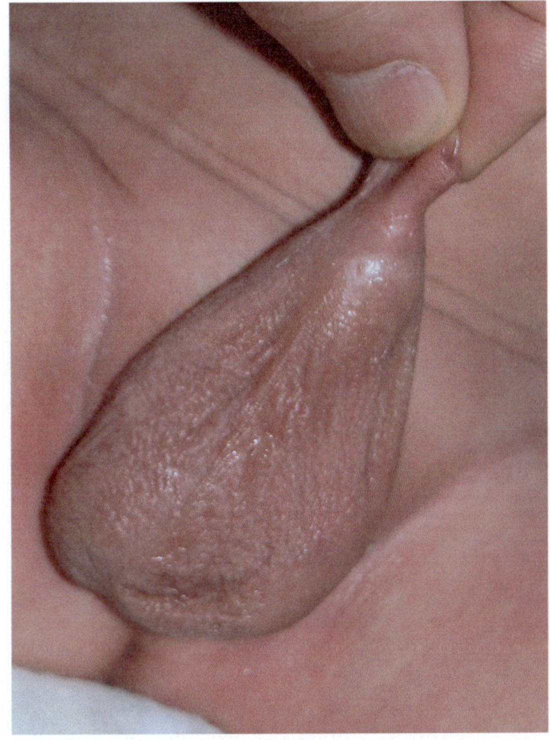

**Historical background**: The condition of buried penis has been recognized for many years but only until recently it has begun to receive proper attention. An early description of the buried penis was mentioned in 1919 by Keyes [3]. PSF was first reported as 'virga palmata' in Italian literature at 1953 [4], and described as a penile deformity in the English language at 1968 [5]. At 1986, Maizels et al. [6] were the first to classify webbed penis.

**Normal anatomy**: Structurally, the normal skin of the scrotum is  continues to the base of the penis, forming a penoscrotal angle of more or less 90°, thus giving way to a hair-free penile dermal coverage (Fig. 13.4). Penile skin is hairless and smooth, while scrotal skin is hair bearing, wrinkled and darker. Dartos fascia and muscle extend smoothly from the scrotum to the penile shaft forming the prepenile muscle, and it is attached to the deep Buck's facia at the root of the penis to create the penoscrotal angle externally and to keep both testicles confined to the scrotal sacs (Chap. 9).

For a normal penile function, the skin that surrounds the shaft of the penis must have a free and absolute mobility, without any pathological anchors to the scrotum, to thus allow a good and complete erection; for a normal sexual performance and sound psychological life. In PSF the man's sexual gratification and self-esteem are strongly affected [7].

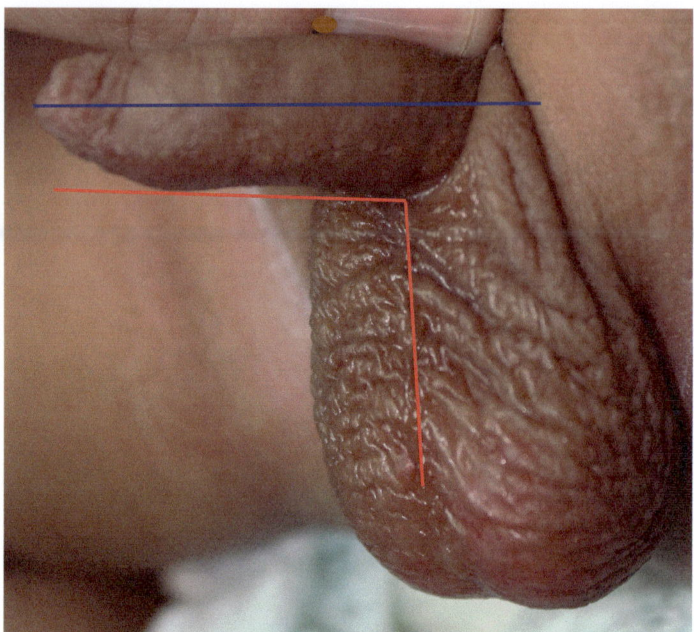

**Fig. 13.4** Normal penoscrotal angle with clear distinction between scrotal and penile skin

**Classifications**: Cohen [8] classified PSF to three grades according to the height where the scrotum is inserted into the penis:

Grade 1: when the folds of the scrotal skin obscure the penoscrotal angle and inserted at the base of the penis.

Grades II: the scrotum inserted at the mid shaft of the penis.

Grade III: the scrotum reaches to the prepuce and usually result in phimosis with inability to protrude the glans (Fig. 13.5).

Mizales et al. [6] referred mainly to the buried penis, and they embarked on excessive deposits of fat and subcutaneous tissue for classification of this anomaly to buried, webbed, trapped and micropenis. Buried penis divided to poor skin suspension and localised fad adiposity at adolescent. They tried to emphasize the anatomical cause in each case, so that the treatment is adequate for each penile alteration.

It is of outmost importance to recognise the level of defective tissue which leads to PSF; either at the skin, dartos or the corpora. Also the extension of penoscrotal fusion will predominates the types of fusion.

So we classified this penoscrotal fusion to:

1. Short median raphe (Fig. 13.6)
2. Fusion without penile webbing (Fig. 13.1).
3. Fusion with webbing; which could be:

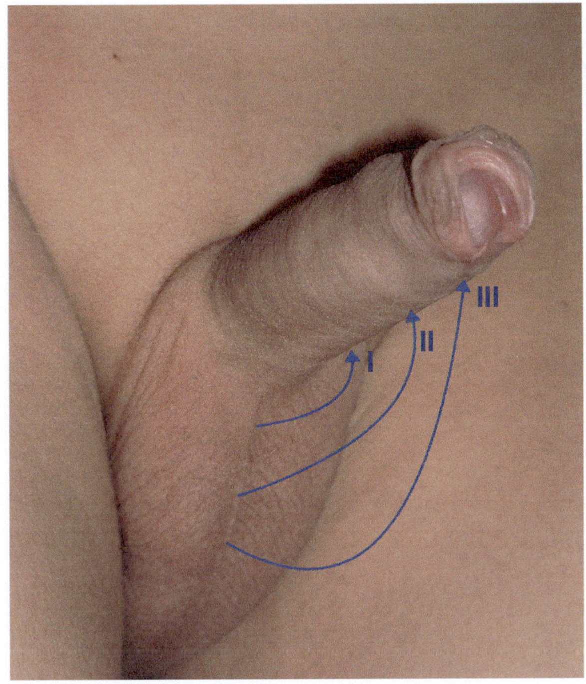

**Fig. 13.5** Grades of PSF after Cohen [8]

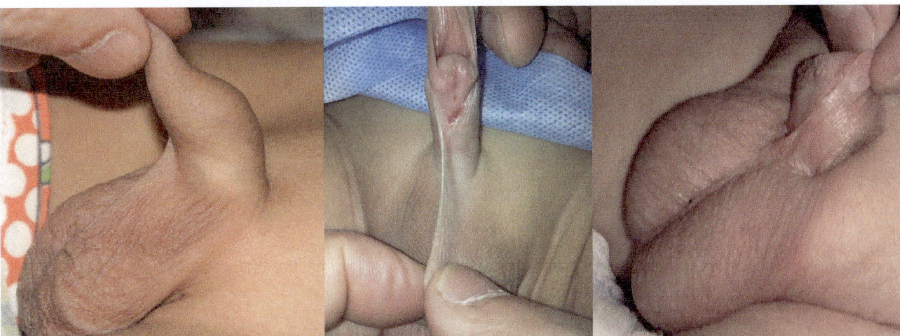

**Fig. 13.6** Different forms of PSF at the level of shortened median raphe, the middle case had a distal hypospadias

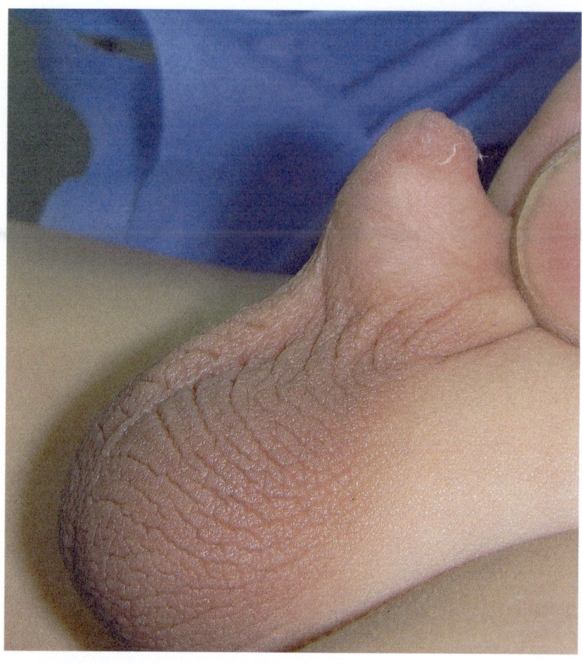

**Fig. 13.7** Central PSF forming web and associated with diminutive penis

A  Central at the midline (Fig. 13.7)
B  Bilateral at both sided of the penis (Figs. 13.8 and 13.9).

**Etiology**: Generally, this condition is the result of combined abnormal penoscrotal skin configuration, abnormal dartos muscle and facia, with inadequate subcutaneous attachment to Buck's fascia, which end with abnormal anchoring of the

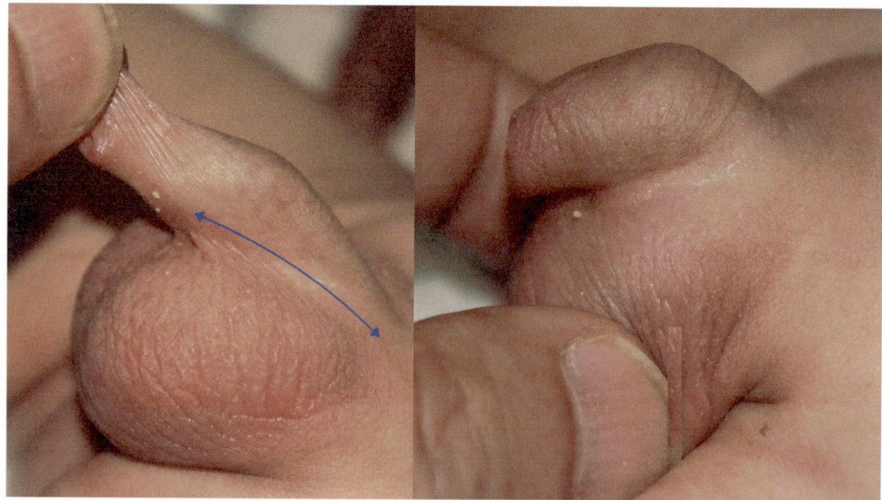

**Fig. 13.8** Bilateral PSF at the both sides of the proximal penile shaft

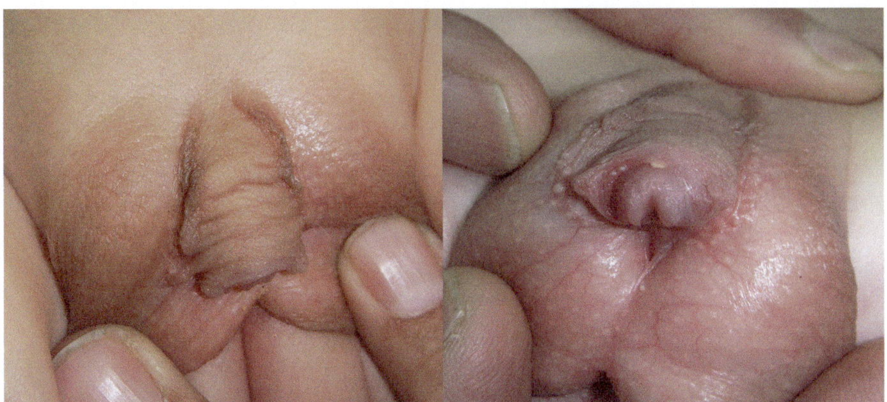

**Fig. 13.9** Severe bilateral penoscrotal fusion with penoscrotal hypospadias

**Fig. 13.10** A rare case of preputial fusion to the scrotum

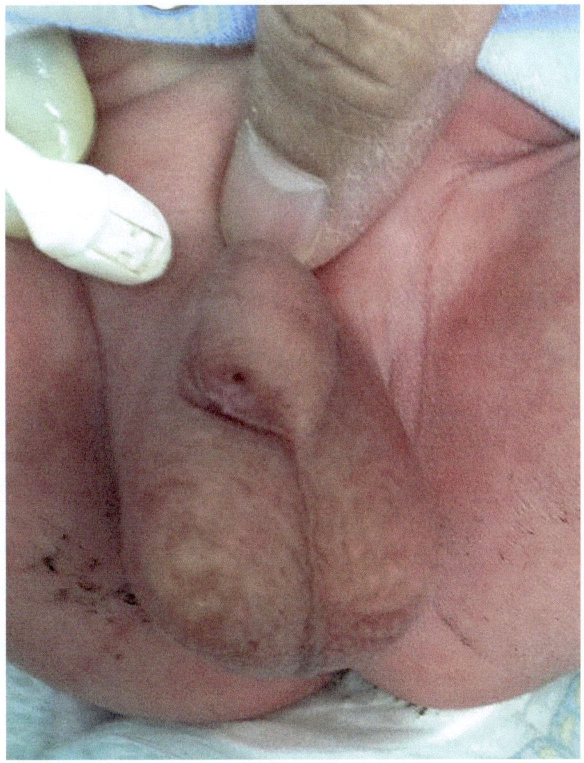

scrotum to the penile skin and obliteration of the normal penoscrotal angle. Some authors have proposed that PSF is secondary to aberrant preputial development, where there is insufficient ventral skin coverage of the penis and, instead, the penis is covered by adjacent scrotal tissue [8], but this not usually the case. Extension of the PSF to the prepuce is a rare finding (Fig. 13.10).

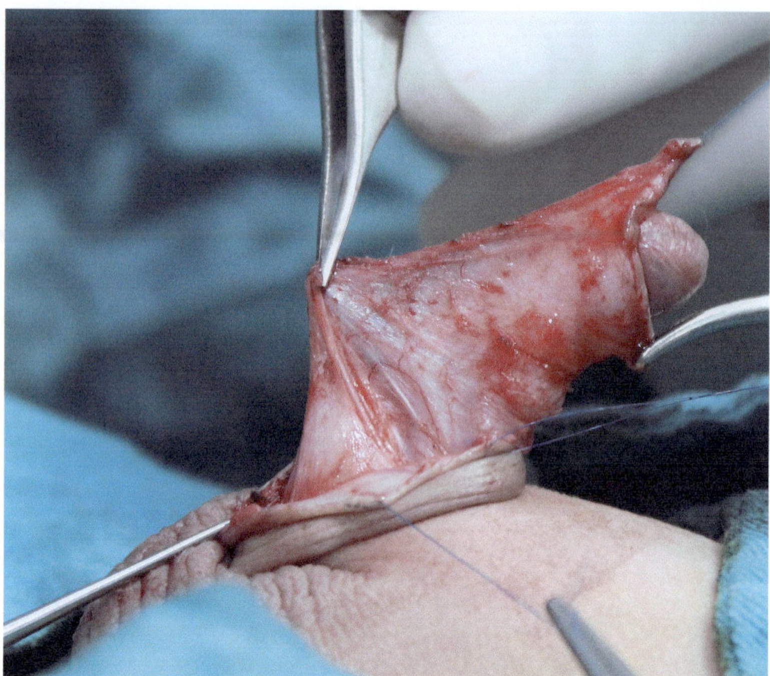

**Fig. 13.11** Dysplastic dartos fascia forming band anchoring the scrotum high in the penile shaft

In most cases of PSF, that we reconstructed, there is an obvious dysplastic dartos fascia and apparent abnormally dartos band (Fig. 13.11). It is recently proved that buried penis is associated with structural anomalies in dartos tissue. Spinoit et al. [9] recognised three different dartos tissue patterns in cases of congenital penile anomalies. Pattern I (normal) consisted of smooth muscle fibers of dartos tissue organized in a parallel configuration in the subcutaneous tissue. Pattern II was characterized by poorly developed and hypotrophic smooth muscle fibers. Pattern III was determined by randomly distributed smooth muscle fibers in the subcutaneous tissue, without parallel configuration. Dartos muscle in 78% of the cases of buried penis were considered abnormal (pattern II in 4 cases and III in 10 cases of Spinoit et al. series of cases). Tack et al. [10] at 2019 found that there is no statistically significant difference in Androgen Receptor (AR) expression in the normal preputial skin on cases of buried penis, but the main limitation of this study that the AR expression was tested only in a tissue unrelated to the pathological one; they only tested the preputial AR, so a further study for evaluation of AR expression in the defective dartos fascia is indicated.

**Associated anomalies**: PSF may be diagnosed as an isolated cases or sometimes it is associated with other malformations such as hypospadias, chordee and true micropenis [11].

Common anomalies associating PSF are:

- Phimosis, which may be secondary to anchoring of the preputial ring to the scrotal tissue [8].
- Micropenis; is commonly associating webbed penis as a primary anomaly, or as a sequelae for the defective penile growth due to abnormal attachment. Micropenis should be differentiated from the objective penile diminutive look, which is due to over growth of the scrotal skin.
- Hypospadias; different grades of hypospadias may be associated with a different forms of PSF [12] (Figs. 13.6 and 13.9)
- Undescended testicle is not commonly reported with PSF.
- The biomedical literature states that PP is infrequently associated with other unrelated pathologies; there is one case described and associated with syndactyly of the left foot [13].
- Webbed penis also reported with autosomal dominant Robinow Syndrome [14].

**Manifestations**: PSF is an under diagnosed pathology, most cases seeking consultation with a different complaints like: micropenis or phimosis. Some cases, specially newborns, may be referred as a case of aphallia or ambiguous genitalia. A considerable number of cases are diagnosed during evaluation for hypospadias repair, or during ritual circumcision. Older children may complain of difficult micturition in the standing position with wetting of their pants. Difficult preputial hygiene and recurrent episodes of balanitis with eventually manifestations of urinary tract infection are a common complaints. Adult will have a painful erection, sexual embarrassment, psychological consequences with a decrease in self-esteem due to shame compared to their peers with an appreciated micropenis, and in advanced cases a sexual dysfunction with penetration during intercourse will supervenes [5]. Very rarely, and could be due to normal pulling up of the suspensory ligaments with the defective ventral penile attachments, to have a PSF with a dorsal curvature instead of the usual ventral bending (Fig. 13.12).

We diagnosed some cases of PSF presented with an abnormally peeping testicles to the root of the penis, secondary to the deficient fascial attachments at the root of the penis (Fig. 13.13). These cases may be diagnosed wrongly as an ectopic testicles, but herein there is only a defect in the deep tissue which allow testicles to move up to the root of the penis. Repositioning of the testicles along the PSF reconstruction with readjustment of a dartos layer at the base of the penis to isolates testes is feasible in such cases.

**Diagnosis**: Diagnosis of PSF is confirmed by physical examination; when the shaft of the penis is lifted up, the obliteration of the penoscrotal angle by a cutaneous fold which extends from the ventral penile skin to the scrotal wall is clearly evident. In some cases, penoscrotal fusion can involve the entire length of the penis up to the preputial skin. Literature describe the importance of diagnosing a PSF before performing a circumcision in countries which are still doing it routinely, since circumcision would further aggravates the condition and its correction, thus promotes the appearance of a micropenis [8, 15]. Penoscrotal fusion, although not

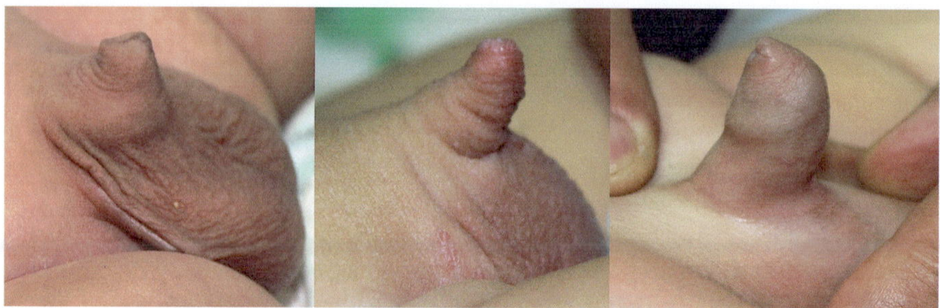

**Fig. 13.12** Rare presentation of PSF with a unusual dorsal curvature

**Fig. 13.13** A case of PSF
with defective fascial
covering of the testicles,
which are easily drawn up at
the root of the penis, and
looks like an ectopic testis

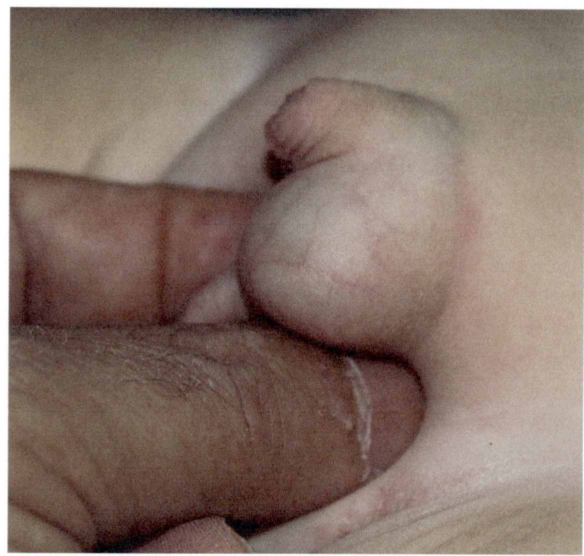

pernicious, certainly presents a grossly abnormal appearance. Early detection will be beneficial to avoid physical and psychological consequences.

**Differential diagnosis**: As mentioned before; PSF should be differentiated from cases of just penile scrotolisation without webbing, (Fig. 13.3) and cases of penile chordee without hypospadias; where the defect is located at the level of the deficient corpora spongiosum [16]. In Fig. 13.14 it is clear that inspite of obvious severe penile chordee, the penoscrotal angle is still preserved without any creeping ectopic scrotal tissue. It should be noted that bilateral hydroceles, hernias, obesity and severe hypospadias may all give a false appearance of penoscrotal fusion. Concealed penis should be differentiated from cases of primary and secondary microphallus; it is easy to estimated accurately the actual size of penis including the hidden proximal part in most cases of PSF (Fig. 13.8).

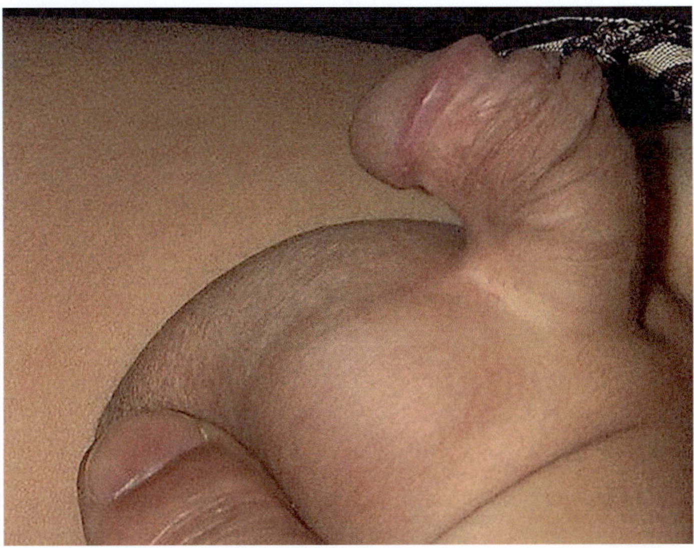

**Fig. 13.14** Isolated penile chordee without hypospadias or PSF; the penoscrotal angle is normal

**Management**: In 1963 Brown stated that webbed penis may resolve at puberty if the testes were normal [17]. But it is difficult to leave a child with a PSF suffering from difficult penile hygiene, inability to micturate standing with the possibility of UTI till puberty. This congenital anomaly and its allies deserve surgical correction at an early age to avoid frustrations and psychological trauma. Waiting for puberty, with its hormonal serge, to fix this problem, has no scientific basis, and on the other hand, the children are aware of their anatomical problem long before they reach puberty, so correction PSF sooner rather than later is our policy in agreement with other authors [18, 19].

Many surgical techniques have been described to resolve this pathology, all with variable cosmetic results. Early descriptions of treatment have included simple incisions to mobilize skin flaps and/ or excise redundant skin, tailored incisions and excisions with multiple Z plasties (whereby skin flaps are mobilized to elongate skin and tissue) [19]. However, some disadvantages have been reported with these techniques. The procedures that are characterized by a vertical suture line crossing the penoscrotal angle can be associated with scar contracture, which interferes with penile erection; skin flaps that are excessively manipulated or stitched are at risk of necrosis with a functional and cosmetic consequences, while some authors believed that multiple Z plasties are unnecessary as PSF penis can be fixed using simple surgery and the skin web is easy to manipulate, moreover, the undesirability of transferring hairbearing skin to the penis has been pointed out [20].

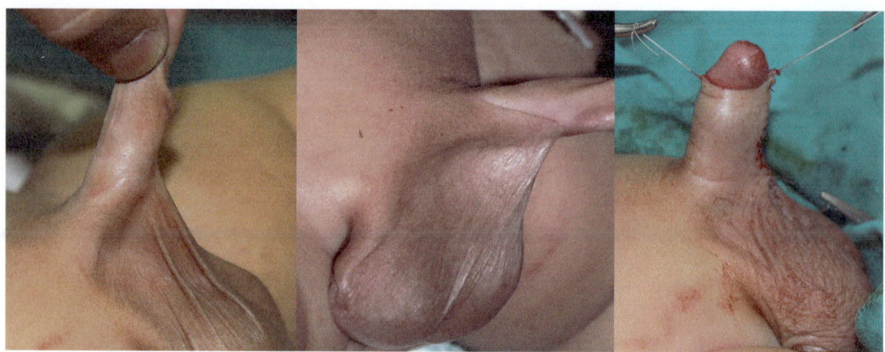

**Fig. 13.15** PSF with high insertion of the scrotum at the distal penile shaft, repaired with restoration of the penoscrotal angle

Proper dissection of the dysplastic dartos bands with restoration of the penoscrotal angle, will gives a good results even with a linear midline incision (Fig. 13.15).

Dilley and Currie [21] described a simple method for reconstructing the penoscrotal angle, which avoids a vertical suture line by using a diamond shaped incision. This diamond is subdivided into four triangles and two triangles on opposite sides are excised. The remaining two triangles are mobilized as simple skin flaps so that the horizontal suture line becomes the new penoscrotal angle.

Topical or systemic testosterone was tried by some authors, it may improve the quality of local tissues and the penile size by stimulating intrinsic penile growth [6]. We advocate topical testosterone before attempting surgery by 4–6 weeks, which results in limited improvement of the penile size.

Cases of PSF associating hypospadias could be reconstructed in two sessions, but one stage repair is also feasible (Fig. 13.16). Bilateral PSF is an uncommon entity, and if the child had normal urethra and corpora, the results of penile release and penoscrotal restoration is excellent (Fig. 13.17).

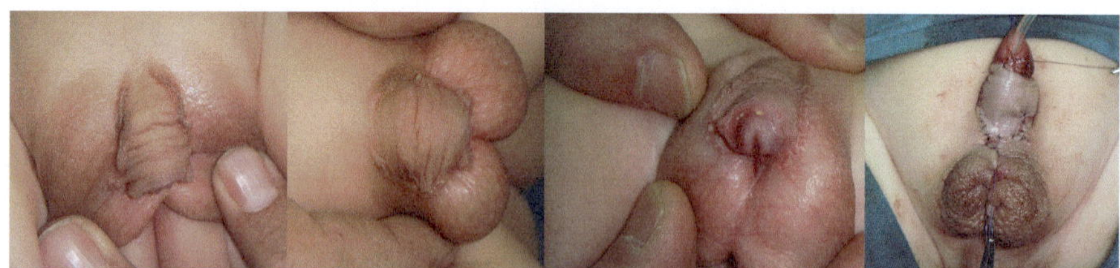

**Fig. 13.16** Bilateral PSF with proximal penoscrotal hypospadias, repaired in one stage with scrotoplasty

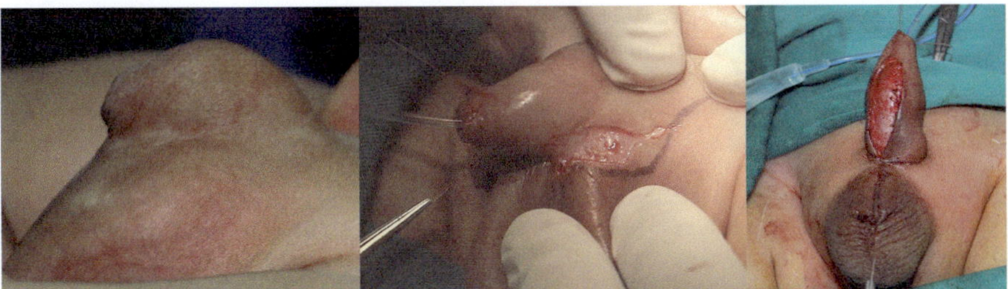

**Fig. 13.17** Another case of bilateral PSF, but with normal urethra, repaired with diamond incision, ended with a midline suture

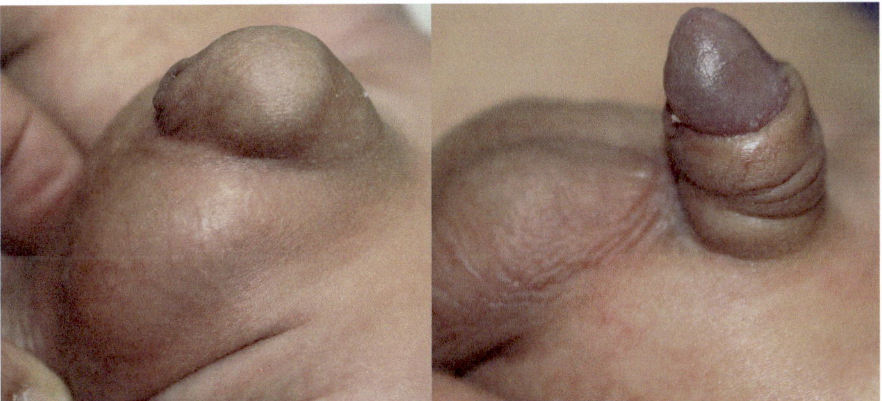

**Fig. 13.18** Prepuce unfurling to correct PSF with an excellent result

Preputial unfurling to correct the buried penis is a simple and useful technique for the patients or parents who will accept the circumcised penis; in this technique the preputial skin is used to replace the deficient ventral penile skin [22]. There are many modification of the primary principle [23]. I think the modified prepuce unfurling is a safe and effective method to correct many cases of buried penis (Fig. 13.18).

# References


1. Chin TW. Buried penis. Formos J Surg. 2016;49:133–5.https://doi.org/10.1016/j.fjs.2016.03.004.
2. Matsuo N, Ishii T, Takayama JI, Miwa M, Hasegawa T. Reference standard of penile size and prevalence of buried penis in Japanese newborn male infants. Endocr J. 2014;61:849–53.
3. Keyes EL. Phimosis-paraphimosis-tumors of the penis. In: Urology. New York: D. Appleton & Co; 1919, Chapt. 67. p. 649.

4. Bisotti P. Suuncasodi: "virgapalmata." Rass Int Clin Terap. 1953;33:452–3.

5. Glanz S. Adult congenital penile deformity. Plast Reconstr Surg. 1968;41:579–80.

6. Maizels M, Zaontz M, Donovan J, Bushnik PN, Firlit CF. Surgical correction of the buried penis: description of a classification system and a technique to correct the disorder. J Urol. 1986;136:268–71.

7. Glanz S. Adult congenital penile deformity. Plast Recons Surg. 1968;41:579–80.

8. Cohen SS. PENE PALMADO: Revista Chilena de Urología. 2002;67(3):195–201.

9. Spinoit AF, Van Praet C, Groen LA, Laecke EV, Praet M, Hoebeke P. Congenital penile pathology is associated with abnormal development of the dartos muscle: a prospective study of primary penile surgery at a Tertiary Referral Center. J Urol. 2015;5(193):1620–4. https://doi.org/10.1016/j.juro.2014.10.090.

10. Tack L, Praet M, Van Dorpe J, Haid B, Buelens S, Hoebeke P, Van Laecke E, Cools M, Spinoit A, Androgen receptor expression in preputial dartos tissue correlates with physiological androgen exposure in congenital malformations of the penis and in controls. J Pediatr Urol. https://doi.org/10.1016/j.jpurol.2019.10.031.

11. Perlmutter AD, Chamberlain JW. Webbed penis without chordee. J Urol. 1972;107:320–1.

12. Dilley AV. Webbed penis. Ped Surg Int. 1999;15:446–8.

13. Masih BK. Webbed penis. J Urol. 1974;111:690–2.

14. Roifman M, Brunner H, Lohr J, et al. Autosomal dominant robinow syndrome 2019. In: Adam MP, Ardinger HH, Pagon RA, et al., editors. GeneReviews®. Seattle (WA): University of Washington, Seattle; 1993–2020. https://www.ncbi.nlm.nih.gov/books/NBK268648/.

15. Redman FJ. A technique for the correction of penoscrotal fusion. J Urol. 1985;133:432–3.

16. Fahmy MA. Penile chordee in congenital anomalies of the penis. Springer International Publishing; 2017. pp. 85–87. https://doi.org/10.1007/978-3-319-43310-3.

17. Brown JJM. The genitourinary system. In: Surgery of childhood. Baltimore: The Williams & Wilkins Co.; 1963, Chapt. 37. p. 1094.

18. Shapiro SS. Surgical treatment of the buried penis. Urol. 1987;30:554–9.

19. Wilson CS, Sallade RL. Webbed penis. Plast Reconstr Surg. 1980;66:453–4.

20. Puri P. Webbed penis without chordee. J Pediatr Surg. 1976;11:125.

21. Dilley AV, Currie BG. Webbed penis. Pediatr Surg Int. 1999;15:447–8.

22. Donahoe PK, Keating MA. Preputial unfurling to correct the buried penis. J Pediatr Surg. 1986;21:1055e105. https://doi.org/10.1016/0022-3468(86)90007-2.

23. Chin TW, Tsai HL, Liu CS. Modified prepuce unfurling for buried penis: a report of 12 years of experience. Asian J Surg. 2015;38:74e78. https://doi.org/10.1016/j.asjsur.2014.04.006.

# Chapter 14
# Bifid Scrotum


**Mohamed A. Baky Fahmy**


**Abbreviations**

| | |
|---|---|
| SSS | Separation of the Scrotal Sac |
| AIS | Androgen Insensitivity Syndrome |
| MR | Median Raphae |
| VEG | Virilization of the external genitalia |
| SMR | Split Median Raphe |

**Synonyms**: Separation of the Scrotal Sac, Scrotal bipartition.

**Definition**: Scrotal midline indentation or cleft with absent scrotal raphe. Bifid scrotum is presented in a wide range of phenotypic forms, and simply classified to partial or complete. Perineal groove is a sulcus of mucosal tissue with clearly defined margins that can be found in the midline anywhere between the vagina and anus in girls, and rarely reported in boys, and if it is extended anteriorly to involve the scrotum it is considered as a partial bifid scrotum. Scrotal dimple is a rare form of minimal partial bifid scrota at the bottom.

## 14.1 Etiology

Bifid scrotum occurs along the same spectrum as penoscrotal transposition, with abnormal positioning of the genital tubercle in relation to the labioscrotal swellings. However, the labioscrotal folds are completely separated, and no median raphe is present in typical form of bifid scrotum. By the end of the sixth week, a down-growth of the urogenital septum reaches the cloacal membrane, dividing it into the urogenital and anal membranes. There are two swellings which become the urogenital swellings anteriorly and the anal folds dorsally, with the perineal body developing


M. A. B. Fahmy (✉)
Al-Azhar University, Cairo, Egypt

between both. Lateral to the urogenital swellings, a pair of the genital swellings develop. During the eighth week of gestation, the urogenital and anal membranes rupture, so that the urogenital sinus and anal canal communicate freely with the amniotic cavity [1]. At the same time the labioscrotal folds of both sides migrate inframedially and fused in male to form both scrotal sacs with a raphe in between, but it kept completely separated in female with the introitus cleft in-between the both labia, without any median raphe. One of the main phenotypic difference between male and female is the closure of the line between the two scrota in male to form the scrotal raphe and the two unfused labia which kept split by the introitus in female (Fig. 14.1). That's why the bifid scrotum is commonly seen in males with AIS.

The urethral folds in male may fail to fuse because of defective caudal-ventral growth of the caudal mesenchyme, which will result in different forms of hypospadia with or without bifid scrotum [3].

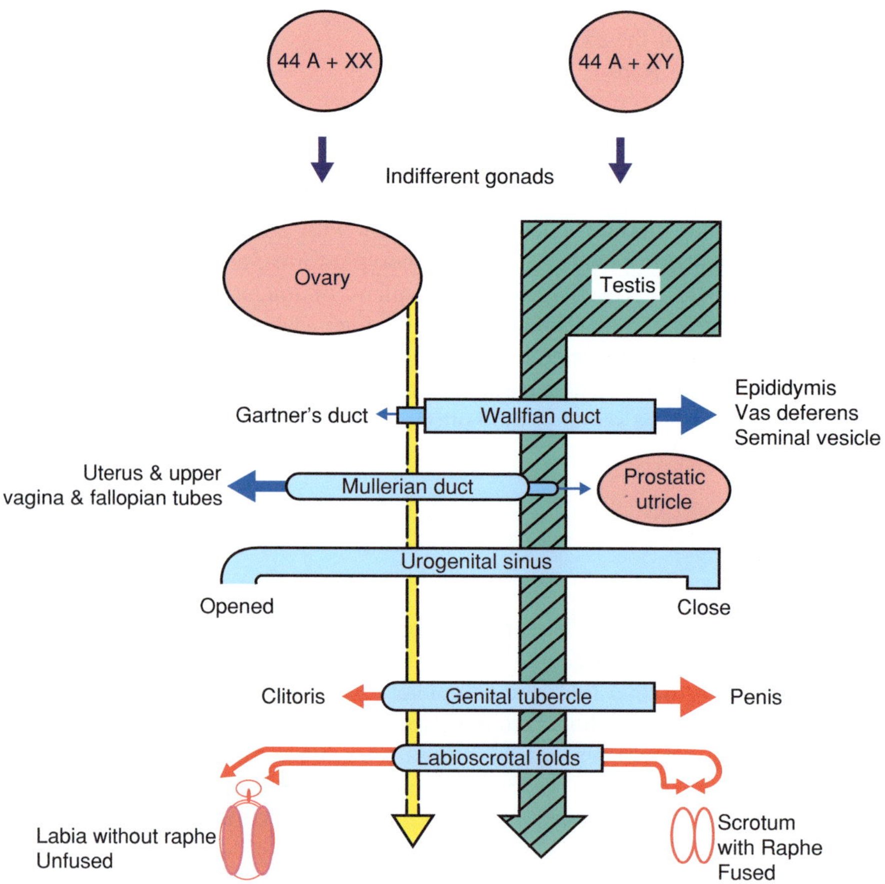


**Fig. 14.1** Genetic and hormonal factors in the normal differentiation of duct systems and external genitalia. (Modified after Tuchmann-Duplessis, 1970 [2])

It is thought that the defects in the median raphe are the result of the failure of the fusion mechanisms of the ventral wall of the abdomen at the caudal end. Such failures of fusion of the ventral wall may occur anywhere from the symphysis menti to the anal margin, which is embryologically extended from the stomodaeum (The oral portion of the digestive tract of an embryo) to the cloaca. The deficiency in closure may be manifest in the infra-umbilical region of the abdomen as extroversion of the bladder, varying degrees of malformation, such as epispadias, open penile urethra delineated below by a crescentic glans and preputial fold or even as two genital tubercles with widening of the pubic bones [4]. A minor degree of deficient ventral wall closure of the median raphe in the penoscrotal region and perineum can also occur as a median raphae canals apparently manifest themselves only after infection. The canals may become so infected without involvement of the urethra [5]. The infection is acquired venereally or transmitted to the sexual partner. Sometimes, in spite of the infection, the condition may go unnoticed because it tends to be mild and painless [6] (Chap. 17).

## 14.2 Manifestations and Classification of Bifid Scrotum

This anomaly may be taken lightly by the examining physicians, but sometimes it may be an indicator for the hypogonadism with deficient androgen receptors or associating other major anomalies. Bifid scrotum may be complete or partial and it could be manifested with a different varieties:-

1. **Complete**: the two scrotal sacs are completely separated widely.
2. **Partial**: superficial or deep depression either separate the whole scrota at the cephalic or caudal ends, so this partial bifid scrotum may be seen as a three subtypes:
   - Total
   - Upper
   - lower

Complete bifid scrotum usually seen with cases of inguinal ectopic scrotum; where the normal and ectopic scrota are separated by a wide distance of normal skin without any raphe in between (Fig. 14.2).

Cases of complete AIS may be presented with either complete or partial bifid scrotum, the later usually seen with a penoscrotal hypospadias and Prader stage 2 and 3 [7] (Fig. 14.3). Incomplete or partial AIS may also presented with a complete bifid scrota and an opened urethra seen caudally to a small phallus (Fig. 14.4). Partially bifid scrotum is more commoner with a very wide varieties; as regard the depth and the extension of clefting, the whole line between the two scrotal sacs may be seen bifid, with even an extension to the perineum, and this considered as a partial total bifid scrotum (Fig. 14.5).

                                                          

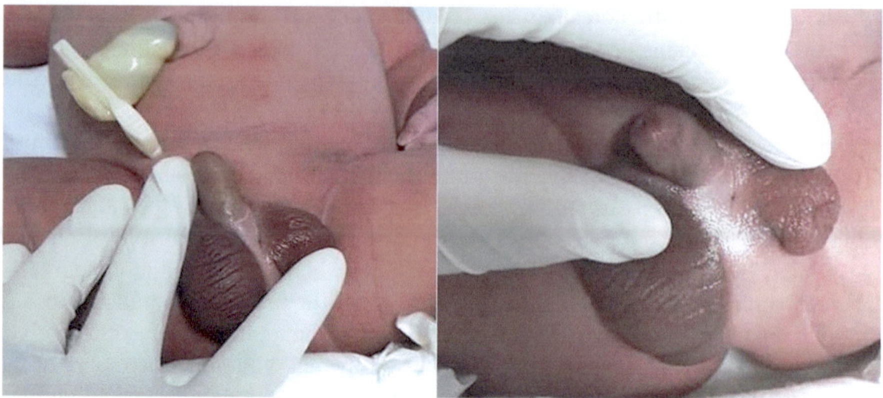

**Fig. 14.2** Left inguinal ectopic scrotum, which is separated from the normal right scrotum by a normal skin

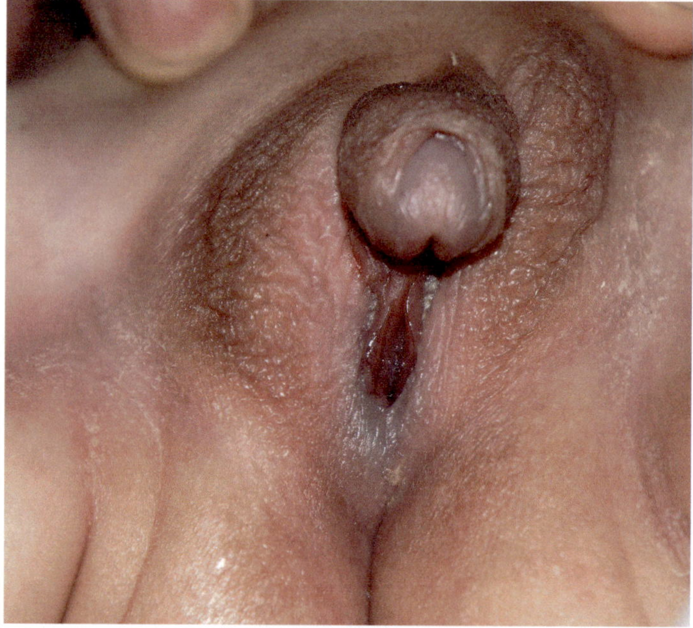

**Fig. 14.3** Complete AIS with a complete bifid scrotum and proximal hypospadias

Failure of the scrotal fusion cranially just lateral to the base of the penis, will results in upper partial bifid scrota (Fig. 14.6). Lowermost failure of scrotal fusion seen frequently with cases of ARM, specially with higher anomalies (Fig. 14.7) Isolated cases of bifid scrotum without any other genital anomalies are usually

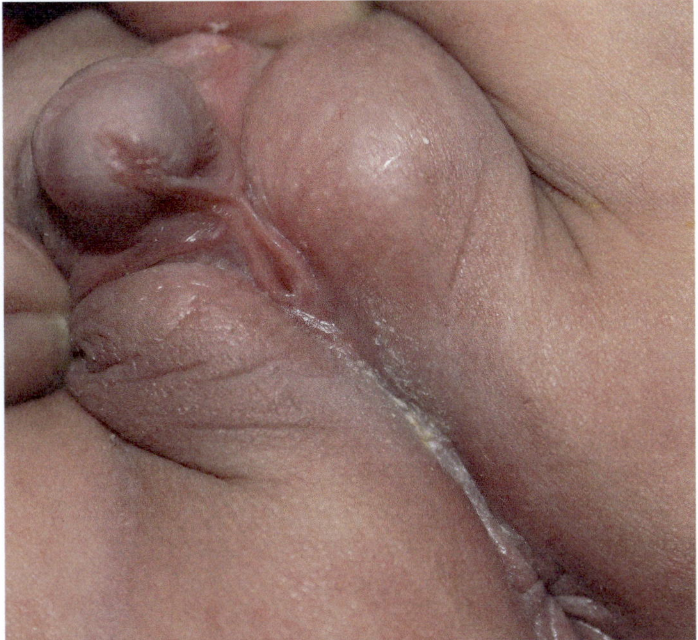

**Fig. 14.4** Partial AIS with bifid scrota, hypospadias and two descended testicles

affecting the upper end of the scrota (Fig. 14.8), or may be manifested as just a widening of the median raphe (Figs. 14.9 and 14.10).

## 14.3 Variants of Bifid scrotum:

1. **Perineal groove:** Failure of midline fusion, caudally to the introitus in female, also referred to as a perineal groove, which is a sulcus of mucosal tissue with clearly defined margins that can be found in the midline anywhere between the vagina and anus. It may also appear as a midline blind fistula in the same areas. It has been associated with an anteriorly displaced anus. It is a rare congenital variant thought to result from a failure of the labioscrotal swellings and perineal raphae to fuse during development. It can be mistaken for genital trauma, raising the concern for the possible sexual abuse of a child [8]. Perineal groove was initially thought to occur only in girls, but in 2003, Chatterjee and colleagues reported a case of perineal groove in a 7-year-old boy with severe penoscrotal hypospadias and a bifid scrotum [9]. At 2009 another case reported in a male child, with severe penoscrotal hypospadias and a bifid scrotum [10].

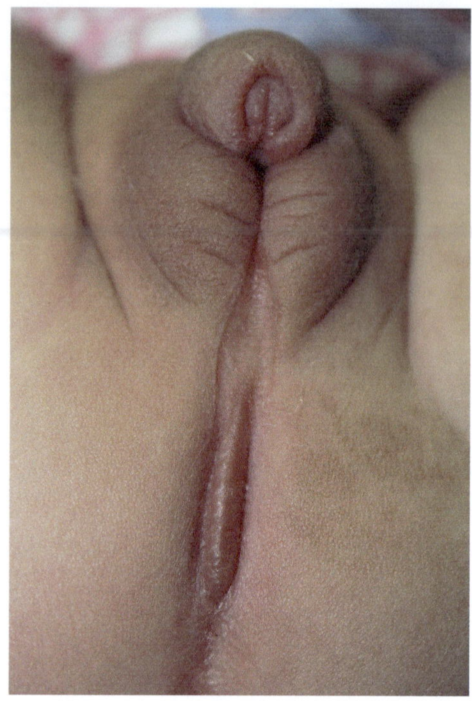

**Fig. 14.5** Partial total bifid scrotum extended to include the perineum in a case of ARM, the cleft perineum considered as a perineal groove

Generally, the congenital failure of midline fusion may be manifested by perineal groove, infantile pyramidal protrusion, prominent median raphe, and diastasis ani. Diastasis ani is a V-shaped or wedge-shaped smooth area in the midline of the perianal skin folds thought to result from the failure of fusion of the underlying corrugator external anal sphincter muscle. Diastasis ani refers to the absence of muscle fibers in the midline of the external anal sphincter which creates a fan-shaped loss of anal folds in the midline. These midline fusion defects show no evidence of scarring [11]. In many cases of imperforate anus there is a wide unfused perineal raphae, which may be extended cranially to be manifested as a partial bifid scrotum. (Fig. 14.5) Two cases of an unusual congenital malformation as an isolated defect at the median raphe covered by colonic mucosa extending from a hypospadiac urethral orifice to the anal orifice had been previously reported [12].

2. **Split median raphe of the penis (SMR):** SMR is thought to be the result of defective fusion of ectodermal tissue in the urethra and scrotum area or of defective growth of the perineal mesoderm around the urethra during gestation. Although SMR associated with other major penile congenital defects like: epispadias, hypospadias, penile torsion, bifid scrotum and chordee. But an isolated SMR is probably underdiagnosed, although it is not a rare malformative condition [13].

3. **Scrotal dimple:** Normal scrotal sacs had a pear like shape, with the left scrotum commonly hanging little bit lower than the right, but without any cleavage or

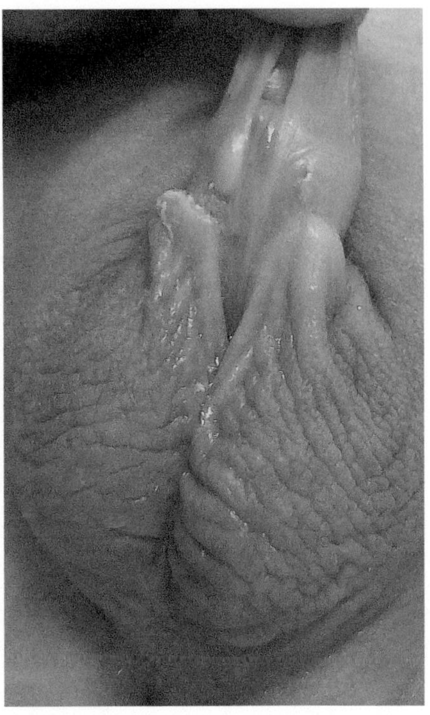

**Fig. 14.6** Uppermost partial bifid scrotum at the base of penis

partition between both sacs at the bottom. Some animals like goats, sheep, bull, white-tailed deer and others have a distinctive scrotal dimple at the bottom of the scrota; which gives it the look of bipartition. Animals which had this dimple as a morphological characteristics for adaptation to desert and semiarid regions, may had this distinctive anatomy to increase the surface area of each testicle exposed to environmental temperature, favouring heat dissipation and improving reproductive efficiency [14] (Fig. 14.11).

Also it was concluded that the spermatogenetic line parameters of sheep with scrotal bipartition were different if compared to those without scrotal bipartition, with greater efficiencies in spermatogenesis yield and Sertoli cells in the sheep with scrotal bipartition, suggesting that these animals present, as reported in goats, better reproductive indices [15].

In human's scrotum the connective tissue fibers of the facial layers intersperse with dartos muscle fibers. This explains dimpling at the lower end of the scrotal septum, which is rarely seen normally in some children. This could be considered as a minimal degree of partial bifid scrotum.

We diagnosed 6 cases with this scrotal dimple without any associated other anomalies, except hypospadias in 2 cases but many cases showed a different forms of local dermatitis at the dimple between the two scrotal sac (Fig. 14.12).

**Fig. 14.7** Partial bifid
scrotum with ARM

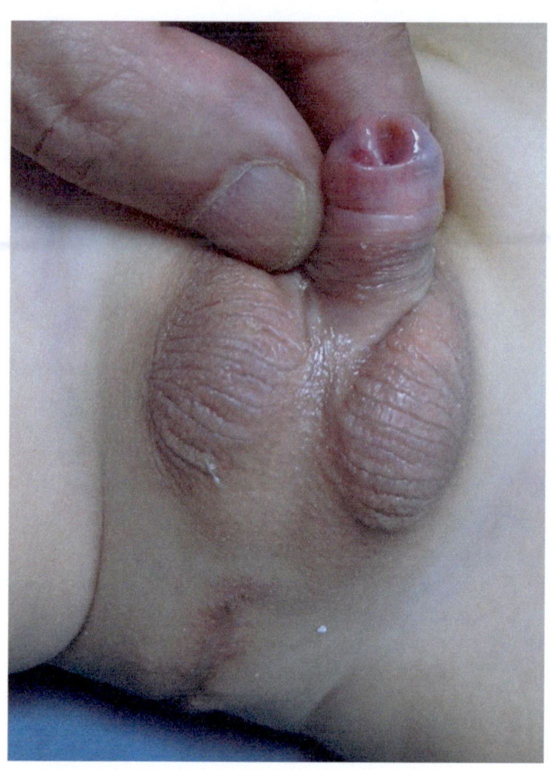

**Fig. 14.8** Bifid scrotum in
the form of widen median
raphe with otherwise normal
genitalia

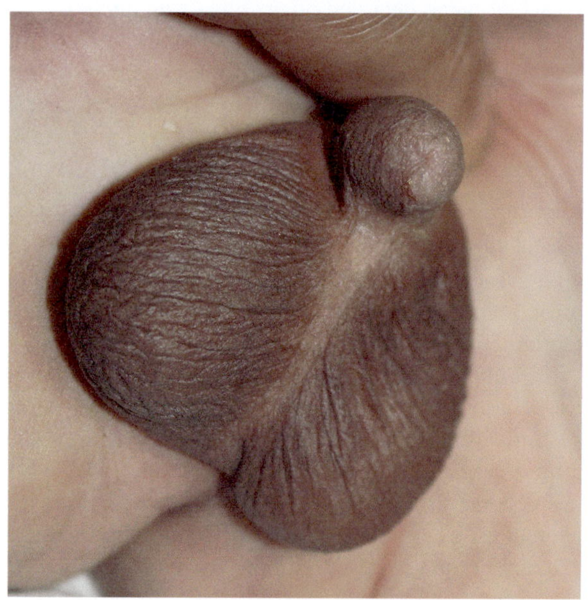

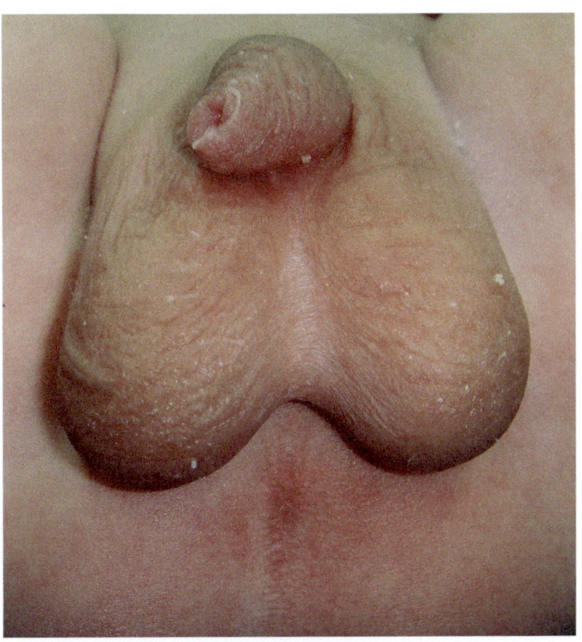

**Fig. 14.9** Widening of median raphe with a lower partial bifid scrotum

Lateral or midline scrotal dimpling may result from shortening of the gubernaculum, both types of dimpling have been observed as an acquired abnormality. A recently appreciated scrotal dimpling may offer a means of earlier diagnosis of testicular torsion in cases of acute scrotum, as dimpling of the scrotum has been described as a physical sign of torsion of the testis. It possibly offers a way to differentiate epididymoorchitis from testicular torsion as a cause of testicular pain in infants. The dimple is apparently produced when the twist causes shortening of the cord and its coverings. In cases of intravaginal torsion of the spermatic cord, and a dimple on the dependent aspect of the scrotum was often noticed if the patient seen early [16].

## 14.4   Associated Congenital Abnormalities

Incomplete penoscrotal transposition defect must be differentiated from a bifid scrotum. Some few cases may had a combination of both anomalies; in such cases the typical labioscrotal migration is defective and the two scrota lack the confluence or conjunction at the median raphe (Fig. 14.13). Accessory scrotum with bifid scrotum and hypospadias are infrequently reported [17].

**Hypospadias and bifid scrotum**: It is reported that approximately 5% of patients with posterior hypospadias have a bifid scrotum [18]. A partially or completely

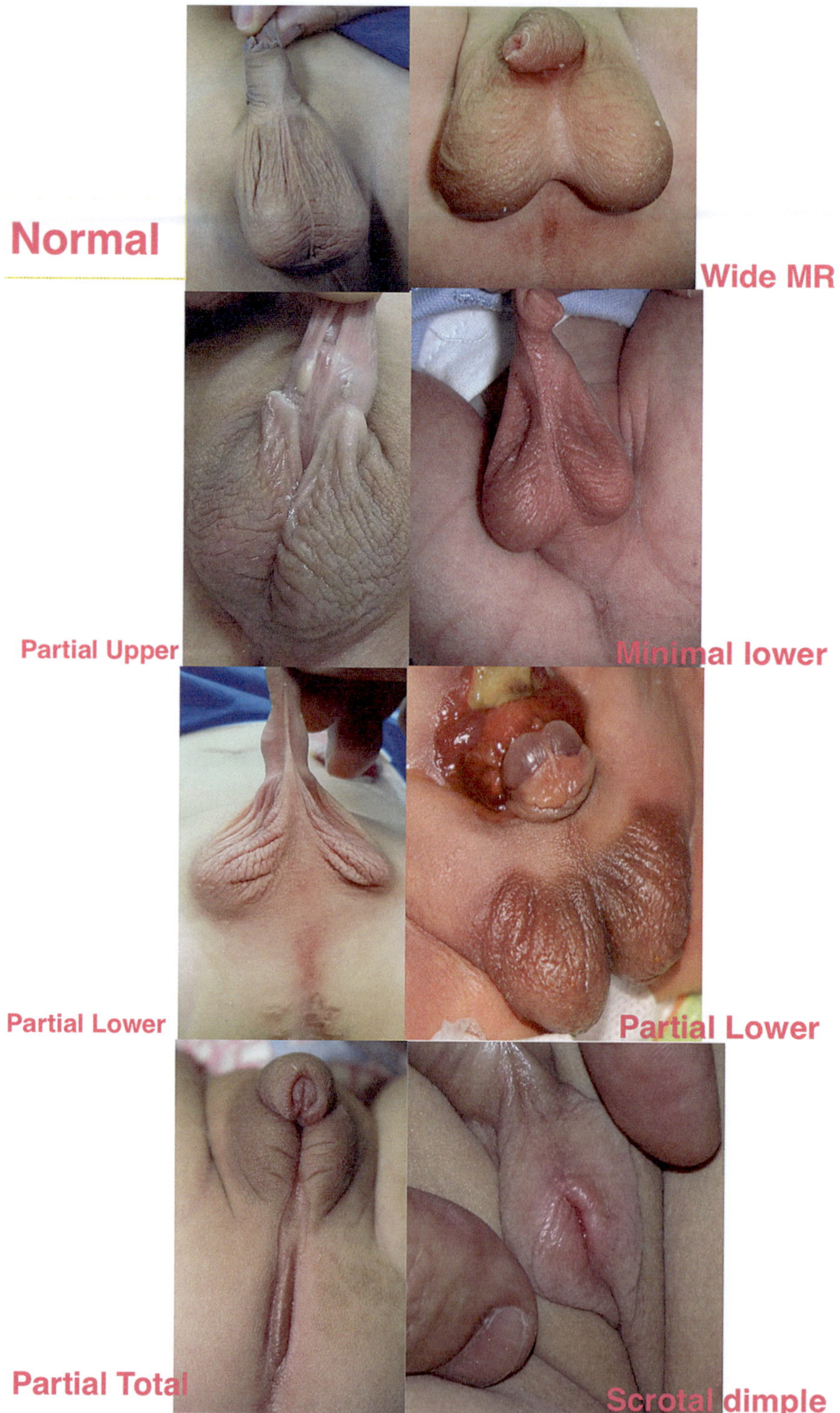


**Fig. 14.10** Collection of a different forms and degrees of bifid scrotum

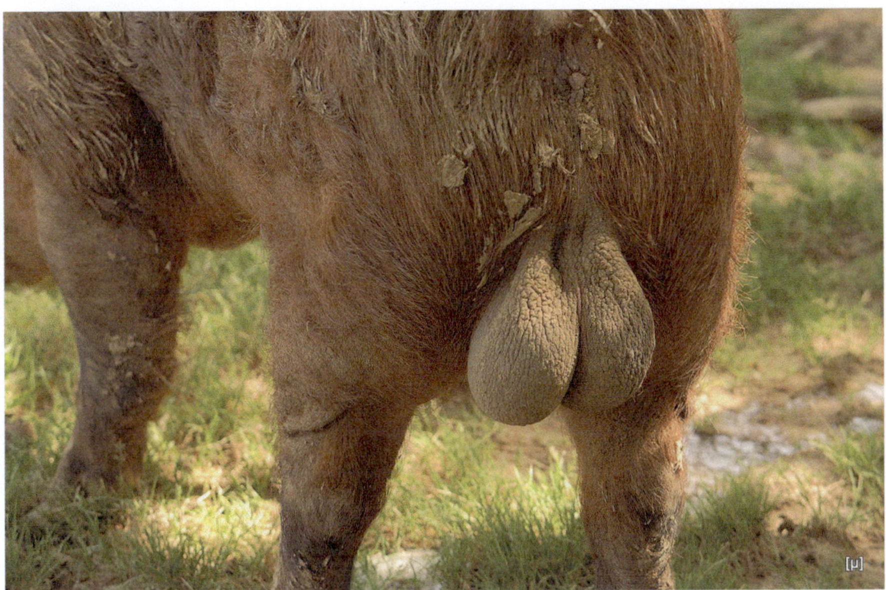

**Fig. 14.11** Normal scrotal dimple (bipartition) in goats

bifid scrotum is occasionally present in proximal forms of hypospadias [19]. Recognition and assessment of the the degree of scrotal cleft and transposition is of utmost importance before committing hypospadias repair (Fig. 14.14).

**Fig. 14.12** Rare case of scrotal dimple in infant, with an obvious dermatitis

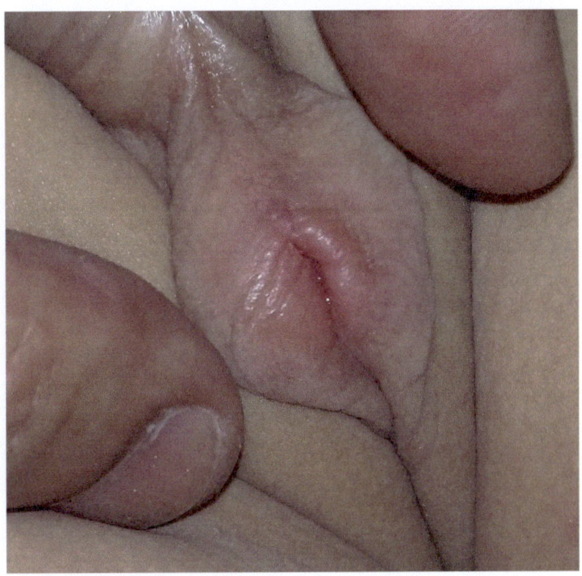

 M. A. B. Fahmy

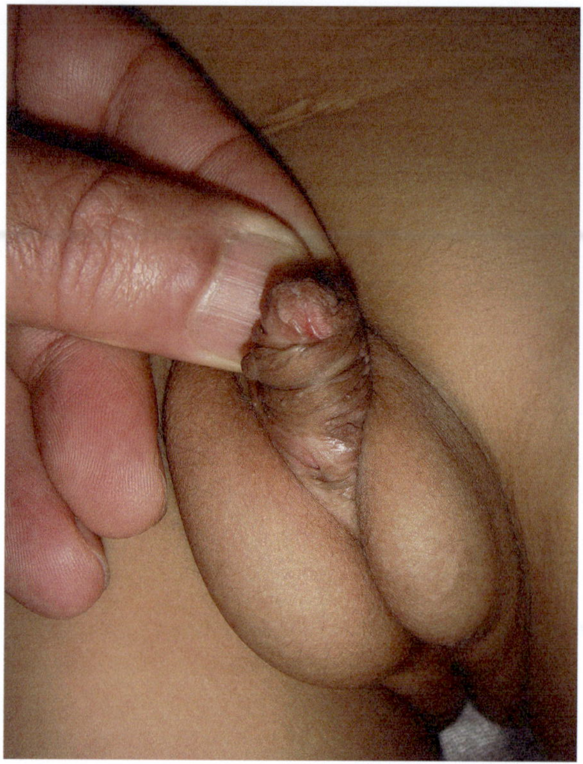

**Fig. 14.13** Partial scrotal transposition, bifid scrota, and proximal hypospadias which was repaired without concerning the abnormal scrotum, and complicated by fistula

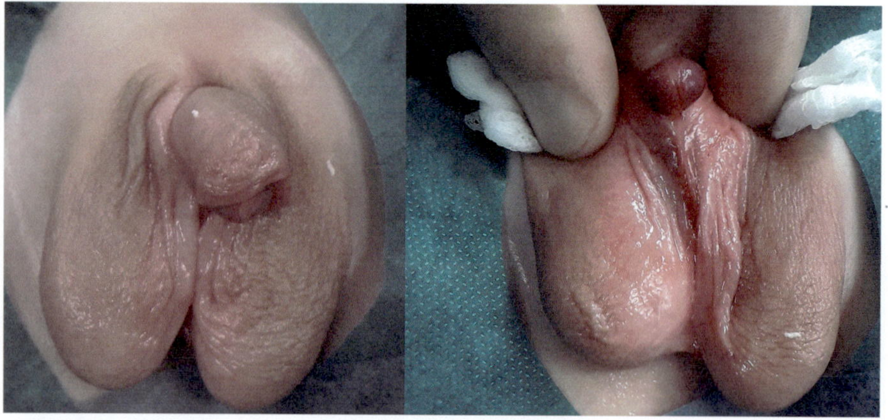

**Fig. 14.14** Proximal hypospadias, deficient corpora spongosium and partially bifid scrotum

Presence of bifid scrotum as a scrotal sac separation (SSS) is a predictive for the need to transect the urethral plate during hypospadias repair, presence of SSS is a marker of the hypospadias severity, and this severity translates into a less usable urethra, and this fairly an obvious clinical feature seems to reflect importance of ventral tissue hypoplasia, which itself correlates with quality of the urethral plate [20] (Fig. 14.14).

**Bifid scrotum with diphallia or pseudo diphallia**: Diphallia or penile duplication is a rare congenital abnormality thought to result from duplication of the genital tubercle or cloacal membrane in the early developmental stages in the uterus. Diphallia are strongly associated with genitourinary and anorectal malformations, most commonly bladder duplication, bifid scrotum, imperforate anus, pubic diastasis and lumbosacral abnormalities [21] (Fig. 14.15).

**Bifid scrotum and bladder exstrophy**: Cases of bladder exstrophy epispadias complex are associated with a wide penoscrotal distance and a distal partially bifid scrotum, which is not rare in such cases (Fig. 14.16).

**Syndromes**: Bifid scrotum had been described along other common or rare syndromes.

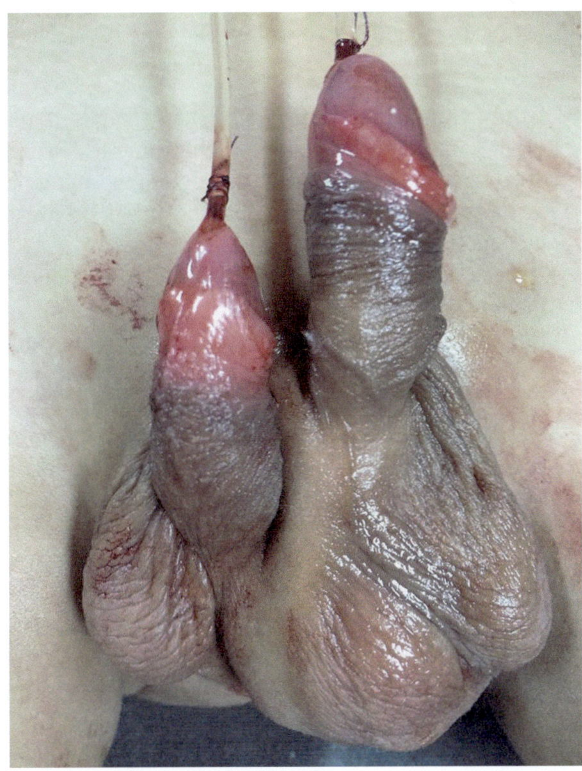

**Fig. 14.15** A rare case of diphallia and the scrota are bifid completely, with a normal skin in between

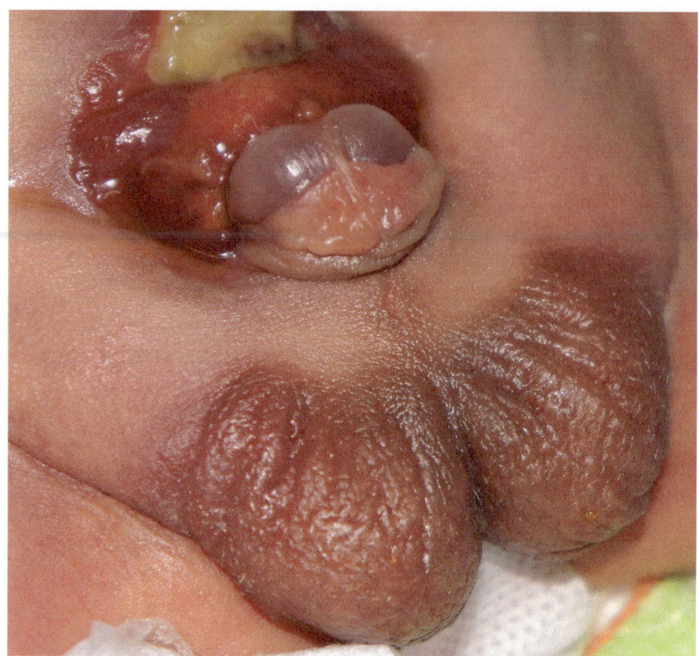

**Fig. 14.16** Partial lower bifid scrota with bladder exstrophy

- Bifid scrotum has been well established as a phenotype of the complete and partial androgen insensitivity syndrome [22] (Figs. 14.3 and 14.4).
- Also virilization of the external genitalia in young girls (VEG) manifests mostly as ambiguity of the genitalia, and in such cases the labia looks like a widely clefted scrota [23].
- Varying degrees of 17, 20-desmolase deficiency, resulting in varied development of external genitalia that ranges from female phenotype to virilization with microphallus, bifid scrotum, perineal hypospadias, and cryptorchidism secondary to insufficient testosterone production during fetal life. The enzyme 17, 20- desmolase cleaves the side chain of 17-hydroxypregnenolone and 17-hydroxyprogesterone to form DHEA and androstenedione, respectively. This enzyme is encoded by a gene that has been mapped on chromosome 10 [24].
- We diagnosed a male child with a chromosomal translocation between chromosomes 11 and 22 at q24 and q12 with female phenotype (Prader scale 1) he had a bilateral undescended dystrophic testicles, and his scrotum is bifid like female (Fig. 14.17).
- In the syndrome of XXXXY male, which constitute a clinical entity distinct from Klinefelter's syndrome, with severe mental retardation, growth retardation, peculiar rounded faces and markedly hypoplastic male genitalia. This hypoplasia consists of small penis, small testes and rudimentary scrotum in more than 80 per cent of cases. Hypospadias, cryptorchidism and bifid scrotum have been

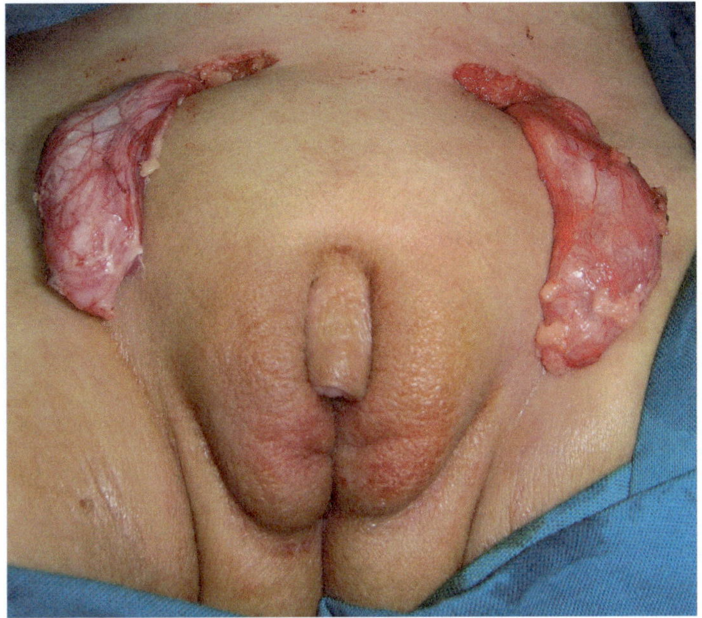

**Fig. 14.17** A male chad a chromosomal translocation between chromosome 11 and 22 at q24 and q12 with female phenotype (Prader scale 0) and a bilateral undescended dystrophic testicles, the scrota are bifid

recorded but not regularly [25]. Fraccaro et al. [26], in the original description of this entity, noted an extremely small penis, bifid scrotum and tiny testes.

- Beare–Stevenson syndrome is rare syndrome characterized by craniosynostosis, acanthosis nigricans, ear defects, broad toes and fingers, prominent umbilical stump, bifid scrotum, cryptorchidism, hypospadias, and ectopic anus [27].
- Popliteal pterygium syndrome (rare autosomal dominant disorder) associated with a wide range of anomalies include cleft palate, cleft lip, spina bifida, bifid ribs, and short sternum. Genital anomalies include cryptorchidism, bifid or ectopic scrotum and ambiguous genitalia in males [28].
- Bardet-Biedl syndrome (BBS), which was first described in 1920, is a pleiotropic disorder characterized by obesity, mental retardation, postaxial polydactyly, and hypogonadism. In 28% of the cases there is a hypoplastic or bifid scrotum; and a small penis [29].

**Investigations**: An inguinoscrotal and renal ulterasound is recommended for cases of bifid scrotum, to locate the testicles properly and to detect any renal abnormalities. With the presence of proximal hypospadias in association with bifid scrotum; we usually recommend an ascending cystourethrogram to evaluate the proximal urethra and to detect any associated prostatic utricle.

**Treatment**: Partial and minimal cases doesn't need any surgical intervention. Usual surgical repair in severe cases includes rotation of two scrotal flaps, joining them in the midline, and vertical skin closure. Additionally, there are surgical techniques such as reorienting the scrotum inferiorly with limited rotation flaps. Surgical repair is usually carried out at the time of hypospadias repair [30]. It is performed in a manner similar to penoscrotal transposition, and rotation of flaps of scrotal tissue may be required. An alternative method is the use of single or multiple Z-plasty procedures to correct the defect [31].

# References


1. Schoenwolf GC, Bieyl SB, Brauer PR, Francis-West P. Larsen's Human Embryology. 4th ed. Philadelphia, PA: Churchill Livingstone; 2008.
2. Tuchmann-Duplessis J, Herbert QS, Haegel S, Pierre T. Organo-genese. 2nd ed. Paris: Masson,1970.
3. Moore KL, Persaud TVN, Torchia MG. The developing human. 10th ed. Philadelphia: Elsevier; 2013.
4. Arey LB. Developmental anatomy: a textbook and laboratory manual of embryology. 7th ed. Philadelphia: WB Saunders; 1966. p. 308–12.
5. Neff JH. Congenital canals and cysts of the genito-perineal raphe. Am J Surg. 1936;31:308. https://doi.org/10.1016/S0002-9610(36)90493-2.
6. Clifford GR, Krieger JN, Rein MF. Gonococcal infection of the median penile raphe. J Urol. 1983;VL(130):138–9. https://doi.org/10.1016/S0022-5347(17)50999-4.
7. Prader A. Genital findings in the female pseudo-hermaphroditism of the congenital adrenogenital syndrome; morphology, frequency, development and heredity of the different genital forms. Helv Paediatr Acta. 1954;9(3):231–48.
8. Sekaran P, Shawis R. Perineal groove: a rare congenital abnormality of failure of fusion of the perineal raphe and discussion of its embryological origin. Clin Anat. 2009;22:823–5. https://doi.org/10.1002/ca.20855.
9. Chatterjee SK, Chatterjee US, Chatterjee U. Perineal groove with penoscrotal hypospadias. Pediatr Surg Int. 2003;19:554–6.
10. Sekaran P, Shawis R. Perineal groove: A rare congenital abnormality of failure of fusion of the perineal raphe and discussion of its embryological origin. Clin Anat (New York, NY). 2009;22(7):823–5.
11. McCann J, Voris J, Simon M, Wells R. Perianal findings in prepubertal children selected for nonabuse: a descriptive study. Child Abuse Negl. 1989;13(2):179–93. https://doi.org/10.1016/0145-2134(89)90005-7.
12. Gangopadhyayl AN, Biswasl SK, Khanna S. Exstrophy of the uroreetal septum-report of two cases and embryological review. Pediatric Surg Int. 1992;7:311–3.
13. Valerio E, Cutrone M. Split median raphe: case series and brief literature review. Pediatr Dermatol. 2014;31:e136–9. https://doi.org/10.1111/pde.12417.
14. Rocha EF, Francelino R, Santos NA, et al. Prevalence of scrotum bipartition in sheep in the Paraiba backwoods Brazil. Anim Reprod. 2018;15:1199–204.
15. Rodrigues RTGA et al. Influence of scrotal bipartition on spermatogenesis yield and sertoli cell efficiency in sheep. Pesq Vet Bras. 2016;36(4):258–62.
16. Ger R. The scrotal dimple in testicular torsion. Surgery. 1969;66:907–8.. PMID: 5356920.
17. Çiftdemir NA et al. Accessory scrotum with bifid scrotum and hypospadias. Turkish J Pediatr Dis. 2013;(1):38–40.

18. Chiang G, Cendron M. Chapter 42—disorders of the penis and scrotum. In: Pediatric urology, 2nd edn. Elsevier; 2010. pp. 544–62. https://doi.org/10.1016/B978-1-4160-3204-5.00042-6.
19. Avellán L. Morphology of hypospadias. Scand J Plast Surg. 1980;14:239–47.
20. Arnaud A, Cyril Ferdynus C, Harper L. Can separation of the scrotal sac in proximal hypospadias reliably predict the need for urethral plate transection? J Pediatr Urol. 2016;12:121.e1e121.e5.
21. Gyftopoulos K, Wolffenbuttel KP, Nijman RJ. Clinical and embryologic aspects of penile duplication and associated anomalies. Urology. 2002;60:675.
22. Perovic S, Vukadinovic V. Penoscrotal transposition with hypospadias: 1-stage repair. J Urol. 1992;148:1510–3.
23. Ekenze SO, Adiri CO, Igwilo IO, Onumaegbu OO. Virilized external genitalia in young girls: clinical characteristics and management challenges in a low-resource setting. J Pediatr Adolesc Gynecol. 2014;27(1):6–9. https://doi.org/10.1016/j.jpag.2013.07.004.
24. Kaufman FR, Costin G, Goebelsmann U, Stanczyk Z, Zachmann M. Male pseudo-hermaphroditism due to 17,20-desmolase deficiency. J Clin Endocrinol Metab. 1983;57:32–6.
25. Cunningham DM, Ragsdale JL. Genital anomalies of an xXx y male subject. J Urol. 1972;(107):872–4.
26. Fraccaro M, Kaijser K, Lindsten J. A child with 49 chromosomes. Lancet. 1960;2:899.
27. Vargas RA, Maegawa GH, Taucher SC, Leite JC, Sanz P, et al. Beare-Stevenson syndrome: two South American patients with FGFR2 analysis. Am J Med Genet A. 2003;121A:41–6.
28. Lees MM, Winter RM, Malcolm S, et al. Popliteal pterygium syndrome: a clinical study of three families and report of linkage to the Van der Woude syndrome locus on 1q32. J Med Genet. 1999;36:888–92.
29. Green JS, Parfrey PS, Harnett JD, et al. The cardinal manifestations of Bardet-Biedl syndrome, a form of Laurence-Moon Biedl syndrome. N Engl J Med. 1989;321:1002–9.
30. Defoor W, Wacksman J. Results of single staged hypospadias surgery to repair penoscrotal hypospadias with bifid scrotum or penoscrotal transposition. J Urol. 2003;170:1585–8.
31. Mokhless I, Youssif M, Eltayeb M, et al. Z-plasty for sculpturing of the bifid scrotum in severe hypospadias associated with penoscrotal transposition. J Pediatr Urol. 2011;7(3):305–9.

# Chapter 15
# Ectopic Scrotum

Mohamed A. Baky Fahmy

**Abbreviations**

CAH   Congenital Adrenogenital Hyperplasia
ARM   Anorectal Malformations

**Definition**: Ectopic scrotum is defined as the presence of the normal hemiscrotum or a scrotal tissue away from its normal location; between the penis and the perineum, with deficiency of one hemiscrotum. Simply it is a congenital anomaly in which the scrotum located in a position away from its normal scene. Ectopic scrotum may be in the form of a well formed scrotal sac or just as a patch of scrotal tissue. Females may be rarely presented with an ectopic scrotal tissue in their labia or distantly.

**Historical background**: Adair and Lewis at 1960 [1] reported the first case of unilateral ectopic scrotum in a 13-month-old clild with a normal left testis and scrotum, but a right scrotum containing a testis situated above the right inguinal ligament; this patient also had a bifid penis (diphallia) and an absent right kidney. Flanagan el al. [2] at 1961 reported a second case in a 6-week-old baby with a normal right testis and scrotum and a left scrotum containing a testis overlying the left external inguinal ring.

**Classifications**: Congenital ectopic scrotum classified into:

Suprainguinal
Perineal
Femoral
Other sites

Suprainguinal type is the most common [3] (Fig. 15.1). Unilateral femoral ectopic scrotum was also reported [4] (Fig. 15.2). Bilateral ectopic scrotum induced in experimental animals, but none of the cases gleaned from the literature reported a

M. A. B. Fahmy (✉)
Al-Azhar University, Cairo, Egypt

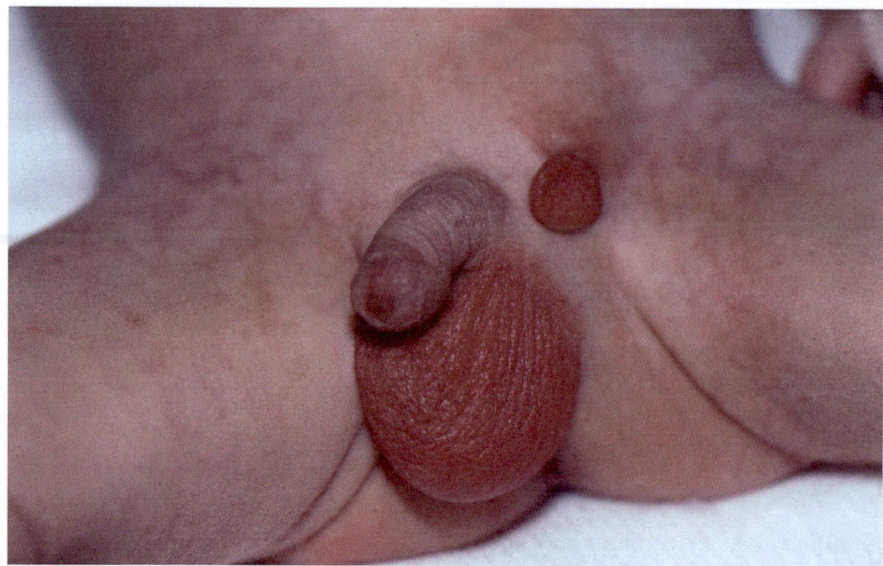

**Fig. 15.1** A small superainguinal ectopic scrotum in a neonate [22]

bilaterality in humans [5]. Redman and Ferguson [6] described a rare case of an unilateral caudal extension of the left hemiscrotum to the perineum in an adult patient who was presented with testicular pain.

**Etiology**: The etiopathogenesis of ectopic testis is controversial, with many divergent explanations; but the most acceptable one is related to abnormal insertion or branching of the gubernaculum. The gubernaculum is a prerequisite embryonic structure for the ultimate location of both the testis and scrotum, its role is complicated by the subsequent differential growth of the labioscrotal folds in which the gubernaculum is stabilized [7]. The precursor of the gubernaculum appears during the 5th to 6th week of human embryogenesis and extends from the urogenital ridge to the mesenchyme of the labioscrotal swellings. If this interaction is disturbed, the result may be a suprainguinal ectopia, unilteral penoscrotal transposition or a perineal scrotum. The descent of the testis outside its normal path with resultant formation of an ectopic scrotum may be explained by a malformed or splitted gubernaculum [8] (Fig. 15.3). Although the bulk of the gubernaculum is contained within the labioscrotal folds, it has been suggested that other gubernacular terminals ("accessory tails") may be directed to secondary sites, thus permitting the formation of an ectopic scrotum. Such appendages may attach either to the medial surface of the thigh or to some other unlikely area [9]. The causes of defective gubernaculum formation could be mechanical, genetic, chromosomal or teratogenic. A mechanical pressure effect on the developing fetus was described [10]. Earlier; Flanagan et al. [2] stated that the defect must be in the movement via either migration or differential growth of the labioscrotal fold itself. While the etiology of

**Fig. 15.2** Right side ectopic
scrotum at the upper thigh

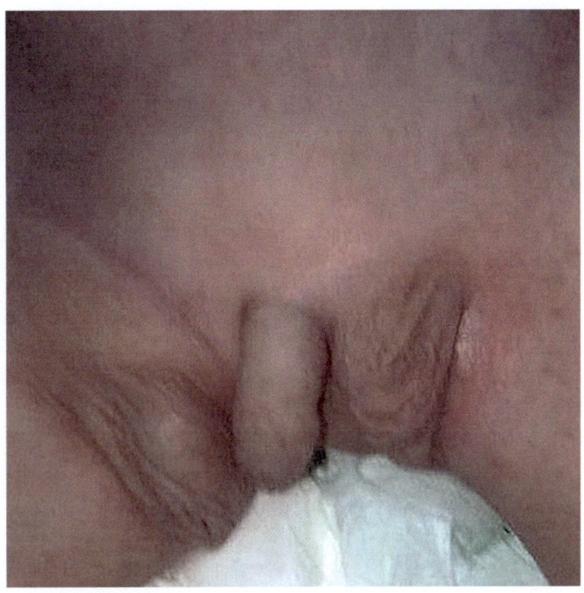

this malformation is likely to be multifactorial, the existence of an inbred strain of rats characterized by a high incidence of an ectopic scrotum suggests a genetic component to this anomaly [5]. Suprainguinal scrotal ectopia in rats may either be unilateral or bilateral [5], whereas bilaterality was not reported in humans. Some cases reported to occur in pregnancies complicated by oligohydramnios and breech presentation. Association of lower spine agenesis with pubic diastasis, may be attributed to more than just a defect that is caused by direct mechanical compressions [10]. Some authors stated that ectopic scrotum may be a single dysmorphogenic event during the late blastogenesis period [11].

O'Rahilly and Müller [4] postulated that any ectopic testis/scrotum was probably due to local fibrosis blocking normal descent. It must be recalled that at approximately 40 days of age, the genital tubercle of the human embryo appears as a mound of tissue bounded by the umbilicus, tail, and thighs. Thus there is ample tissue in its lateral and cranial components for a "cone-shaped" or a "many-tailed" gubernaculum to have the potential for multiple connections, providing a simple, although erroneous, explanation for the variety of ectopic scrota. Other hypotheses postulate a congenital obstruction of the 'secondary external inguinal ring' with a subsequent dislocation of the testis to an ectopic location, and subsequently the ipsilateral scrotum became ectopic [12].

**Clinically**: Recently most cases of ectopic scrotum are diagnosed early after delivery, and some cases may raise the confusion of intersex. A unilateral suprainguinal smaller scrotum without testicular contents, but a normal bilateral scrotal sacs are usually seen as a common presentation (Fig. 15.1). Sometimes the suprainguinal ectopic scrotum contains a testis or has one in the immediate vicinity, such ectopia is

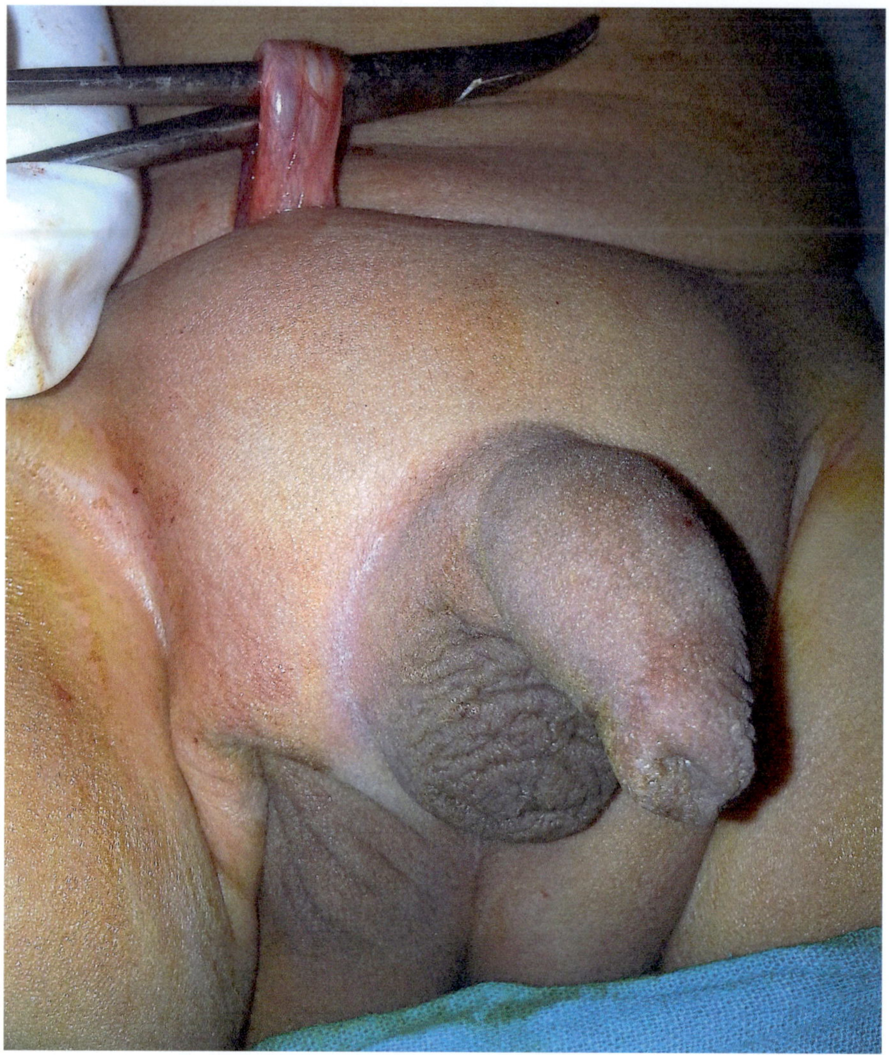

**Fig. 15.3** 8 months old boy with an ectopic perineal scrotum over an ectopic testicle, with an abnormal long gubernaculum inserted in the ectopic scrotum

often associated with ipsilateral upper urinary tract anomalies, which were not reported in the rat model of Ikadai et al. [5]. Ectopic scrotum may be detectable over a perineal ectopic testes with a normally located empty scrotum (Fig. 15.3).

The descent of the testis outside its normal path with resultant formation of an ectopic scrotum may be explained by a malformed or split gubernaculum [13]. Redman and Ferguson at 2005 [6] described a rare case of unilateral caudal extension of the left hemiscrotum to the perineum in an adult patient, ectopic scrotum in this case was described as a factor in the origin of orchalgia and discomfort.

As a suprainguinal ectopic scrotum can be seen in males, so in females a labium majorum may be similarly displaced in an ectopic position, where the normal labia may be even absent, and an extra suprainguinal ectopic labia had been also reported with ARM [14]. Scrotalization of the normally located labia in female is commonly associated with over androgen stimulation; as in most cases of Congenital Adrenogenital Hyperplasia (CAH), where the labia major looks like scrotum. The untreated newborn girl with CAH usually exhibits an ambiguous genitalia with an enlarged clitoris and scrotalization of the labia majora (Prader IV) [15], in such cases the labia looks like a well formed scrotum (Fig. 15.4). Cases of Turner's

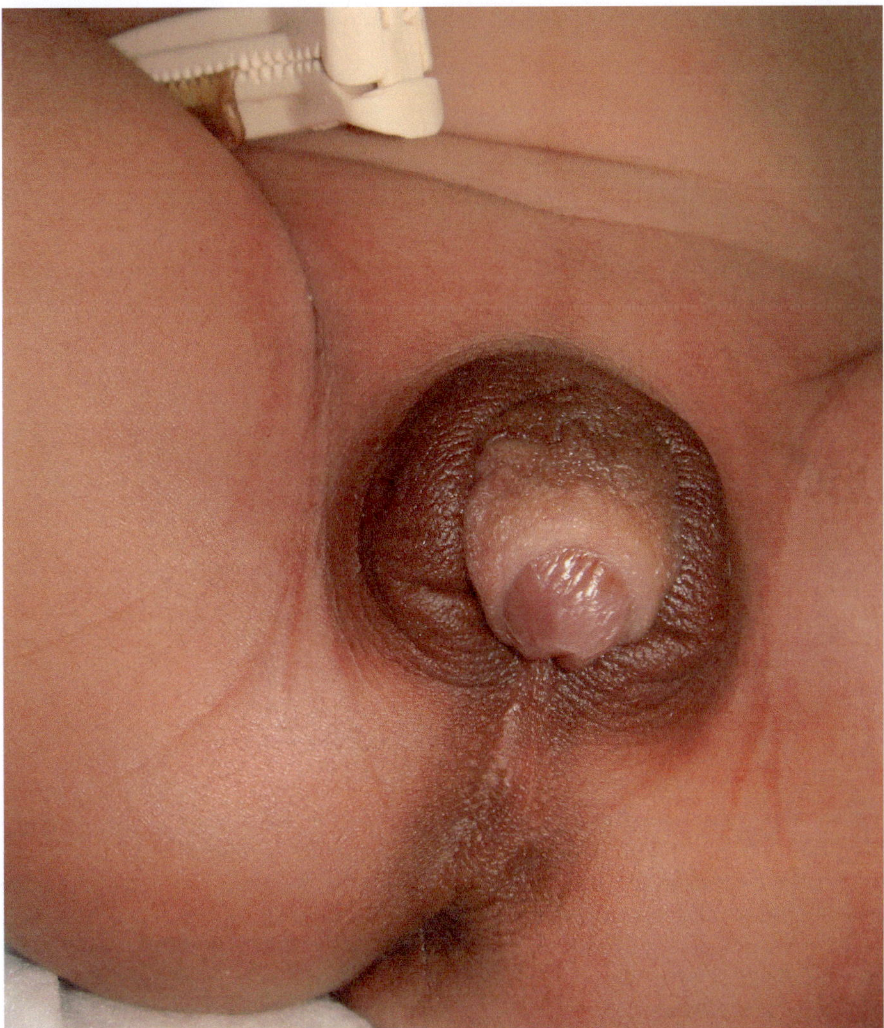

**Fig. 15.4** Labial scrotalization and clitoromegaly in a XX girl with CAH

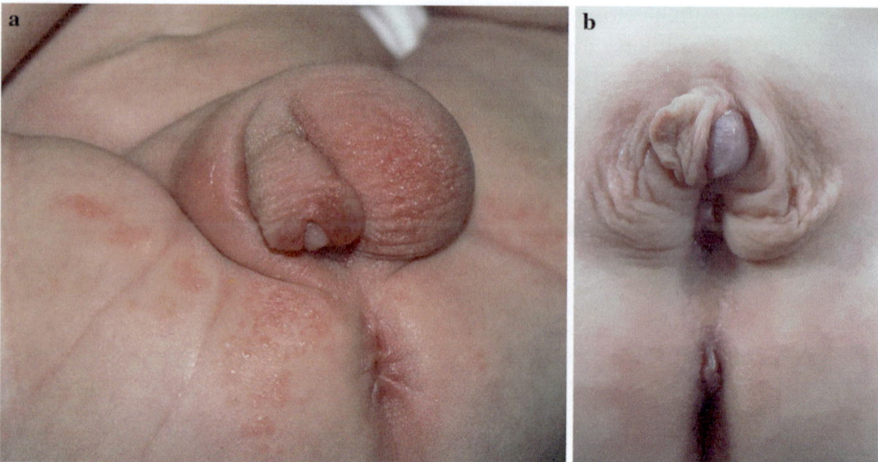

Fig. 15.5 **a** A rare case of unilateral scrotalization in a neonate diagnosed to have Turner's syndrome, **b** bilateral labial scrotalization in Turner's syndrome, a clitoromegaly is also obvious

Fig. 15.6 A normal neonate girl with a scrotalization patch of the right labia without any obvious underling etiology

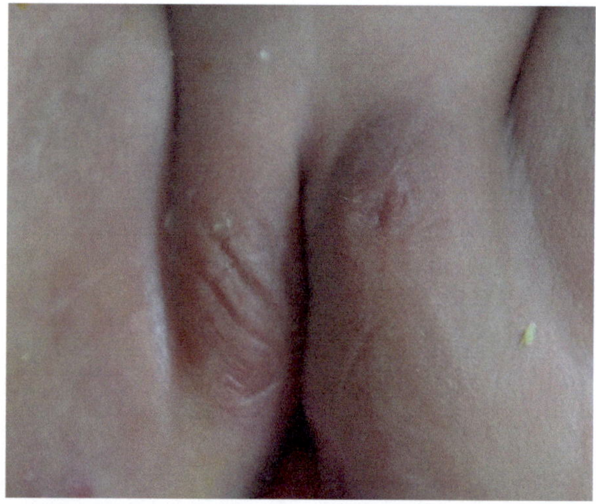

syndrome may presented with a uni or bilateral labial scrotalization, as a sequence to defective feminization, such cases were not reported before (Fig. 15.5).

Localised patches of labial skin looking like the scrotum is a rare idiopathic anomaly, but it may be a manifestation of virilization (Fig. 15.6).

Neonate female, specially the post mature may have transitory, superficial intraepidermal furrows, they are likely related to the long permanence in a moist environment and the consequent maceration; the presence of more or less deep furrows could also be due to the relaxation of the skin after the regression of hormone dependent hypertrophy during the intrauterine life, which is known as the

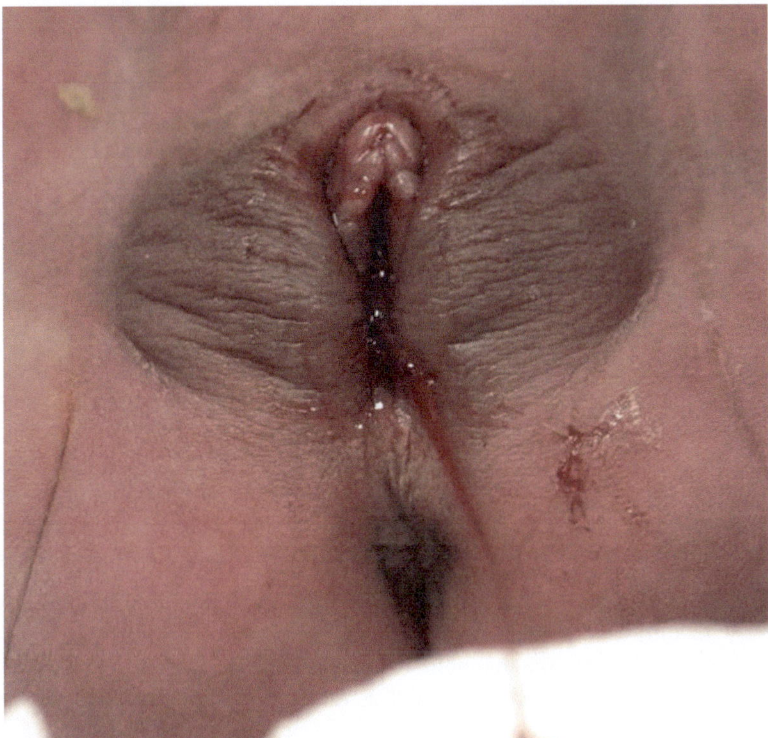

**Fig. 15.7** A normal post-term (post mature) neonate with deep labial furrows; giving the labia major the semblance of scrotum

miniature puberty secondary to maternal hormones [16]. In such cases the labia look like scrotum (Fig. 15.7).

**Differential diagnosis**: Ectopic scrotum should be differentiated from cases of accessory scrotum; as the former cases are usually associated with a major renal anomalies, so it should be detected early. Table 15.1 gives the main points of differentiation between both anomalies. Ectopic scrotum should also be differentiated from cases of penoscrotal transpositional anomalies, specially the unilateral cases (Chap. 12).

**Associated anomalies**: Ipsilateral testicle with ectopic scrotum is usually undescended or ectopic (Fig. 15.3). There is a possible causal interrelationship between upper urinary tract anomalies and the ipsilateral gubernaculum, which might result in the formation of a suprainguinal ectopic scrotum. This does not appear plausible when one postulates a similar causation for a bi- or unilateral femoral ectopic scrotum [7]. Renal agenesis or dysplasia was always ipsilateral to ectopic scrotum. In one review, 70% of boys with a suprainguinal ectopic scrotum, they exhibited ipsilateral upper urinary tract anomalies, including renal agenesis, renal dysplasia,

**Table 15.1** Main differences between ectopic and accessory scrota

|  | Accessory scrotum | Ectopic scrotum |
| --- | --- | --- |
| Normal scrotum | Always present | Always deficient or absent |
| Etiology and pathogenesis | Abnormal labioscrotal folds division and intervening perineal swelling | Abnormally inserted gubernaculum |
| Relation to testicle | Not closely related | Mainly related to cryptorchidism or ectopic testicle |
| Associated Perineal mesenchymal swelling | Cardinal combination | Not common |
| Associated renal anomalies | Not detectable | Commonly associated |

and ectopic ureter [8]. Different forms of ARM are commonly had an ectopic scrotum in both male and female [14, 17]. Patent urachus, bladder exstrophy, cleft lip or palate, spina bifida and leg deformities are a reported associating anomalies [18].

**Investigations**: Patients with an ectopic scrotum should undergo upper urinary tract imaging with ultrasonography basically, with the possible indication for a further investigations modalities like magnetic resonance or renal isotope scanning. Female with an ectopic labia or persistent labial scrotalization should be investigated for any underlying virilization anomalies i.e. CAH, or an androgen secreting tumors.

**Management**: Scrotoplasty and orchiopexy may be performed at 6 to 12 months of age or earlier if other surgical procedures are necessary for an associated anomalies [19]. The recommended intervention is a single stage rotational flap reconstruction with orchidopexy, as it is feasible and should be considered. The management of ectopic scrotum includes one-stage repair (simultaneous scrotoplasty through scrotal transposition and orchiopexy) without sacrificing scrotal tissue, while preserving and relocating the testis. Also one-stage repair for infrainguinal ectopic scrotum with penoplasty for penile torsion is possible without any postoperative complication [20]. Two-stage repair (orchiopexy with subsequent scrotoplasty or scrotoplasty with subsequent orchiopexy), with a rotation flap and excision of defective ectopic scrotal tissue is also reported [21].

# References

1. Adair EL, Lewis EL. J Urol. 1960;84:115.
2. Flanagan MJ, McDonald JH, Krifer JH. J Urol. 1961;86:273.
3. Palmer LS, Palmer JS. Management of anormalities of the external genitalia in boys. In: Wein AJ, Kavoussi LR, Partin AW, Peters CA, editors. Campbell-Walsh Urology. 11th ed. Philadelphia: Elsevier; 2016. p. 3382.

4. O'Rahilly R, Müller F. Human embryology and teratology. New York: Wiley-Liss; 1992. p. 219–21.
5. Ikadai HC, Ajisawa K, Taya, Imamichi T. Suprainguinal ectopic scrota of TS inbred rats. J Reprod Fertil. 1988;84:701–7.
6. Tedman JF, Ferguson SF. Unilateral perineal ectopic scrotum resulting in debilitating orchalgia: diagnosis and management. J Urol. 2005;(173):104–5. https://doi.org/10.1097/01.ju.0000146671.36646.26.
7. Hoar R, Calvano CJ, Reddy PP, Bauer SB, Mandell J. Unilateral suprainguinal ectopic scrotum: the role of the gubernaculum in the formation of an ectopic scrotum. Teratology. 1998;57:64–9.
8. Elder JS, Jeffs RD. Suprainguinal ectopic scrotum and associated anomalies. J Urol. 1982;127:336–8.
9. Wahyudi I, Ardianson I, Gerhard D, Situmorang R, Rodjani A. One stage rotation flap scrotoplasty and orchidopexy for the correction of ectopic scrotum: a case report. Urology Case Reports
10. Volume 25, July 2019, https://doi.org/10.1016/j.eucr.2019.100886.
11. Bawa M, Garge S, Sekhon V, Rao K. Inguinal ectopic scrotum, anorectal malformation with sacral agenesis and limb defects: an unusual presentation. J Korean Pediatr Surg. 2015;21(2):32.
12. Punwani VV, Wong JS, Lai CYH, Chia CY, Hutson JM. Testicular ectopia: why does it happen and what do we do? J Pediatr Surg. 2017;52:1842–7.
13. Snell RS. Clinical embryology for medical students. Boston: Little, Brown and Company; 1975. p. 235.
14. So EP, Brock W, Kaplan GW. Ectopic labium and VATER association in a newborn. J Urol. 1980;124:156–7.
15. New MI, Wilson RC. Steroid disorders in children: congenital adrenal hyperplasia and apparent mineralocorticoid excess. Proc Natl Acad Sci. 1999;96(22):12790–7. https://doi.org/10.1073/pnas.96.22.12790.
16. Cutrone M, Milano A, Rovatti G, Bonifazi E. Genital and anal anatomical variants. Eur J Pediat Dermatol. 2013;23:29–45.
17. Spears T, Franco I, Reda EF, Hernandez-Graulau J, Levitt SB. Accessory and ectopic scrotum with VATER association. Urology. 1992;40(4). https://doi.org/10.1016/0090-4295(92)90385-A.
18. Chiang G, Cendron M. Disorders of the penis and scrotum. In: Gearhart JP, Rink RC, Mouriquand P, editors. Pediatric Urology. 2nd ed. Philadelphia: Saunders Elsevier; 2010. p. 553.
19. Palmer LS, Palmer JS. (146) Management of Abnormalities of the External Genitalia in Boys. Campbell Walsh Wein Urology, 12th edn. www.elsevier.com/books/campbell-walsh-urology/partin/978-0.
20. Hisamatsu E, Shibata R, Yoshino K. Surgical correction of ectopic scrotum and penile torsion in a 5-year-old boy. Indian J Urol. 2019;35(4):299–300. https://doi.org/10.4103/iju.IJU_160_19.
21. Daniel G, Coleman R. Staged rotation flap scrotoplasty and orchidopexy in a patient with inguinal ectopic scrotum. J Surg Case Rep. 2015:2015.
22. Singh RR, Seager RL, Shibu M, Misra D, Joshi A. Ectopic scrotum: single stage rotational flap reconstruction with orchidopexy. J Pediatr Surg Case Rep. 2020;58. https://doi.org/10.1016/j.epsc.2020.101469.

# Chapter 16
# Accessory Scrotum

**Mohamed A. Baky Fahmy**

## Abbreviations

AS     Accessory Scrotum
FIF     Fetus in Fetu
ARM   Anorectal Malformation

**Definition**: Accessory scrotum is the rare presentation of the scrotal skin or scrotal sac outside its normal location, in either the perineum or elsewhere, without any included testicular tissue, in addition to a normally developed scrotum in its normal position, it differs from ectopic scrotum; which defined as the existence of the normal scrotal tissue outside its normal location with a deficient normal one. (Figs. 16.1 and 16.2) Such rare cases diagnosed by existence of scrotum-like tissues similar to the scrotum macroscopically and histopathologically, AS does not contain testicular tissue, but presents as an isolated, rugae sac with tunica beneath the scrotal dermis. Perineal lipoma or rarely other mesenchymal tumors are more often observed in concomitant with AS [1]. It has been postulated that similar pathology is responsible for the accessory labioscrotal fold (labium majorum) which seen rarely in females [2] (Fig. 16.3). On rare occasions, a perineal lipomas can coexist also in female patients with an accessory labioscrotal fold. An ectopic scrotolized skin affecting the labia major is a more commoner anomalies in females.

**Combination with a perineal swellings**: When accessory scrotum is accompanied with a perineal lipomatous mass, the two lesions are so contiguous. AS is usually attached to a lipomatous mass as a pedunculated skin tag or an incompletely separated protruding second nodule [3] (Fig. 16.4). In a review of 43 cases of AS by Murase et al. [4] a contiguous subcutaneous tumor had a high incidence in association with AS, most of them were lipoma (72.5%) other less common swellings are hamartoma, fibroma and lipoblastoma.

M. A. B. Fahmy (✉)
Al-Azhar University, Cairo, Egypt

     215
M. A. B. Fahmy (ed.), *Normal and Abnormal Scrotum*,
https://doi.org/10.1007/978-3-030-83305-3_16

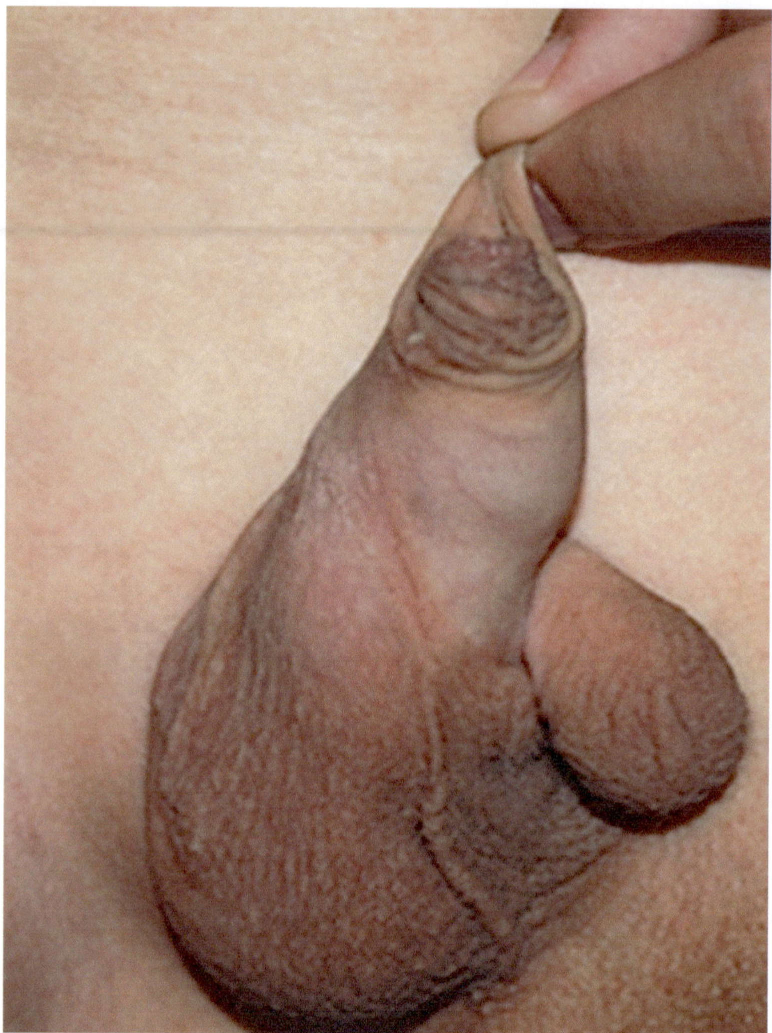

**Fig. 16.1** Left lateral accessory scrotum with left undescended testicle, with deviation of the penile raphae to the right side. From Ref. [10] with a kind permission from Dr. Zoran Gucev

**Classifications**: Accessory scrotum has been classified into two main subtypes, depending on its location: the mid-perineum type and the lateral type [5] (Figs. 16.1 and 16.2).

AS usually associating cases of diphallia. Other extremely rare phenotype of AS with bifid scrotum and penoscrotal hypospadias had been reported. Very rarely (few case reports) the AS presented as a remote scrotum-like protuberance in the back or the buttock, and it is considered as a back variant of AS.

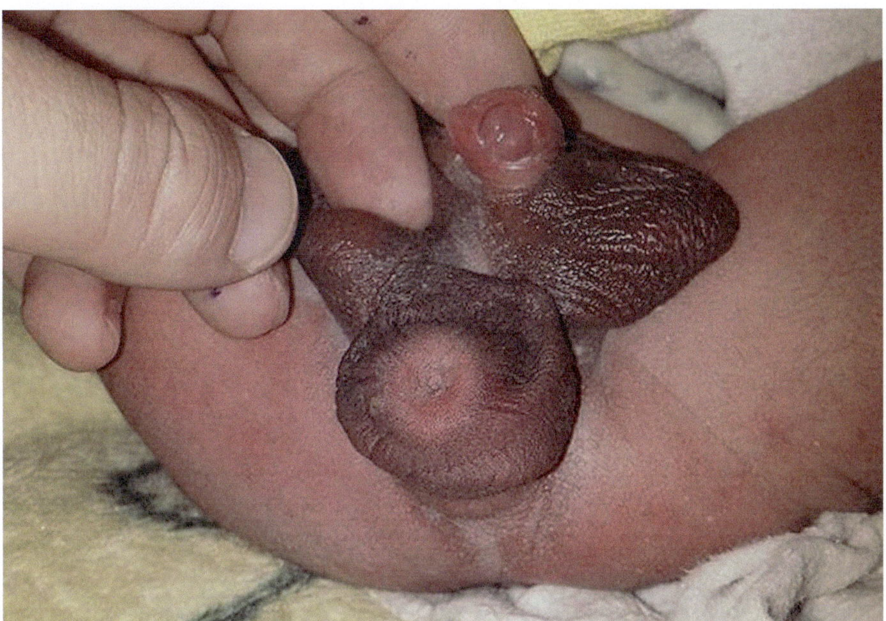

**Fig. 16.2** Accessory scrotum at the perineum with a normal scrotum and penis, but with ARM

**Associated anomalies**: Interestingly, and without clear explanation; there is no renal anomalies were identified in the reported cases of AS. Perineal lipoma is the more often pathology observed in combination. Other associated scrotal anomalies include: bifid scrotum, scrotal transposition, and diphallia, which are not rare with AS [6, 7].

**Penile anomalies**: Many cases reported with a normally-situated external genitalia and urethra, but penile torsion, hypospadias are the most common association. Complete absence of the median scrotal raphe is also common with AS, it is likely that the splitting and posterior migration of the accessory penoscrotal tissue during early gestation may interfere with the development of the anorectum and the development and fusion of the genital folds, which accounting for these findings [8] (Fig. 16.1). One case had been reported with an associated bifid scrotum and diphallia, and another case had glandular hypospadias [7]. Maldescended testicles are also common, (either in the form of cryptorchidism or ectopic testicle), inguinal hernia, and bladder exstrophy had been also reported. Theoretically, with the simultaneous development of the scrotum and the anus, it is possible that the association of accessory scrotum with anorectal malformation may not occur by chance; they probably represent simultaneous developmental events [9]. Accessory scrotum and pseudodiphallia have a high incidence of association with ARMs (Figs. 16.2 and 16.6).

**Skeletal anomalies**: Tibial atresia [10], and other multiple skeletal anomalies had been reported [11].

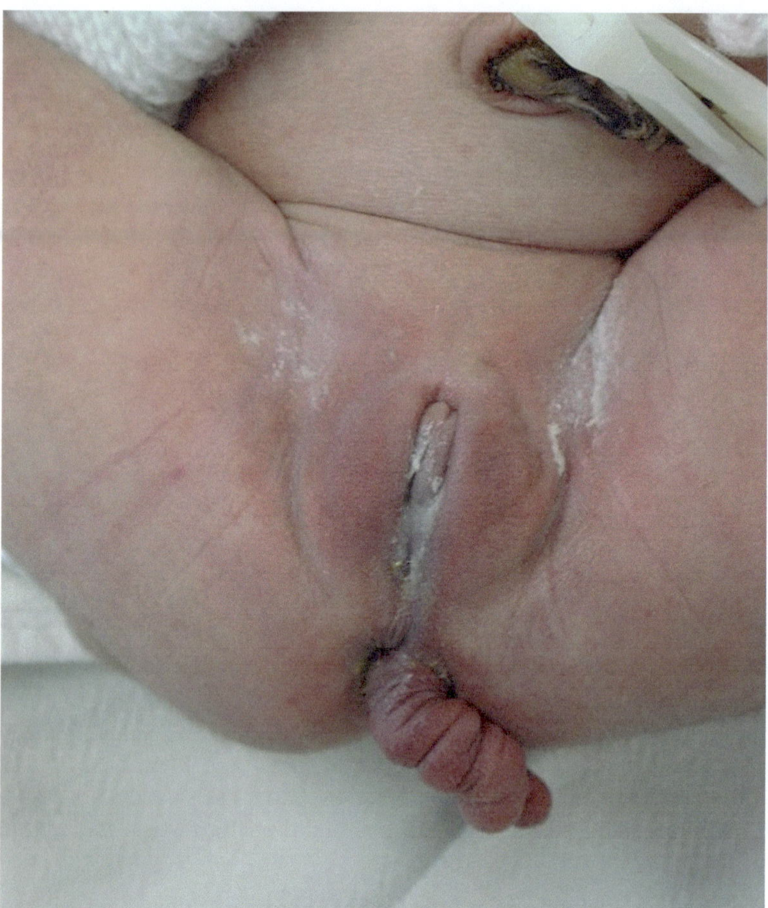

**Fig. 16.3** Neonate girl with a perianal swelling resembles the scrotum

**Systemically**: few cases of AS were reported with the popliteal pterygium syndrome [12] (Fig. 16.5).

Only one case had been reported with a retrocerebellar arachnoid cyst and penoscrotal transposition [6]. Szylit et al. [13] reported at 1986 the first patient with both a Becker's nevus and an accessory perineal scrotum, postulating that both anomalies were a result of both embryologic abnormalities and grow up later on by androgenic stimulation. Becker's nevus was originally described as an acquired hyperpigmented, hypertrichotic macule with androgen receptors in high concentrations like that in scrotal skin.

**Pathogenesis**: A review of the literature does not provide enough informations on the confirmed causative mechanism for the occurrence of accessory scrotum. The most accepted etiopathogenetic hypothesis for this condition is that an abnormal migration of labioscrotal swelling mainly due to distention of an associated lipoma

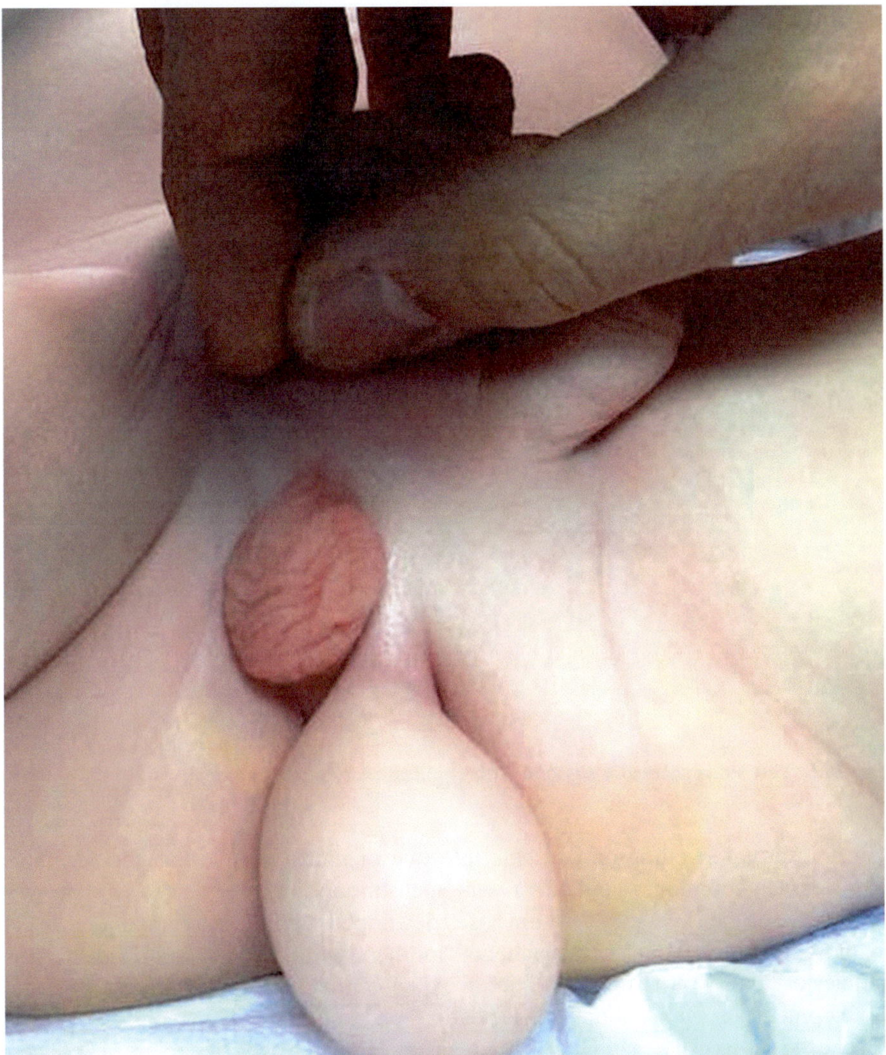

**Fig. 16.4** Perineal accessory scrotum over a pedunculated perineal lipoma

or compression by the foetus's heel in utero [12]. Takayasu et al. [14] have hypothesized that a mid-perineum AS may result from a triple primordial analogous of the labioscrotal swelling or from a teratomatous structure. Lamm et al. [15] suggested that the lateral type of AS might represent a duplication or division of the ipsilateral labioscrotal swelling. Coupris and Bondonny [16] proposed abnormal division of the labioscrotal swelling as the causative factor for the occurrence of accessory scrotum. Sule et al. [5] suggested that the abnormal mesenchymal tissue (including lipoma, lipoblastoma and hamartoma) in the perineal region could divide

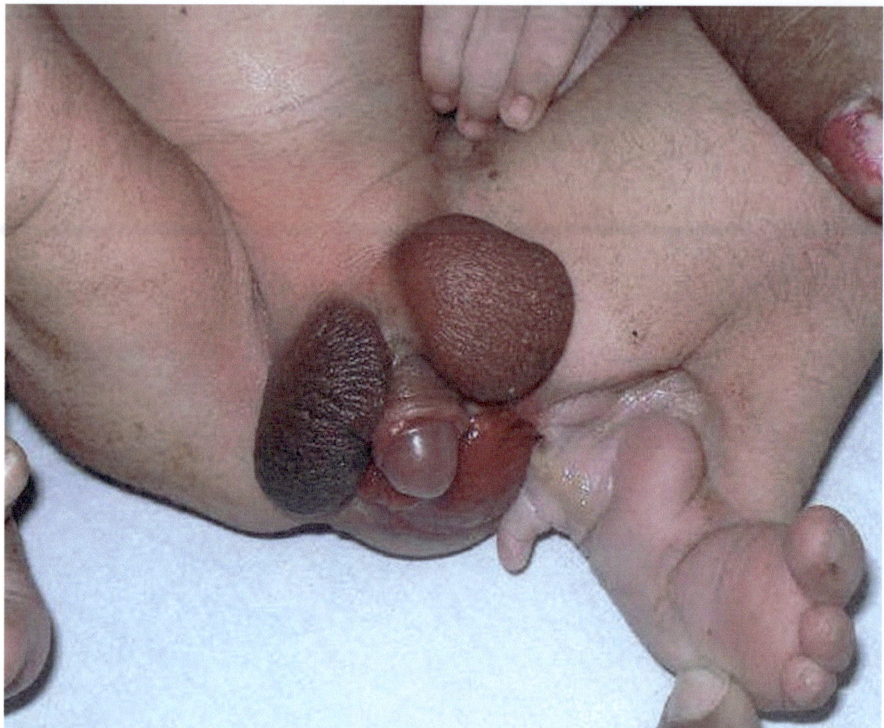

**Fig. 16.5** Left sided accessory scrotum with popliteal pterygium syndrome

the labioscrotal swelling on one side into two or more parts so that the accessory scrotum was commonly coincident with such tumors, that seemed to explain why about 83% of the accessory scrotum cases developed with mesenchymal tumors [4]. In most literature, none of the patients' mothers with AS had complicated pregnancies or history of harmful gestational exposure that might have predispose to the development of such anomalies. Detection of uncommon cutaneous hamartoma (Becker's nevus) that has been shown to contain androgen receptors in concentrations similar to those in genital skin in combination with AS, raised the possibility of over androgenic stimulation as a possible cause of the last anomaly [13].

**Fetus in fetu (FIF):** There are few cases reported with an accessory small penis and scrotum on the buttock, lumbar or posterior thoracic regions, which considered as an accessory small penis with well-formed glans, urethral meatus, and scrotum over the swelling. There were no formed testes [17].

Scrotal tissue of such cases is reported as an AS, which could be considered either as a fetus in fetu (FIF), pseuodotail, pseudo duplication or a hamartoma. If the accessory swelling only looks like the phallus it is called pseudophallia. The most widely accepted theory is that FIF results from the unequal division of the totipotent cells of a blastocyst. The smaller twin then gets incorporated within the normally developing twin by unknown mechanisms. The most common site of FIF is the retroperitoneum, unlike teratoma, which often occurs in the lower abdomen and pelvis [18, 19].

**Pseudotail**: Pseudotail is a dermal appendage arising from the lumbosacral region with spinal dysraphism containing bone, cartilage, notochord or spinal cord tissues. Sometimes a phallus or a scrotal like structure is appreciated in such cases, and this considered as an AS at a remote sites [20].

Pseudoduplication of the external genitalia is also extremely uncommon; it is probably best regarded as a localized or unsuccessful form of caudal duplication or twinning. Most similar cases consist of an accessory scrotum alone, which in itself is an extremely rare condition [21] (Fig. 16.6).

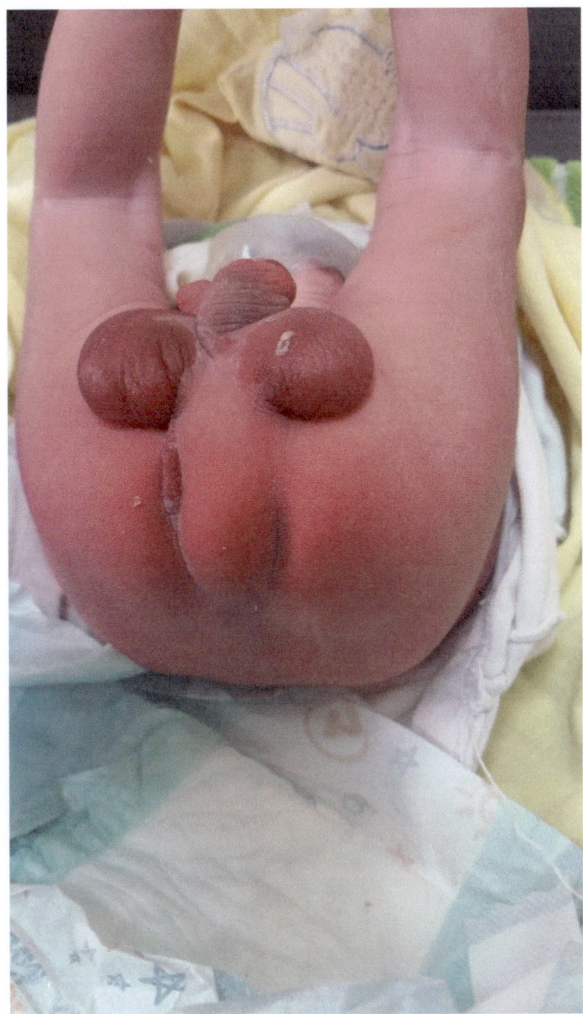

**Fig. 16.6** A case of penile duplication and scrotal duplication; which could be considered as an AS with a high ARM, this photo provided by Dr. Ahmed Maher Ali (Maher et al.) Assistant lecturer of pediatric surgery at Assiut University Hospital [7]

                                                          

Hamartoma is another variant of pseudodiphallia, where there is a rudimentary atrophic penis existing independently of the normal penis [22] (Fig. 16.7). The most likely explanation for the embryogenesis of this abnormality is that during early gestation an embryonic tissue with the potential to develop into the skin of the phallus, scrotum, and anal region splits and migrates posteriorly.

**Manifestations**: The manifestations were consistent with the described pathogenesis hypothesis. AS usually seen in combination with other anomalies or at least with a perineal swelling, most of it were lipoma which consisted of only adipocytes. In the two cases presented by Zhong et al. [23] there are soft fibroma composed mainly of collagen and fibroblasts, isolated fibroma seldom arises in children, especially in the perineal region. AS is usually configured as a rounded or pear like soft or firm structure, but there is no explanation why the abnormal extra scrotum

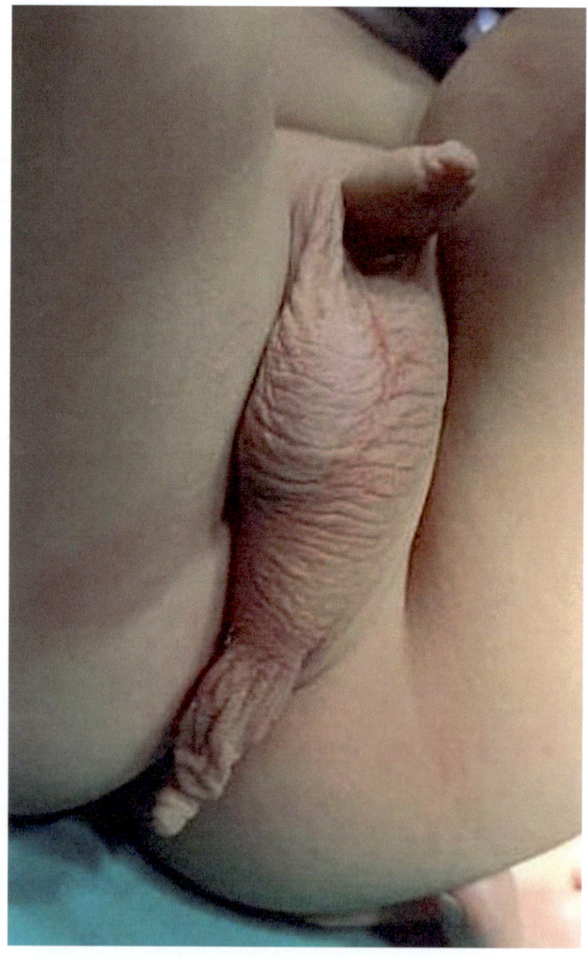

Fig. 16.7 A case of accessory scrotum, which configured as a pseudophallus, this photo kindly provided by Dr. Ali Aliu and Dr. Isber Ademaj, University Clinical Center of Kosovo. Pediatric surgery clinic in Prishtina

takes the shape of the phallus. (Fig. 16.7) Prenatal diagnosis of AS is possible as reported since 1999 by Özcan et al. [9]. Many cases may be roughly diagnosed after delivery as an ambiguous genitalia or intersex, but careful examination will reveal the normal scrotum and penis, AS with or without hypospadias.

**Differential diagnosis**: In literatures, specially in case reports, their is a misleading between accessory and ectopic scrota. Actually in some cases it is difficult to have a definite discrimination between the two anomalies. As the pathogenesis of both conditions is different; the ectopic scrota usually secondary to abnormal migration or insertion of the gubernaculum, while the AS is commonly combined with a mesenchymal perineal swellings. So we adopt the main differences between these two conditions is the presence of a normal scrota with an extra scrotal swelling in AS and deficient normal hemiscrotum in ectopic cases. Also ectopic scrotum usually presented as a small patch of skin and rarely seen as a pendulous swelling.

**Investigations**: Magnetic resonance imaging is usually requested to diagnose the nature and extension of the accompanying perianal swelling, usually the mass was homogenous with high signal intensity on T1- and T2-weighted images in cases of lipoma. Cases with suspected skeletal, spinal or neurological associated anomalies should be investigated accordingly and individually.

The histopathological findings of the surgically excised extra scrotum showing the scrotal skin with underlying dartos facia and muscle fibers, the excised accompanying swelling also revealed that the majority of the main mass consisted of mature adipose tissue, muscle fibers and scattered neural tissue in the fibrous septal wall [24].

**Management**: Surgery was the only treatment option. AS is treated with complete surgical excision. Careful and detailed histological examination for AS and the combined mesenchymal swellings is mandatory. The other urogenital anomalies would require additional corrective surgery. Surgical excision of the AS and corrective surgical interventions should be planned for neonates for the near future, as they are not urgent.

# References


1. Chatterjee S, Gajbhiye V, Nath S, Ghosh D, Chattopadhyay S, Das SK. Perineal accessory scrotum with congenital lipoma: a rare case report. Case Rep Pediatr. 2012:757120–2. https://doi.org/10.1155/2012/757120.
2. Numajiri T, Nishino K, Sowa Y, Konishi K. Congenital vulvar lipoma within an accessory labioscrotal fold. Pediatr Dermatol. 2011;28:424–8. https://doi.org/10.1111/j.1525-1470.2011.01237.x.
3. Amann G, Berger A, Rokitansky A. Accessory scrotum or perineal collision-hamartoma: a case report to illustrate a misnomer. Pathol Res Pract. 1996;192:1039–43.
4. Murase N, Uchida H, Hiramatsu K. Accessory scrotum with perineal lipoma diagnosed prenatally: case report and review of the literature. Nagoya J Med Sci. 2015;77(3):501–6.

5. Sule JD, Skoog SJ, Tank ES. Perineal lipoma and the accessory labioscrotal fold: an etiological relationship. J Urol. 1994;151(2):475–7. https://doi.org/10.1016/s0022-5347(17)34996-0.
6. Kawa G, Kawakita S, Ohara T, Matsuda T. Accessor scrotum with penoscrotal transposition and retrocerebellar arachnoid cyst. Int Urol. 1997;4:327–8.
7. Ahmed Maher Ali. Tarek Abdelazeem Sabra, Hussein Ibrahim, Mahmoud Mostafa: newborn with complete double penis and two separate scrotums: a case report. Int J Surg Case Rep. 2020. https://doi.org/10.1016/j.ijscr.2020.11.002.
8. Chadha R, Gupta S, Mahajan JK, Kothari SK. Two cases of pseudoduplication of the external genitalia. Pediatr Surg Int. 2001;17:572–4.
9. Özcan C, Celik A, Erdener A. Accessory perineal scrotum associated with anorectal malformation. BJU Int. 1999;83:729–30.
10. Gucev Z, Castori M, Tasic V, Popjordanova N, Hasani A. A patient with unilateral tibial aplasia and accessory scrotum: a pure coincidence or nonfortuitous association? Case Rep Med. 2010:4 p. https://doi.org/10.1155/2010/898636.
11. Kendirci M, Horasanli K, Miroglu C. Accessory scrotum with multiple skeletal abnormalities. Int J Urol. 2006;13:648–50. https://doi.org/10.1111/j.1442-2042.2006.01362.x.
12. Cunningham LN, Keating MA, Snyder HM, et al. Urological manifestations of the popliteal pterygium syndrome. J Urol. 1989;141:910–2.
13. Szylit J, Grossman M E, Luyando Y, Olarte M and Naglar M. Becker's nevus and an accessory scrotum. J Am Acad Dermatol. 1986;14:905–907.
14. Takayasu H, Ueno A, Tsukada O. Acdessory scrotum: a case report. J Urol. 1974;112:826–7.
15. Lamm DL, Kaplan GW. Accessory and ectopic scrota. Urology. 1977;9(2):149–53. https://doi.org/10.1016/0090-4295(77)90185-6.
16. Coupris L, Bondonny JM. The accessory scrotum. Apropos of 2 cases. Chir Pediatr. 1987;28(1):61–3.
17. Wang YZ, Cao L, Cai C. Accessory penis and scrotum in a male infant. J Child Sci. 2017;7:e24–6. https://doi.org/10.1055/s-0037-1604158.
18. Tiwari C, Shah H, Kumbhar V, Sandlas G, Jayaswal S. Fetus in fetu: two cases and literature review. Dev Period Med. 2016;20(03):174–7.
19. Kubo T, Eto H, Inoue T, Tanaka H, Amano M. Case of accessory scrotum with hamartoma located in sacrococcygeal region: the first report. J Dermatol. 2020;47:e248–9. https://doi.org/10.1111/1346-8138.15338.
20. Raines MD, Wills ML, Jackson GP. Imperforate anus with a rectovestibular fistula and pseudotail: a case report. J Med Case Rep. 2010;7(4):317.
21. Vilanova X, Raventos A. Pseudodiphallia, a rare anomaly. J Urol. 1954;71: 338±346
22. Daut WW, Daut RV. Accessory scrotum, posteriorly located. Review of the literature and report of case. J Iowa Med Soc. 1949;39:194–200.
23. Zhong L, Zou X Sun J. Two cases of accessory scrotum with soft fibroma in neonates. Indian J Surg. 2020. https://doi.org/10.1007/s12262-020-02241-8.
24. Ramzisham AR, Thambidorai CR. Perineal hamartoma with accessory scrotum, anorectal anomaly, and hypospadias-a rare association with embryological significance: case report. Pediatr Surg Int. 2005;21:478–81.

# Chapter 17
# Scrotal Median Raphe Anomalies

Mohamed A. Baky Fahmy

## Abbreviations

| | |
|---|---|
| GMR | Genital Median Raphe |
| SR | Scrotal Raphe |
| AGD | Anogenital distance |
| IPM | Intact Prepuce Megameatus |
| MAIS | Mild Androgen Insensitivity Syndrome |
| MRC | Median Raphe Cyst |

## 17.1  Normal Scrotal Raphe

**Definition**: Raphe means a line of fusion of the two halves of various symmetrical body parts, and the term median raphe refers to the perineal raphe, which is also known as the median raphe of the perineum; and it is divided anatomically to: penile raphe, scrotal and perineal raphae. This line starts just anterior to the anus and extends through the scrotum, continuing on the ventral surface of the penis and prepuce; it is usually darker in colour than the surrounding skin; specially in coloured men, generally it is deep pink or brown and usually devoid of hair (Fig. 17.1).

Genital Median Raphe (GMR) is a result of a fetal developmental phenomenon; whereby the labioscrotal folds migrate infromedially toward the midline and fuse, to form this line which represents the superficial effects of the midline fusion of ectoderm along these areas, as development progresses, the ectodermal edges of the urethral groove begin to fuse to form the median raphe. This embryological line or ridge may be subjected to a various anomalies, which not well known by many

M. A. B. Fahmy (✉)
Al-Azhar University, Cairo, Egypt

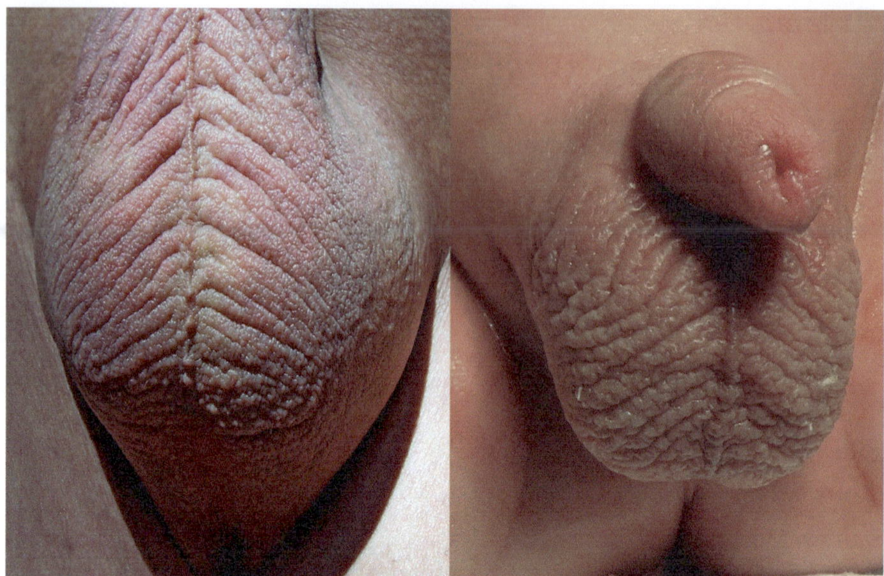

**Fig. 17.1** Normal scrotal raphe in adult and child

practitioners, and can thus pass unnoticed, specially in children. The raphe is characterized by dense fibrovascular tissue with a conspicuous parallel and longitudinal orientation. It may for some time reveal a groove in the midline, in which some pseudostratified columnar epithelium may extend from the margins of the urethra. So raphe is an epithelial-mesenchymal interaction (a subcutaneous fibrous plate), it has been hypothesized that the delayed fusion is under control of androgen hormone [1] (Chap. 8).

As a derivative of the cloaca and supportive mesenchymal structures, the anogenital region demonstrates from the beginning of its development with a special histological features in the structure of the epidermis and its appendages and in the presence of fascial tissue instead of the usual dermis and subcutaneous tissues [2]. The septum of the scrotum is a vertical layer of fibrous tissue that divides the scrotum into two compartments. It consists of flexible connective tissue, and its structure extends to the skin surface as the scrotal raphe. It is an incomplete wall of connective tissue and nonstriated dartos muscle fibers dividing the scrotum into two sacs, each containing a testis. (Fig. 17.2).

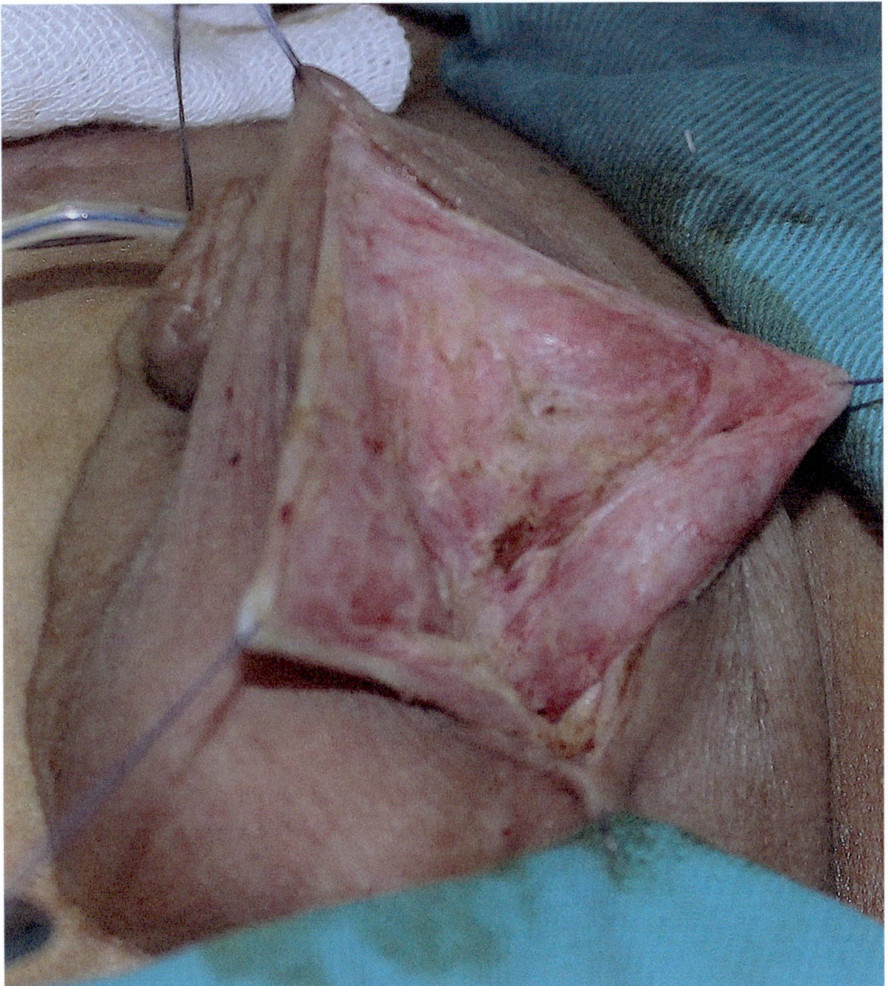

**Fig. 17.2** Scrotal raphe from inside; showing the scrotal septum during surgery via the raphe incision

## 17.2   Significance of GMR Anomalies

GMR is a midline structure, but its deviation to one side is considered as a sign indicating other undetectable anomalies, and during the last decade there were many publications concerned with the significance of raphe deviation in norm and diseased, Neff at 1936 [3] was the first one who draw the attention about the importance of raphe anomalies. It becomes crucial to examine GMR in every baby to detect any obvious or hidden congenital genitourinary anomalies, as such anomalies of GMR are not so rare as thought before, and some anomalies may necessitate surgical correction. Pathology of the GMR anomalies may be simple, carries no direct impact on the child health and in many occasions it needs no surgical intervention, but its significance mainly comes from the serious associated anomalies, which are usually hidden and may be only disclosed after detection of GMR anomalies; as in cases of IPM for example [4]. Also recently, with the advance in ultrasound techniques, median raphe could be visualised accurately antenatally as an indictor not only for sex determination, where the male fetus was recognised by the scrotal sacs separated by an echogenic median raphe, but also it may gives a hint about any associated anomalies; like hypospadias [5]. As we will see from the wide range of GMR anomalies, such anomalies may be used in the future for more detection and diagnosis of other congenital genitourinary anomalies antenatally. In a survey of 2880 babies aged from 1 day to 7 weeks we detected an overall incidence of raphe anomalies of about 2%, with a wide spectrum ranging from simple anomaly like prominent raphe to raphe cysts and canals [6]. An extensive study of the complex histological composition of the median raphe in human embryo, with a special reference to the embryonic differential development between male and female raphae was published by Zhe et al. [7].

## 17.3 Anoscrotal Distance (Anogenital Distance)

The Anogenital distance (AGD)  has been suggested to represent a phenotypic signature reflecting in-utero androgen action, and it may have impaction throughout life. It is longer in males than in females in both rodents and humans. It is suggested that boys born with cryptorchidism or hypospadias have shorter AGD, and cross-sectional studies have found an associations between shorter AGD and lower testosterone levels, poorer semen quality, and infertility in adult men [8].

Table 17.1 refer the wide variations of different opinions of publications concerned with the AGD and its relation to hypospadias and undescended testis [9–14].

**Table 17.1** AGD, hypospadias and undescended testis

| Title | Year of publication | Ref |
|---|---|---|
| Caucasian male infants and boys with hypospadias exhibit reduced anogenital distance | 2012 | [9] |
| Shorter anogenital distance correlates with undescended testis: a detailed genital anthropometric analysis in human newborns | 2013 | [10] |
| Anogenital distance and penile length in infants with hypospadias or cryptorchidism: comparison with normative data | 2014 | [11] |
| Shorter anogenital distance correlates with the severity of hypospadias in pre-pubertal boys | 2016 | [12] |
| Prenatal Anogenital Distance Is Shorter in Fetuses With Hypospadias | 2017 | [13] |
| Shorter anogenital and anoscrotal distances correlate with the severity of hypospadias: A prospective study | 2017 | [14] |

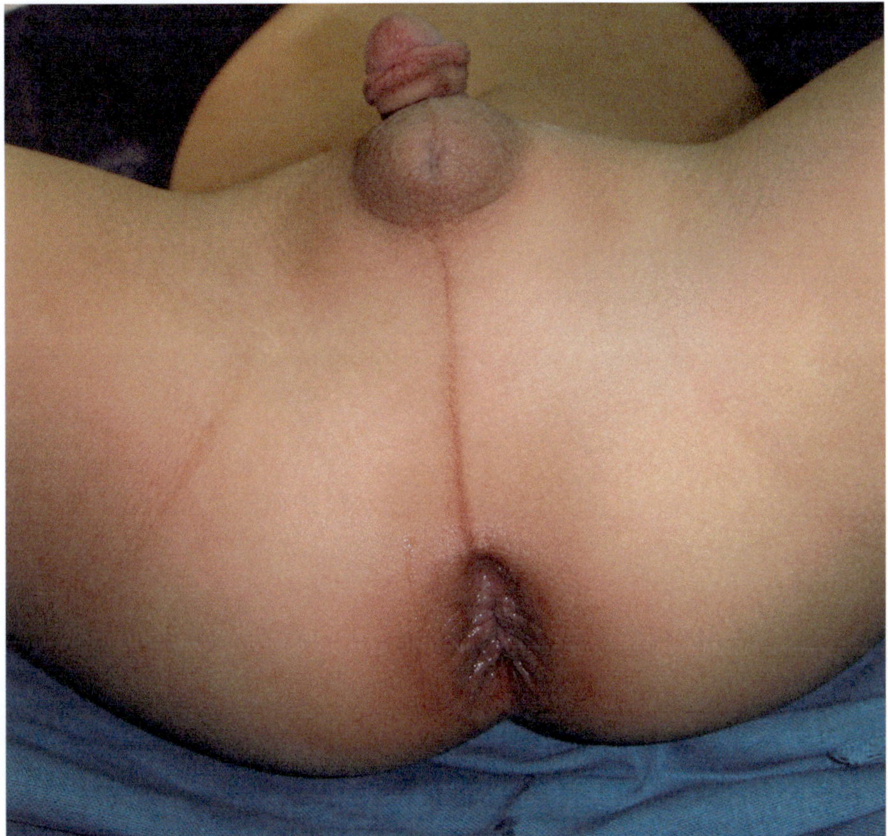

**Fig. 17.3** Very wide AGD in a normal child, aged 2 years old

Normal scrotum is very rarely seen more cephalically or caudally positioned, but we encountered may cases with a wide AGD (wider separation of the scrotum from the anus) in a completely normal children (Fig. 17.3), and this may be attributed to a posteriorly positioned anus, other than an anteriorly positioned scrotum. In the other way around this distance may be normally shorter than usual without any associated anomalies. Detailed abnormal scrotal position was discussed in Chap. 12.

## 17.4  Common Scrotal Raphe Anomalies

**1. Absent Scrotal Raphe**: Absent median raphe either in the scrotum alone or with deficient penile raphe is rarely seen in a normal male. (Fig. 17.4) In our series of cases diagnosed with raphe anomalies; three babies were detected to have no median raphe and 2 of them had also a hypospadias [6]. Absent median raphe is reported in associated with transverse testicular ectopia, where both testes were

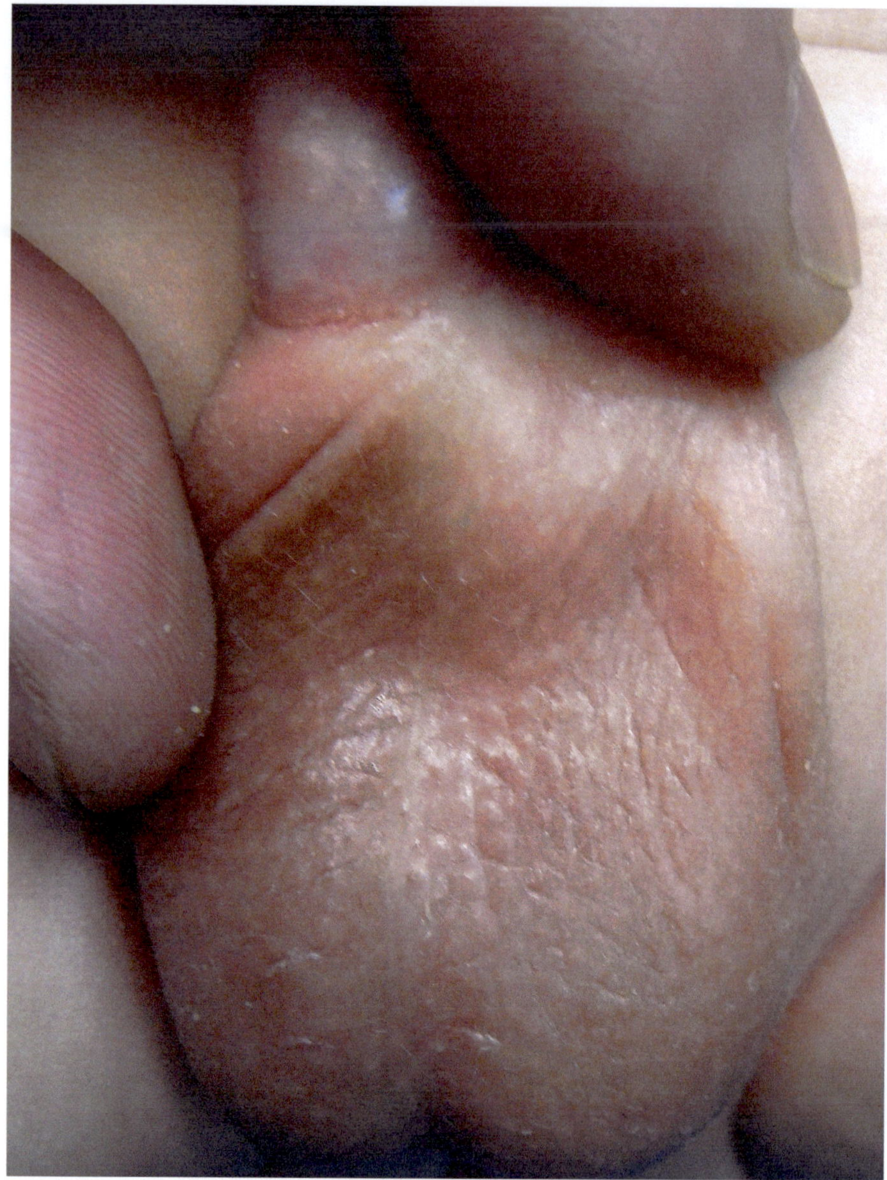

**Fig. 17.4** Absent scrotal raphe in otherwise normal child

normal in size, shape and signal intensity, and there was a single scrotal sac and no median raphe was appreciable [15]. Such cases may also have no scrotal septum in association with absent raphe. Also in some cases of perineal ectopic testis the scrotal raphe is also absent, but on the other hand we diagnosed many other cases of perineal ectopic testicles with a well demarcated scrotal raphe. (Figs. 17.5 and 17.6) Sometimes when the median scrotal raphe is absent then there is a very high likelihood incidence of severe urinary tract anomalies, including absent kidneys (renal dysplasia or agenesis) [16]. A combination of penile agenesis, imperforate anus, and absence of the scrotal and perineal raphae is an ominous physical finding

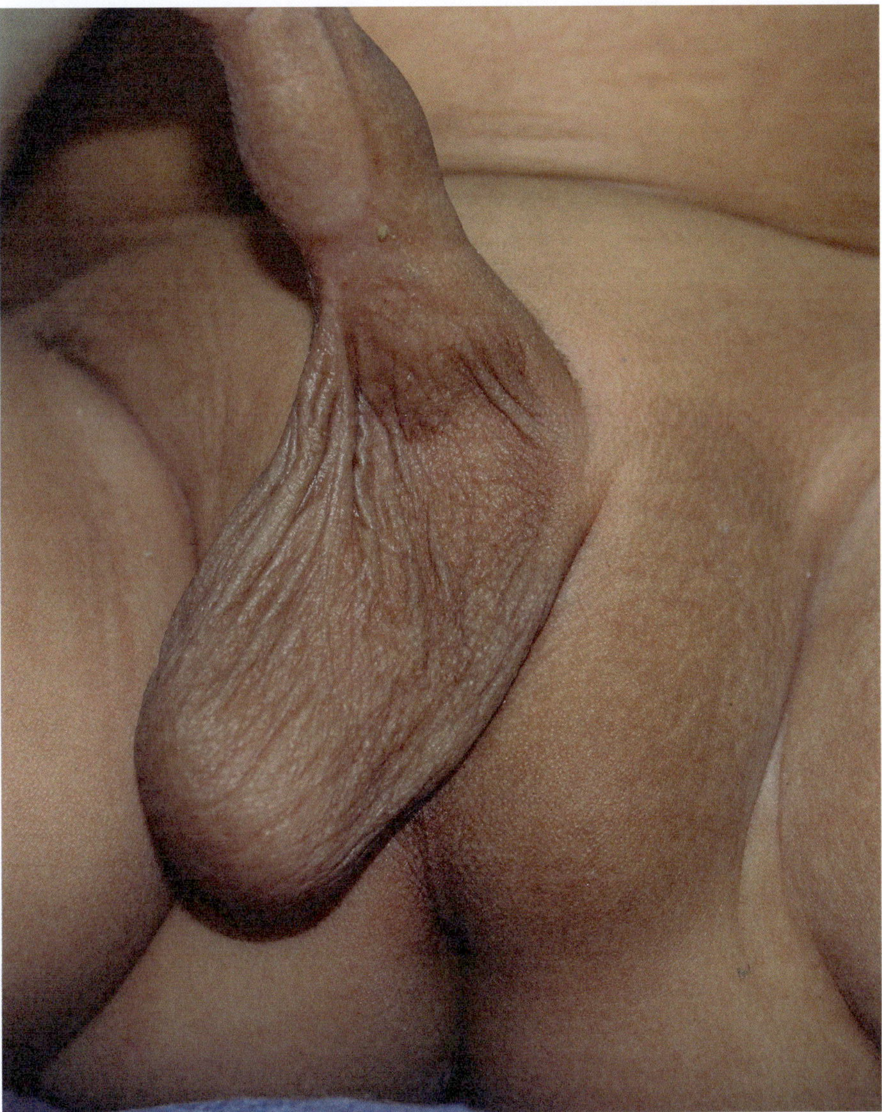

**Fig. 17.5** An absent scrotal raphe in association with a left sided perineal ectopic testis

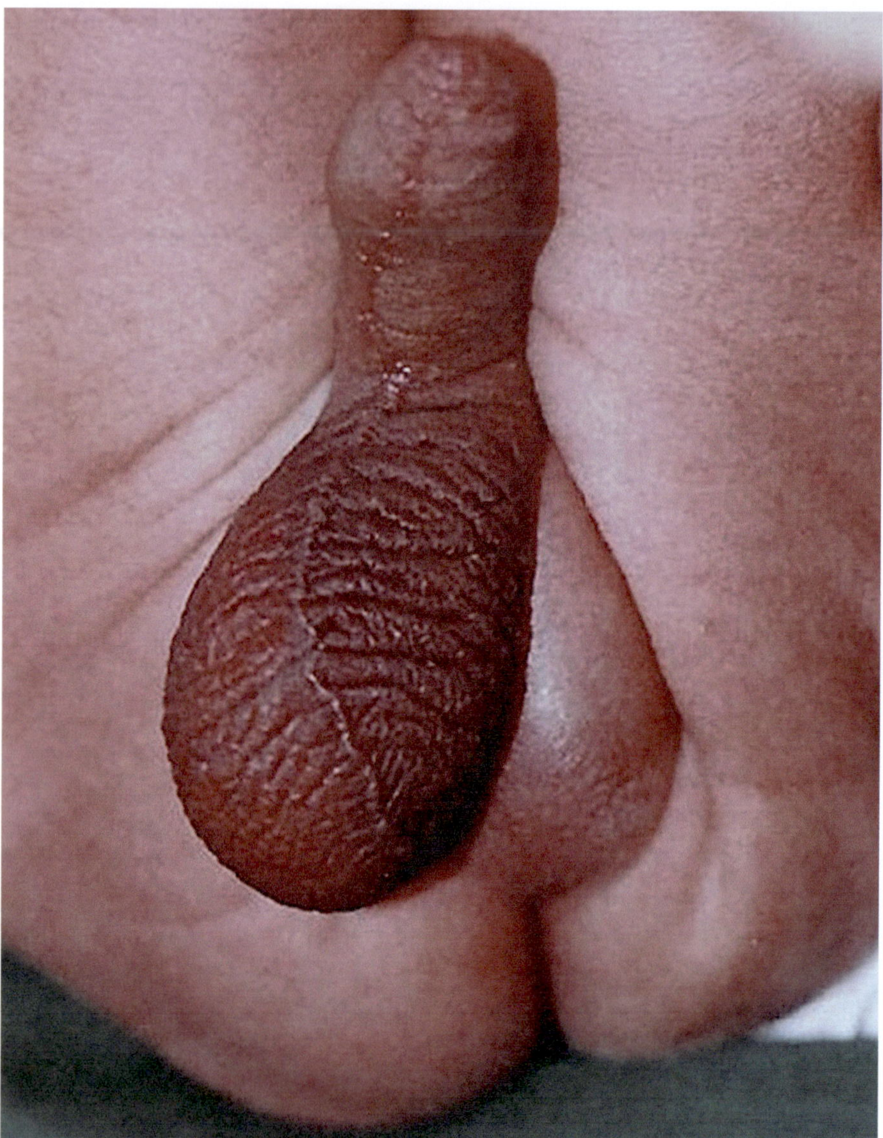

**Fig. 17.6**  A case of left perineal ectopic testicle with a preserved scrotal raphe

indicative of severe renal anomalies, which in all cases have been incompatible with extrauterine survival [17]. It is worthy to mention that scrotal raphe is usually preserved in cases of scrotal hypoplasia and unilateral scrotal agenesis, but cases of bilateral scrotal agenesis had no scrotal raphe (Chap. 11).

**2. Scrotal Raphe deviation**: Deviation of median raphe mainly seen in the penile raphe, and very rarely encountered in the scrotum. False impression of the raphe deviation may be appreciated in cases of the scrotal asymmetry (Chap. 18). Mohan et al. [18] demonstrate a significant association between hypospadias and deviation of the penoscrotal raphe. Consideration should be given to whether include this finding within the other spectrum of abnormalities seen in hypospadias or not. Examination of the penoscrotal raphe is simple to perform and could aid in the early diagnosis of children with milder forms of hypospadias. In a study of 80 children with hypospadias and 80 control cases, deviation of the median raphe was observed in 88.8% and 13.7% of cases, respectively. A deviation to the right is more likely to be associated with hypospadias than a deviation to the left [18] (Fig. 17.7).

GMR deviation to one side, may be also a significant sign for detection of other rare cases of IPM, a variant of hypospadias with an intact normal prepuce, raphe deviation detected in 75% of cases of IPM in our series, and this will be helpful medically and medicolegally for surgeons and practitioners doing circumcision for infants, specially in countries which still practising circumcision for all infants with a religious background [4]. Deviation of the meatus always was noted with deviation of the median raphe and it was found in 2.2 per cent of Ben-Ari et al. [19] study of 274 neonates, where deviation of the median raphe without deviation of the meatus was found in 27 newborns (10%).

The distal end of scrotal raphe along with the perineal raphe may show deviation to one side in association with different forms of anorectal malformations, at the meantime other forms of scrotal raphe anomalies are not rare with imperforate anus (Fig. 17.8).

**3. Hyperpigmentation**: Normally, and specially in coloured males, the median raphe is slightly darker than the rest of the scrotal skin. Pathologically hyperpigmented scrotal raphae are usually associated with other raphe anomalies like wide raphe or deviated raphe, and again this anomaly may be an indication for a hidden IPM, as we can see in Fig. 17.9; the scrotal raphe is wider than normal and hyperpigmented, and once the prepuce retracted an obvious megameatus was detectable.

We have a case of prominent hyperpigmented scrotal raphe diagnosed with an evident penile rotation. (Fig. 17.10) Hyperpigmented raphe should be differentiated from the minute pigmented raphe cysts, which will be discussed later.

**4. Prominent median raphe:** Scrotal raphe may looks so prominent, and this prominence may be in the form of a raised raphe above the surrounding scrotal skin, wide raphe, or a hyperpigmented raphe. Such anomalies are not rare in association with different forms of hypospadias (Fig. 17.11). Cases of Mild Androgen Insensitivity Syndrome (MAIS) which presented phenotypically as a male patients whose external genitalia are underdeveloped or who have subtle genital alterations such as hypospadias are commonly had a prominent midline raphe of the scrotum

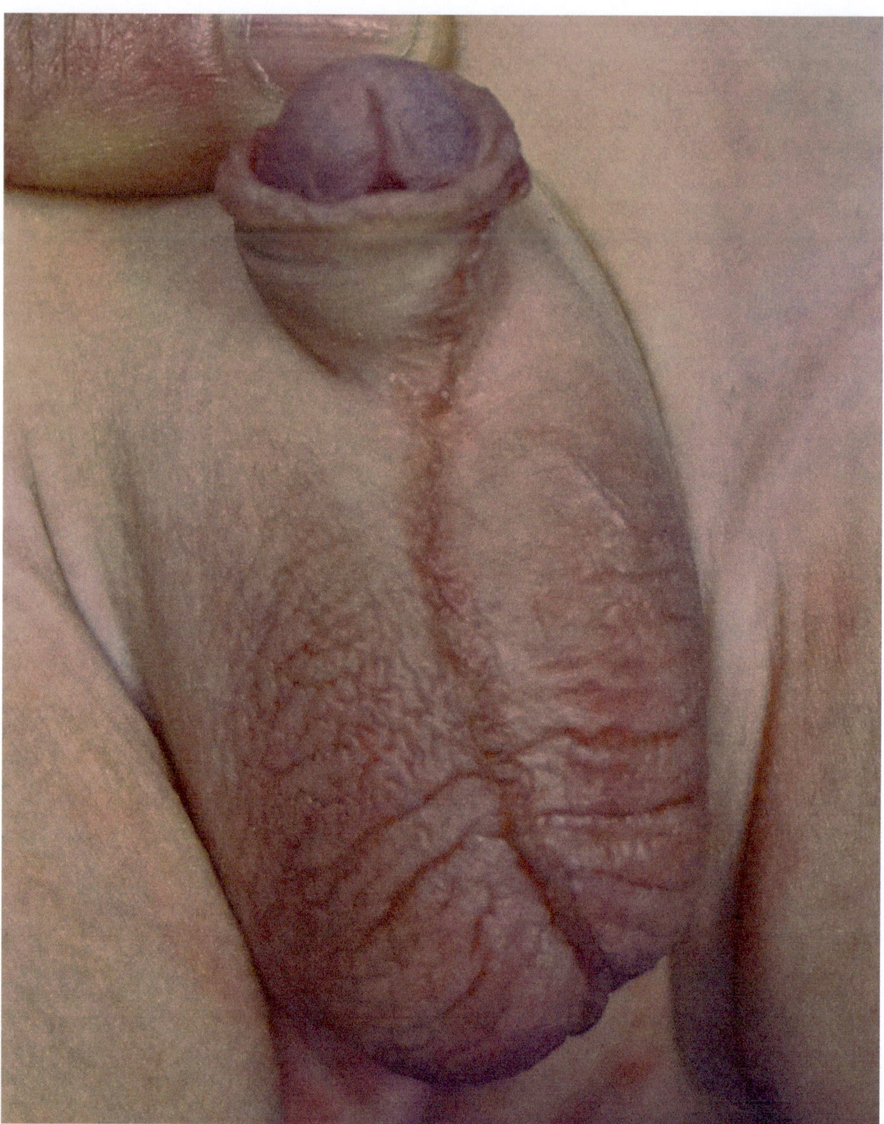

**Fig. 17.7** Left sided penile raphe deviation associating a case of coronal hypospadias

[20]. This raphe prominence may looks like a mucosal groove covered by urethral epithelium as in cases penoscrotal or more proximal cases of hypospadias, which are common with MAIS (Fig. 17.12). Also prominence of the scrotal raphe may be seen as a midline ridge of skin (Fig. 17.13).

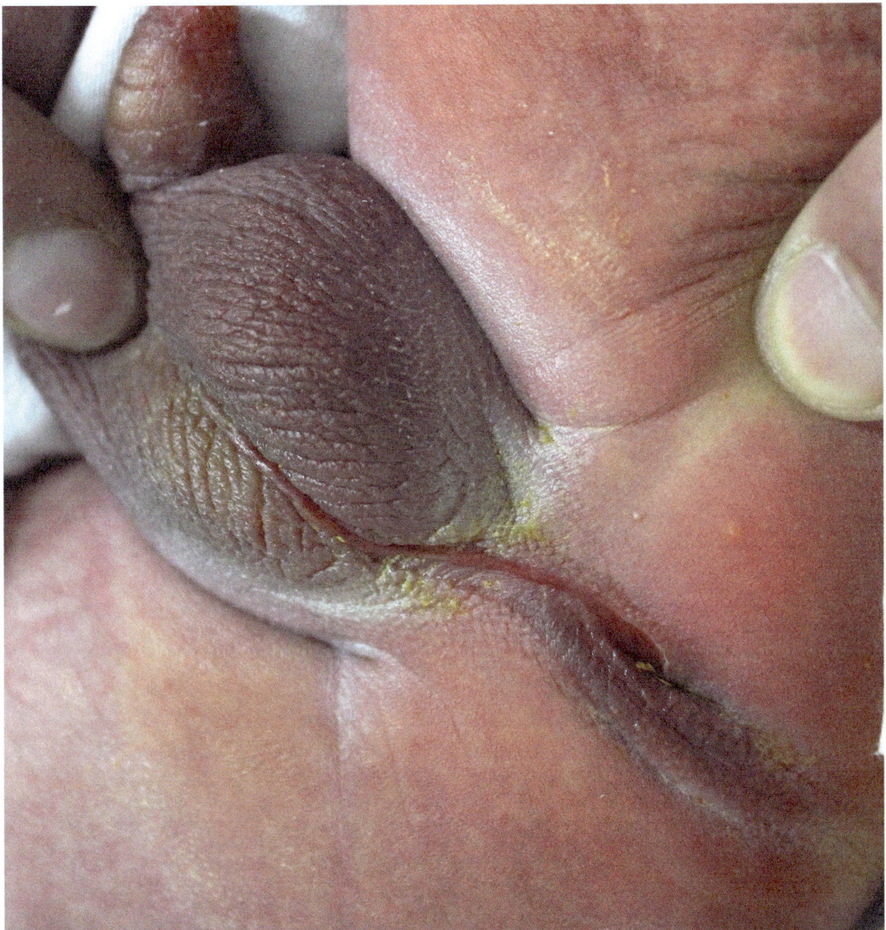

**Fig. 17.8** An interesting case of high anorectal malformation with a left sided deviation of the caudal end of scrotal and perineal raphae

**5. Wide median raphe**: Splitting of the median raphe was probably due to the defective proper fusion of ectoderm. Also partial failure of closure occurs because of the failure of maturation of the midline mesodermal components. If raphe widening is so evident; we may have a bifid raphe, which if subsequently so severe it may end with a different degrees of bifid scrota (Chap. 14).

**6. Bifid Scrotal Raphe**: Bifid or splitted scrotal raphe is the minimal degree of the bifid scrotum, it is commonly seen with different forms of ARMs, Androgen insensitivity and hypospadias (Fig. 17.14).

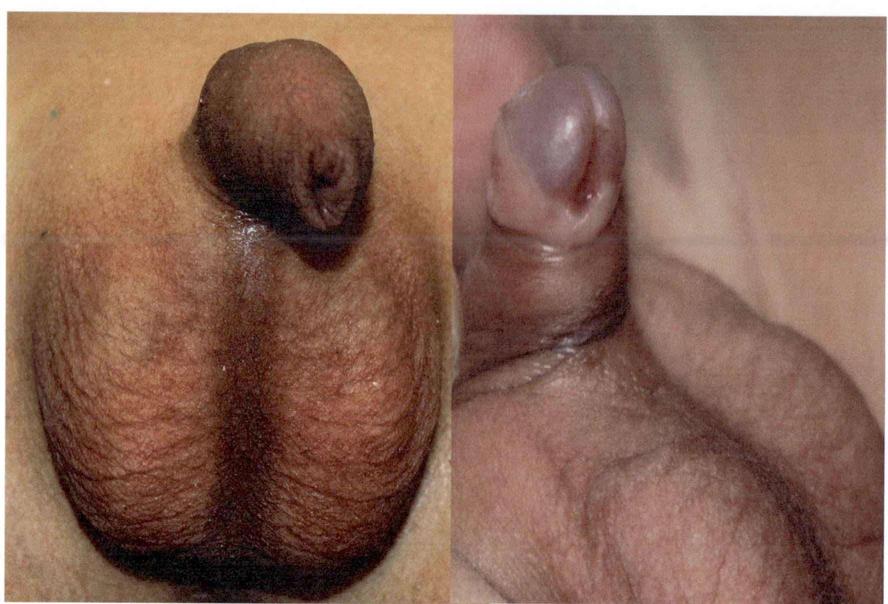

**Fig. 17.9** Wide hyperpigmented scrotal raphe associating an IPM

**7. Short raphe leads to webbed penis**: Short contracted raphe with a defective penoscrotal junction may be manifested as a sort of webbed penis which may be due to loss of the normal dartos muscle and facia (Fig. 17.15).

**8. Beaded Median Raphe "Scrotal pearl"**: Rare cases of brown fine darker nodules replacing the normal smooth line of median raphe had been reported, and this could be a normal variant, or a variation of minute penile cysts with the same pathology and etiology, it is usually presented as an indurated cord prominence along the line of the median raphe of the scrotum, but may be extended caudally to the perineum (Fig. 17.16). We diagnosed few cases in association with anorectal malformation. Pearls of meconium can be seen on the raphe of the scrotum and are considered as a sign of low presentation of an anorectal malformation [21]. Such anomaly may be attributed to an epithelial overgrowth and the meconium may be trapped before closure of the genital folds via an anocutaneous fistula in anorectal malformation. Sometimes it looks like a black ribbon because it is full of meconium. These features are externally visible and help diagnosis of a perineal fistula. Scrotal pearls without an anorectal malformation, which are usually whitish in colour, are very rare in infants and designated as median raphe cysts of the

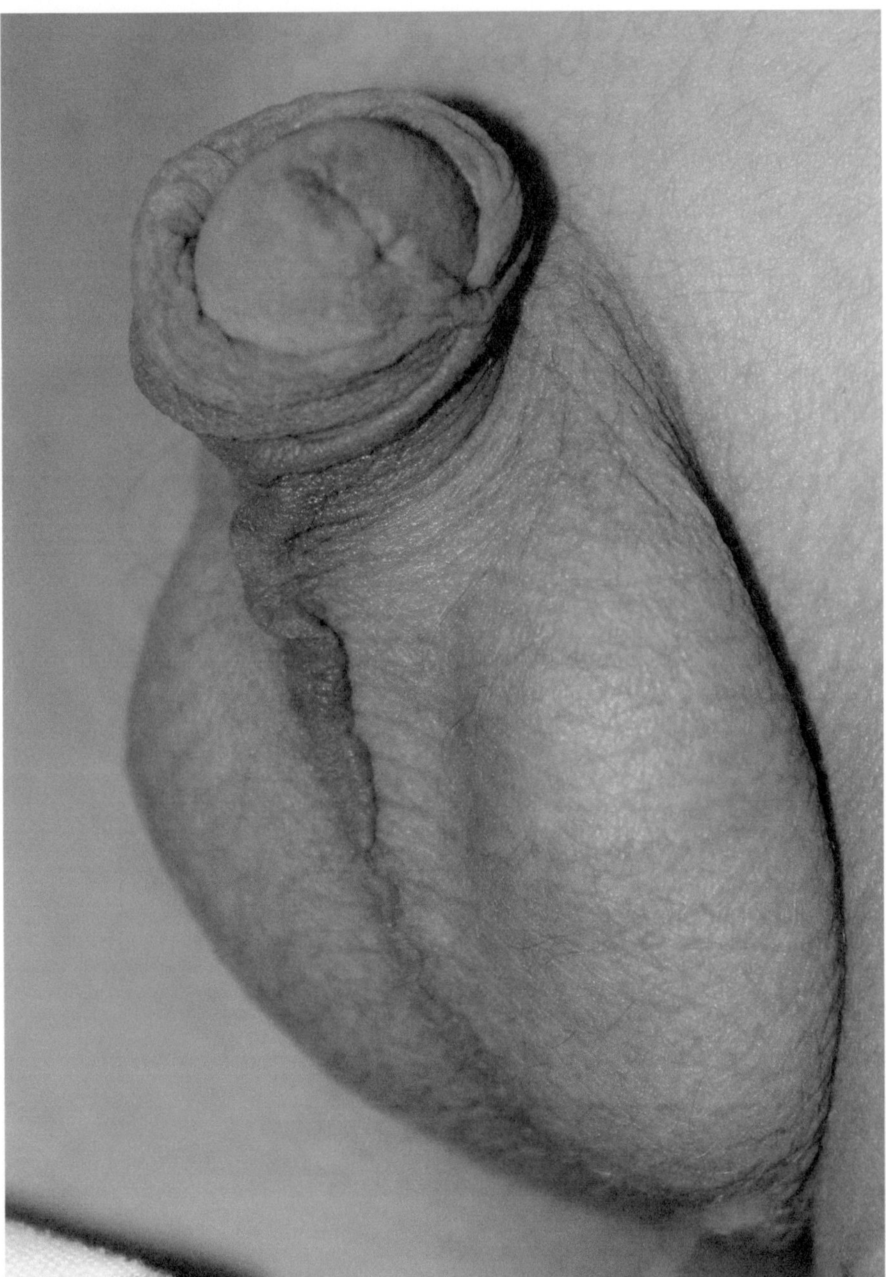

**Fig. 17.10** Hyperpigmented raised scrotal raphe with a significant left sided penile rotation

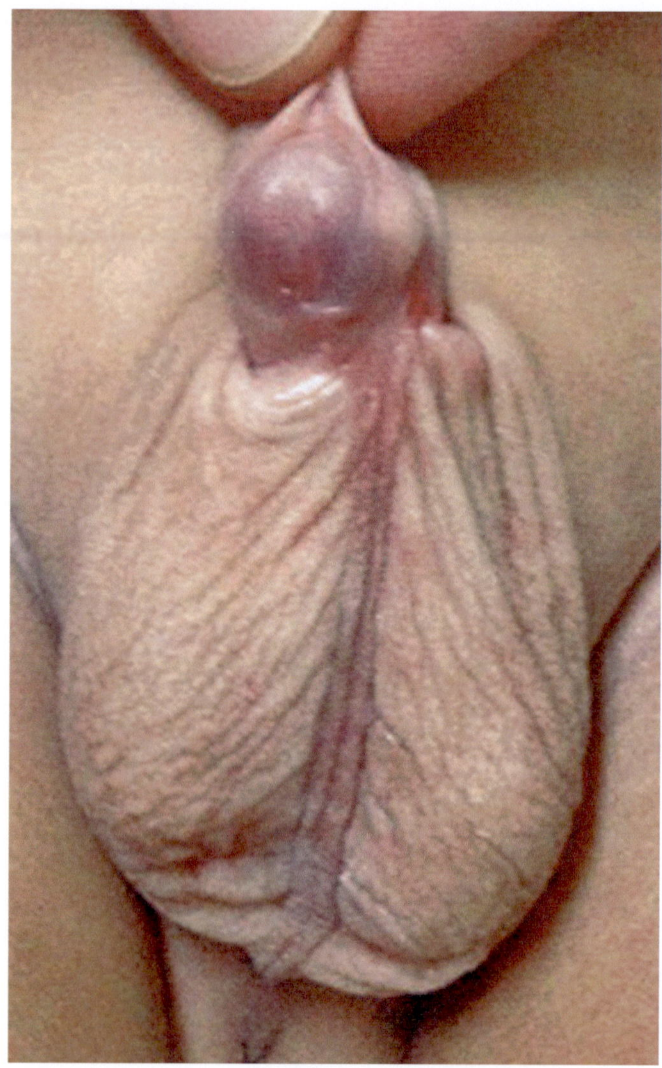

**Fig. 17.11** Hyperpigmented wide scrotal raphe with hypospadias

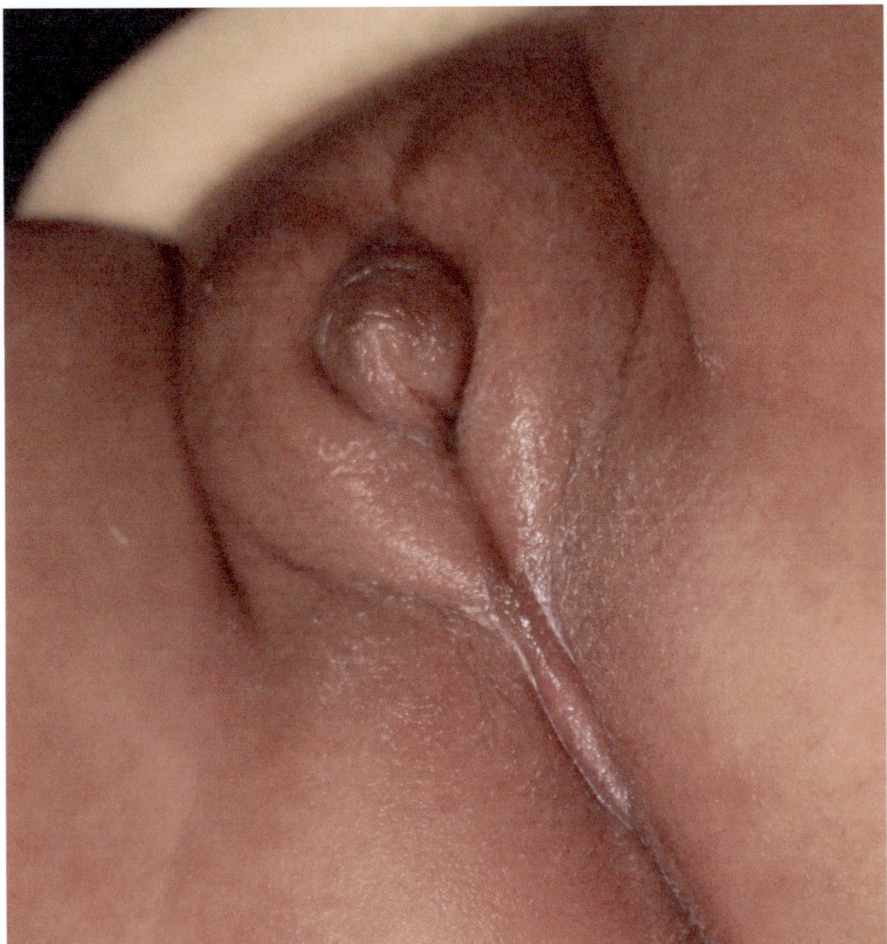

**Fig. 17.12** Wide scrotal raphe in a case of mild androgen insensitivity syndrome, the marked hypogonadism and defective scrotal rugae are also evident

perineum. It may also be considered as a minute inclusion cysts [21] (Fig. 17.17). Nothing surgical is required for such cases, only a through examination to rule out any associated anomalies, family assurance and follow up. Other congenital abnormalities such as blind-ending canals opening onto the penile surface must be differentiated.

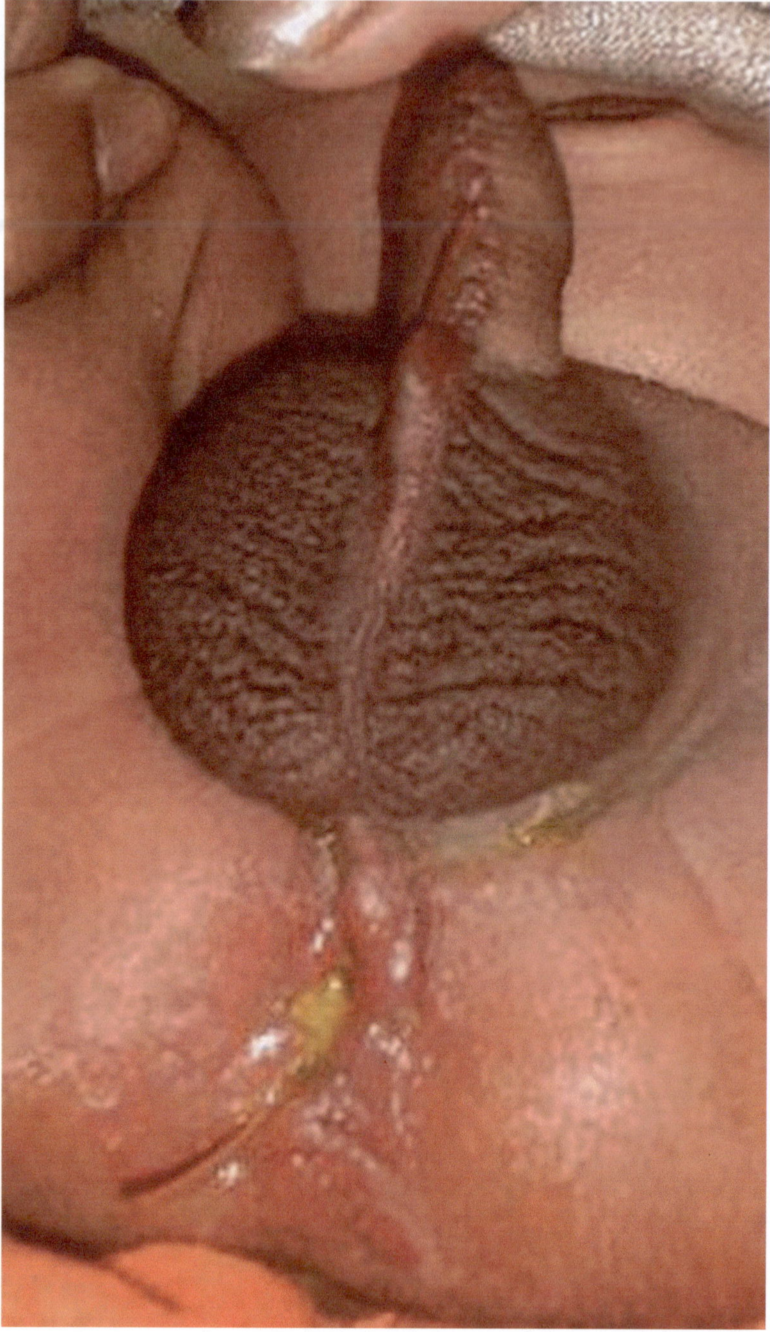

**Fig. 17.13** A neonate with a raised scrotal and proximal raphae looks like a ridge, with an imperforate anus

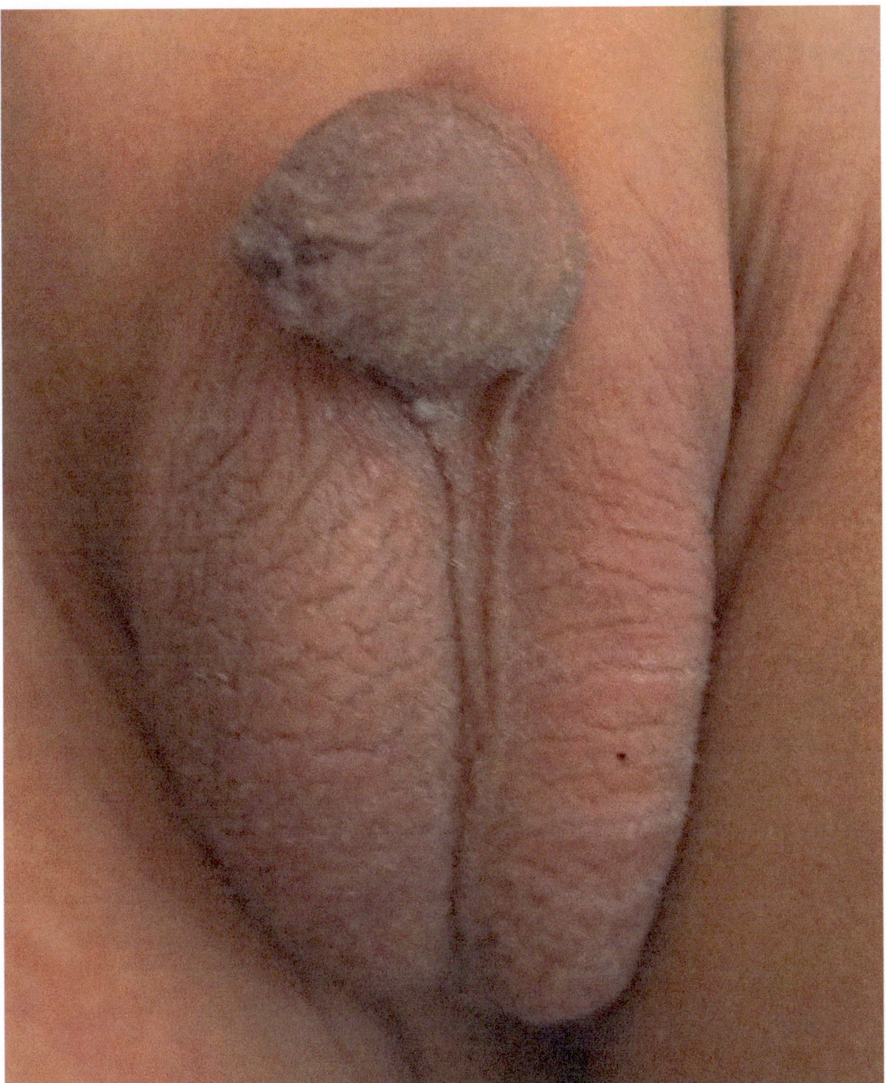

**Fig. 17.14** Minimal bifid scrotal raphe just posterior to the root of the penis

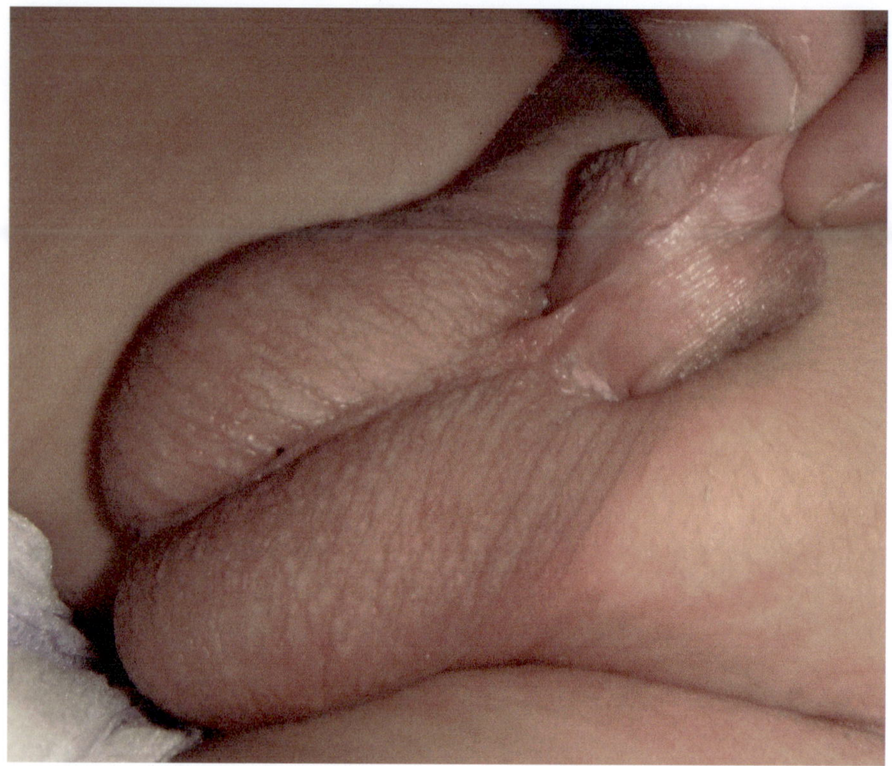

**Fig. 17.15** A contracted short raphe manifested as a webbed penis

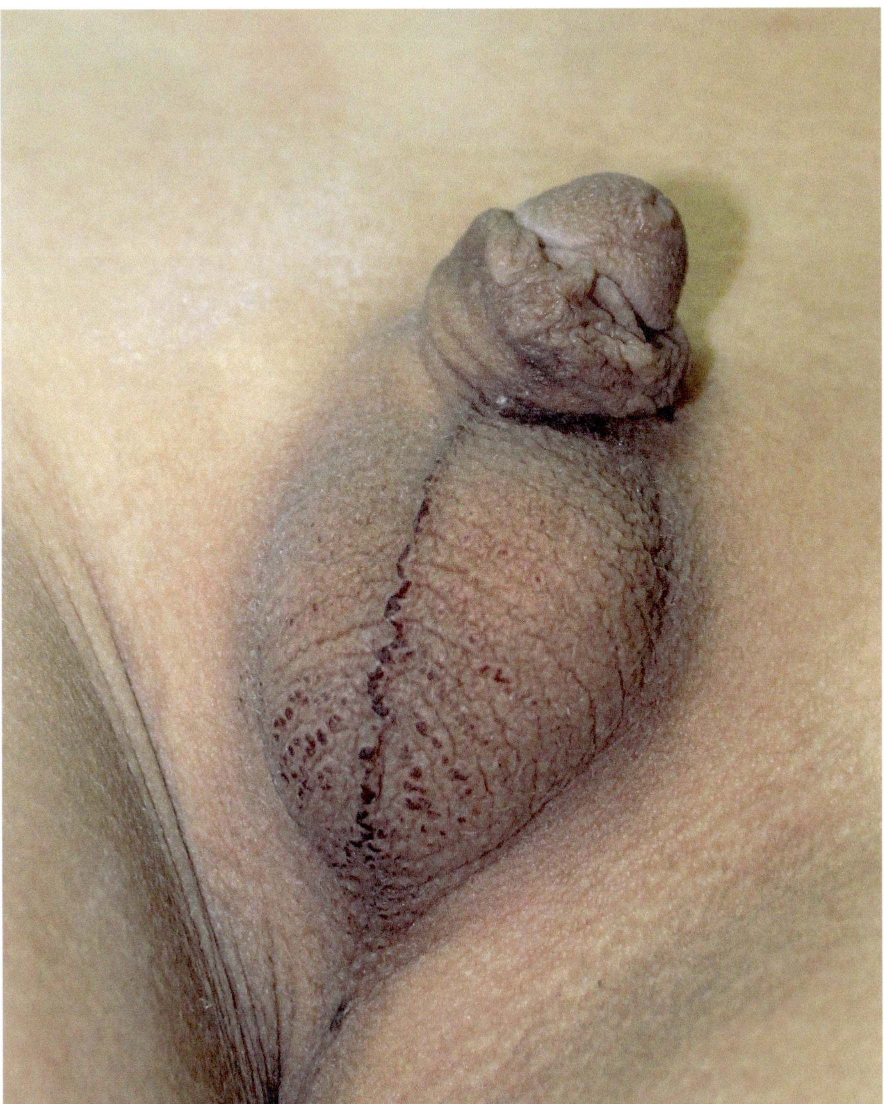

**Fig. 17.16** Brownish beaded median scrotal raphe

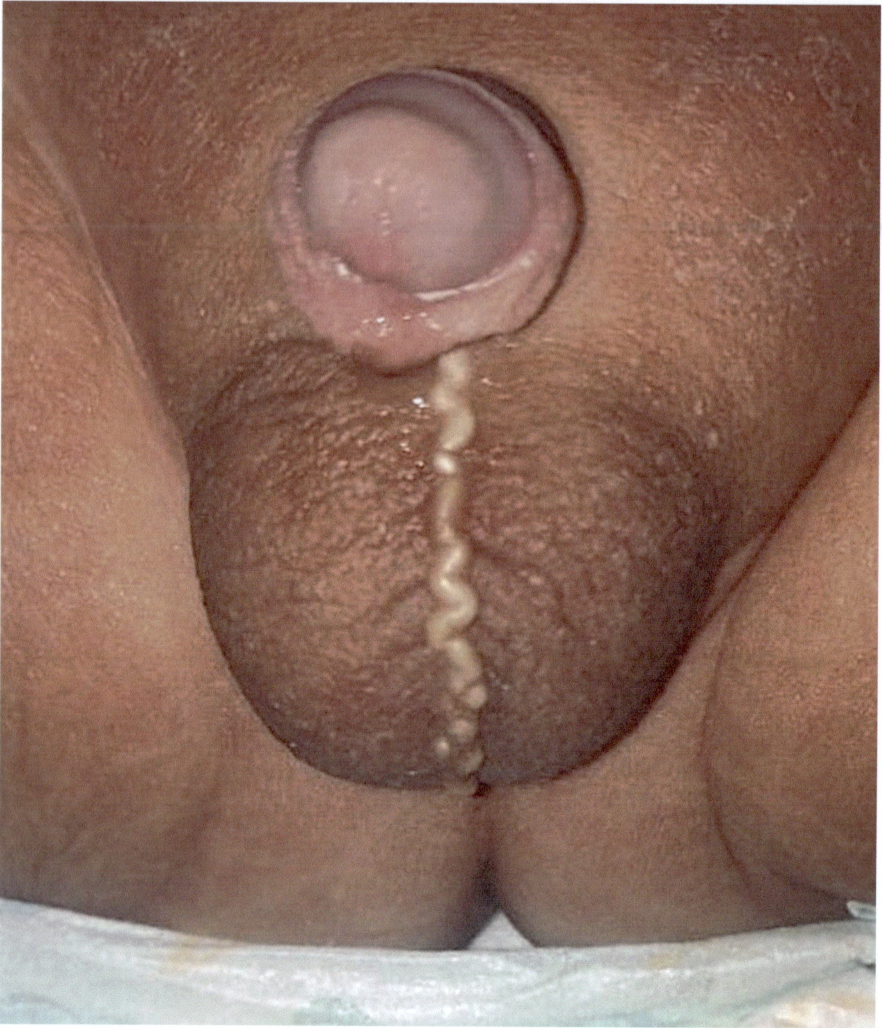

**Fig. 17.17** Whitish scrotal pearl

## 17.5 Median raphe cyst (MRC)

**Nomenclature:** MRC also known as cloacogenic cyst and genitoperineal raphe cyst, if the cyst is presented as a threadlike canal of the raphe it is called a median raphe canal, and if it is presented at the tip of the penis; it is called parameatal raphe cyst. These congenital lesions are generally asymptomatic and hence may be under-reported. As early as 1895; Mermet [22] reviewed 23 cases in which cysts and fistulas along the perineal raphe had become infected and thus called attention to their existence. This author laid special stress on the anomalous nature of the condition.

The true incidence of MRC in infants is not known. In a large series of patients, 25% of cases were younger than 10 years of age, and only one infant was reported to have a scrotal MRC [23]. But we diagnosed some cases during neonatal survey.

MRC may be detected along the genital raphe from the tip of the penis and caudally to the anus; that usually appears as a cystlike or canallike lesion. MRC of the perineum is a rare anomaly that usually presents with solitary, multiple or canal-like watery cysts, it is not rare to have a perineal MRC filled of meconium in association with anorectal malformations. (Fig. 17.18) Such cases should be differentiated from the rare cases of pigmented MRC, where the presence of melanocytes may mimic the colour of the meconium filled cysts.

**Etiology**: This cyst are due to tegumentary formation that arises as a result of "tissue trapping" during midline fusion of the ectoderm. It could be a simple skin pathology or might represent major abnormalities like hypospadias or other urethral anomalies [24].

Two different theories were described regarding the etiology:

1. They arise from epithelial rests incidentally from incomplete closure of the urethral or genital folds.
2. They develop from split off outgrowths of embryologic epithelium after primary closure of the folds.

Shao et al. [23] have published their case series of median raphe cysts, in 2012; 25,5% of the cases were under 10 years old. The localisation of the cysts were ranging from the urinary meatus to the perineum.

**Pathogenesis**: Based on the histopathological findings median raphe cysts can be classified into 4 types: urethral, epidermoid, glandular and mixed type. The urethral type is lined with pseudostratified columnar epithelium (uroepithelium), epidermoid type with squamous stratified epithelium, and mixed type with both epithelia. The most common type is reported as urethral, followed by the epithelial and mixed forms [25]. A medium raphe cyst with ciliated lining cells has been also reported, although it would appear that this cell type had been previously recognized in these lesions [26].

MRCs are either dermoid or mucoid, depending on their embryology or epithelial lining. Very rarely, the basal epithelial lining of the cysts may contain melanocytes, imparting a brown-black pigment to the lesion. Very rarely the median raphe cyst may be presented as a perineal polyp [27].

Ectodermal canals involving part or all of the raphe had been reported for the first time at 1924 by Rupel E [28], and it is considered as an extension of multiple raphe cysts with the same pathology.

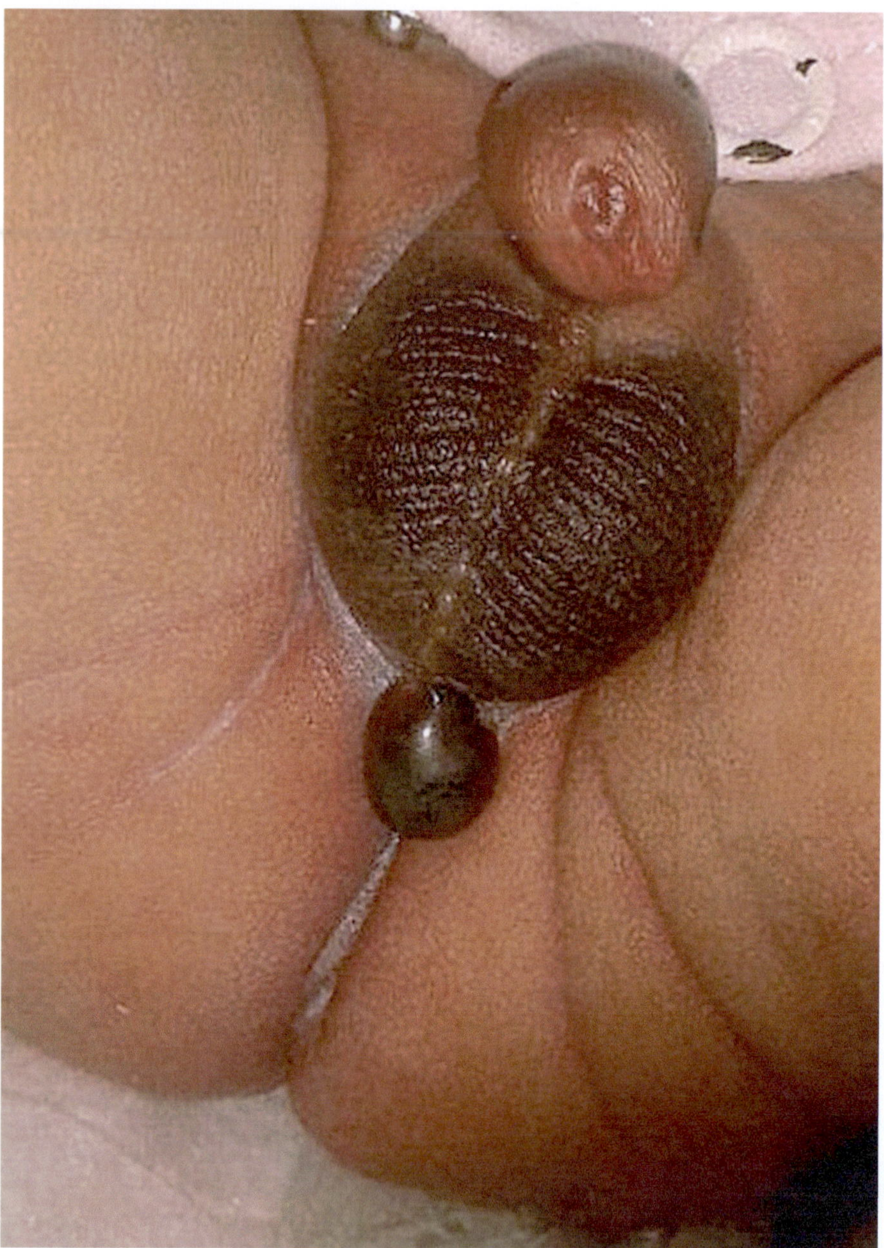

**Fig. 17.18** A neonate with imperforate anus and meconium filled median raphe cyst just caudal to the scrotum

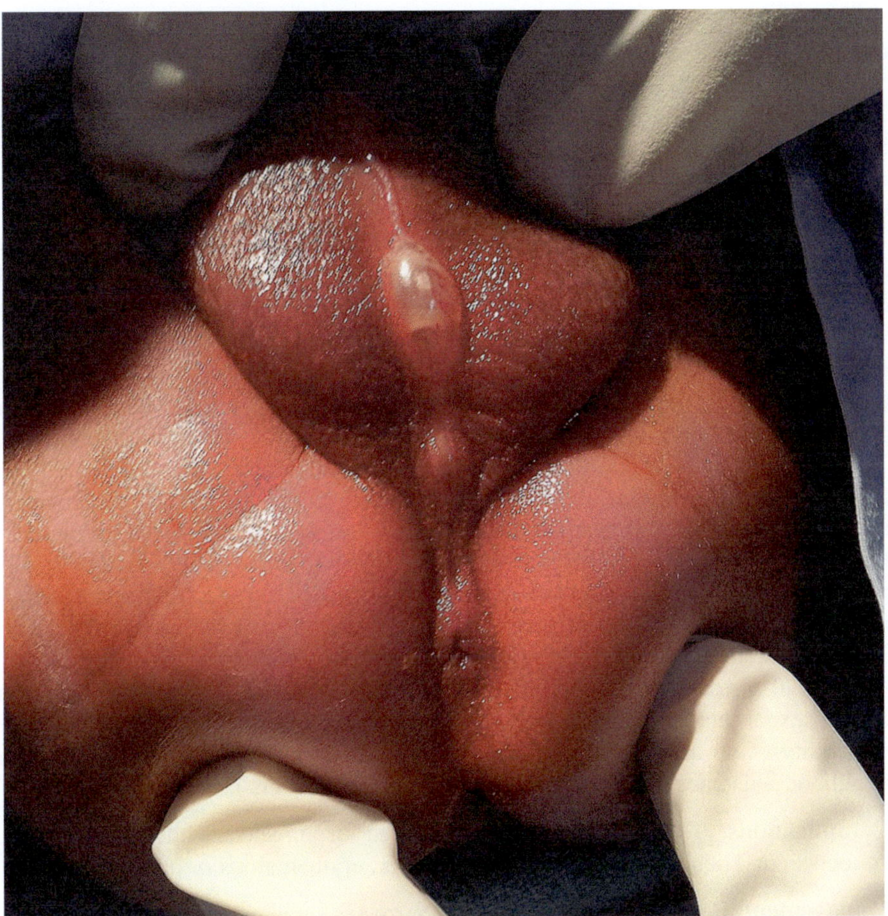

**Fig. 17.19** A neonate with a clear fluid filling a canal like defect in the median raphe of the scrotum and perineum

Canal like structure filled with a clear mucous fluid due to failure of fusion of the median raphe is very rarely encountered with cases of ARM. (Fig. 17.19).

**Clinically**: The cyst is generally solitary, with the penile shaft being the most common location, multiple small cysts are also documented. The average size in children is around 1 cm, but larger size cysts are also reported. The diagnosis is mostly clinical and confirmed histologically.

In some cases the diagnosis may be difficult, or needs be differentiated from other conditions such as epidermal cyst, molluscum contagiosum, syringoma, steatocystoma, glomus tumor, dermoid cyst, urethral diverticulum, and pilonidal cyst when it presents in the scrotal region [29].

There is little confusion with sebaceous cysts; which is usually easily distinguishable. Common pyogenic infections as well as specific venereal and acid-fast bacilli infections must be considered, and there is no explanation why these cysts are vulnerable to gonorrhoea infection either as an isolated cyst infection or along urethral affection [30].

Steatocystoma multiplex is a disorder of pilosebaceous unit that occur as sporadic or an autosomal dominant fashion. The condition presents with development of sebum filled dermal cysts (benign sebaceous gland tumour).

MRCs are usually nontender and asymptomatic but can be complicated with rupture, sinus formation, calcification and secondary bacterial infections [31]. The median raphe cyst appears as skin coloured to translucent cystic papule, nodule, or cord like/linear lesion located in the midline from the urethral meatus to the anus. This cysts typically present in adolescents and sometimes in adulthood [32]. Pigmented median raphe cysts with melanosis are uncommon. The cause of pigmentation is not fully understood, this pigmentation may be due to the presence of lipochrome or the presence of melanocytes. This pigmentation was due to the presence of melanocytes and melanophages as proved on the light and electron microscopic results [33]. Some cases may be detected early in the neonates with ARM, the combination of both cystic lesion and cord like structure is not rare. (Fig. 17.20) Presentation at old age usually comes to medical attention due to pain during sexual intercourse, or after severe infection. It is crucial to consider the rare possibility of an association between median raphe cyst and faecal fistula, and a likelihood existence of a MRC covering the ostium of this fistula. (Fig. 17.21).

**Complications**: The cyst may be traumatised or infected with staphylococci, gonococci or Trichomonas and present as tender, erythematous or purulent nodules.

**Management**: Reassurance is adequate if the cyst is small and asymptomatic, but if family worries about the cyst nature or the surgeon is not confident about the diagnosis; surgical excision is indicated, and if the cyst infected, systemic antibiotics to cover S. aureus and/or N. gonorrhoea are indicated. If there are a symptomatic or a cosmetic concern, surgical excision and primary closure is indicated [34]. Complete surgical excision has the advantage of allowing all ectopic tissue to be removed, thereby reducing the risk of recurrence.

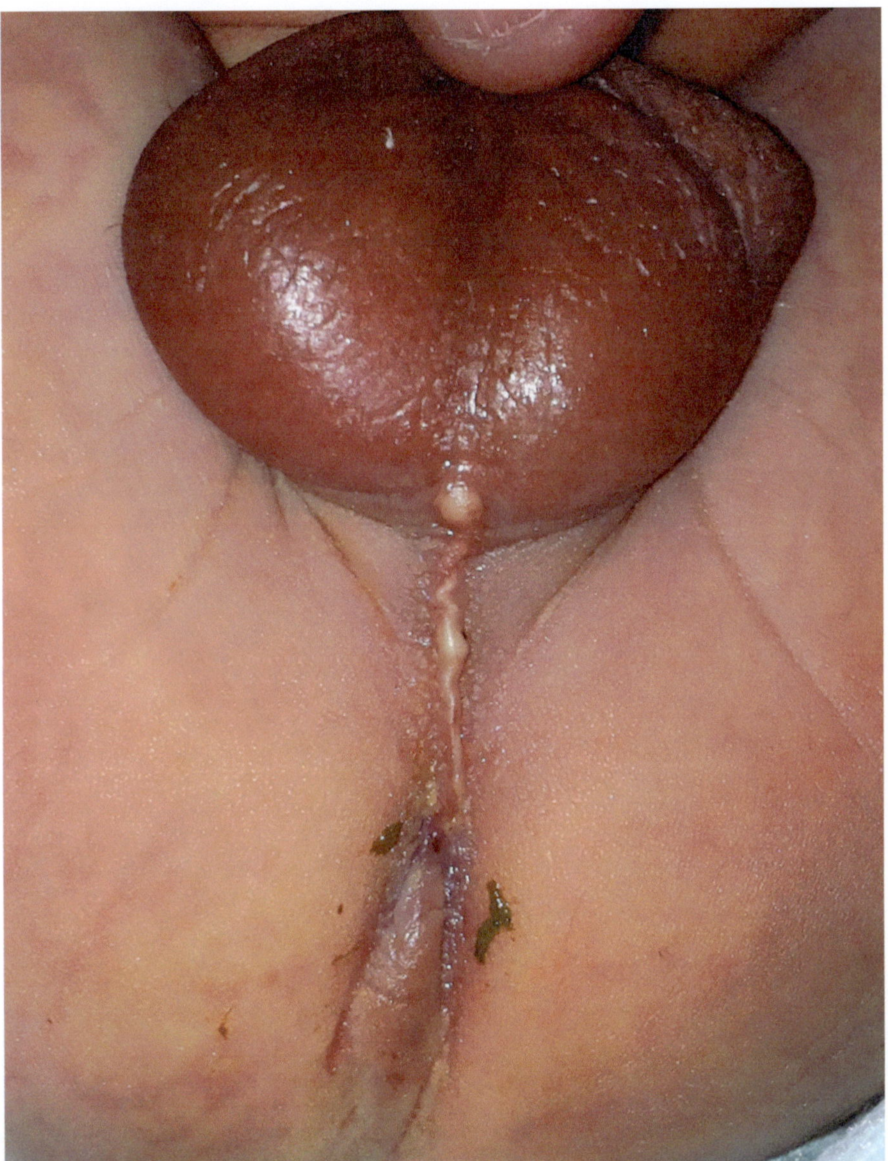

**Fig. 17.20** A neonate with high form of ARM presented with a combined scrotal median raphe cyst and another multiple minute cysts looks like cord structure at the perineal raphe

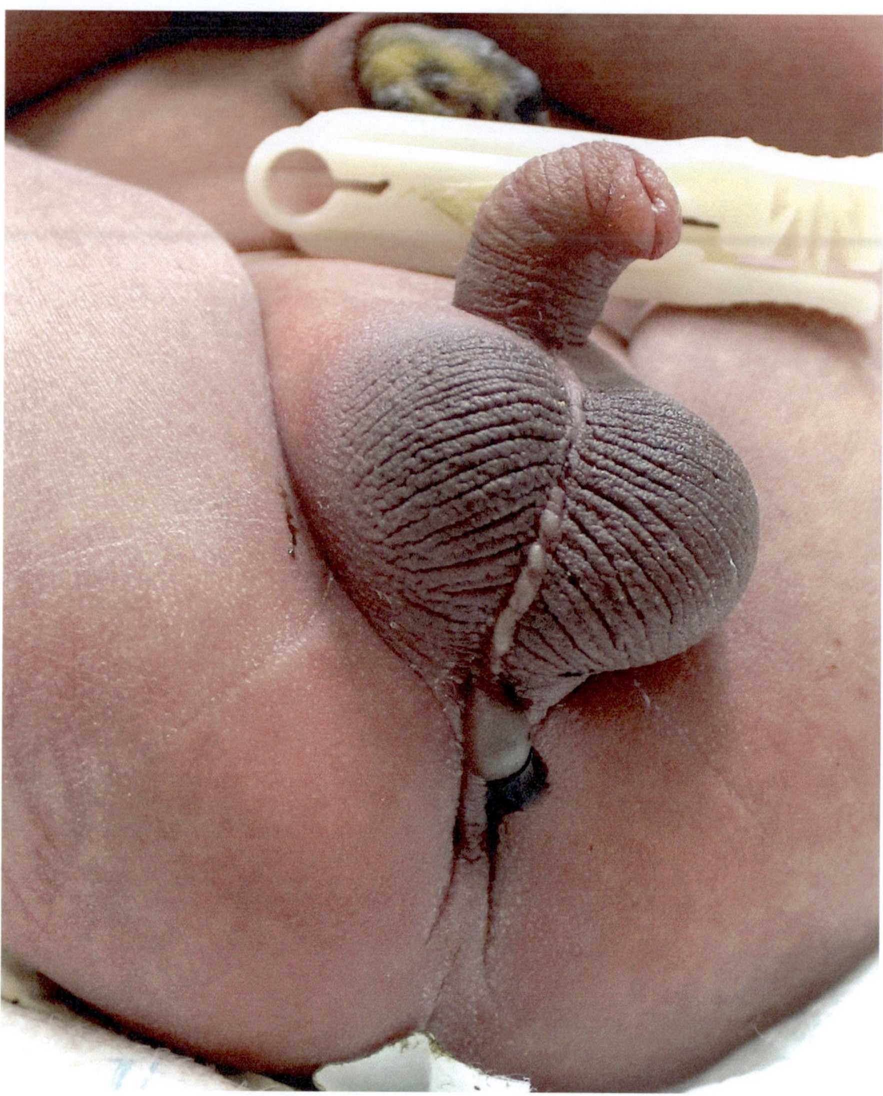

**Fig. 17.21** A cord like MRCs in the scrotum and a perineal meconium filled cyst covering an outer opening of a faecal fistula

## 17.6  Rare Scrotal Raphe Anomalies

- Hypopigmentation of the median raphe are commonly an acquired phenomenon secondary to lichen sclerosis or other perineal or scrotal dermatosis (Chap. 26). Congenital scrotal hypopigmentation in the form of vitiligo is very rare.
- Congenital scrotal sinuses are an extremely rare midline raphe anomalies, few cases were published in the literature up to date. Etiology is similar to the perineal midline cystic defects, as it is believed that during the early embryogenesis the rape sinus may arise from trapped epithelial cells as a result of incomplete closure of epithelial folds. Diagnosis depends on the physical

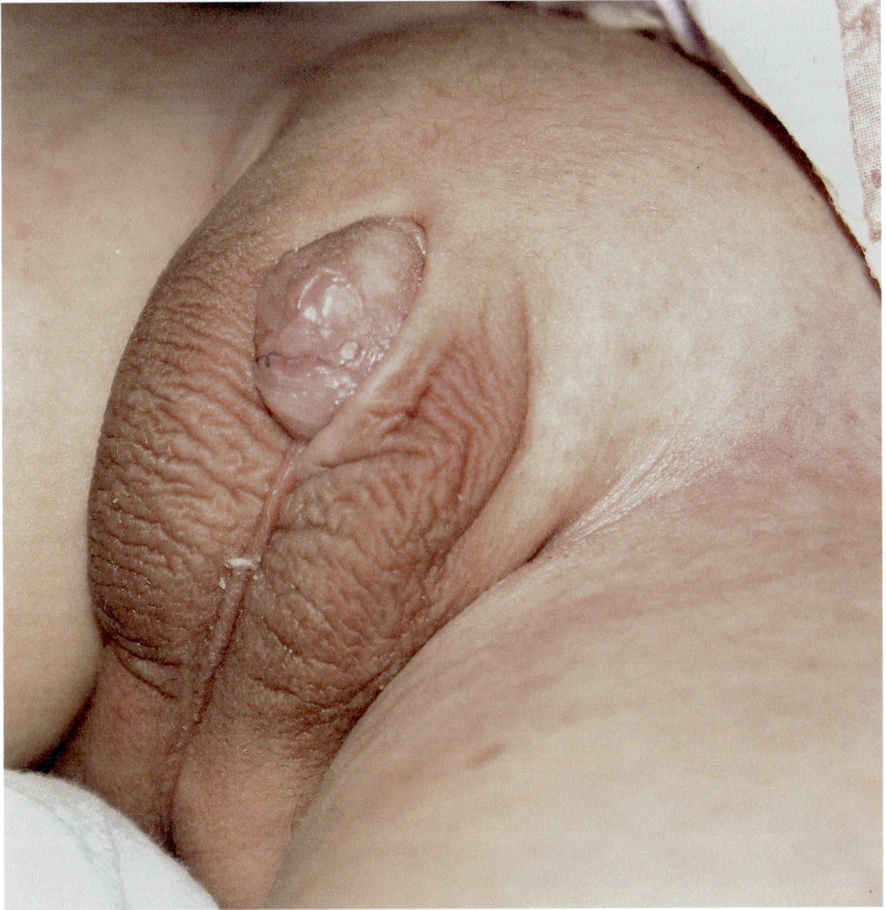

**Fig. 17.22**  A rare case of a congenital adhesion between the tip of the prepuce and the scrotal raphe

examination and some radiological investigations such as ultrasonography or contrast studies. The only treatment is total excision of the sinus structure both for cosmetic reasons and the prevention of probable future complications, the excised specimen should be examined histological to confirm the diagnosis and to rule out other possibilities [35].

- Very rarely there is an congenital adhesion between the scrotal raphe and the tip of the prepuce leads to anchoring the tip of the penis to the scrotum and requiring an urgent release [36] (Fig. 17.22).
- Scrotal horn: A cutaneous horn, is a hard, conical projection composed of compacted keratin that resembles animal's horn. They commonly occur on sun-exposed areas, it is extremely rare in genital area, few cases arising from the penis or the prepuce are reported [36]. The first case in the English literature of a cutaneous horn arising from the scrotal skin is recently reported by John et al. [37], a non-tender curved, yellow–brown, horn-like projection was diagnosed arising from the median raphe of the scrotum. If a suspicion about malignancy raised; the histopathological examination confirm the presence of a verruciform architecture with tiers of parakeratosis in association with hypergranulosis and koilocytes, and excluding any dysplastic changes [37].

# References


1. Baskin LS, Erol A, Jegatheesan P, Li Y, Liu W, Cunha GR. Urethral seam formation and hypospadias. Cell Tissue Res. 2001;305:379–87.
2. Van der Putte SCJ. The development of the perineum in the human. Adv Anat Embryol Cell Biol. 2005;177:1–131.
3. Neff JH. Congenital canals of the genito perineal raphe. Am J Surg. 1936;31:308–15.
4. Fahmy MA, El Shenawy A, Altramsy A, et al. Penile median raphe anomalies as an indicator of megameatus intact prepuce anomaly in children undergoing routine circumcision. Pediatr Urol. 2018. https://www.ncbi.nlm.nih.gov/pubmed/30096348.
5. Chitayat D, Glanc P. Diagnostic approach in prenatally detected genital abnormalities. Ultrasound Obstet Gynecol. 2010;35:637–46.
6. Baky Fahmy MA. The spectrum of genital median raphe anomalies among infants undergoing ritual circumcision. J Pediatr Urol. 2013;9(6):872–7. https://doi.org/10.1016/j.jpurol.2012.11.018.
7. Jin ZW, et al. Perineal raphe with special reference to its extension to the anus: a histological study using human fetuses. Anat Cell Biol. 2016;49:116–24. https://doi.org/10.5115/acb.2016.49.2.116.
8. Eisenberg ML, Jensen TK, Walters RC, Skakkebaek NE, Lipshultz LI. The relationship between anogenital distance and reproductive hormone levels in adult men. J Urol. 2012;187:594–8.
9. Hsieh MH, Eisenberg ML, Hittelman AB, Wilson JM, Tasian GE, Baskin LS. Caucasian male infants and boys with hypospadias exhibit reduced anogenital distance. Human Reprod (Oxford, England). 2012;27:1577–80.
10. Jain VG, Singal AK. Shorter anogenital distance correlates with undescended testis: a detailed genital anthropometric analysis in human newborns. Human Reprod (Oxford, England). 2013;28:2343–9.

11. Thankamony A, Lek N, Carroll D, Williams M, Dunger DB, Acerini CL, et al. Anogenital distance and penile length in infants with hypospadias or cryptorchidism: comparison with normative data. Environ Health Perspect. 2014;122:207–11.
12. Singal AK, Jain VG, Gazali Z, Shekhawat P. Shorter anogenital distance correlates with the severity of hypospadias in pre-pubertal boys. Human Reprod (Oxford, England). 2016;31:1406–10.
13. Gilboa Y, Perlman S, Kivilevitch Z, Messing B, Achiron R. Prenatal anogenital distance is shorter in fetuses with hypospadias. J Ultrasound Med. 2017;36:175–82.
14. Cox K, Kyriakou A, Amjad B, O'Toole S, Flett ME, Welsh M, et al. Shorter anogenital and anoscrotal distances correlate with the severity of hypospadias: a prospective study. J Pediatr Urol. 2017;13:57.e1–.e5.
15. Gutt AA, Pendharka PS. Transverse testicular ectopia associated with persistent Mullerian duct syndrome. Br J Radiol. 2008;81:176-e8.
16. Srinivasan J, McDougall P, Hutson JM. When is 'intersex' not intersex? A case of penile agenesis demonstrates how to distinguish non-endocrine disorders in neonates with genital anomaly. J Paediatr Child Health. 2003;39(8):629–31.
17. Berry SA, Johnson DE, Thompson TR. Agenesis of the penis, scrotal raphe, and anus in one of monoamniotic twins. Teratology. 1984;29:173–6. https://doi.org/10.1002/tera.1420290204 .
18. Mohan A, Ashton L, Dalal M. Deviation of the penoscrotal median raphe: Is it a normal finding or within the spectrum of hypospadias? Indian J Plast Surg. 2014;47(01):92–4. https://doi.org/10.4103/0970-0358.129630.
19. Ben-Ari J, Merlob P, Mimouni F, Reisner SH. Characteristics of the male genitalia in the newborn: penis. J Urol. 1985;134(3):521–2.
20. Melo KF, Mendonca BB, Billerbeck AE, et al. Clinical, hormonal, behavioral, and genetic characteristics of androgen insensitivity syndrome in a Brazilian cohort: five novel mutations in the androgen receptor gene. J Clin Endocrinol Metab. 2003;88:3241–50.
21. Soyer T, Karabulut A, Boybeyi O, Günal Y. Scrotal pearl is not always a sign of anorectal malformation: median raphe cyst. Turk J Pediatr. 2013;55:665–6.
22. Mermet P. Les kystes congénitaux du raphe' gènito-pèrinèal. Rev de chirurg. 1895;15:382.
23. Shao IH, Chen TD, Shao HT, et al. Male median raphe cysts: serial retrospective analysis and histopathological classification. Diagn Pathol. 2012;7:121.
24. Sarch RG, Golitz LE, Sausker WF, Kreye GM. Median raphe cysts of the penis. Arch Dermatol. 1979;115:1084–6.
25. Krauel L, Tarrado X, Garcia-Aparicio L, et al. Median raphe cyst of perineum in children. Urology. 2008;71:830–1.
26. Romani J, et al. Median raphe cyst of the penis with cilicated cells. J Cutan Pathol. 1995;22:378–81.
27. Scelwyn M. Median raphe cyst of the perineum presenting as a perianal polyp. Pathology. 1996. 28, May:201–3.
28. Rupel E. Epidermal canals infected with gonococci. Surg Gynec Obstet. 1924;39:636–8.
29. Lamb Ohn H. Congenital epidermal canals of the perineal raphe. Arch Dermatol Syphilol. 1943;47(1):74–81.
30. Clifford GR, Krieger JN, Rein MF. Gonococcal infection of the median penile raphe. J Urol. 1983;130(1):138–9.
31. Karawita A, Ranawaka RR. Genital dermatoses. In: Ranawaka RR, Kannangara AP, Karawita A, editors. Atlas of Dermatoses in pigmented skin. Singapore: Springer;2021. https://doi.org/10.1007/978-981-15-5483-4_38.
32. Navalón-Monllor V, Ordoño-Saiz MV, Ordoño-Domínguez F, et al. Median raphe cysts in men. Presentation of our experience and literature review. Actas Urol Esp. 2017;41(3):205–9. https://doi.org/10.1016/j.acuro.2016.06.008.
33. Urahashi J, et al. Pigmented median raphe cysts of the penis. Acta Derm Venereol. 2000;80:297–8.

34. Verma SB. Canal-like median raphe cysts: an unusual presentation of an unusual condition. Clin Exp Dermatol. 2009;34:e857–8.
35. Can Demïrtürk H, Günşar Cü, Berkan Usta I, Gizem Özamrak B. Giant congenital scrotal sinus. J Pediatr Surg Case Rep. 2020. https://doi.org/10.1016/j.epsc.2020.101516.
36. Fahmy MAB. Rare preputial anomalies. In: Normal and abnormal prepuce. Cham: Springer;2020. p. 141–9.
37. John J, Mngqi N, Morse N, Lazarus J, Kesner K. Cutaneous horn arising from the scrotum. J Clin Urol. 2020:2051415820939459. https://doi.org/10.1177/2051415820939459.

# Chapter 18
# Scrotal Asymmetry

Mohamed A. Baky Fahmy

## Abbreviations

BWS   Beckwith-Wiedemann syndrome
DSD   Disorders of Sex Development
DSP   Daily Sperm Production
AIS    Androgen Insensitivity Syndrome

**Nomenclature**: Scrotal asymmetry also known as scrotal ptosis, and sagging Scrotum.

**Historical background**: Astley Cooper at 1830 was well aware of the differences in height of the testes, although he did'nt comment on differences in size. Scrotal asymmetry inspired biologist and artists along the mankind history. Accuracy of scrotal size and position is noticeable in ancient Egyptian sculptures and Greek classical and pre-classical art, which took great care and attention to anatomical details, sculptors correctly portrayed the right testicle as the higher, but then incorrectly portrayed the left testicle as visibly larger [1] (Figs. 18.1and 18.2) The scrotal asymmetry is obvious in David masterpiece of Renaissance sculpture created in marble between 1501–1504 by the Italian artist Michelangelo (Fig. 18.3).

Biological symmetry can be thought of as a balanced distribution of duplicate body parts or shapes within the body of an organism. Importantly, unlike in mathematics, symmetry in biology is always approximate. For example, plant leaves—while considered symmetrical—rarely match up exactly when folded in half. Symmetry is one class of patterns in nature whereby there is near-repetition of the pattern element, either by reflection or rotation. The relationship of symmetry to aesthetics is a complex phenomena. Humans find bilateral symmetry in faces physically attractive; it indicates health and genetic fitness. Opposed to this is the tendency for excessive symmetry to be perceived as boring or uninteresting. People

M. A. B. Fahmy (✉)
Al-Azhar University, Cairo, Egypt

    255
M. A. B. Fahmy (ed.), *Normal and Abnormal Scrotum*,
https://doi.org/10.1007/978-3-030-83305-3_18

                                                                                            M. A. B. Fahmy

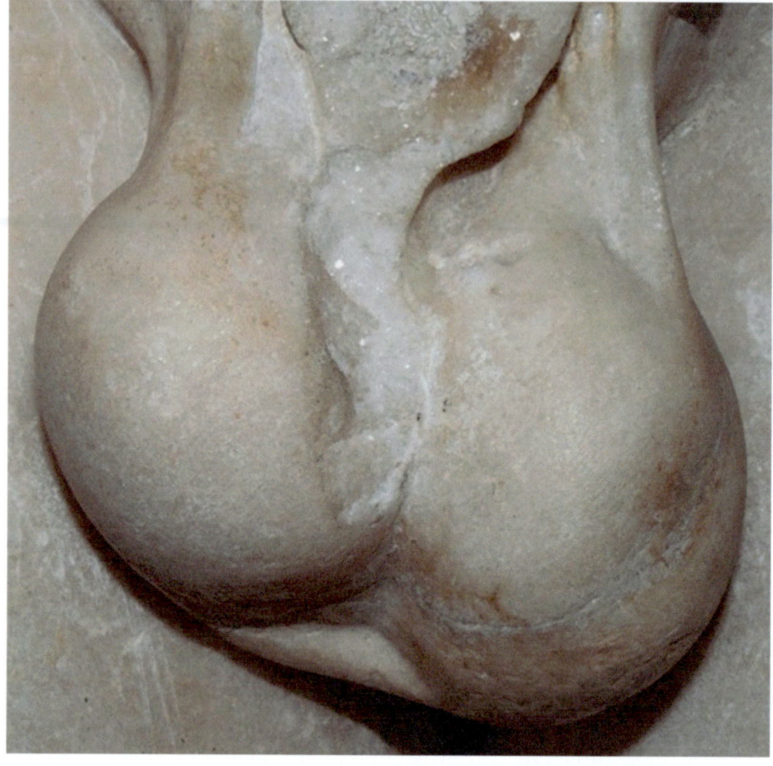

**Fig. 18.1** Ingrid Berthon-Moine's Marbles series features closely cropped images of Ancient Greek male statue testicles

usually prefer shapes that have some symmetry, but enough complexity to make them interesting [2]. Although asymmetry is typically associated with being unfit, but this not always the case; biologists consider that some species have evolved to be asymmetrical as an important adaptation, as some owls which have asymmetrical size and positioning of ears, allowing them to determine precisely the location of prey.

The presence of these asymmetrical features requires a process of symmetry breaking during development, both in plants and animals; symmetry breaking occurs at several different levels in order to generate the anatomical asymmetry which we observe. These levels include asymmetric gene expression, protein expression, and activity of cells. It seems that scrotal asymmetry is a normal beneficial phenomena of the mankind. Scrotal asymmetry could be an inherited phenomenon in its creation, or secondary to the testicular asymmetry.

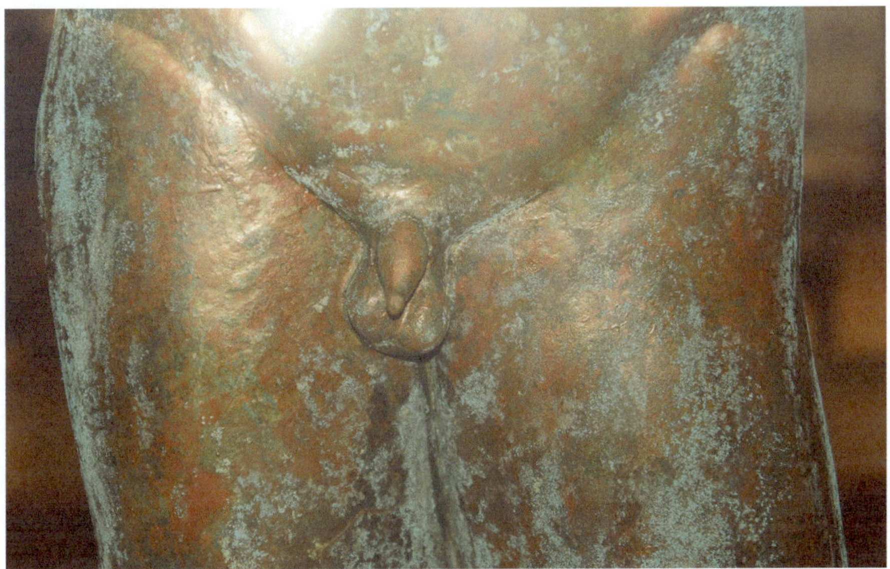

**Fig. 18.2** Apollo bronze status (30 BC-313 AD), Roman era, From the Egyptian museum, with the right scrotum higher than the left with uncircumcised penis

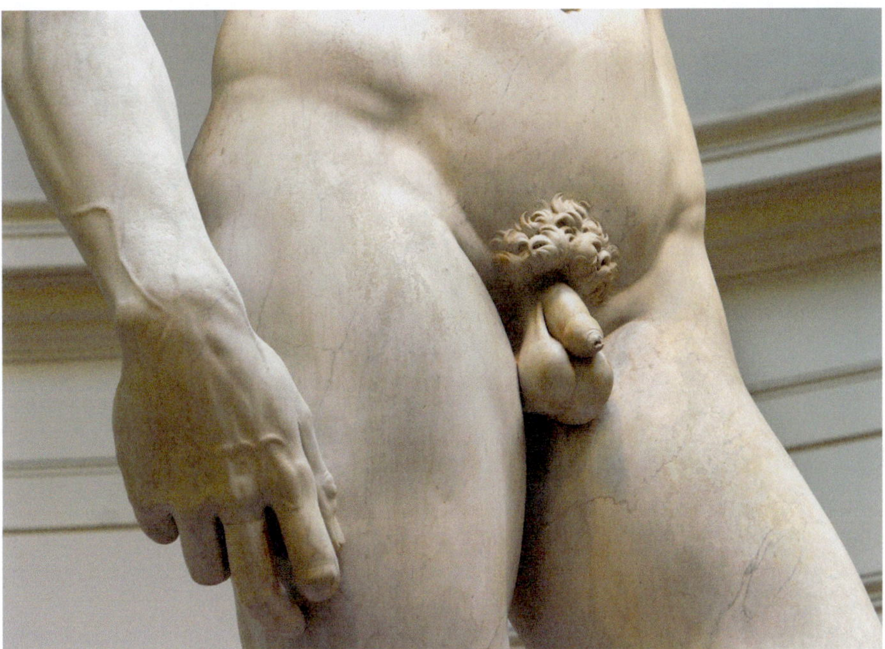

**Fig. 18.3** David sculpture created in marble between 1501 and 1504 by the Italian artist Michelangelo, with intact prepuce and higher, smaller right scrotum

## 18.1 Physiological Scrotal Asymmetry

Genital asymmetry has been reported in lower animals, including the gonads of horseshoe bats, oxen and chicks and the penises of certain flies, i.e. Drosophila melanogaster [3]. Scrotal asymmetry could be a reflection of the testicular asymmetry, but many authors consider testicular and scrotal asymmetry as a same; Chang et al. [4] founded that the right testis was the higher in 62% of 486 men, and the left testis is higher in 27%, the two being equal in height in the remaining 11%. Antliff and Shampo at 1959 [5] found an essentially similar result in 386 men, the right testis being higher in 65% and the left higher in 22%. Chang et al. [4] found that the average weights of the right and left testes were 9.95 and 9.36 g respectively, and the volumes are 9.69 and 9.10 cc, the differences being highly significant statistically (The normal average weight of the testicle is variable; but it ranges from 10 to 15 g). The densities are thus 1.0268 and 1.0286, a difference that is unlikely to be significant. Mittwoch [6] found a similar relationship in human foetuses, and showed that the right ovary also tends to be the larger. This difference is also found in many animal species.

Genital asymmetry also varied, to a small degree, as a function of handedness. Like right-handers, nonright-handers were more likely to have a left inclination than a right inclination, but this trend was not so pronounced. The asymmetry typically occurred in the left direction, and this pattern occurred in both right- and nonright-handers [7]. Asian/Oriental populations have been reported to have testicles substantially smaller than Whites/Caucasians. Whether such a size difference, along with additional differences in genital morphology that may occur across race/ethnicity, accounts for these differences is unknown [7].

Most researchers reported genital asymmetry mainly in adults, considering this phenomena only after puberty. Most of neonates had an equally positioned scrota (Fig. 18.4). But observing and following up of normal children and infants may reveals a scrotal asymmetry at younger ages, in the same way as in adults (Fig. 18.5). We found that most cases of dominant lower right scrotum (reverse to the common attitude) usually had an accompanying sort of genitourinary anomalies (Fig. 18.6).

## 18.2 Impact of Testicular Asymmetry

Clinicians must be aware about the phenomena of scrotal asymmetry; firstly to assure the worried parents about the normal variations of the testicular sizes among their children and to pick up the pathological cases with abnormal scrota or testicles in adult patients. Scrototestical asymmetry is not a simple morphological feature between both sides, it may had a clinical and pathological impaction, although little is known about the fractional functional difference between two testicles, but there

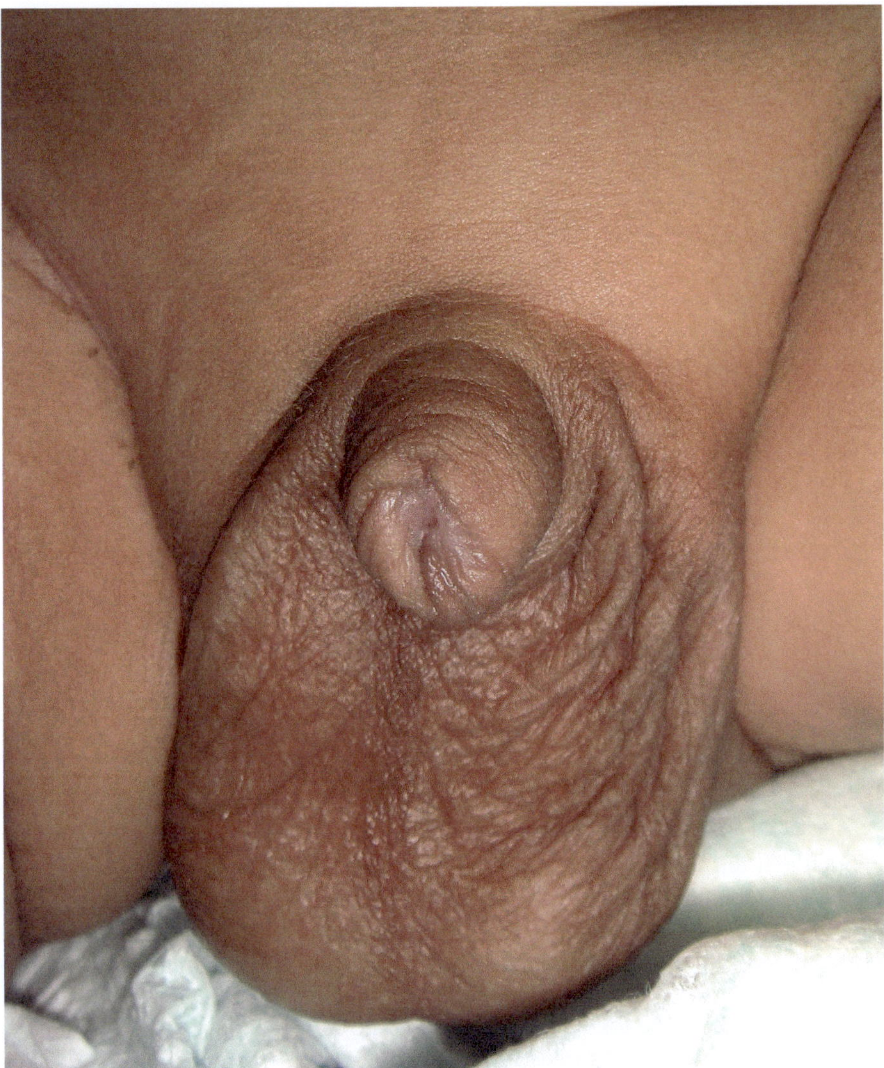

**Fig. 18.4** A neonate with symmetrical scrota and testicles

are some reports describing functional asymmetry of the normal testes, with the right side being less functioning than the left side [8].

The right testis showing a greater response either to luteinizing hormone (LH) deficiency treatment or to hemicastration than the left gonad. The left testis is more vulnerable to congenital anomalies than the right, and in humans, there is a greater incidence of cryptorchidism and varicocele on the left side [9]. Johnson et al. [10] in a study of 132 testes obtained at autopsy within 24 h of sudden death,

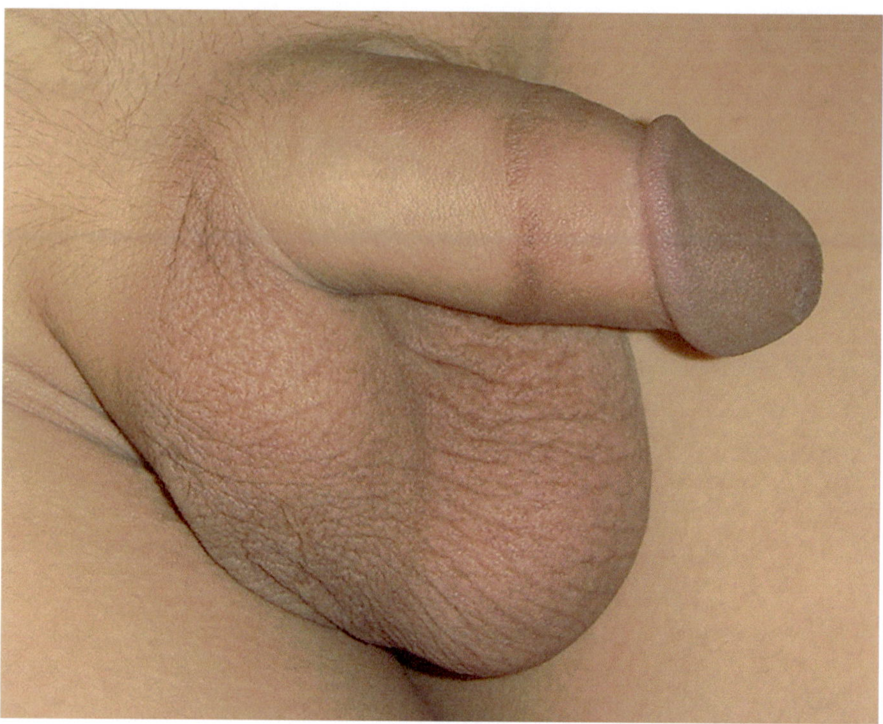

**Fig. 18.5** 6 years old boy with an obvious higher right testicle inside a smaller scrotum in comparison to the left side

reported that left testis is smaller than the right, they studied the changes between both sides; including both the total testis weight and the weight of the testicular parenchyma. Specifically, total testicular weight and testicular parenchyma weight were reported; and they found a total 10% lower on the left than on the right side. In the same report, the values of daily sperm production (DSP)/testis were positively correlated with both the total testis weight and the weight of testicular parenchyma and they found a 13% lower on the left side. Therefore, the smaller testis produces fewer spermatozoa. Testicular carcinoma may reflect lateral body asymmetry, where the larger testis that is the right may be more likely to be affected by cancer than the smaller [11]. In a large study involving over 250,000 cancer patients, a significant difference in cancer incidence by laterality was reported for all sites studied, including the breasts, lungs, kidneys, testes, and ovaries. Specifically, testicular cancer was found to be commoner in the right testis when compared with the left and a similar mass difference was also reported, with the right testis being larger, suggesting that tissue mass is an important contributor to asymmetry in testicular cancer incidence. Patients with left testicular carcinoma also showed significantly better survival rates than those with contralateral disease [12]. Stone et al. [13] in conducting a survey of 1116 cases of testicular neoplasms in Australia,

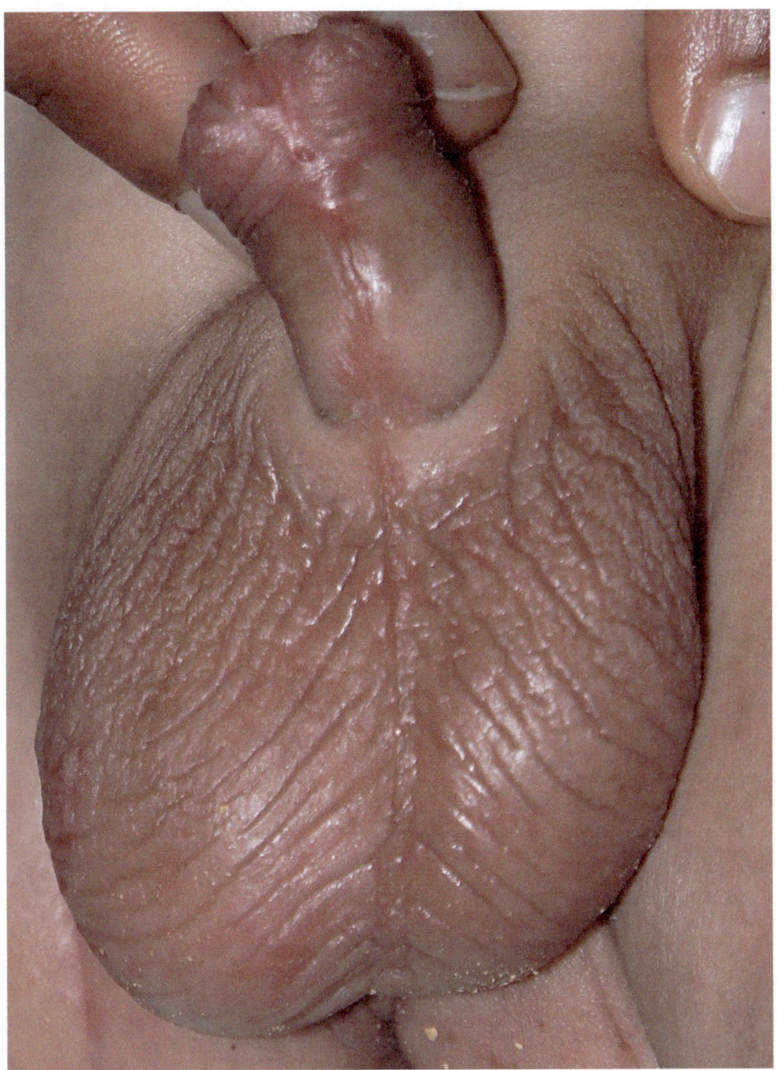

**Fig. 18.6** An infant with right side lower scrotum, but a coronal hypospadias is an associate

they reported a ratio of right to left-sided tumors of 54:46, suggesting an etiological connection between maldescent and laterality of germ cell neoplasms.

Genital and other body symmetry (e.g. handedness and cerebral asymmetry) may, in part, reflect a common prenatal hormonal origin. Differences in testes size have also been related to cognitive skills. Kimura et al. [14] reported that men with a larger right testis were found to perform relatively better on certain spatial tasks, the so-called "masculine" tasks when compared to men with a larger left testis performing better on "feminine" tasks. Thermal asymmetry of the human scrotum was also reported by a French study [15].

**Explanation**: This asymmetry is an interesting phenomenon, for which many explanations have been proposed, but the exact cause is not clear. Some authors however reject a simple mechanical explanation which would say that the heavier of the two organs is pulled to the lower position by the action of gravity, for in both adults and foetuses it is clear that the right testicle is both the heavier and also the greater in volume; that is the larger and heavier is also the higher.

**Embryological explanation**: Evidence from hermaphrodites indicates that growth favours the development of the testes on the right and ovaries on the left side [6]. The left testis descends in advance of the right, or that the left spermatic cord is longer because of the association of the left testis with the more cranially situated left kidney. In human fetuses, the right testicle seems to develop more quickly than the left, with the left side usually hanging lower than the right, due to a greater length of the spermatic cord.

The venous drainage of the testes commenced by the spermatic veins, i.e. the right vein joining the inferior vena cava at an acute angle and the left joining the left renal vein at right angles, with the accompanying disadvantage of increasing the resistance to the venous return from the left side. There is a general agreement that on account of this increased resistance and a consequent vascular stasis in the tributaries of the left spermatic vein, the left testis hangs slightly lower than the right. The right testis is in fact generally heavier and bulkier than the left.

Testicular asymmetry has been also attributed to more well-developed and greater flexion of the muscles on one side of the lower abdomen relative to the other side and/or the different length, angle and source of the blood vessels supplying the two testicles. Interestingly, varicoceles, when they occur in men, are also usually left-sided, a pattern that has been attributed to the characteristics of the blood vessels supplying the two testicles [4].

**Physiological role of scrotal asymmetry**: Normal scrotal asymmetry may had a role in testicular thermal regulation; as the left side was lower than the right side of scrotum. And the left side had more contact area with the groin than the right side. It seemed that the heat-dissipation area of the left side of scrotum was decreased by contacting with groin. On the other hand, most skin surface in the right side of scrotum was exposed to ambient air. So testis descent asymmetry is evolved to enable more effective cooling of the testicles by increasing the total scrotal skin surface area [16].

Also, it is assumed that one testis is typically lower than the other to avoid compression in the event of impact, during walking and in case of exposure to trauma.

**Investigations**: Investigations are not required for cases of normal scrotal asymmetry, but if there is any suspicious about abnormal scrotal wall or contents; a careful examination and investigations are mandatory, specially to rule out varicocele at adolescents. Simply the physician have to differentiate between physiological and pathological scrototesticular asymmetry at different ages. Although ultrasonography represents the primary imaging modality in the investigation of scrotal diseases, magnetic resonance imaging (MRI) has emerged as an important supplemental diagnostic tool [17].

## 18.3  Pathological Scrotal Asymmetry

Pathological scrotal asymmetry is an abnormal condition where the scrotum is enlarged asymmetrically secondary to a either a unilateral localised pathology in the scrotal wall, scrotal sac contents or secondary to a generalised body asymmetry.

**Aetiology**

- Pathological asymmetry of the genitalia seen in disorders of sex development (DSD) with mixed chromosomes, where mosaicism in the sex chromosomes leads to gonadal and genital duct asymmetry, rather than an even mixture of different cells. Asymmetry is more common in mixed gonadal dysgenesis (45,X/46,XY DSD) and in ovo-testicular DSD; in such cases the right side recognized to be more masculine than the left side, with a descended testis in the right hemiscrotum and an undescended intra-abdominal left ovary, ovotestis or streak gonad [18].
- Cases of partial androgen insensitivity syndrome may be presented with scrotal asymmetry, secondary to unilateral ill-developed scrotum (Fig. 18.7). Subsequently, all cases of unilateral scrotal agenesis or hypoplasia are considered as a cases of primary pathological scrotal asymmetry ( Chap. 11)
- In Beckwith-Wiedemann syndrome (BWS); which is an overgrowth chromosomal disorder characterized by macrosomia, macroglossia, organomegaly and developmental abnormalities (in particular abdominal wall defects, sometimes in the form of exomphalos), caused by alterations in growth regulatory genes on chromosome region 11p15.5, which is subjected to genomic imprinting. Genitally there is a diminutive penis with anteriorly displaced scrotum in 57% of the males cases [19]. Children with BWS and hemihypertrophy of one body side, may have an isolated asymmetry of one body part, such cases will have a scrotomegaly of the affected side, usually the left. (Fig. 18.8)
- Hemihyperplasia, also known as hemihypertrophy, is an asymmetric overgrowth of one or more body parts that is more pronounced than what can be accounted for by normal physiologic variation (arbitrarily defined as <5%). Hemihyperplasia results from an overgrowth of cells rather than an increase in individual cell size, the term hemihyperplasia is more accurately descriptive and preferred [20]. Scrotal asymmetry may be presented in such cases in the affected body side.

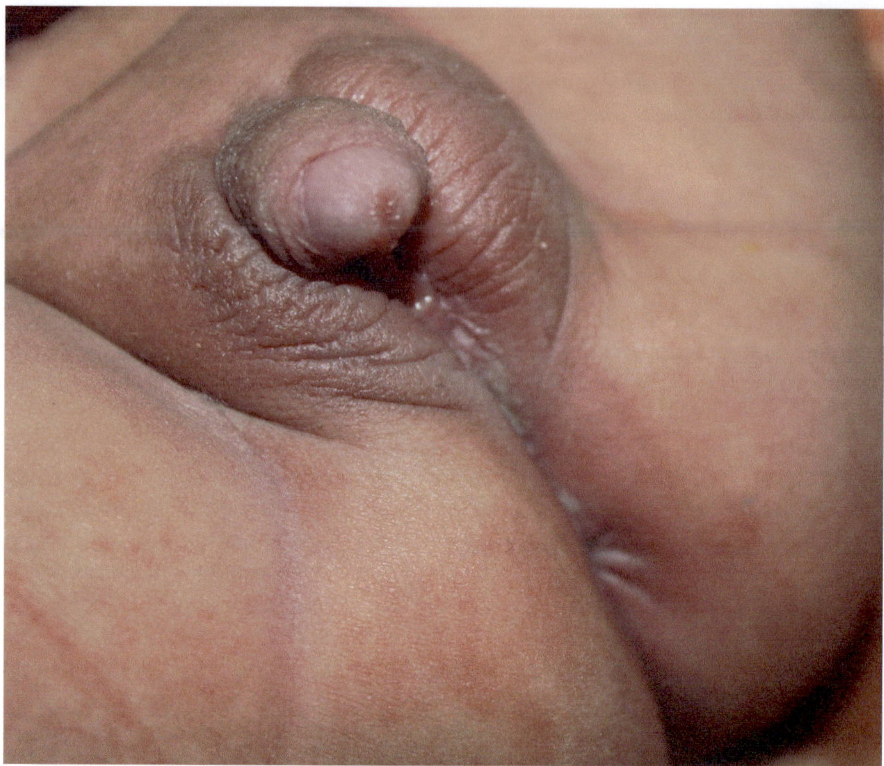

**Fig. 18.7** Right sided small hypoplastic scrotum and small testicle in a case of incomplete AIS

- Scrotal asymmetry could also be seen if one scrotal side had an atrophic testis; which may be lost congenitally (Anorchia) or after intrauterine or neonatal torsion, so the other normal side will show a compensatory hypertrophy of both the testicle and scrotum. (Fig. 18.9)
- Some primary cases of an acquired scrotal asymmetry are detected in elder man, where the asymmetry related to aging due to decreased dartos and cremasteric muscles tone and gravity's dependent stretching, which may affect one side over the other, but generalised symmetrical scrotal enlargement (usually called scrotomegaly or scrotal ptosis) is more commoner. Even though, there is no consensus in literature about what is considered a "normal hanging" scrotum or an abnormal scrotomegaly.
- Secondary scrotal asymmetry is completely different from the previously described entity of physiological asymmetry; such cases showed a marked difference in sizes between both sided with a bizarre contour (Fig. 18.10). These cases are very common and seen if one side increases in size or the other side is

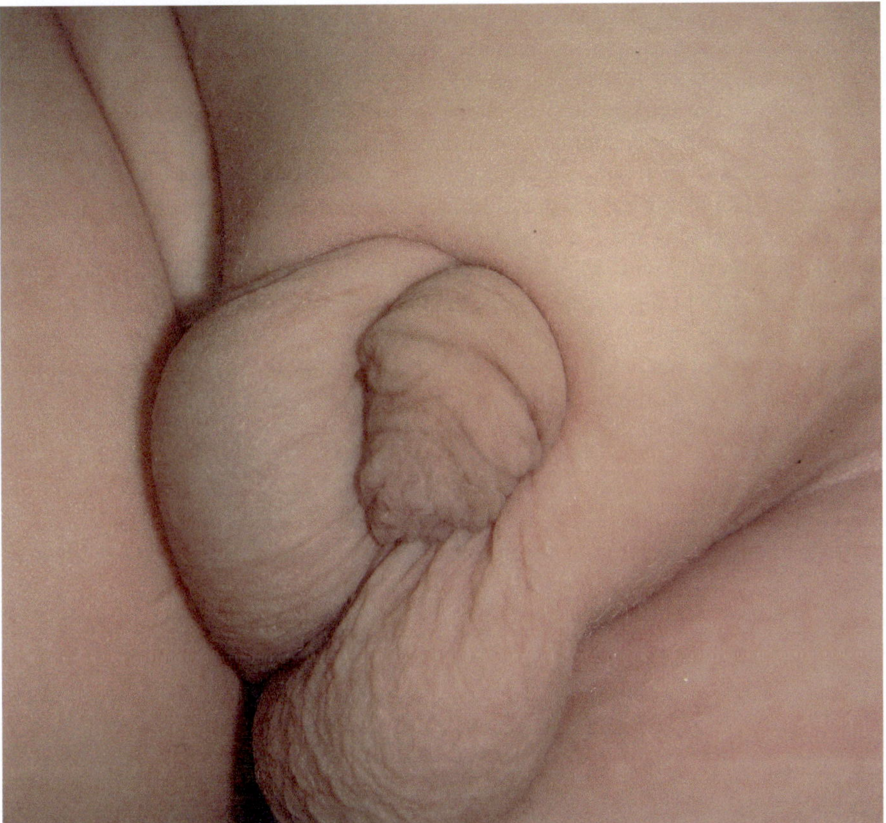

**Fig. 18.8** Differential growth of the both scrotal sided in association with left sided hemihypertrophy in a case of BWS

smaller due to deficiency of one or more of its structures, i.e. in all cases of unilateral pathology affecting any of the testicle, its coverage, or scrotal skin; like hernia, hydrocele, varicocele, undescended testicle, lymphedema, different scrotal cysts and swellings. (Chapter 22)

**Clinically**: Patients with abnormally lax scrota can complain of discomfort while wearing loose and short clothes, walking, doing sports and during intercourse. Thomas and Navia [21] defined "low hanging scrotum" as an enlarged and redundant scrotal bag hanging more than 1 or 2 cm below the tip of the flaccid penis. The representation of a "young hanging" and aesthetically pleasing scrotum coincides approximately with the distal penis in a standing position.

**Treatment**: In many occasions; exclusion of any underlying pathology, family or patient assurance is enough to alleviate patient's concern. All cases secondary to other pathologies will usually return to normal once the defect managed. Bothersome scrotomegaly and aesthetic scrotoplasty techniques still remain as entities which are poorly addressed in international literature. Treatment of severe or troublesome cases is mainly surgical through scrotoplasty or scrotal rejuvenation, some authors reporting the use of absorbable suspension sutures [22]. Ehle et al. [23] described the resection of excessive scrotal tissue using a posterior W-shaped incision for patient with idiopathic congenital dysmorphic megascrotum. But a vertical skin resection pattern is better than a horizontal one because it restores the scrotum in a more anatomical and aesthetically pleasant way, by placing the resultant scar in the median raphe. This would also theoretically allow better preservation of scrotal sensitivity, as the genital branch of the genitofemoral nerve and the ilioinguinal nerves run from lateral to medial.

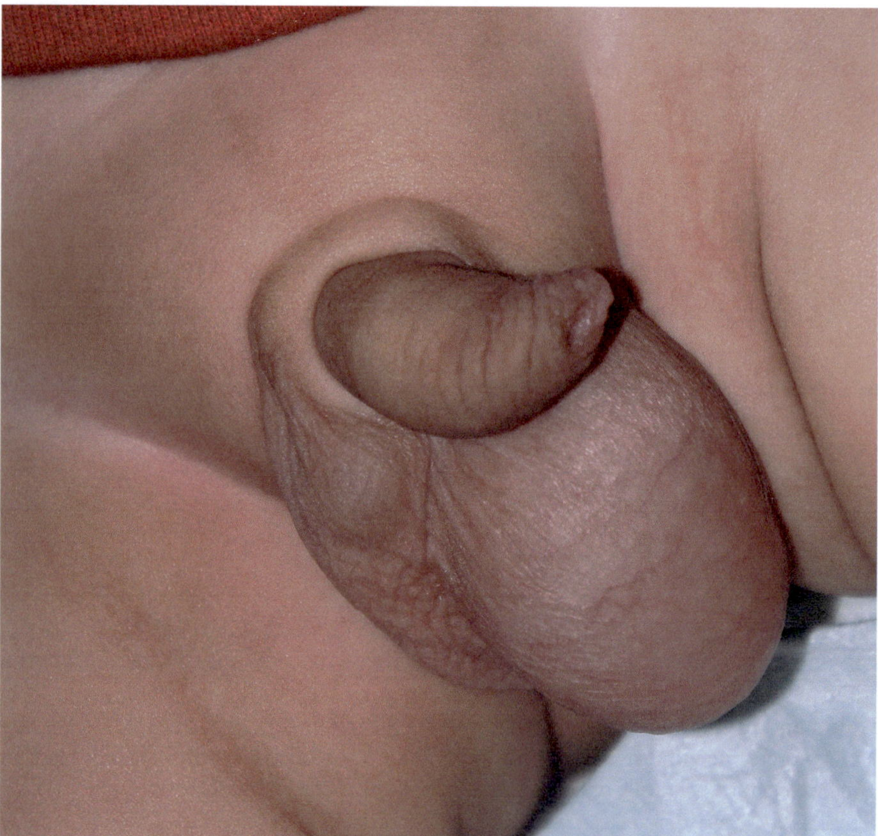

**Fig. 18.9** An infant with a congenital small right testicle with a compensatory left side hypertrophy which is manifested as asymmetry

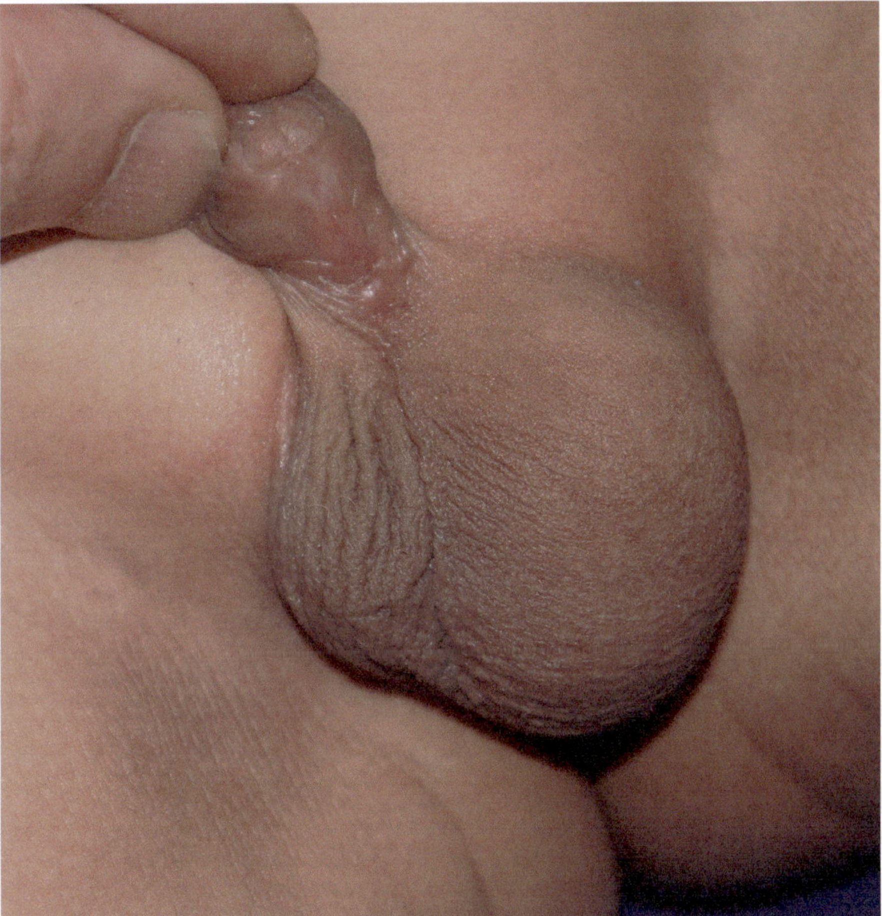

**Fig. 18.10** Secondary scrotal asymmetry in an infant with right sided undescended testicle and marked difference between both sided

# References

1. McManus. Right-left and the scrotum in Greek sculpture. Laterality. 2004;9(2):189–99.
2. Grammer K, Thornhill R. Human (Homo sapiens) facial attractiveness and sexual selection: the role of symmetry and averageness. J Compar Psychol. (Washington, D.C.). 1994;108 (3):233–42. https://doi.org/10.1037/0735-7036.108.3.233.
3. Morgan M, et al. Embryology and inheritance of asymmetry. In: Harnard S, Goldstein L, Jaynes J, et al., editors. Lateralization in the nervous system. New York, NY, USA: Academic Press; 1977. p. 173–94.
4. Chang RH, Hsu FK, Chan ST, et al. Scrotal asymmetry and handedness. J Anat. 1960;94:543–8.
5. Antliff HR, Shampo DR. Causative factors for the scrotal position of the testis. J Urol. 1959;81:462–3.

6. Mittwoch U. Ethnic differences in testicle size: a possible link with the cytogenetics of true hermaphroditism. Hum Reprod. 1988;3:445–9.
7. Bogaert AF. Genital asymmetry in men. Hum Reprod. 1997;12(1):68–72.
8. Gerendai I, Halalász B. Asymmetry of the neuroendocrine system. News Physiol Sci. 2001;16:92–5.
9. Gerendai I, Halasz B. Asymmetry of the Neuroendocrine system. News Physiol Sci. 2001;16:92–5.
10. Johnson L, Petty CS, Neaves WB. Influence of age on sperm production and testicular weights in men. J Reprod Fert. 1984;70:211–8.
11. Kostoff RN. Bilateral asymmetry prediction. Med Hypotheses. 2003;61:265–6.
12. Roychoudhuri R, Putcha V, Møller H. Cancer and laterality: a study of the five major paired organs (UK). Cancer Causes Control. 2006;17:655–62.
13. Stone JM, Cruickshank DG, Sandeman TF, et al. Laterality, maldescent, trauma and other clinical factors in the epidemiology of testis cancer in Victoria Australia. Br J Cancer. 1991;64:132–8.
14. Kimura D. Body asymmetry and intellectual pattern. Personal Indiv Differ. 1994;17:53–60.
15. Bengoudifa B, Mieusset R. Thermal asymmetry of the human scrotum. Human Reprod. 2007;22:2178–82.
16. Song GS and Seo JT. Relationship between ambient temperature and heat flux in the scrotal skin. Int J Androl. 2007;32:288–94. https://doi.org/10.1111/j.1365-2605.2007.00848.x.
17. Aganovic L, Cassidy F. Imaging of the scrotum. Radiol Clin North Am. 2012;50:1145–65.
18. Hutson JM, Warne GL, Grover SR. Disorders of sex development: an integrated approach to management. Berlin: Springer; 2012.
19. Hatada I, Mukai T. Genomic imprinting and Beckwith-Wiedemann syndrome. Histol Histopathol. 2000;15:309–12.
20. Arora MV, Choubey MS, Saikia M, Fotedar S. Congenital hemihyperplasia with hemipigmentation: a rare presentation. J Anaesthesiol Clin Pharmacol. 2015;31(2):253–5. https://doi.org/10.4103/0970-9185.155161.
21. Thomas C, Navia A. Aesthetic scrotoplasty: systematic review and a proposed treatment algorithm for the management of bothersome scrotum in adults. Aesth Plast Surg. 2020. https://doi.org/10.1007/s00266-020-01998-3.
22. Cohen PR. Nonsurgical rejuvenation of scrotal laxity: the sutures can raise by orienting threads in an upward manner (SCROTUM) procedure. Skinmed. 2019;17:118–20.
23. Ehle JJ, Hutcheson JC, Snyder HM 3rd, Cooper CS. Idiopathic congenital dysmorphic megascrotum. Urol Int. 2000;65:218–9.

# Chapter 19
# Scrotoschisis

**Mohamed A. Baky Fahmy**

**Abbreviation**

ETE   Extracorporeal testicular ectopia

**Synonymous:** Extracorporeal testicular ectopia, Eviscerated testicle, Testicular exstrophy, Congenital rupture of the scrotum, and Bubonoschisis.

**Definition:** Scrotoschisis is a congenital defect on the scrotal wall through which one or both testes are extruded and become extracorporeal, lying outside the scrotal cavity. The term has been used for testes extruding through scrotum or through an inguinal canal defect, although in this case the term bubonoschisis would be more appropriate [1].

**Pathogenesis:** Many theories have been proposed to explain the etiology and pathogenesis of this condition, but none is entirely proved. An underlying preceded meconial periorchitis is the best theory available with some substantial evidences [2]. The proposed pathophysiology is the late rupture of the scrotal skin secondary to an inflammatory reaction caused by exposure to meconium extruded from a minute intestinal perforation, which may heal later on, and meconium trickled to the scrotum during fetal life through the patent processus-vaginalis, as many cases reported a histological evidence of meconium in the scrotum. Meconium residual have been described in the scrotal wall for three of the infants reported and one case of contralateral meconial periorchitis, diagnosed at 4 months of age as a paratesticular calcified mass, which has been reported by Chun et al. [3]. An association of scrotoschisis with jejunal atresia, which was reported by Salle et al., also supports this theory [4]. The absence of intestinal abnormalities in most diagnosed infants

M. A. B. Fahmy (✉)
Al-Azhar University, Cairo, Egypt

    269
M. A. B. Fahmy (ed.), *Normal and Abnormal Scrotum*,
https://doi.org/10.1007/978-3-030-83305-3_19

can be explained by fetal cicatrisation of the proposed original intestinal lesion without sequelae [5].

Against this concept are the other reports, which failed to demonstrate evidence of meconium peritonitis. Also the site of defect described in meconium-associated evisceration is anteromedial in the scrotum, but in many other cases the defect was detected at the base of the scrotum, or the inguinal region, which suggesting other etiology [6]. Chun et al. [3] noted that experimental studies in rats showed that excision of future scrotal skin inhibited gubernacular migration, and leading to ipsilateral testicular ectopia. This suggests that a normally developed scrotum is required to guide gubernacular migration before testicular descent. They further suggested that since, in scrotoschisis, the defect is medial, the scrotal skin required for gubernacular descent may arise more laterally or posteriorly. Gongaware et al. [7] suggested the failure of differentiation of scrotal mesenchyme which leaving a defect where gubernaculum was covered only by a thin layer of epithelium. Lack of sufficient supporting structure in the scrotal wall results in rupture or a sort of avascular necrosis leading to the scrotal defect. Early amnion rupture or the adhesion/band spectrum is often cited as a probable factor in scrotoschisis. Aberrant amnion bands, strands, or sheets can cause disruption of morphogenesis in the abdominal wall, limb or a digit, and the same pathology may affect the scrotum and leads to disruption of its integrity and end with scrotoschisis [8]. In his study, Davies [9] postulated that the amnion band sequence mechanism could have played a causative role in this abnormality.

External mechanical compression due to arthrogryposis is also suggested as a cause of scrotoschisis by Lais et al. [10] in their article. Iatrogenic injury is a potential cause and could be concurrently associated if obstetrical difficulties were encountered during labor, mostly if completed by cesarean section [11]. Aseptic reaction of the exposed tissue, similar to the serosal changes seen in gastroschisis, which appear to be secondary to chemically-induced inflammation [12]. It is thus likely that the parietal defect is the primary lesion and the testis descends through it to becomes extracorporeal [5].

Concisely scrotoschisis could be due to:

Meconium periorchitis.
Failure of differentiation of scrotal mesenchymal layers.
Avascular necrosis of scrotal overlying epithelium.
Amniotic band.
Chemically induced scrotal wall inflammation.
External mechanical compression effect due to arthrogryposis.
Iatrogenic injury.

**Types**: The scrotoschisis could be:

- Unilateral
- Bilateral

According to the site of extrusion; scrotoschisis could be:

- Scrotal (Fig. 19.1)
- Inguinal "bubonoschisis" (Fig. 19.2)

The constant site of the ruptures (medial and cranial scrotal wall) might be related to the anatomic location of the patent process vaginalis (anteromedial to the cord and the testis). The testis eviscerates through an opening high on the anterior wall of the scrotum. This can be considered as extracorporeal testicular ectopia (ETE) or bubonoschisis according to the site of extrusion, respective to the location of the defect. Most reported cases are unilateral, but bilateral scrotoschisis were also reported [13].

**Diagnosis**: The testicle, epididymis, and part of the cord which looks as a one amalgamated mass were commonly extruding through a small defect in the scrotal wall or the inguinal canal at the level of the superficial inguinal ring, covered with a thick fibrotic layer resembling what we see occasionally in cases of gastroschisis. (Fig. 19.1). The cord is usually normally long and if the cord and testicular coverages are distinguishable; the processus vaginalis is usually intact, there was no hernial sac or penile anomalies reported in any case till now. The scrotal wall defect is usually smaller than the diameter of the extruded testicle, which means that the defect happened early in pregnancy, but rarely the defect seen widely opened. The scrotum was although empty but well formed and around the same size as the contralateral side. During a physical examination, it is fundamental to rule out testicular torsion, which is a common complication due to lack of testicular anatomical attachments.

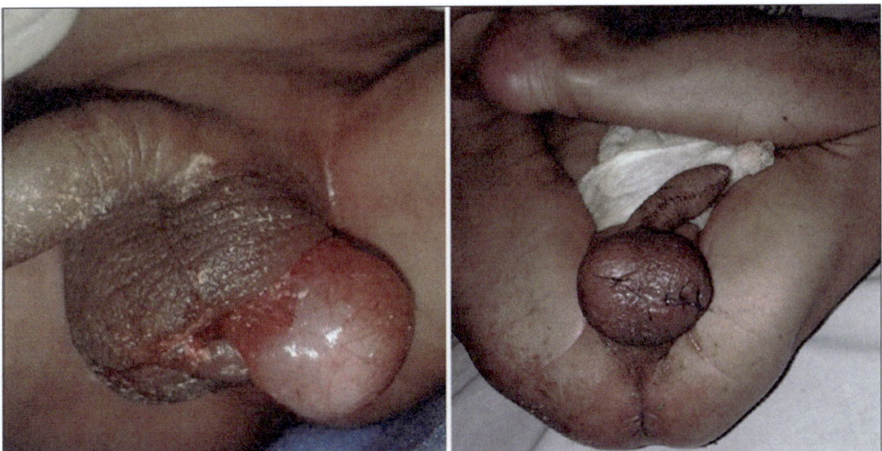

**Fig. 19.1** Left side scrotoschisis repaired in two layers transversally

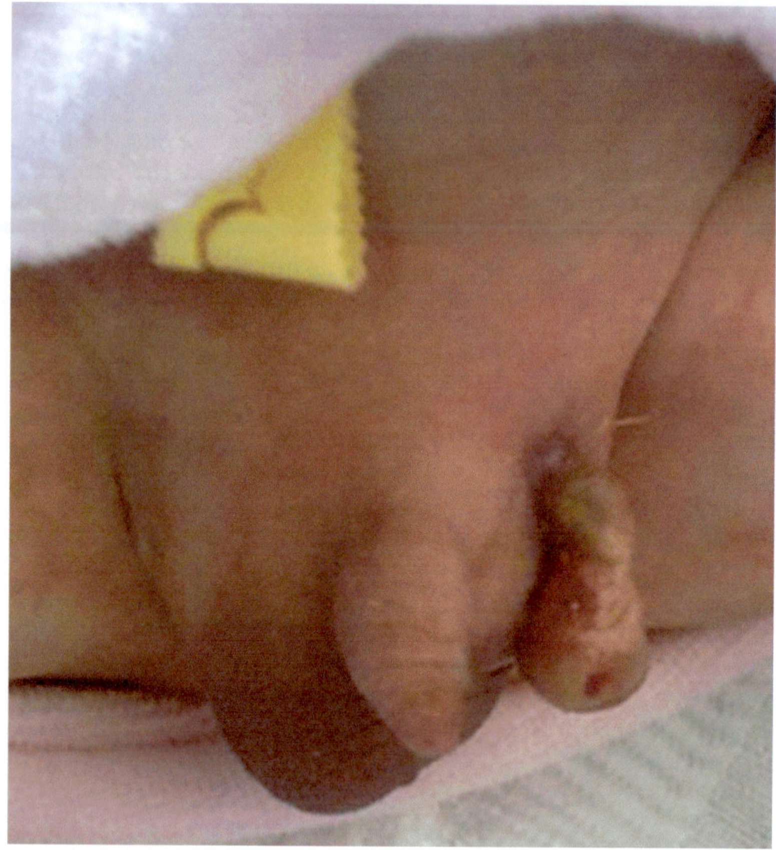

**Fig. 19.2** A neonate with a left sided bubonoschisis

**Investigations**: Plain X ray abdomen, and a whole abdomen ultrasound is mandatory to diagnose any associated bowel perforation, peritonitis or other congenital anomalies.

**Associated Anomalies**: Most cases of scrotoschisis are unilateral and affect normal males. One case was reported with an association between jejunal atresia and scrotoschisis [4]. There have been some reports on cases associated with intestinal atresia, Beckwith–Wiedemann syndrome, ruptured omphalocele and meconium periorchitis. Some patients present with an associated testicular torsion [14].

**Complications**: Testicular torsion may occur, as in the study by Ameh et al. [14] which may results in gangrene of the testis, if the management delayed. Testicular torsion may be a complication other than an association. If the processus vaginalis ruptured it may pave a way for the pathogens to reach the peritoneum and results in peritonitis.

**Treatment**: Early management is substantial, such cases are a semi-urgent condition which should be managed immediately if it presents in the delivery room. Scrotoschisis is treated by returning the testis to the scrotal sac followed by orchidopexy. Immediate repair of the defect in layers (two planes) under general anesthesia is the stander management, the defect could be closed horizontally or vertically after orchidopexy (Fig. 19.1).

Some authors reported repair under local anesthesia within a few hours after birth, which is feasible with good healing [15]. Broad-spectrum antibiotics should be commenced immediately on diagnosis.

If the general situation of the baby or the hospital facilities doesn't permit immediate repair; frequent cleaning and dressing with antiseptics and systemic broad spectrum antibiotic are mandatory to avoid local testicular infection and systemic peritonitis [13]. Another approach reported with a simple dressing and leaving the defect to heal by secondary intention. Postoperative follow-up should not be discontinued until verification of two symmetric, vital, and normally growing testes. A further research is recommended to study the effect of scrotoschisis on fertility.

# References


1. Haidar AM, Gharmool BM. Extracorporeal testicular ectopia through inguinal canal: a case report. J Neonat Surg. 2013;2(1):10.
2. Kojori F, DeMaria J. Scrotoschisis associated with meconium periorchitis. J Pediatr Urol. 2007;3(5):415–6.
3. Chun K, St-Vil D. Scrotoschisis associated with contralateral meconium periorchitis. J Pediatr Surg. 1997;32(6):864–6.
4. Salle JL, de Fraga JC, Wojciechowski M, Antunes CR. Congenital rupture of scrotum: an unusual complication of meconium peritonitis. J Urol. 1992;148(4):1242–3.
5. Shukla RM, Mandal KC, Roy D, Patra MP, Mukhopadhyay B. Scrotoschisis: an extremely rare congenital anomaly. J Indian Assoc Pediatr Surg. 2012;17(4):176–7. https://doi.org/10.4103/0971-9261.102342.
6. Jesus LE, Dekermacher S, Filho JA, Rocha LJ. Scrotoschisis: An extremely rare congenital uropathy. Urology. 2012;79:219–21.
7. Gongaware RD, Sussman AM, Kraebber DM, Michigan S. Scrotoschisis as a mechanism for extracorporeal testicular ectopia. J Pediatr Surg. 1991;26(12):1430–1.
8. Smith DW. Early amnion rupture spectrum. In: Smith DW, editor. Recognizable patterns of human malformations. 3rd ed. Philadelphia: WB Saunders; 1982. p. 488–96.
9. Davies MR. Scrotoschisis—a case of congenital "shameful exposure of the testes". Pediatr Surg Int. 1994;9:146–7.
10. Lais A, Serventi P, Caione P, Ferro F. Arthrogryposis as a possible mechanism of scrotoschisis acquired in utero. Pediatr Surg Int. 1994;9:605–6.
11. Premkumar MH, Colen JS, Roth DR, Fernandes CJ. Could Scrotoschisis Mimic an Iatrogenic Injury? A case report. Urology. 2009;73:795–6.
12. Kluck P, Tibboel D, van der Kamp AWM, et al. The effect of fetal urine on the development of the bowel in gastroschisis. J Pediatr Surg. 1983;8:47–50.
13. Fahmy MAB. Scrotum. In: Rare congenital genitourinary anomalies. Berlin, Heidelberg: Springer; 2015. https://doi.org/10.1007/978-3-662-43680-6_4.

14. Ameh EA, Amoah JO, Awotula OP, Mbibu HN. Scrotoschisis, bilateral extra-corporeal testicular ectopia and testicular torsion. Pediatr Surg Int. 2003;19(6):497–8.
15. Premkumara M H, Colen SJ, Roth DR, Fernandes CJ. Could Scrotoschisis mimic an iatrogenic injury? A case report. Urology. 2009;(73), Issue 4:795–6.

# Chapter 20
# Scrotal Calcinosis

Mohamed A. Baky Fahmy

**Abbreviations**

ISC   Idiopathic scrotal calcinosis
TM    Testicular microlithiasis

## 20.1   Definition

ISC is described as a skin condition of multiple hard, painless, asymptomatic cutaneous nodules within the scrotal wall and without detectable abnormalities in the calcium/phosphorous metabolism.

**Synonymous**
It is also known as a idiopathic calcinosis cutis. But scrotal pearl or scrotal calculi is a different entity, which is defined as a freely mobile calcified bodies lying between the layers of the scrotum.

Testicular microlithiasis (TM) is rare condition characterized by presence of multiple, small, uniform-appearing echogenic foci of less than 3 mm without acoustic shadowing in the seminiferous tubules, which may be indicative of degeneration of the testicular parenchyma.

## 20.2   Historical Background

Scrotal calcinosis is first described by Lewinski over a century ago [1]. This disorder is named as idiopathic scrotal calcinosis by Shapiro et al. in 1970 [2].

M. A. B. Fahmy (✉)
Al-Azhar University, Cairo, Egypt

© The Author(s), under exclusive license to Springer Nature Switzerland AG 2022
M. A. B. Fahmy (ed.), *Normal and Abnormal Scrotum*,
https://doi.org/10.1007/978-3-030-83305-3_20

## 20.3 Clinically

These lesions are usually multiple and bilaterally distributed in the scrotum, only few case of a unilateral form has been published in the English literature [3]. Lesions presented as a multiple brown and indolent nodules, of varying size, number and form without any discharge or inflammatory reaction. These lesions are located within the dermis, tend to grow slowly in number and size, and contain chalky material corresponding to calcium deposits.

A penile extension has been reported for multiple scrotal calcinosis nodules, which may causing sexual discomfort, and may had impact on the patient's quality of life. Lesion size ranges from a few millimetres to several centimetres (Fig. 20.1).

Patients with dark skin are probably more susceptible to have nodular calcifications, suggesting an ethnic susceptibility [4]. Patients are usually young men, aged 20–40 years old but children and older men have also been affected (Fig. 20.2), they usually have multiple (up to 50) long-standing, firm to hard nodules varying in size from a few millimetres up to 3 cm. The overlying skin is usually intact and hypopigmented; specially in a dark skin patients, but it may ulcerate releasing cheesy material. Occasionally, a single hard nodule may be present. There is one case reported as an extensive ISC, which was associated with vitiligo [5].

On the other hand scrotal calculi are a benign entities, which are thought to represent freely mobile calcified bodies lying between the layers of the tunica vaginalis of the testes. Some recent studies revealed that the prevalence of scrotal calculi was very high in some specific populations [6]. Scrotal calcinosis lesions may be complicated by a secondary inflammation or it may be infected following trauma.

## 20.4 Etiopathogenesis

Scrotal calcinosis occurs in two settings: calcification of pre-existing epidermal or pilar cysts, and calcification of dermal connective tissue in the absence of cysts (idiopathic scrotal calcinosis). The hypothesis for the later form favours origin from eccrine duct milia because of immunoreactivity for carcinoembryonic antigen, a marker for eccrine sweat glands. A published study indicated that the idiopathic form may be related to trauma [7]. The idiopathic character was previously approved by Song et al. [8], who analysed more than 50 nodules of scrotal calcinosis, and concluded that the common characteristic is a calcified dystrophy of epidermal cysts. Other authors supported the calcified dystrophy of the dartos muscle [9]. Dubey et al. [10] after histological examination using Von Kossa staining revealed a basophilic, calcified deposit in the scrotal dermis and the calcinosis nodules that is surrounded by giant cell granulomas in an intense foreign body inflammatory reaction (Fig. 20.3).

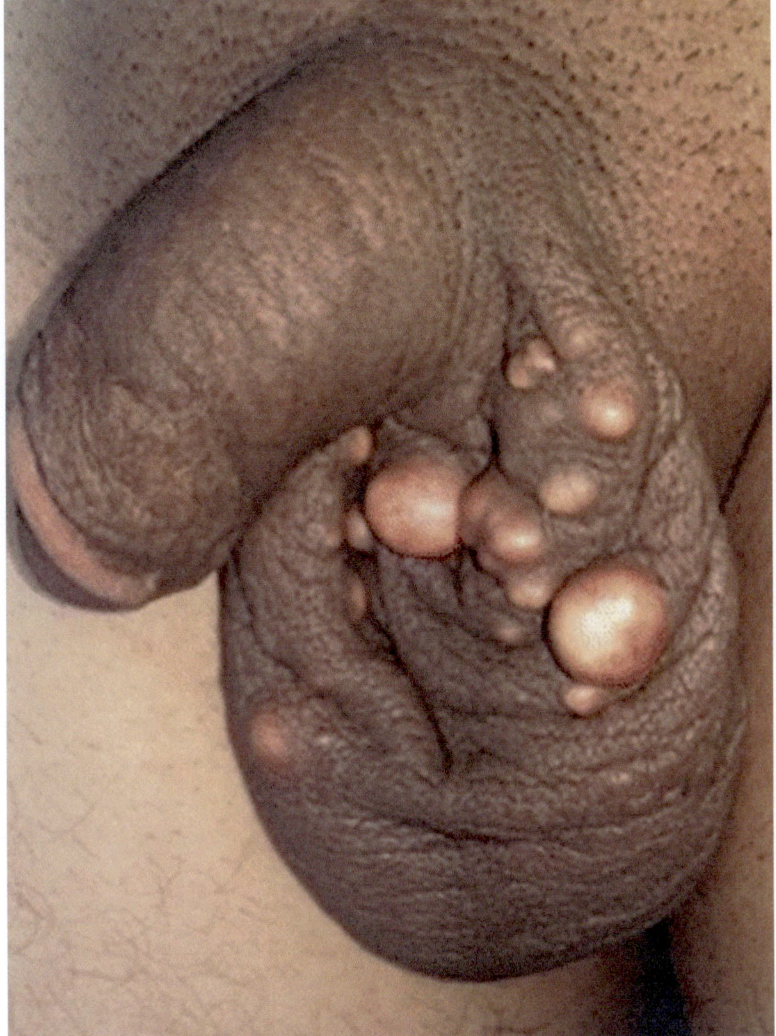

**Fig. 20.1** Calcified nodules of the scrotum measuring 5–15 mm. This photo reproduced after a kind permission from Dr. Omar Karray, Urology Unit, Interior security forces hospital [19]

Saladi et al. [11] classified scrotal calcinosis according to the proposed causal mechanisms into:

- Calcific degeneration of epidermoid cysts
- Dystrophic calcification of dartos muscle
- Calcification of eccrine sweat ducts
- Idiopathic/undetermined (most cases).

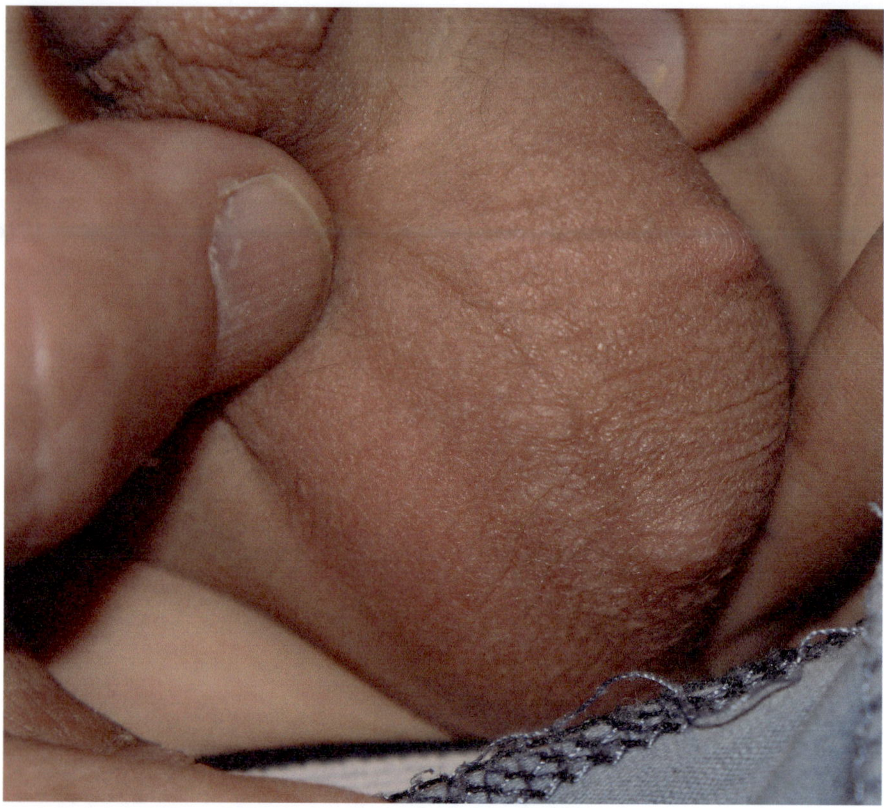

**Fig. 20.2** Rare case of multiple nodules of idiopathic calcinosis in the scrotum of 4 years child confined to one side

Scrotal calculi may develop as a sequela to hematomas or inflammatory changes within the scrotum or loose bodies from torsion and infarction of the appendix of the testis or epididymis.

Also there are several theories about the origin and causes of testicular microlithiasis have been reported, but the exact etiology is still remains unclear. Previous studies have reported an association between TM and testicular germ cell tumors and carcinoma in situ. In addition, an association between TM and infertility has been also reported. Although real impact of TM in children is still a matter of debate, it has been described in previous reports that the incidence of TM is high in some congenital disorders, such as undescended testicle, Down's syndrome, Klinefelter syndrome, McCune-Albright syndrome and Peuzt-Jeghers syndrome, which may be associated with testicular impairment and infertility [12].

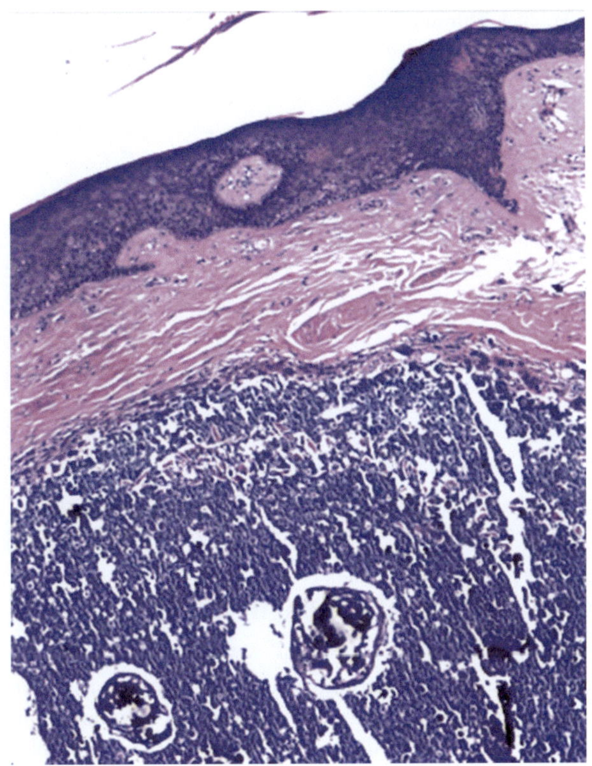

**Fig. 20.3** Histopathology of a calcified scrotal nodules composed of amorphous basophilic material (H&E)

## 20.5   Diagnosis

Diagnosis of scrotal calcinosis is clinically accomplished with confirmation by plain X ray, also ultrasound may be helpful; specially to rule out any other associated testicular pathology (Fig. 20.4). Imaging studies such as CT scans will show calcifications in the scrotal wall, but are usually not needed [13]. Biochemical tests for the calcium, phosphorous and parathyroid hormones level showed be done for every patient; specially the younger one, they are usually of normal values. Histologically, scrotal calcinosis lies within the dermis and contains granules and globules of hematoxylinophilic calcific material. It may or may not be accompanied by giant cell granulomatous inflammation and recognizable cyst wall fragments. It is plausible that idiopathic scrotal calcinosis represents an end-stage phenomenon of numerous old undetectable epidermal cysts that over time have lost their cyst walls [8].

**Fig. 20.4** Ultrasound of adult
testicle with extensive
microliathiasis

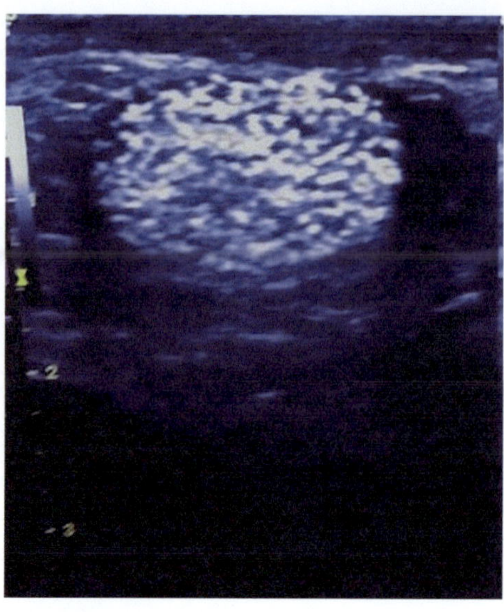

## 20.6   Differential Diagnosis

Scrotal calcinosis should be differentiated from other rare cases of scrotal nodules;
like fibroma, neuroma and granuloma. Median raphe cysts and swelling are classically confined only to the redline [14]. Theoretically, it may be necessary to
differentiate non-calcified epidermoid cysts from other nodular calcifications.
Epidermoid cysts corresponding to yellowish nodules of variable sizes with a relatively soft consistency, and nodular calcifications corresponding to very hard
marble-like nodules (Chap. 17). Of course scrotal nodules should be differentiated
from testicular calcification and microlithiasis; which may be associated with impaired testicular function. It is characterized by multiple, small, uniform-appearing
echogenic foci of less than 3 mm without acoustic shadowing in the seminiferous
tubules, which may be indicative of degeneration of the testicular parenchyma [15].

## 20.7   Treatment

Treatment may be unnecessary for asymptomatic lesions, but surgery is indicated
for infected, recurrent, or extensive lesions with a subtotal excisions of the scrotal
wall. Also surgery is usually indicated in patients presented with voluminous
lesions carrying a psychological and a sexual prejudice. Surgery is the traditional
treatment for ISC, as it allows a histopathological examination and confirmation of
the diagnosis. However, newer treatments, such as ablative lasers, have been proposed with a good results. The $CO_2$ super pulsed laser is reported as a fast and
effective way to treat ISC and may be an alternative to traditional surgery [16].

The total excision of calcified nodules may ignore small lesions, and there is potential for recurrence. Recently, Noël et al. [14] proposed a one-stage technique used mainly for giant nodules with a considerable skin defect. An elliptic resection is performed after making an incision centered on the median raphe and a thorough dissection of the scrotal dermis from the dartos muscle, allowing more pertinent detection of small nodules than the classical resection of nodules detectable on the surface of the skin. This technique is a particularly attractive procedure because the vascularization provided by the external pudendal artery is peripheral. The aesthetic result is better after a median raphe incision and a fine dissection conserving the integrity of the skin integumentary capillaries. Few cases of recurrence have been reported, which seems to be related to neglected fine tiny nodules that increase in size later. No cases of malignant transformation have been reported [17]. But many cases; specially at older age may confuse with neoplastic lesion, and the proper diagnosis could be only reached after excision and biopsy [18].

# References


1. Lewinski HM. Lymphangioma der Haut mit verkalktem Inhalt. Virchows Arch Pathol Anat. 1883;91:371–4.
2. Shapiro L, Platt N, Torres-Rodriguez VM. Idiopathic calcinosis of the scrotum. Arch Dermatol. 1970;102(2):199–204.
3. Hwang C, Kim YJ, Lee Y, Seo YJ, Park JK, Lee JH. A case of unilateral scrotal calcinosis. Clin Exp Dermatol. 2010;35(4):e159–60.
4. Angamuthu N, Pais AV, Chandrakala SR. Calcinosis cutis: a report of four cases. Trop Dr. 2003;33:50–2.
5. Sara M, Dergamoun H, Karima S, Laila B. Case of extensive scrotal calcinosis associated with vitiligo. BMJ Case Rep. 2020;13(9). https://doi.org/10.1136/bcr-2020-238695.
6. Artas H, Orhan I. Scrotal calculi. J Ultrasound Med. 2007;26:1775–9.
7. Swinehart JM, Golitz LE. Scrotal calcinosis. Dystrophic calcification of epidermoid cysts. Arch Dermatol. 1982;118:985–8.
8. Song DH, Lee KH, Kang WH. Idiopathic calcinosis of the scrotum: histopathologic observations of fifty-one nodules. J Am Acad Dermatol. 1988;19:1095–101.
9. Pabuççuoglu U, Canda MS, Guray M, et al. The possible role of dartoic muscle degeneration in the pathogenesis of idiopathic scrotal calcinosis. Br J Dermatol. 2003;148:827–9.
10. Dubey S, Sharma R, Maheshwari V. Scrotal calcinosis: idiopathic or dystrophic? Dermatol Online J. 2010;16:5.
11. Saladi RN, Persaud AN, Phelps RG, Cohen SR. Scrotal calcinosis. Is the cause still unknown? J Am Acad Dermatol. 2004;51:97.
12. Nakamura M, et al. Prevalence and risk factors of testicular microlithiasis in patients with hypospadias: a retrospective study. BMC Pediatr. 2018;18:179. https://doi.org/10.1186/s12887-018-1151-6.
13. Grenader T, Shavit L. Scrotal calcinosis. N Engl J Med. 2011;365(7):647.
14. Noël B, Bron C, Künzle N, De Heller M, Panizzon RG. Multiple nodules of the scrotum: histopathological findings and surgical procedure. A study of five cases. JEADV. 2006;20:707–10. https://doi.org/10.1111/j.1468-3083.2006.01578.x.
15. Drut R, Drut RM. Testicular microlithiasis: histologic and immunohistochemical findings in 11 pediatric cases. Pediatr Dev Pathol. 2002;5(6):544–50.

M. A. B. Fahmy


16. Cannarozzo G, Bennardo L, Negosanti F, Nisticò SP. $CO_2$ laser treatment in idiopathic scrotal calcinosis: a case series. J Lasers Med Sci. 2020;11(4):500–1. https://doi.org/10.34172/jlms.2020.79.
17. Sugihara T, Tsuru N, Kume H, Homma Y, Ihara H. Relapse of scrotal calcinosis 7 years after primary excision. Urol Int. 2014;92(4):488–90.
18. Akhtar K, Warsi S, Rab AZ, Sherwani RK. Scrotal calcinosis mimicking malignancy—a rare case presentation. IP J Diagn Pathol Oncol. 2020;5(1):99–101.
19. Karray O, Dhaoui A, Boulma R, et al. Scrotal calcinosis: two case reports. J Med Case Rep. 2017;11:312. https://doi.org/10.1186/s13256-017-1451-8.

# Chapter 21
# Scrotal Vascular Anomalies

Mohamed A. Baky Fahmy

## Abbreviations

AVMs      ArterioVenous Malformations
ISSVA     International Society for the Study of Vascular Anomalies
MALT      Minimal access laser therapy
Nd:YAG    Neodymium:yttrium-aluminum-garnet
LC        Lymphangioma circumscriptum

## 21.1  Hemangiomas

Hemangiomas are benign vascular malformations of enlarged dysplastic vascular channels with abnormal growth and proliferation of the endothelial cells. It is the most common tumors of infancy; affecting 1–3% of neonates and 10% of children by the age of 1 year [1]. After an initial proliferating phase, it many undergoes complete regression with fibrosis. The color depends on its location; hemangiomas involving the papillary dermis (superficial hemangiomas) are red, but those in the reticular dermis and subcutaneous fat are usually blue or colorless (deep hemangiomas). Large segmental hemangiomas may be associated with regional congenital anomalies.

Before 1982, the term "hemangioma" was used to encompass a wide range of vascular outgrowths, independent of clinical manifestations, natural history, or embryological origin. Subsequently, at 1982 Mulliken and Glowacki [2] proposed

**Electronic supplementary material** The online version of this chapter (https://doi.org/10.1007/978-3-030-83305-3_21) contains supplementary material, which is available to authorized users.

M. A. B. Fahmy (✉)
Al-Azhar University, Cairo, Egypt

the first biological classification for vascular birthmarks; based on their clinical behavior and endothelial cell characteristics into two groups: hemangiomas and vascular malformations. More recently the International Society for the Study of Vascular Anomalies (ISSVA) devised a multidisciplinary etiopathogenesis based approach to classify benign vascular anomalies into tumors and malformations; vascular tumors subdivided to: benign, local aggressive and malignant, while vascular anomalies subdivided into: simple, combined, of major vessels and associating other anomalies [3] (Table 21.1).

The etiopathogenesis based classification has major therapeutic and prognostic implications, hence the management of vascular anomalies has been evolving continuously. Surgical resection, embolization or sclerotherapy are the preferred treatment modalities for vascular malformations (VM), while beta-blockers, sclerosing therapy and steroids have a curative role in proliferative endothelial tumor-like hemangioma. Recently there has been a shift from surgery to pharmacotherapy in the treatment of hemangiomas; as Beta- blockers are now the first line modality for treating infantile hemangiomas requiring systemic therapy. For congenital hemangiomas, a wait and watch is often the best treatment, but surgery and Minimal Access Laser Therapy (MALT) are used for problematic cases only. Surgical excision with or without embolization, sclerotherapy, and pulsed dye laser is the common therapy used to manage vascular malformations in many centers [4].

Hemangiomas of the scrotal wall are rare vascular malformations, which often show extension to the penis and into the perineum. Involvement of the thigh, anterior abdominal wall, and, occasionally, deep organs such as the rectum and sigmoid colon have been described [5] (Fig. 21.1).

Localised small scrotal haemangioma confined to the scrotum with minimal extension to the root of the penis is not rare and in early infancy it is liable for ulceration, infection and a profound secondary bleeding (Figs. 21.2 and 21.3).

These lesions are congenital but are usually not diagnosed until the teenage years or young adulthood. Those lesions presented early are appreciated as a faint blue patch or a soft blue mass.

**Cavernous hemangioma**: Scrotal arteriovenous malformations (AVMs) are generally uncommon, there are only several case reports in the literature. It is characterised by large feeding vessels, hypervascularity, numerous arteriovenous connections around the nidus, early venous filling and washout in angiography. VMs can be also subdivided into either slow-flow (capillary, lymphatic, venous) or fast-flow (arterial, arteriovenous) type [5].

Cavernous hemangiomas, are much less common in genital area, and are probably more appropriately classified as a vascular malformation. They may be detected at birth or later in life. It tends to enlarge gradually and should be treated with care. Physical examination reveals a "bag of worms" sensation similar to that of a varicocele, although the lesions tend to be firm and do not decompress when the patient is recumbent. An associated superficial lesions like verruca or warts are not rare (Fig. 21.4).

**Table 21.1**  A recent classification of vascular malformation guided by The International Society for the Study of Vascular Anomalies (ISSVA) classification

Classifications of vascular anomalies

| Vascular tumors | Vascular malformations | | | | |
|---|---|---|---|---|---|
| Benign<br>Locally aggressive<br>Malignant | Simple | Combined | | of major vessels | With other syndromes |
| | | Types | Abbreviations | | |
| | Capillary malformations<br>Lymphatic malformations<br>Venous malformations<br>Arteriovenous malformations<br>Arteriovenous fistula | 1. Capillary-venous malformation | VVM | | |
| | | 2. Capillary-lymphatic malformation | CLM | | |
| | | 3. Capillary-arteriovenous malformation | CAVM | | |
| | | 4. Lymphatic-venous malformation | LVM | | |
| | | 5. Capillary-lymphatic-venous malformation | CLVM | | |
| | | 6. Capillary-lymphatic-arteriovenous malformation | CLAVM | | |
| | | 7. Capillary-venous-arteriovenous malformation | CVAVM | | |
| | | 8. Capillary-lymphatic-venous-arteriovenous m | CLVAVM | | |

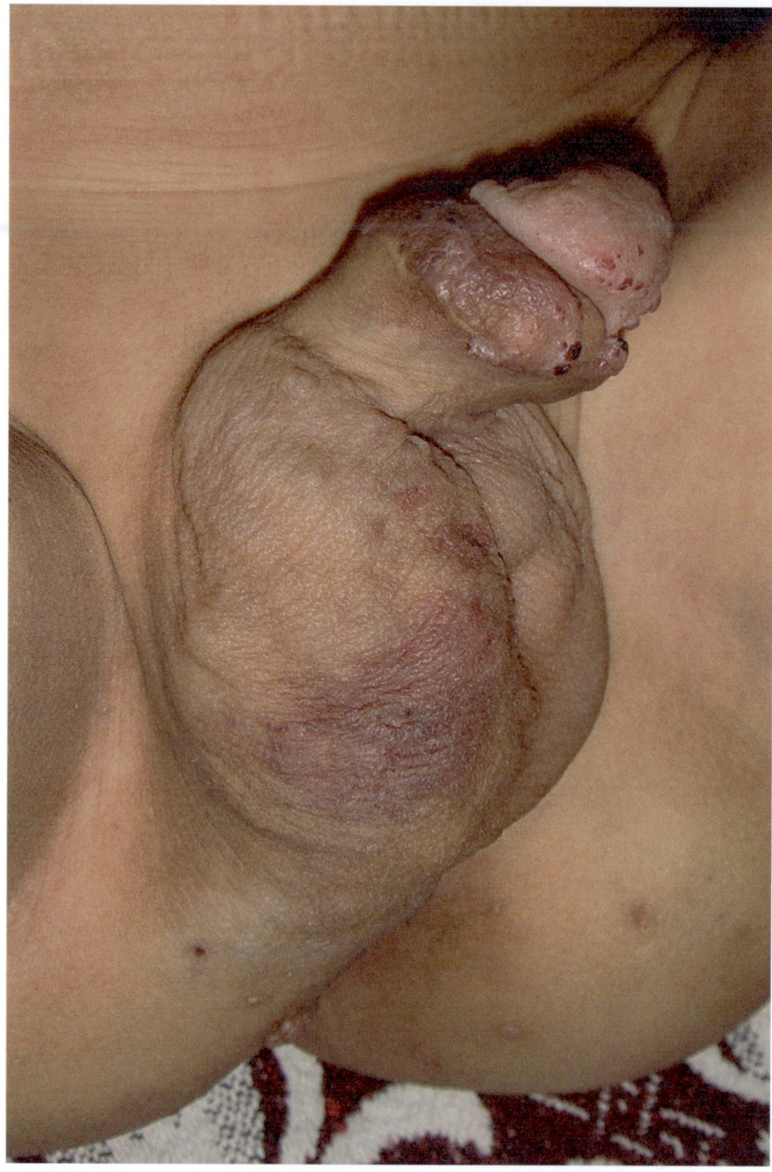

**Fig. 21.1** Scrotal haemangioma with extension to the perineum and penile skin

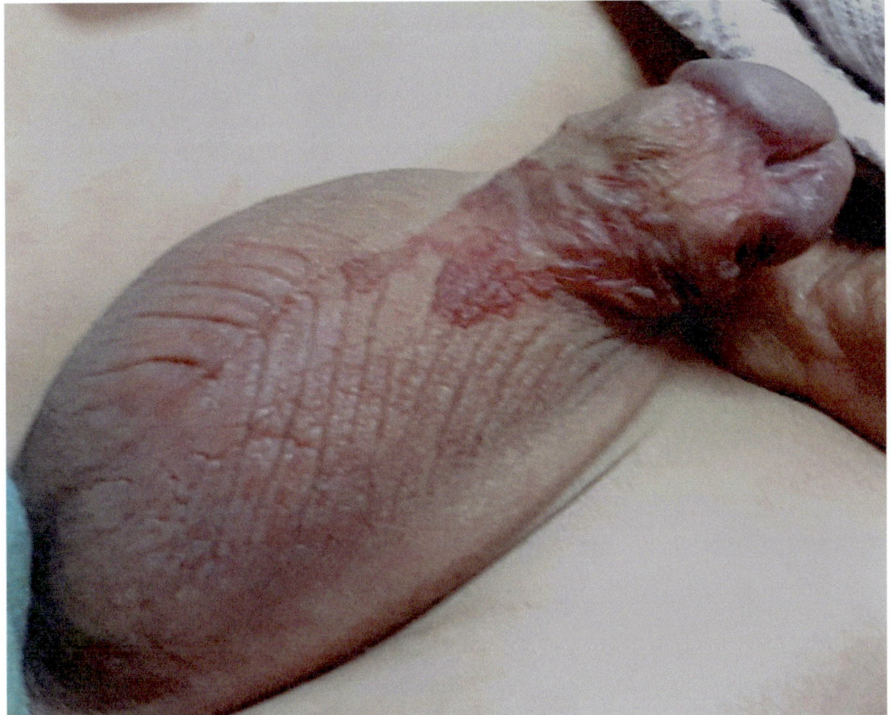

**Fig. 21.2** Superficial scrotal haemangioma with extension to the root of the penis

Both genital haemangiomas and AVVs may be diagnosed along other syndromes of vascular malformations like Klippel-Trénaunay-Weber syndrome; which is a triad of cutaneous vascular malformation, most commonly in the form of nevus flammeus, in combination with soft tissue and bone hypertrophy. This anomaly manifests at birth, usually involving a lower extremity, but it may also involves the trunk, upper limb or the face. Abdominal wall and genitalia are affected in 3% of the cases. These vascular lesions have a propensity to bleed; in a review of 214 patients from a single institution, Husmann et al. [6] found that 30% of the confirmed cases had a genitourinary involvement. Also, penoscrotal area may be affected along the VMs of Kasabach-Merritt syndrome which is a rare type of vascular lesions with peculiar characteristics based upon three basic findings; enlarging haemangioma, thrombocytopenia and consumption coagulopathy [7].

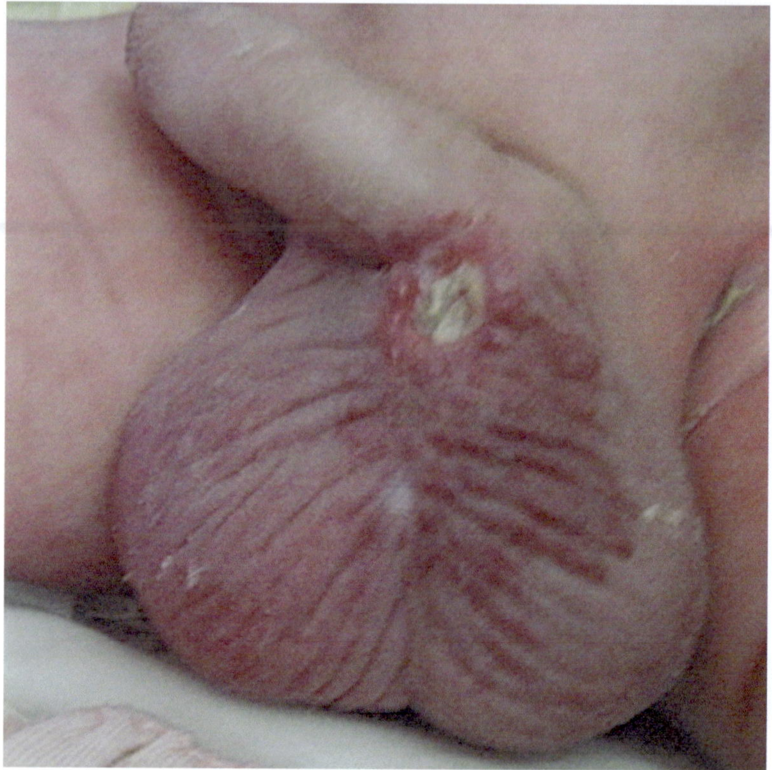

**Fig. 21.3** Scrotal haemangioma in a neonate with deep ulceration and infection

Precise surgical excision of the scrotal VM with primary scrotal reconstruction is possible as a one stage procedure, but extensive VM of the scrotum may deserve a preceded tissue expansion before attempting removal of the defective scrotal skin. Other cases with an extensive scrotal skin involvements may deserve skin grafting or local flap reconstruction (Fig. 21.5).

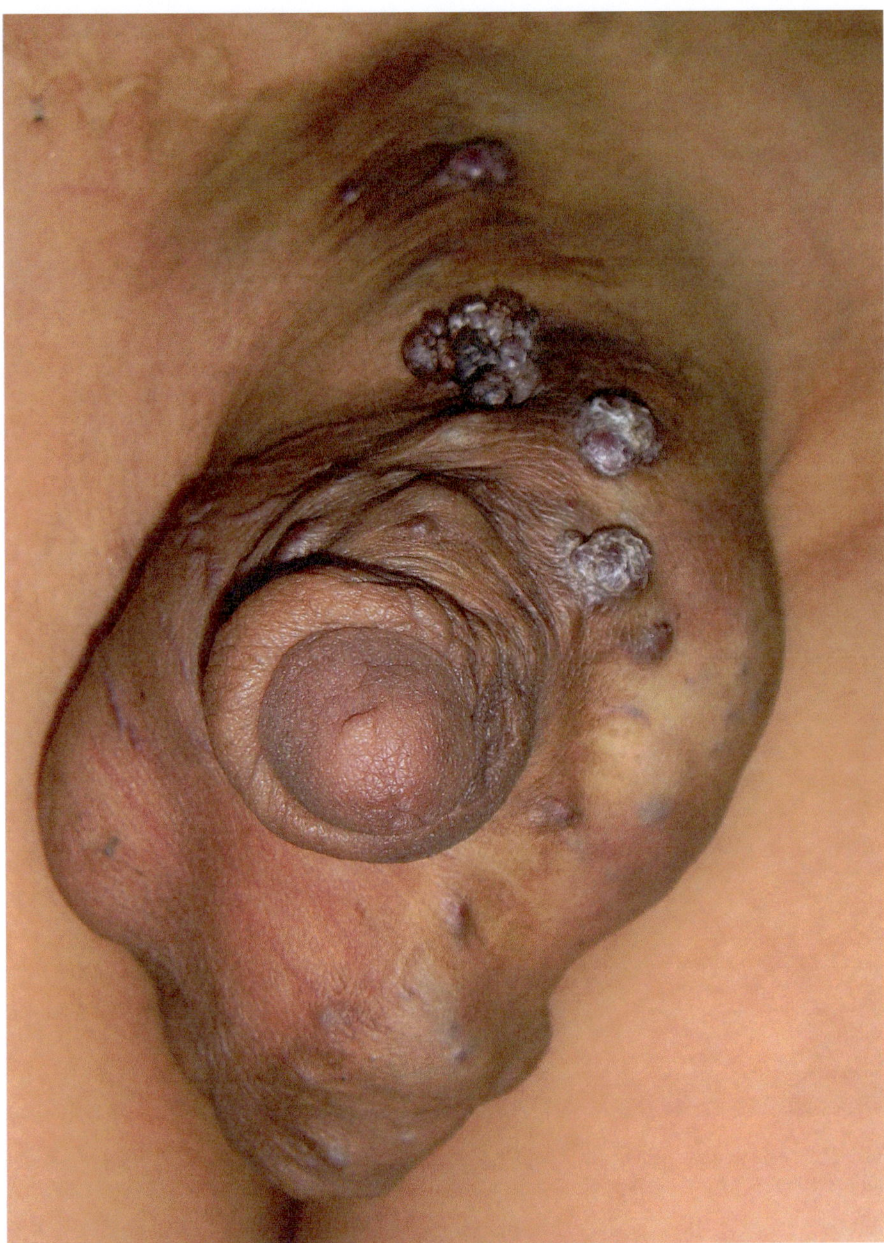

**Fig. 21.4** Extensive arteriovenous malformation of the scrotum; mainly in the left side with a multiple superficial penile lesions; looks like verruca

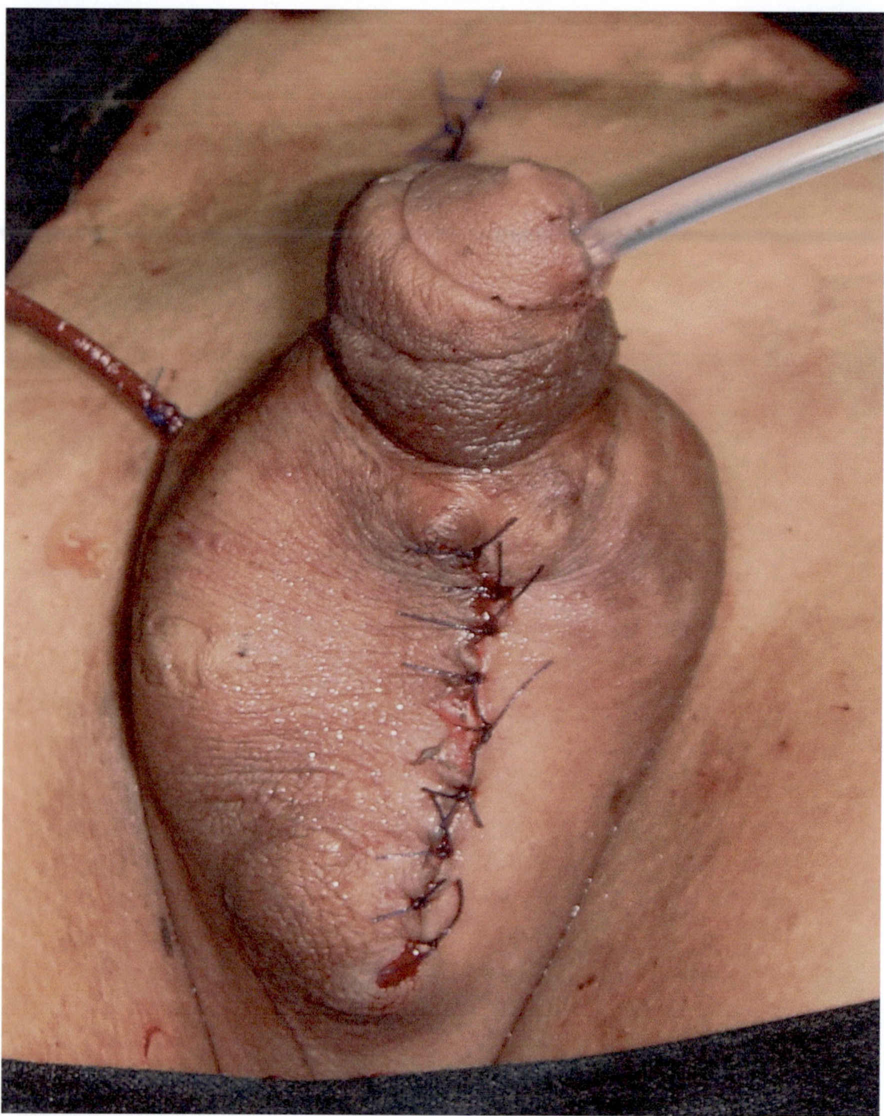

**Fig. 21.5** The same patient in Fig. 21.4 after primary excision of the scrotal vascular malformation

**Scrotal lymphangiomas** are very rare benign congenital soft tissue tumors of the lymphatic system that should be included in the differential diagnostic considerations for clarifying the acute scrotum and unclear cystic scrotal masses. Typically, they appear as painless scrotal swelling, and should be excluded preoperatively by radiographic imaging. Recurrences can only be reliably prevented through complete surgical resection.

**Nomenclature**: Lymphangioma scroti, Lymphangioma circumscriptum.

**Definition**: Large, irregular vascular spaces (similar to cavernous hemangioma and may resembles cysts) lined by one or two layers of flattened, bland epithelial cells with various amounts of fibrous stroma separating the cysts into cavities. Cystic and cavernous lymphangiomas are usually considered the same entity.

Lymphangioma circumscriptum (LC) is a term used for hamartomatous abnormality of the lymphatic channels of the skin, which can be encountered anywhere in the body. It is an uncommon skin condition characterized by large muscular-coated lymphatic cisterns that lie deep within the subcutaneous tissue and communicate with dilated dermal lymphatics. Patients suffer from edema, or a grouped vesicles resembling frog spawn and rarely the patients may poses a troublesome variable amounts of lymphatic fluid leakage from the affected skin. These swellings frequently have accompanying verrucous alterations of variable colours giving them a warty appearance and, if there is significant hyperkeratosis, the swelling may clinically resemble condyloma acuminata (Figs. 21.6 and 21.7 and Video link).

Lymphangiomas are characterized by lesions that are thin-walled cysts; these cysts can be macroscopic, as in a cystic hygroma, or microscopic manifested as a diffuse scrotal thickening. Most lymphangiomas are benign lesions that result only in a soft, slow-growing, "doughy" mass. It is thought to be the result of early developmental malformations, where, due to unknown etiology, the lymph fails to drain into the central lymphatic channels and accumulates in the lymphatic vessels [8]. Since they have no chance of becoming malignant, lymphangiomas are usually treated for cosmetic reasons, and surgical removal is the only efficacious therapeutic approach and is the best way to achieve a definitive diagnosis in those patients.

The intrascrotal localisation of lymphangioma in children is uncommon, especially when the lymphangioma does not depend on testicular structures. The majority of lymphangiomas (90%) develop during the first two years of life and 50% are present at birth. They are usually multi-cystic lesions lined by one or two layers of cells with various amounts of fibrous stroma separating the cysts into cavities [9]. Histopathologic features include numerous cystic lymphatic spaces lined with a flattened endothelium in the dermis. There may be overlying hyperkeratosis, acanthosis, haemorrhage, and mononuclear inflammatory cells.

A cystic lymphangioma usually presents as a painless mass that progressively enlarges over time. Occasionally, it presents with an acute onset of pain and sudden rapid enlargement, this commonly occurs after a haemorrhage within the cyst, which may be spontaneous or following injury, an inflammation or a disruption of the balance between lymphatic production and drainage.

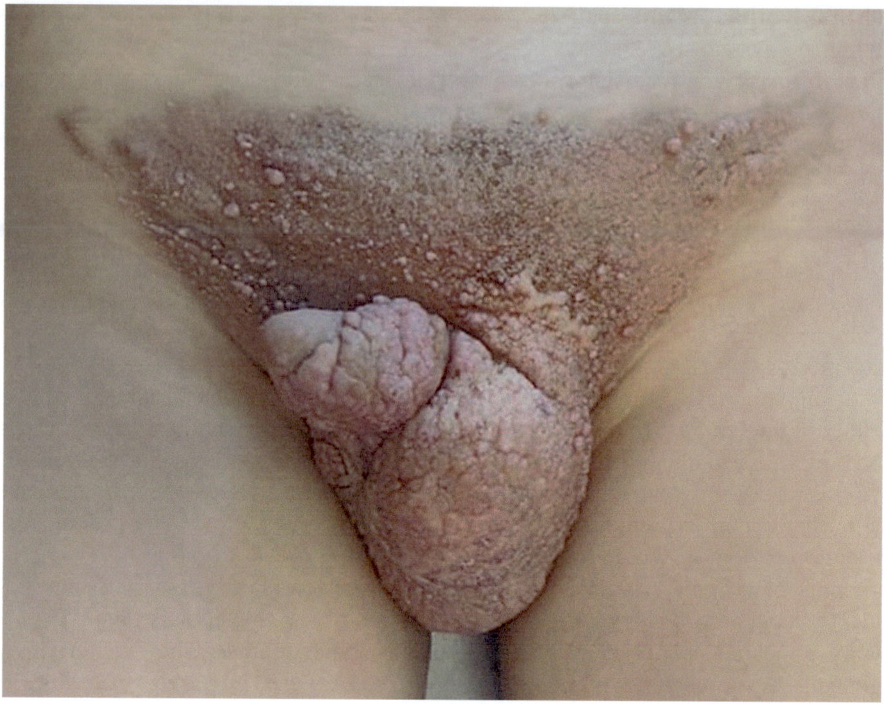

**Fig. 21.6** A rare case of lymphangiomatous malformation of the scrotal, penile and suprapubic skin; leaking a lymphatic fluid. (Video link) The photo and the video are provided by Dr Isber Ademaj, MD, Pediatric Surgeon, University Clinical Center of Kosovo, after parents consent

Lymphangiomas are traditionally classified as capillary (circumscriptum), cavernous and cystic, this classification cannot be generally applied as commonly all types co-exist in the same lesion [9].

The most common type, is the benign dilatation and malformation of inner lymphatic channels located in the deep dermal and subcutaneous tissues. The disease often affects the proximal portions of the extremities, but scrotal, vulvar, and mucosal lesions are rare. Lymphangioma circumscriptum is more common in women than in men. It can occur at any age, but usually appears at or soon after birth [10].

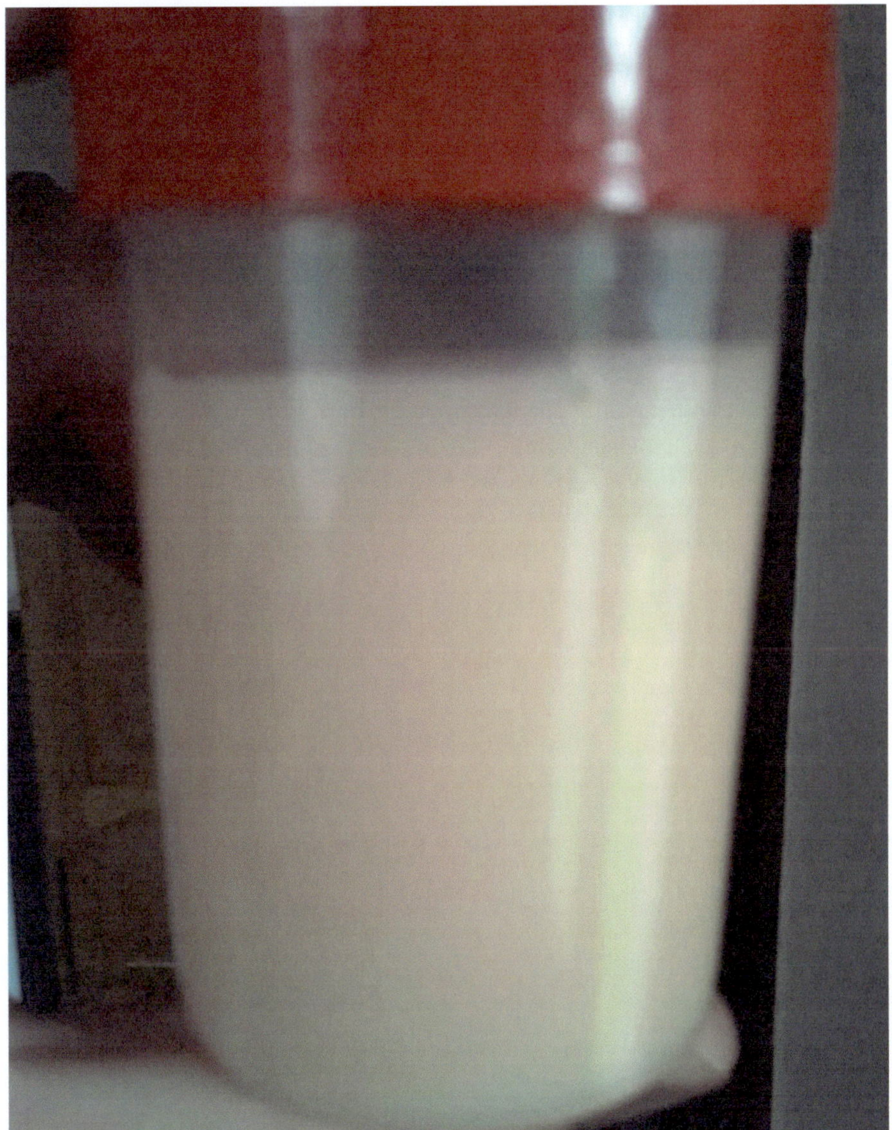

**Fig. 21.7** Daily lymph drainage from the patient with genital lymphangioma in Fig. 21.6

**Investigations**: Both hemangiomas and lymphangiomas may be superficial (cutaneous) or deep (subcutaneous) or may have both superficial and deep involvement. In lesions with deep components, imaging is indicated to determine the extent of the lesion, to detect any associated abnormalities, and to help plan therapy and follow-up. On sonography, scrotal wall hemangiomas present with a heterogeneous echo texture and increased through-transmission, showing septa and enlarged vascular spaces. Ultrasonography combined with Doppler examination can provide important insights, useful to the differential diagnosis and surgical approach of these lesions. Color Doppler sonography is usually the imaging modality of choice in patients with scrotal conditions and is frequently able to establish a firm diagnosis. Computed tomography (CT) or magnetic resonance imaging (MRI) may be indicated in complex cases and may be specifically needed in some cases [11].

**Differential diagnosis** should include other cystic lesions of these regions such as teratomas, enlargement of rete testis, intra- or extra-testicular dermoid and epidermoid cysts, hydroceles, hernias, spermatoceles and varicoceles. As the penis and scrotum are rarely involved with lymphangioma circumscriptum and, when occasionally seen at the anogenital region, it may easily misdiagnosed as genital warts, which differs completely in its treatment (Fig. 21.8).

Scrotal cystic lymphangioma should be differentiated from the rare Angiokeratomas of Fordyce, which are well-circumscribed, vascular lesions characterized by red or blue papules (i.e., dilated vessels). They are commonly

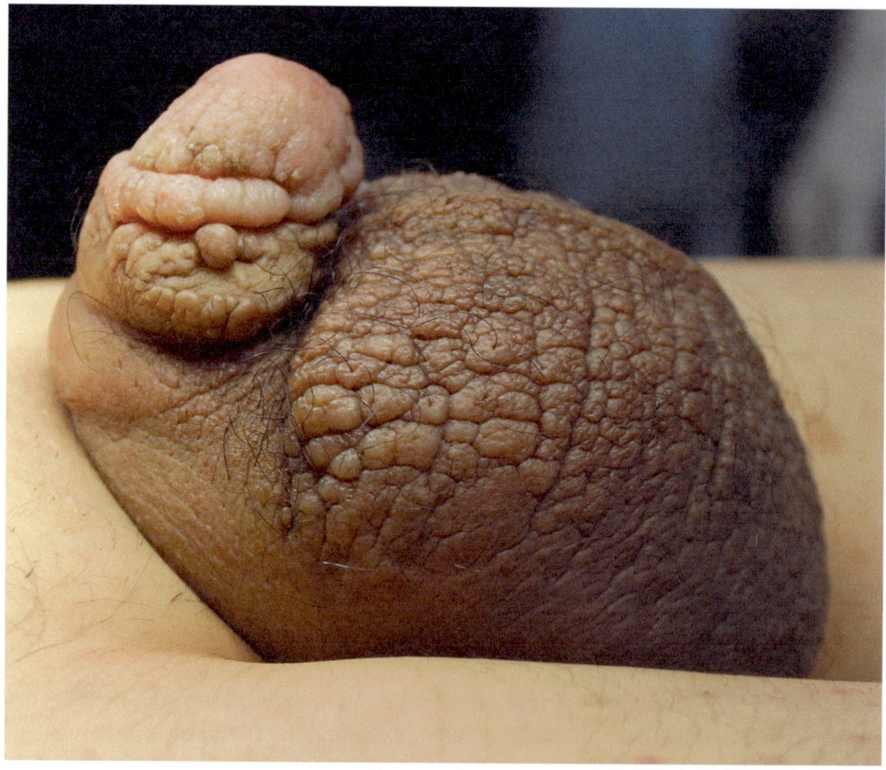

**Fig. 21.8** A case of long standing minute lymphangioma circumscriptum affecting the scrotal and penile skin; misdiagnosed as genital warts

associated with severe varicosity or varicocele. Patients often report bleeding after sexual intercourse or excoriation of the lesions [12].

Also, Steatocystoma multiplex which is characterized by multiple dermal cysts involving the pilosebaceous units, it may mimic the cystic lymphangioma. The dermal cysts may be localized or widespread, and asymptomatic or present with inflammatory symptoms. Histopathology show well-encapsulated cysts with a well formed cyst walls [13].

Recurrence of cystic lymphangiomas is a frequent complication when complete excision is not achieved. Because lymphatics are located within the dermis layer of the skin and the underlying dartos fascia, the complete excision of the subcutaneous tissues along with superficial lesions is vital in preventing recurrences. Surgical excision is the most effective method for treating extensive or deeply placed lesions [14]. Cases with an extensive scrotal lymphangioma involving the whole scrotum should be treated with a total scrotectomy down to the external spermatic fascia of the scrotum and Buck's fascia of the penis, then a split-thickness skin grafts, or a rotation flap reconstruction is indicated to cover the bared testicles [15]. Some cases of lymphangioma circumscriptum with a widespread lesions reported with an excellent symptomatic relief after treatment with the CO2 laser [16].

**Scrotal lymphedema** is a disease that leads to important functional, aesthetic and psychosocial impairments.

**Nomenclature**: Scrotal elephantiasis.

According to the World Health Organization, more than a billion people are still at risk of endemic lymphatic filariasis in 80 countries. The main causative agent is *Wuchereria bancrofti* and the main vector is the *Culex* mosquito [17]. Penoscrotal elephantiasis is not an uncommon clinical picture that may arise as an idiopathic primary lesion or as a symptom of many other diseases; it is usually a sequela of a recurring inflammatory process, eczema or malignancy. Elephantiasis often occurs after radical operations in the pelvic region. Displacement of lymphatic pathways leads to a local edema which over the course of time may leads to a considerable increase in volume of the patient's genitals or other affected parts.

The diagnosis of elephantiasis is not difficult, but it is much more difficult to determine which disease has caused this obstruction of the lymphatic pathways. If it is a reversible stage; the object of treatment is to remove the obstruction and reinstate the physiological lymph flow.

Secondary scrotal elephantiasis is generally encountered in endemic filariasis areas. It is usually caused by an extrinsic or intrinsic lymphatic obstruction. It poses etiologic, therapeutic, cosmetic and psychological problems. the scrotal elephantiasis is variable in size and is covered with a thick skin that loses its elasticity. On the other hand scrotal elephantiasis is often idiopathic despite the prevalence of this pathology in the filarial endemic areas. At the stage of penoscrotal elephantiasis, the research of microfilaria is often negative [18]. Idiopathic scrotal lymphedema is commonly seen in children at their first two years, involves the penis, prepuce and the scrotum (Fig. 21.9).

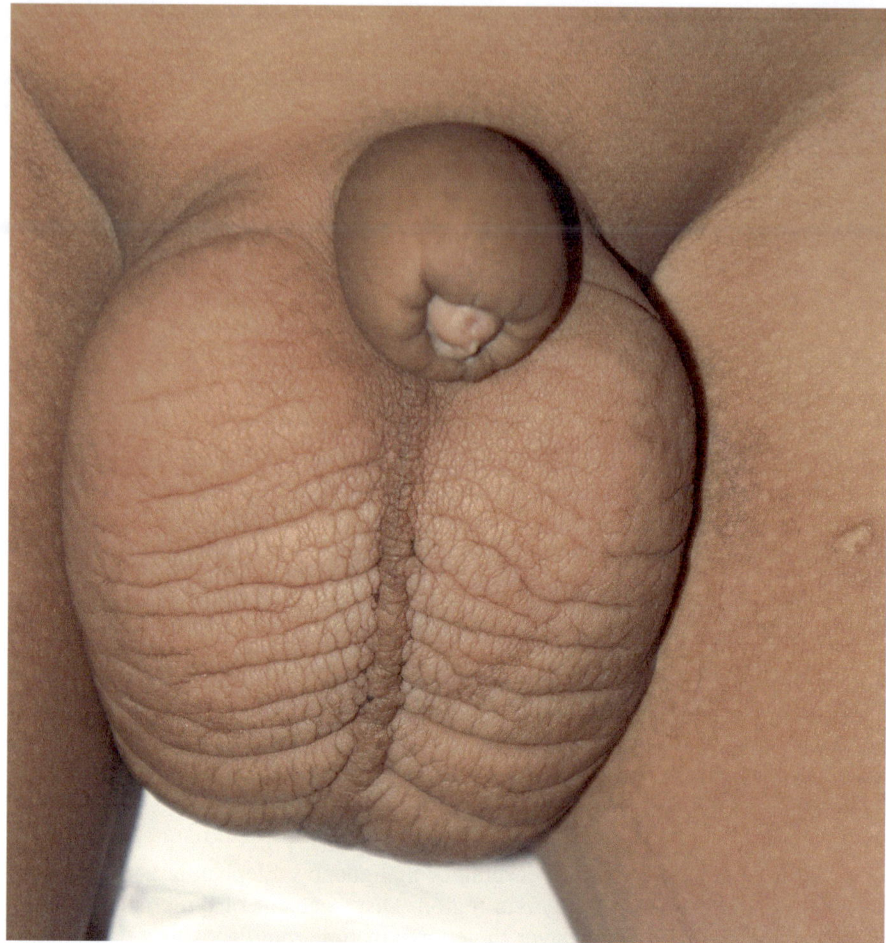

**Fig. 21.9** Idiopathic penoscrotal elephantiasis in a circumcised child

**Symptoms**: Symptoms include pain, swelling, bleeding and infertility at older ages. The scrotum became as a stiff fixed mass, which constituted a disability, limiting patient walk, physical and sexual activity [19]. Sometimes a characterized large grants lymphangitis presented as huge mass with a hypertrophy of the external genitalia that disables and suspends all the patient activities.

**Investigations**: Initial investigations include search for the primary cause, exclude secondary affection by filariasis. Ultrasound examination is essential, which demonstrates arterialised venous flow and low-resistance, high-velocity arterial flow. MRI is helpful, although angiography is the gold standard in the characterisation and management, if it is feasible [8].

**Treatment**: The treatment remains controversial, surgical measures are indicated with varying technics based on the volume of the mass and the experience of the surgeon [19].

Surgical treatment consisted of the removal of the scrotal mass with preservation of both testicles. The cosmetic and penile functional outcomes were usually good [20].

Conservative measures such as administration of anti-inflammatory drugs and diuretics, physical measures such as baths, massage and treatment of the underlying disease may be considered. On progression to irreversible elephantiasis a chronic lymphatic edema occurs for which conservative measures will be unsuccessful. For such cases; excision and amputation of the affected penoscrotal region is recommended in order to eliminate the functional disabilities. Surgical-ablative treatment approaches that have been described for the surgical treatment of penoscrotal edema have existed since the nineteenth century. Most procedures, however, neglect the introduction of a new lymphatic drainage, but a new technique for plastic reconstruction of the soft tissue defect caused by radical resection using a myocutaneous gracilis muscle flap, may ensures adequate lymphatic drainage into the deep muscle compartment of the thigh [21].

# References


1. Eivazi B, Werner JA. Management of vascular malformations and hemangiomas of the head and neck—an update. Curr Opin Otolaryngol Head Neck Surg. 2013;21:157–63.
2. Mulliken JB, Glowacki J. Hemangiomas and vascular malformations in infants and children: a classification based on endothelial characteristics. Plast Reconstr Surg. 1982;69:412–20.
3. ISSVA Classification of Vascular Anomalies ©2018 International Society for the Study of Vascular Anomalies. https://issva.org/classification. Accessed Mar 2021.
4. Rastogi K, Singh L, Khan NA, et al. Benign vascular anomalies: a transition from morphological to etiological classification. 2020.https://doi.org/10.1016/j.anndiagpath.2020.151506.
5. Ergeun O, Ceylan BG, Armagan A, Kapucuoglu N, Ceyhan AM, Perk H. A giant scrotal cavernous hemangioma extending to the penis and perineum: a case report. Kaohsiung J Med Sci. 2009;25:559–61.
6. Husmann D, Rathbun S, Driscol D. Klippel-Trénaunay syndrome: treatment of genitourinary sequelae [abstract]. J Pediatr Urol. 2005;1:161.
7. Hall GW. Kasabach-Merritt syndrome: pathogenesis and management. Br J Haematol. 2001;112:851–62. https://doi.org/10.1046/j.1365-2141.2001.02453.x.
8. Pui MH, Li ZP, Chen W, et al. Lymphangioma: imaging diagnosis. Aust Radiol. 1997;41:324–8.
9. Al-Jabri T, Gruener AM. A rare case of lymphangioma of the scrotum in a 3 year old boy: a case report. Cases J. 2009;2:183.
10. Patel GA, Schwartz RA. Cutaneous lymphangioma circumscriptum: frog spawn on the skin. Int J Dermatol. 2009;48(12):1290–5.
11. Conzi R, Damasio MB, Bertolotto M, Secil M, Ramanathan S, Rocher L, Cuthbert F, Richenberg J, Derchi LE. Sonography of scrotal wall lesions and correlation with other modalities. J Ultrasound Med. 2017;36:2149–63. https://doi.org/10.1002/jum.14257.

12. Trickett R, Dowd H. Angiokeratoma of the scrotum: a case of scrotal bleeding. Emerg Med J. 2006;23(10):e57.
13. Senel E. Question: can you identify this condition? Steatocystoma multiplex. Can Fam Physician. 2010;56(7):667.
14. Vikicevic J, Milobratovic D, Vukadinovic V, et al. Lymphangioma scroti. Pediatr Dermatol. 2007;24:654–6. https://doi.org/10.1111/j.1525-1470.2007.00557.x.
15. Wong R, Melnyk M, Tang SS, Nguan C. Scrotal lymphangiomatosis: a case report. Can Urol Assoc J. 2012;6(1):E11.
16. Treharne LJ, Murison MSC. $CO_2$ laser ablation of lymphangioma circumscriptum of the scrotum. Lymphat Res Biol. 2006;4(2):101–3.
17. Rimtebaye K, Jalloh M, Zarif Agah Tashkand A, Danki Sillong F, Niang L, Gueye SM. Giant penoscrotal elephantiasis: a case report. Open J Urol. 2015;5:109–13.https://doi.org/10.4236/oju.2015.58017.
18. Tazi MF, Mellas S, Ahallal Y, Khallouk A, El Fassi MJ, Farih MH. Penoscrotal ephantiasis, diagnosis and management (about 3 cases) (L'éléphantiasis pénoscrotal, diagnostic et prise en charge (à propos de 3 cas)). Andrologie. 2009;19:108–12. https://doi.org/10.1007/s12610-009-0020-4.
19. Dekou A, Konan PG, Yao B, Vodi C, Fofana A, Manzan K. Idiopathic penoscrotal ephantiasis. A new case and review of the literature (Éléphantiasis pénoscrotal idiopathique: Une nouvelle observation et revue de la littérature). Can Urol Assoc J. 2013;7:E29–32.
20. Häcker A, Hatzinger M, Grobholz R, Alken P, Hoang-Böhm J. Scrotal lymphangioma—a rare cause of acute scrotal pain in childhood. Aktuelle Urol. 2006;37(6):445–8.
21. Schusterman MA, Robb GL, Tadjalli HE. Advances in reconstruction for cancer patients. In: Pollock RE, editor. Surgical oncology. Cancer treatment and research, vol. 90. Boston, MA: Springer; 1997. https://doi.org/10.1007/978-1-4615-6165-1_4.

# Chapter 22
# Acute Scrotum

Lisieux Eyer de Jesus

**Abbreviations**

AS    Acute scrotum
TT    Testis torsion
ATT   Appendix testis torsion
OE    Orchiepididymitis
DUS  Doppler ultrasound
US    Ultrasound

The expression "acute scrotum (AS)" describes a cluster of different pathologies presenting scrotal pain. The causes vary in incidence according to age (testis torsion —TT—predominate in neonates and adolescents and appendix testis torsion—ATT —in school-aged children). Depending on age distribution AS cohorts may show a predominance of orchiepididymitis (OE) (adult cohorts), ATT (predominantly pre-pubertal pediatric cohorts) or TT (cohorts showing predominance of adolescents and young adults) [1]. In children and adolescents, "surgical" causes largely predominate and OE account only for circa 1/5 of the cases.

Despite not being the most common, TT is the most morbid condition related to AS, and is a surgical emergency: postponing treatment for more than 6 h after the beginning of the pain episode risks testicular infarction and loss of the gonad. AS is an active area of litigation concerning Pediatric Surgery and Urology. AS cases are the third most common diagnosis in claims involving adolescents in the United States and the 12th most common cause linked to successful litigation claims against NHS/United Kingdom [2].

The main causes of AS are:

L. E. de Jesus (✉)
Fellow Brazilian College of Surgeons, Brazilian Association of Pediatric Surgeons, Pediatric Surgeon Federal Fluminense University and Servidores do Estado Federal Hospital/Ministry of Health, Rio de Janeiro, Brazil

© The Author(s), under exclusive license to Springer Nature Switzerland AG 2022    299
M. A. B. Fahmy (ed.), *Normal and Abnormal Scrotum*,
https://doi.org/10.1007/978-3-030-83305-3_22

1.  Testicle torsion (TT)
2.  Appendix testis torsion (ATT)
3.  Orchiepididimytis (OE)

However, the list of rarer possible causes of AS is extensive:

1.  Testicular trauma and/or hematocele
2.  Vasculitides affecting the testis and/or the scrotum (Henoch-Schonlein purpura, IgA vasculitis, Kawasaki disease)
3.  Pyocele/scrotal abscess/scrotal infections including necrotizing fasciitis (Fournier's gangrene)
4.  Idiopathic scrotal edema
5.  Inguinal hernia strangulation complicated with testicular ischemia
6.  Tense hydroceles/acute hydroceles
7.  Adrenal hemorrhage (in neonates)
8.  Meconial peritonitis (in neonates)
9.  Renal vein thrombosis (mainly in neonates)

The objective of this chapter is to describe the main causes of AE, emphasizing the most relevant and frequent conditions.

## 1.  Testicle torsion

A very clear description of an episode of testicular torsion has been published by Ombrédanne as soon as 1927 [3], but the anatomical cause of the disease, which usually affects both gonads, was only evidenced in the 1960s by Richards Lyon [4]. This finding changed the paradigm of the disease, leading to the adoption of BILATERAL orchidopexy as the state of the art for treatment. A 40% probability of asynchronous contralateral torsion is assumed in patients that are not submitted to contralateral orchidopexy after a TT episode.

The need to educate physicians and the population about the urgency to evaluate any patient presenting acute scrotal pain was soon recognized. Legal problems leading to the prosecution of health personnel accused of misdiagnosis, diagnostic and treatment delay, causing gonadal loss, imposed aggressive surgical protocols, and refinement of diagnosis.

A normal testis is fixed to the posterior scrotal wall, while the vaginal layer surrounds the rest of the gonad's surface. The usual cause of a TT is the intravaginal rotation of a testicle that is not posteriorly fixed to the scrotal wall and remains free into the scrotum, suspended exclusively by the spermatic cord (bell clapper malformation, which usually affects both sides) (Fig. 22.1). The single presence of the bell clapper malformation does not determine the occurrence of TT: an autopsy study involving men without a TT history detected a 12% incidence of bell clapper malformation [2]. The connection of the free testis to the cremaster fibers that form a muscular layer over the spermatic cord also play a part in the pathophysiology of the condition, as a sudden, forceful, and/or asynchronous contraction of this muscle may induce twisting of the gonad, as the cremaster muscular fibers derive from

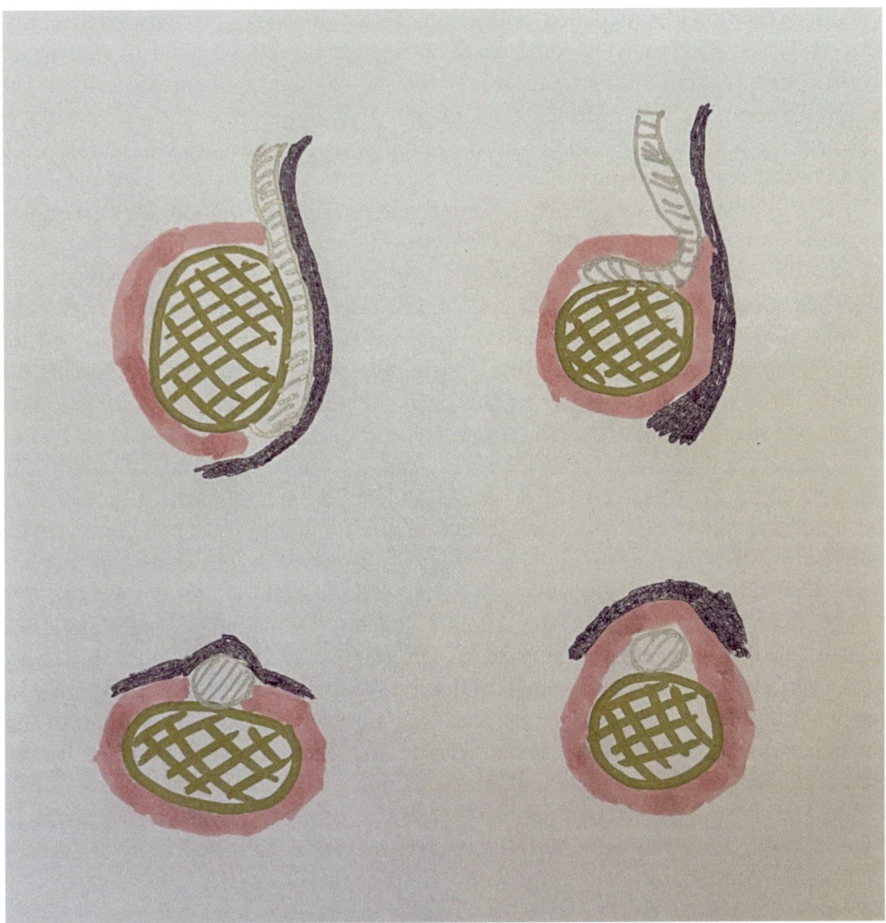

**Fig. 22.1** Normal testicle: upper left (sagittal cut), lower left (transversal cut). Bell-clapper deformity: upper right (sagittal cut), lower right (transversal cut). Legend: testicle (gold), epididymis/vas deferens (silver), vaginal layer (pink), scrotal skin (purple) (drawing by the author)

various layers of the abdominal wall muscles and distribute along the cord in a spiral pattern.

Nocturnal erections, protective reflexes and a cold environment may induce a forceful cremasteric contraction, which may explain the higher incidence of TT in winter [5, 6].

The absence of testicular posterior fixation gives rise to one of the most prominent clinical signs that raise the suspicion of testicular malfixation (bell clapper deformity): the longest axis of the affected testicles assumes a horizontal position in the scrotum in a standing patient, especially in post-pubertal males, after the testicle grows to adult proportions.

Absent fixation also explains the torsion of cryptic testes (that twist over an axis formed by the cord and the gubernaculum testis) and extravaginal torsion in the fetus/neonate, as the normal fixation between the vaginal layer and the scrotal wall is usually complete only after 10 days of life.

A torsion between the testicle and the epididymis is extremely rare and depends on a lax testicular mesentery.

The TT determines a sequence of venous and arterial obstruction, also depending on the presence of a "complete" (360°) twist, the number of twists and "tightness" of turns of the cord. The affected gonad suffers progressive ischemia, leading to the sequential destruction of germinal epithelium, Leydig cells, and, finally, testicular necrosis and atrophy. The irreversibility of the ischemic process depends on the duration of the episode: reversibility is highly probable in a 6 h interval, but chances worsen progressively after this time period. Testicular necrosis is almost always the result after 24 h.

TT affects approximately 1:4000 males, with an annual incidence of 0.004% for children under 18 years-old [7] or 4.5/100000 < 35 years-old men [2]. The incidence of the disease is bimodal, affecting preferentially neonates (intrauterine extravaginal torsion due to immaturity, affecting normally descended testes) and post-pubertal adolescents (intravaginal torsion due to bell clapper deformity).

The main characteristic of the disease (except for neonates—see later) is a sudden and very intense scrotal pain episode. Pain may irradiate to the ipsilateral tight, lumbar, or inguinal region. Abdominal pain is also possible, mainly in pre-pubertal males, and frequently causing diagnostic delay, especially if the physician does not include a systematic genital examination in his/her routine physical examination for acute abdominal pain.

Most episodes are nocturnal and may wake the patient up. Spontaneous erections ("wet dreams"), sexual activity, and trauma may also induce TT by a forceful cremasteric contraction.

Some patients (6–63%) describe previous ipsi or contralateral episodes of scrotal pain with spontaneous resolution [8], suggesting that in carriers of bell clapper deformity episodes of torsion with spontaneous resolution may occur. The diagnosis of those patients before an episode of persisting TT is problematic, as there are no image exams that are able to diagnose the presence of the malformation [8]. The only valuable information to confirm this suspicion is the detection of horizontal lying highly mobile testes in those patients, when standing. The sum of a trustable history of repetitive episodes of testicular pain with spontaneous resolution and horizontal-lying testes authorizes the indication of orchidopexies as prophylaxis of TT.

Nausea and reflex vomit may associate. Fever or urinary symptoms are not to be expected. A history of contralateral urgent orchidopexy or the presence of contralateral atrophy after an untreated pain episode enhances the suspicion of TT. The finding of an atrophic testis associated with a previous undiagnosed AS episode entails the indication of contralateral orchidopexy as soon as possible.

The physical examination should be repeated in supine and standing position. Both gonads and testicular cords should be examined in detail. A twisted testis is usually edematous, hardened, extremely painful and positioned high in the scrotum (Brunzel's sign, "*testis redux*") (Fig. 22.2). The affected gonad and/or the contralateral testicle exhibit a horizontal position, most notable in the orthostatic position and in post-pubertal adolescents (Angell's sign). The examiner may palpate a "naked", free and mobile lower testicular pole, due to the lack of gonadal fixation, in early cases. In patients that are examined very early after the establishment of the torsion, a umbilication presenting in the caudal aspect of the scrotum may be seen (Ger's sign), but this is very uncommon in practice. Palpation of the epididymis out of its usual posterior position is helpful, but not definitive, as the epididymis may be posterior after a 360° rotation. As the disease progresses, local inflammatory changes follow, with scrotal edema and secondary hydrocele. In late cases, after definitive gonadal necrosis and before late atrophy, pain resolves, and the patient may present as a "testicular tumor" (pseudotumoral presentation). The description of a previous pain episode and scrotal ultrasound are the key to the differential diagnosis between late TT and testicular tumors. This is very important because a correct diagnosis allows to protect the contralateral still unaffected gonad from a future torsion episode and spares the patient an oncological approach to a pseudotumoral ischemic testicle.

The absence of the cremasteric reflex is typical of TT, and is valuable for the differential diagnosis of AS, as it is usually present in cases of ATT and in most cases of OE. The absence of cremasteric reflex in a patient presenting AS points to TT as the most probable diagnosis (OR 47.6) [9, 10]. Also, in TT cases the elevation of the affected testicle does not bring relief, which usually happens in OE cases (Prehn's sign).

Some authors have proposed the usage of clinical scores to estimate the probability of TT as the cause of AS. One of those, TWIST (testicular work-up for ischemia and suspected torsion) proposes to consider the presence of testicular edema (2 points), hardness (2 points), vomits/nausea (1 point), high-lying testis (1 point) in patients presenting acute scrotal pain. Patients summing more than 5 points are considered high risk and emergency surgery is indicated (without any complementary exams). The score proved to be highly specific, and the positive predictive value for TT was 93.5% [11, 12].

The difficulties involving the availability of expert sonologists, leading to delays in treatment while waiting for diagnostic confirmation suggest that real-time ultrasound performed by the emergencist (point-of-care ultrasound) should be tested as a supportive approach to the differential diagnosis of TT. This has been tested recently in a 120 AS cohort (12 TT). The correct final diagnosis could be reached in 70% of cases. All TT cases were identified, with one false positive (an ATT case, with 100% negative predictive value and 92.3% positive predictive value), saving an hour between admission and surgery [13].

Considering that the patients should ideally be operated in a maximal interval of 6 h since the beginning of symptoms and that the surgery used to treat TT is low risk in healthy patients, with low morbidity and rare complications, it is accepted that complementary exams can and should be waived if not immediately available. In other words, in cases of high level of suspicion of TT, the physician is authorized

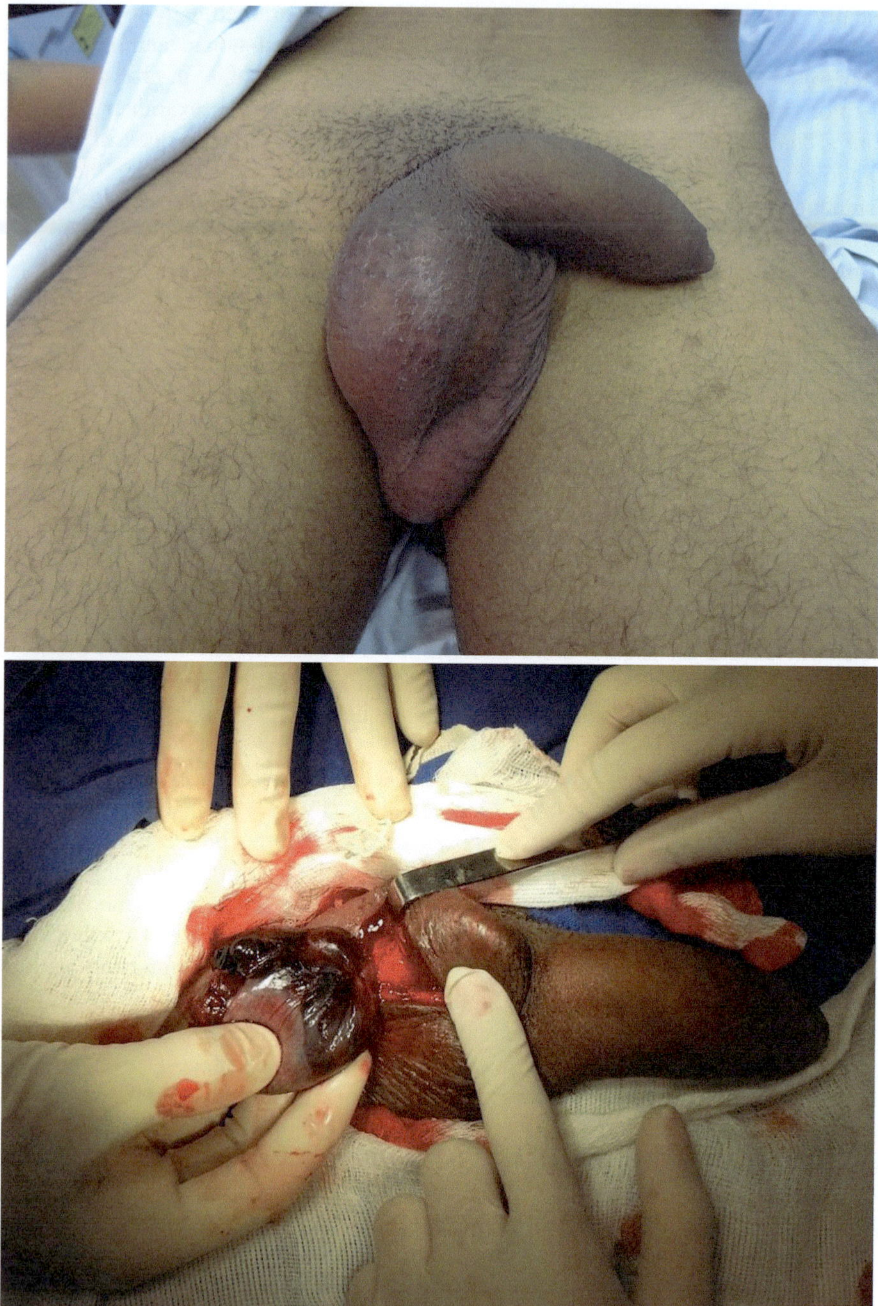

**Fig. 22.2** Testicular torsion. Upper picture: elevated and augmented testis. Lower picture: Aspect of the testis and cord rotation in surgery (from the author's archive)

to operate despite not proving his/her hypothesis with complementary exams, especially if the duration of the episode is close to complete the "safe" period of 6 h. As a matter of fact, to NOT operate emergently on a suspect of a TT in due time may be considered malpractice. The delay time to get a doppler ultrasound after emergency evaluation has been recently estimated as approximately 3.5 h in a Canadian paper (surgery was done after a mean 5.1 h after being admitted to the emergency department) [10].

Doppler ultrasound (DUS) is the most used (and most useful) exam to confirm TT. The ultrasonographic aspect of the affected testis varies depending on the interval since the establishment of ischemia. In the first 6 h, the organ parenchyma is normal. From 6 to 24 h, the organ is usually hypoechogenic and increased in volume. After 24 h the testicular parenchyma is heterogeneous and secondary hydroceles are common. Parenchymal heterogeneity has been related to necrosis [10]. Very late presentations (pseudo tumoral) show heterogeneous augmented testes with calcifications. A post-ischemia atrophic testicle is typically hypoechoic and smaller, associated to a hyperechoic epididymis.

The epididymis is also swollen and heterogeneous, hyperechogenic with radiating hypoechoic bands, eventually difficult to be separated from cord structures. The ultrasound technician should also examine the spermatic cord, from the inguinal region down: during a TT episode the spiraled cord corresponding to the region of the twist ("whirlpool sign") or a heterogeneous "pseudo tumor" representing the edematous distal cord ("boggy pseudo mass") can be directly detected [2].

A doppler evaluation is fundamental for the diagnosis of the testicular ischemia caused by absent arterial irrigation of the testis (Fig. 22.3). The interpretation of the exam is more difficult in small testicles. In protracted cases the secondary inflammatory reaction is characterized by peri-testicular hypervascularization, which can be confounded with a normal testicular flow. The sensitivity of US/doppler for the diagnosis of TT varies from 82 to 100% and specificity may reach 98.8% [7]. Positive predictive value has been proposed as very high, but some authors suggest a lower negative predictive value [14], possibly associated to false negative diagnoses attributable to peri-testicular augmented flow.

Testicular scintigraphy was used to detect the absence of vascularization of the affected testis: the diseased organ does not capture the intravenous radioisotope. A peri-testicular "halo" formed by augmented captation of the isotope in inflamed tissues is typically seen, while the normal testis shows similar captation to the neighboring tissues. The exam is rarely available in due time, exposes the patient to radiation, is difficult to interpret in small testicles, and is rarely used to confirm TT diagnosis contemporaneously.

Magnetic resonance imaging (MRI) with intravenous contrast can diagnose TT, using the same theoretical basis of scintigraphy (the absence of captation of intravenous contrast by the ischemic testis) [15]. It has recently been suggested that MRI can indirectly show a bell-clapper malformation, in the presence of hydrocele (demonstrating the absence of posterior fixation and a free-lying testis) [16]. MRI, however, is costly and not readily available in most institutions.

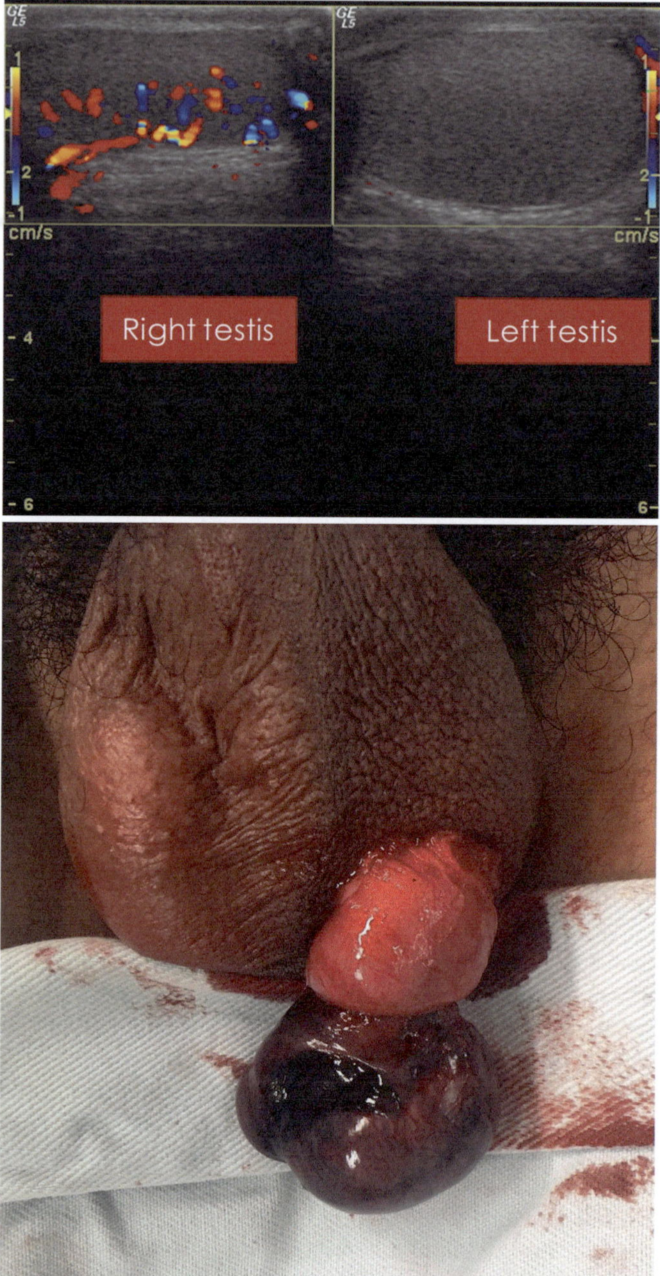


**Fig. 22.3** TT affecting the left side. Normal vascularization at the right side, absent vascularization at the left side (upper picture). Aspect of the testis in surgery (lower picture) (case from Dra. Tatiana Fazecas, MD)

Preliminary studies have examined the possible relevance of transcutaneous near-infrared spectroscopy to detect lower oxygen saturation levels in the torsed testis. The method seems promising both in animal research and in a pilot study in humans [2]. Other exams may be used for differential diagnosis, such as ultrasound of kidneys/bladder, urinary tests, and dosing acute inflammatory markers to exclude urinary tract infections associated with OE, urinary tract malformations and vasculitides [17].

The treatment of TT is an EMERGENCY (except for very protracted cases), surgical (usually as an emergency surgery, demanding ipsilateral resolution of the case and contralateral orchidopexy as soon as possible). Even contemporaneously, the literature shows variable proportions for gonad salvation, usually half to two-thirds of the affected gonads, and late atrophy is common [18]. The prognosis for pre-pubertal patients is worse. Some authors described that the loss of the gonad approximately doubles for pre-pubertal children, possibly due to atypical presentations (mainly abdominal pain) and/or low levels of suspicion [19]. Those numbers depend deeply on the timeliness of the patients' presentation to medical evaluation and on their timely transfer to get surgery. Recent papers showed that a relatively small proportion of the patients present to a physician before 6 h after the emergence of pain and parents complain that they had never been educated about the possibility of a TT and its consequences [20]. Also, diagnostic errors made by non-experts were common, especially misdiagnosing OE, leading to serious extension of the episode before treatment by surgeons/urologists (mean delay time to the right diagnosis 84.4 h) [21]. The education of the patients, parents and non-expert physicians, especially those involved in primary care and non-referral emergency units, including specifically designed campaigns, may help to get early diagnosis and surgery, resulting in better salvation numbers.

Non-surgical detorsion of the cord is a classical maneuver described in 1893 [22], and has been revisited recently, associated to simultaneous doppler-ultrasound to attest to the resolution of the ischemic process.

The rotation of a twisted testes is usually "towards the inside" (clockwise in the right, anticlockwise in the left), so de-rotation maneuvers are "towards the outside" (in the direction of the thigh, from medial to lateral, "open-book" way). The twisted testis may show more than one rotation and some testis twist in the opposite direction (circa 1/3 of the patients) [7, 23], so that the physician must be sure to have fully undone the cord's twists. The expression of a successful maneuver is the immediate resolution of pain and the immediate restoration of flow by doppler ultrasound.

De-rotation maneuvers have been criticized due to the need of doppler/US to secure the resolution of ischemia and to the persistent need to operate to avoid other episodes and to fixate the other testis. Modern authors, however, argue that de-rotation buys time. De-rotation maneuvers may be extremely useful if there is no prompt availability of surgery/anesthesia and in patients presenting prohibitive risks for emergency surgery. De-rotation is most effective and efficient in early cases, before the establishment of edema and secondary hydrocele. Subsequent urgent bilateral fixation is needed as soon as possible. Detorsion auxiliary maneuvers under DUS control have been described recently as effective in 75% of the cases attempted, with higher effectivity in early cases and potential to increase gonadal salvation [24–26].

Surgical treatment of TT after the neonatal period involves trans-scrotal incisions. Most authors prefer a raphe longitudinal incision to access both testes, but some opt for bilateral incisions to get bilateral orchidopexies (in the bottom of the scrotum or using Bianchi's upper-lateral incision). The affected testis is exposed, de-rotated, and observed for 5–10 min in a warm environment. If the organ recovers a normal aspect, fixation follows. In cases of undoubtful necrosis, orchiectomy is usually done. In doubtful cases, the modern approach is to make a long longitudinal incision of the albuginea layer, in order to relieve intratesticular pressure (compartment syndrome) and to cover this incision with a vaginal patch, before fixation. This approach has proved to save some gonads after protracted ischemia [27–29].

As previous worries about possible contralateral damage by immunological mechanisms when conserving a borderline viable testicle has not been proved, the contemporaneous tendency is to be conservative, but black/hemorrhagic testicles more than 5 min after de-torsion (suggesting hemorrhagic necrosis), heterogeneous parenchyma on pre-operative ultrasound, absence of bleeding after incising the albuginea, and episodes with >12 h duration are related to late atrophy [30].

There are a lot of methods for testicular fixation, but unabsorbable material and at least two stitches are preferable, in order not to allow a torsion pivot to form. Some authors fix the testis using a sub-dartos pouch, similar to the technique routinely used to treat cryptorchidism. THE CONTRALATERAL TESTIS MUST BE PEXED IN ANY TT CASE, including cases of post-ischemic testicular atrophy.

Post-operative complications are uncommon. Repetitive episodes of torsion after fixation are rare (0.3%) [31]. Fertility in men affected by unilateral TT (treated either with orchiectomy or orchidopexy) is comparable to the normal population [32].

Time for insertion of substitutive testicular prosthesis in orchiectomy or total atrophy cases is controversial. Many suggest to insert the prostheses only after puberty, in order to avoid a small prosthesis that will need to be changed later in the case of pre-pubertal children. It has been suggested that the insertion of a prostheses in emergency conditions, in the presence of gonadal necrosis, may have a high risk of infectious complications and extrusion. However, some argue that psychological aspects of an empty scrotum have to be considered, and that simultaneous insertion of a prosthesis and orchiectomy is safe [33]. Complications may be more frequent if the insertion of a testicular prosthesis is decided after a long delay time [34].

Perinatal TT patients are a special cohort. They are a minority of TT affecting topical testes, are typically extra-vaginal and usually happen during the third trimester of intra-uterine life, mostly affecting term neonates. Most cases exhibit irreversible late ischemia (histologically calcification, fibrosis, necrosis, and syderophages are usually described after orchidectomy [35]). Bilateral cases are uncommon (circa 1/5 of the cases), 67% asynchronous [2]. A recent metanalysis shows that salvation of the affected gonads is unusual (7.7%, 2/3 of those documented as post-natal episodes) [36].

In typical cases the babies present unpainful augmentation of scrotal volume ("pseudotumoral"), a firm testis, and scrotal discoloration (bluish/violaceous/pale) from birth. Ultrasound shows a heterogeneous non-vascularized testis with hypoechogenic areas, calcifications, and secondary hydrocele. Acute/treatable TT caused by bell clapper malformation, is uncommon in newborns (less than a quarter of AS cases in this age) [37], presenting as irritability, inconsolable crying and a painful swollen testis. Those cases need emergency surgery and should be treated as typical TT. A previous description of a normal testis by the pediatrician is useful to suggest an acute episode of TT.

The level of urgency involved is controversial: as presentation is usually late, an emergency surgery is debatable. On the other side, if there is any doubt about the possibility of a recoverable organ/recent torsion episode emergency surgery is recommended. Most surgeons argue for urgent surgery, intending to fix and protect the other side from future problems, to detect synchronous previously undetected contralateral torsion and to possibly save some gonads, although uncommon. Those who disagree depart from considering the risk of anesthesia in neonates and the rarity of acute/recent torsion in this population.

An inguinal incision is used in those cases. Contralateral fixation is arguable, as immaturity is the cause for extravaginal TT, and the normal fixation is usually complete after the first 10 days of life. This aspect remains controversial, and many authors opt for contralateral fixation to get better chances of contralateral protection, considering the low risks associated to an orchidopexy, the possibility of an unknown bell-clapper contralateral malformation and the potential disastrous consequences of an eventual contralateral problem [38].

## 2. Appendix testis torsion

ATT commonly affects Morgagni's hydatid, the appendix testis located near the upper pole and the epididymis (Fig. 22.4). The patients are mostly pre-pubertal (6–12 years-old predominate): ATT is the most common cause of acute scrotum in pre-pubertal children [39]. The main symptom is acute pain, usually less intense than in TT and without irradiation. More mature children may locate the pain on the upper pole of the testis. Children presenting ATT usually do not present nausea and vomits.

Physical examination may evidence a painful distinct mass on the upper pole of the testis, independent of the testis per se, but the progression of the disease frequently complicates the exam, as edema and secondary hydroceles superimpose. In children, especially those with fair and thin scrotal skin and without severe scrotal edema a dark "dot" may be seen transcutaneously, representing the ischemic appendix testis. Transillumination may also help to individualize the mass near the testicular upper pole (Fig. 22.5). In ATT the cremasteric reflex is preserved and the cord is normal to palpation. Doppler ultrasound shows the twisted appendix near the epididymis/superior pole of the testis (a heterogeneous "salt and pepper" oval avascular mass with posterior acoustic reinforcement, hypoechogenic in the earlier

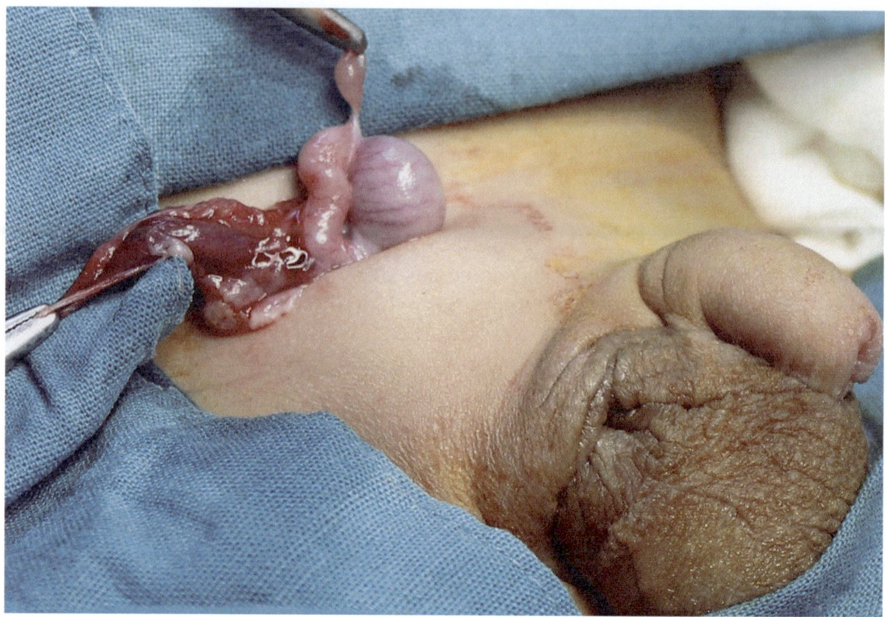

**Fig. 22.4** Morgagni's hydatid, the most common form of testis appendix (Dr. Mohamed Fahmy, personal archive)

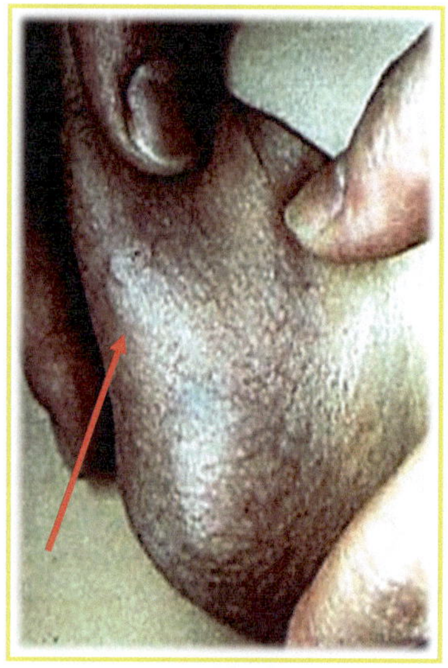
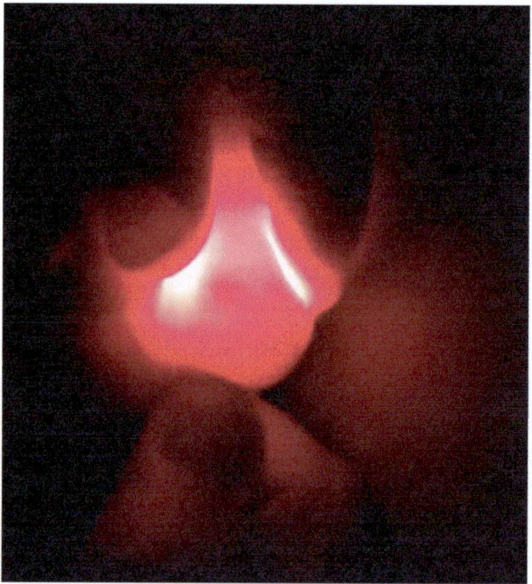

**Fig. 22.5** ATT, blue-dot sign as seen in physical examination (left, red arrow) and by scrotal transillumination (right) (case from Dr. Samuel Dekermacher, MD)

cases—echogenicity tends to be higher in later cases) with a normal testicular flow (Fig. 22.6) [40, 41].

Treatment may be surgical (trans-scrotal exeresis of the twisted appendix testis) or conservative (pain treatment and rest). Protracted pain is frequent in cases conservatively treated (approximately a third of the patients) [31]. In some cases the twisted appendix auto-amputates and turns into a freely mobile palpable scrotal calcified nodule, also shown in ultrasound (Fig. 22.5). Metachronous contralateral ATT is very uncommon (2.6%) [31].

### 3. Orchiepididimytis

OE may be related to viral diseases, lower urinary tract malformations and/or urethral obstructions causing urinary tract infections or urine reflux towards vas

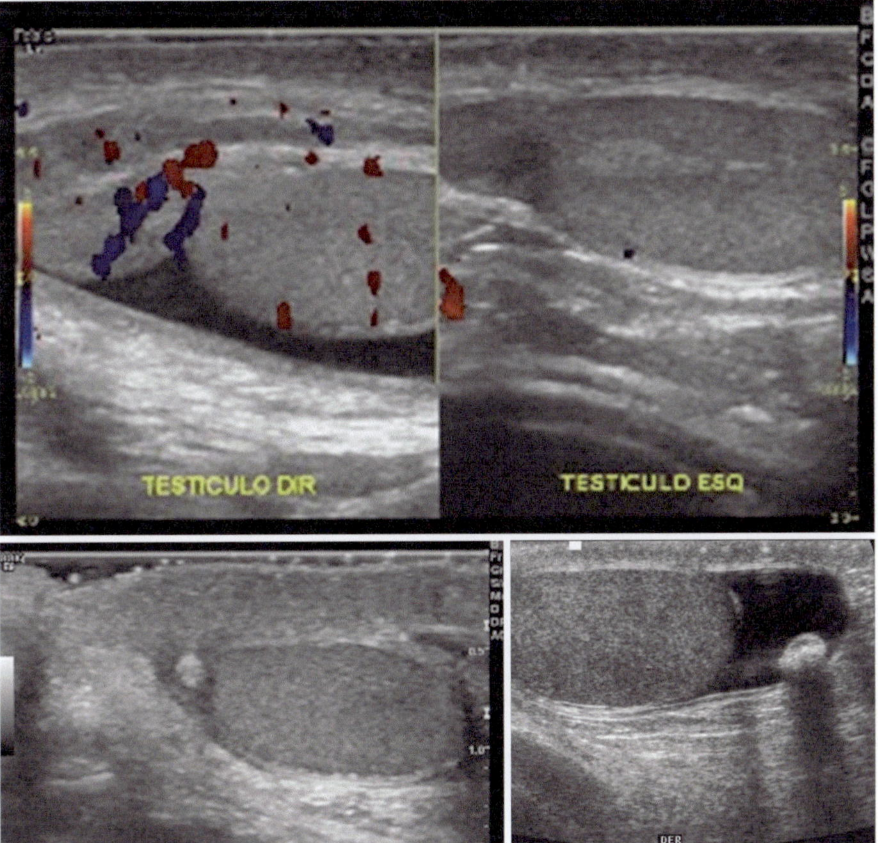


**Fig. 22.6** ATT affecting the right side, acute phase (augmented heterogeneous isoechoic appendix testis) (upper picture) and medium term control (hyperechogenic remnant of the appendix testis) (lower left) and late control, with scrotal "calculus" (lower right) (case from Dra. Tatiana Fazecas, MD)

deferens (chemical orchiepididymitis) and voiding dysfunction with incoordination in pre-pubertal children (causing urine reflux under pressure to the vas deferens). In adolescents, sexually transmitted diseases are also to be considered. The incidence of OE in adolescents is estimated in 1.2 cases/1000 patients/year [42].

Mumps is a classical cause of OE, presenting 3–7 days after the typical clinical manifestations of the disease, and is most frequent in post-pubertal boys. 20% of the patients show bilateral affection and 30% may present late partial atrophy of the organ [43]. Mumps orchitis is rarer nowadays due to vaccination. Other viral diseases (especially paramyxo, adeno, and enteroviruses and influenza) may show similar clinical manifestations. Viral orchitis has recently been described in an adolescent after SARS-COV2 infection [42].

In OE cases the affected testis is indurated, painful, and swollen. The epididymis is also edematous and painful to palpation, as well as the cord. There is no abnormality in the organ position and the pain may be eased by elevation of the testis (Prehn's sign). Pain is usually subacute and progressive. Scrotal edema and associated hydrocele are frequent. Some patients present fever. Pyuria is common and dysuria may associate.

US/doppler shows augmented testis AND epididymis, scrotal edema, and secondary hydrocele. In the doppler evaluation, there is an augmented flow to the testis and the epididymis (Fig. 22.7).

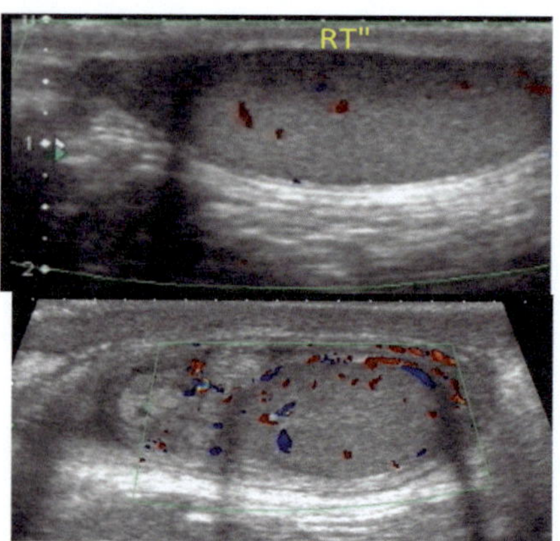
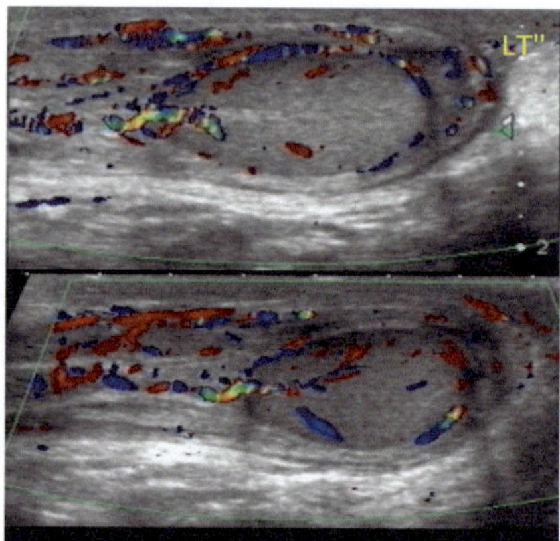


**Fig. 22.7** Epididymitis. Doppler ultrasound, showing hypervascularization of the affected (left) testis (upper picture) (case from Dra. Tatiana Fazecas, MD and Dr. Samuel Dekermacher)

Treatment is non-surgical with anti-inflammatories, antibiotics (in patients presenting associated urinary tract infections), elevation of the testicle, rest, and treating voiding dysfunction/urinary tract malformation, whenever present.

4. Other miscellaneous conditions

Testicular trauma is a commonly alleged cause for AS. Patients frequently attribute pain to a recent relatively minor trauma (especially falls, fights against other children, and sports trauma). A wrong diagnosis of post-traumatic orchitis is a common mistake in TT cases. As a matter of fact, testicular trauma very rarely causes AS, as the testicles are highly mobile and rarely exposed to significant blunt trauma. Conversely, testicular trauma may be a CAUSE for TT, by inducing a forceful sudden defensive reflex cremasteric contraction. Ultrasound is extremely useful to exclude significant testicular trauma, presenting rupture/discontinuity of the albuginea, heterogeneous parenchyma, abnormal contour of the gonad, testicular hematomas, and hematocele [44].

Idiopathic scrotal edema is a relatively uncommon acute condition presenting edema and hyperemia involving the scrotal skin/subcutaneous tissue. The hyperemia usually extends to the adjacent skin (inguinal and genital). Some children have a previous history of allergy. There is no testicular pain and the testis/cord are normal to exam. Ultrasound shows exclusively scrotal/inguinal edema, with normal testis, epididymis, and cord. Idiopathic scrotal edema often regresses spontaneously. Regression may be accelerated by anti-hystaminics and/or steroids.

Neonatal adrenal Hemorrhage (presenting as volume augmentation and scrotal discoloration) [45], meconial peritonitis (presenting as scrotal calcified tumors [46]) and left renal vein thrombosis (causing secondary thrombosis of the gonadal vein) [47, 48] should be considered in the differential diagnosis of AS in neonates, but those patients usually show comorbidities, including prematurity and/or perinatal complications and clinical signs of the primary disease that associates with the scrotal signs.

Henoch-Scholein purpura and other vasculitides are rare diseases, often preceded by an infection that may affect the testis. The clinical manifestations are characterized by acute pain, due to small areas of testicular infarction, secondary to the primary affection, that may be bilateral and associate to scrotal edema. Those patients usually show symptoms of their primary disease (classically purpura, arthritis and abdominal pain), but occasionally the testicular affection presents as the initial manifestation. The differential diagnosis is important for those patients, as they exhibit higher risks for surgery and anesthesia in the presence of complications of the vasculitis (carditis, renal affection, pulmonary disease). Treatment of acute scrotum secondary to vasculitides is conservative, associating the treatment of the primary disease to symptomatics.

A torsion of an epidydimal cyst or epididymal appendix (Fig. 22.8) is a rare cause of AS, and is very difficult to differentiate from TAT [49]. Torsion of the epididymis per se is uncommon.

Strangulated hernias are frequently associated to testicular ischemia, by compression of the vascular structures of the cord (Fig. 22.9). The diagnosis is usually

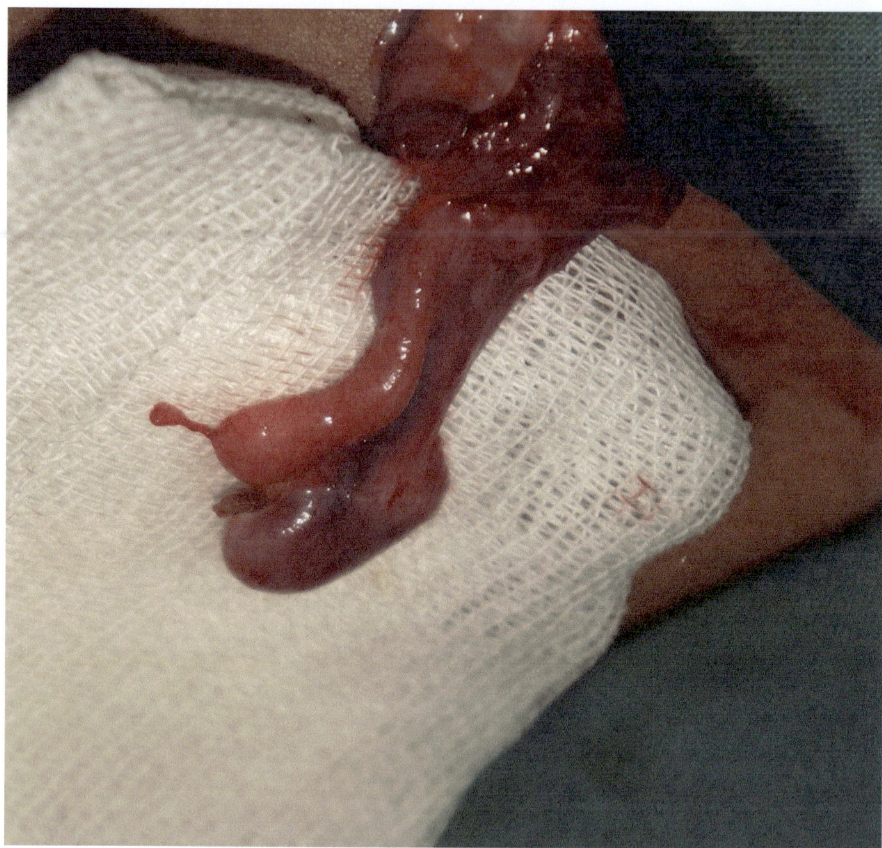

**Fig. 22.8** Torsion affecting an epididymal appendix (Dr. Mohamed Fahmy, personal archive)

obvious, and treatment relies on the resolution of the strangulation episode by taxis maneuvers and surgery. An important observation is that in some cases protracted testicular ischemia (by direct compression of the vessels, vascular spasm or vascular trauma during cord manipulation) may be irreversible and lead to progressive atrophy of the gonad. If this risk is predictable the parents must be informed, in order to avoid medicolegal problems.

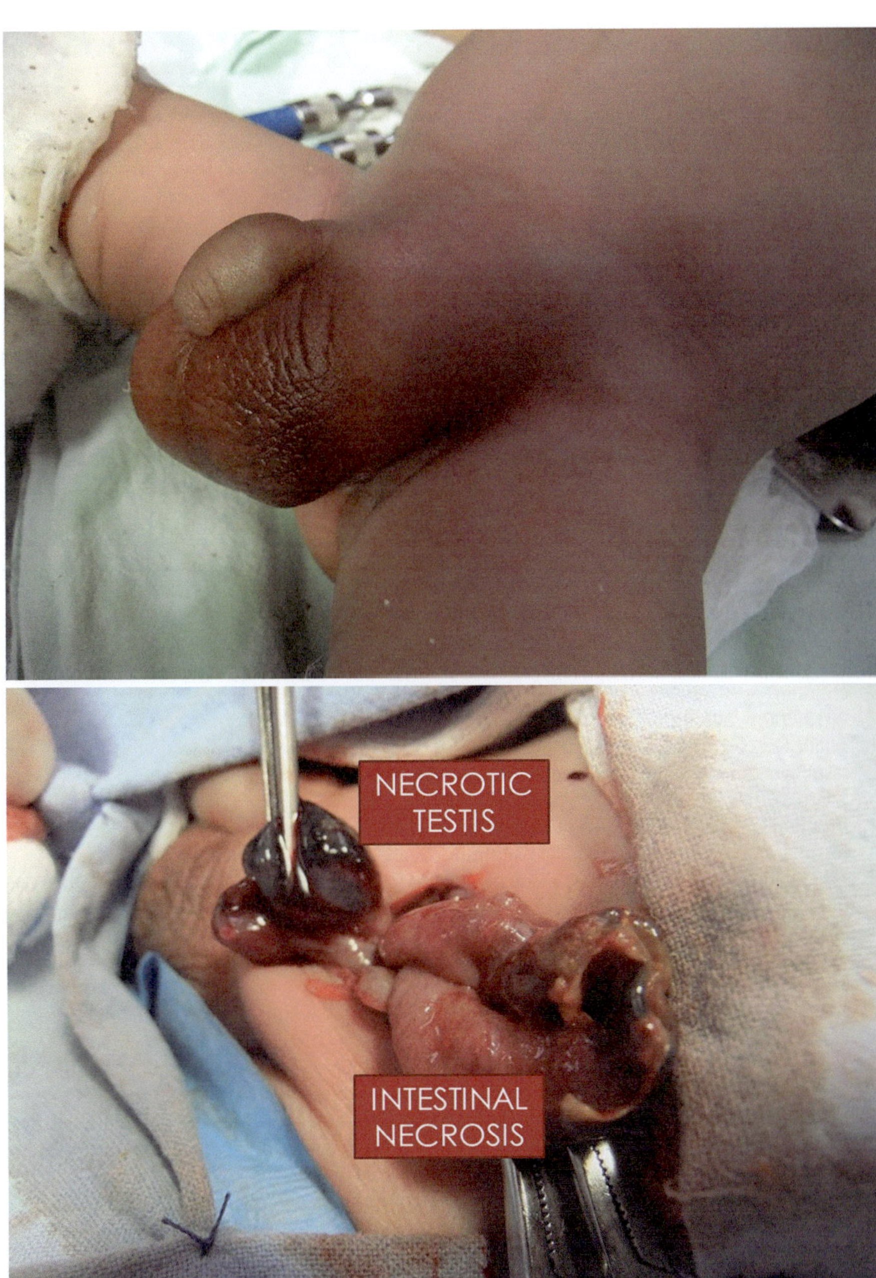


**Fig. 22.9** Strangulated inguinal hernia. Patient diagnosed after 18 h. Upper picture: diffuse hyperemia of scrotal and inguinal skin, indurated and edematous testicle. Lower picture: necrotic testicle and area of intestinal necrosis (case from the author's archive)

# References


1. Murphy F, Fletcher L, Pease P. Early scrotal exploration in all cases is the investigation and intervention of choice in all cases of acute pediatric scrotum. Pediatr Surg Int. 2006;2:413–6.
2. Dajusta D, Granberg CF, Villanueva C, Baker LA. Contemporary review of testicular torsion: new concepts, emerging technologies and potential therapeutics. J Pediatr Urol. 2013;9:723–30.
3. Ombredanne L. "Torsion testiculaire". In: Ombrédanne L, editor. Précis Clinique et opératoire de chirurgie infantile. Paris: Livraria Masson et Cie Ed; 1927.
4. Lyon RP. Torsion of the testicle in childhood: a painless emergency requiring contralateral orchiopexy. JAMA. 1961;178:702–5.
5. Molukwu CN, Somani BK, Goodman CM. Outcomes of scrotal exploration for acute scrotal pain suspicious of testicular torsion: a consecutive series of 173 patients. BJU Int. 2011;107:990–3.
6. Pogorelic Z, Mustapic K, Jukic M, Todoric J, Mrklic I, Messtrovic J, et al. Management of acute scrotum in children: a 25-year single center experience on 558 pediatric cases. Can J Urol. 2016;23:8594–601.
7. Bowlin PR, Gatti JM, Murphy JP. Pediatric testicular torsion. Surg Clin North Am. 2017;97:161–72.
8. Kadish HS, Bolte RG. A retrospective review of pediatric patients with epidydimitis, testicular torsion and torsion of testicular appendages. Pediatrics. 1998;102:73–6.
9. Lemini R, Guana R, Tommasoni N, Mussa A, Di Rosa G, Schleef J. Predictivity of clinical findings and doppler ultrasound in pediatric acute scrotum. Urol J. 2016;13:2779–83.
10. Liang T, Metcalfe P, Sevcik W, Noga M. Retrospective review of diagnosis and treatment in children presenting to the pediatric department with acute scrotum. Am J Roentgenol. 2013;200:w444–9.
11. Sheth KR, Keays M, Grimsby GM, Granberg C, Menon VS, DaJusta DG, et al. Diagnosing testicular torsion before urological consultation and imaging: validation of the TWIST score. J Urol. 2016;195:1870–6.
12. Frohlich LC, Paydar-Darian N, Cilento BG Jr, Lee LK. Prospective valication of clinical score for males presenting with an acute scrotum. Acad Emerg Med. 2017;24:1474–82.
13. Friedman N, Pancer Z, Savic R, Tseng F, Lee MS, Mclean L, et al. Accuracy of point-of-care ultrasound by emergency physicians for testicular torsion. J Pediatr Urol. 2019;15(608):e1-6.
14. Nason GJ, Tareen F, McLoughlin D, McDowell D, Cianci F, Mortell A, et al. Scrotal exploration for acute scrotal pain: a 10-year experience in two tertiary referral pediatric units. Scand J Urol. 2013;47:418–22.
15. Makela E, Lahdes-Vasama T, Ryymin P, kahara V, Suvanto J, Kangasniemi M, et al. Magnetic resonance imaging of acute scrotum. Scand J Surg. 2011;100:196–201.
16. Tokuda B, Kiba M, Yamada K, Nagano H, Miura H, Goto M, et al. The split sign: the MRI equivalent of the bell clapper deformity. Br J Radiol. 2019;92:20180312.
17. Mestrovic J, Biocic M, Pogorelic Z, Furlan D, Druzijanic N, Todoric D, et al. Differentiation of inflammatory from non-inflammatory causes of acute scrotum using relatively simple laboratory tests: prospective study. J Pediatr Urol. 2013;9:313–7.
18. MacDonald C, Kronfli R, Carachi R, O'Toole S. A systematic review and metanalysis revealing realistic outcomes following paediatric torsion of testes. J Pediatr Urol. 2018;14:503–9.
19. Goetz J, Roewe R, Doolitle J, Roth E, Groth T, Mesrobian HG. A comparison of clinical outcomes of acute testicular torsion between prepubertal and postpubertal males. J Pediatr Urol. 2019;15:610–6.
20. Ubee SS, Hopkinson V, Srirangam SJ. Parental perception of acute scrotal pain in children. Ann R Coll Surg Engl. 2014;96:618–20.
21. Kumar V, Matai P, Prabhu SP, Sundeep PT. Testicular loss in children due to incorrect early diagnosis of torsion. Clin Pediatr (Phila). 2020;59:436–8.

22. Nash WG. Acute torsion of spermatic cord: reduction: immediate relief. Br Med J. 1893;3:742–3.
23. Hosokawa T, Takahashi H, Tanami Y, Sato Y, Ishimaru T, Tanaka Y, et al. Diagnostic accuracy of ultrasound for the directionality of testicular rotation and the degree of spermatic cord twist in pediatric patients with testicular torsion. J Ultrasound Med. 2020;39:119–26.
24. Uribe AS, Perez JIG, Rueda FV, Rodriguez MRI, Pascual FJM, Sanchez SDR, et al. Manual detorsion and elective orchiopexy as an alternative treatment for acute testicular torsion in children. Cir Pediatr. 2019;32:17–21.
25. Vasconcelos-Castro S, Flor-de-Lima B, Campos JM, Soares-Oliveira M. Manual detorsion in testicular torsion: 5 years of experience at a single center. J Pediatr Surg. 2020;55:2728–31.
26. Dias Filho A, Rodrigues O, Riccetto C, et al. Improving organ salvage in testicular torsion: comparative study of patients undergoing vs not undergoing preoperative manual detorsion. J Urol. 2017;197:811–7.
27. Chu DI, Gupta K, Kawal T, Van Batavia JP, Bowen DK, Zaontz MR, et al. Tunica vaginalis flap for salvaging testicular torsion: a matched cohort analysis. J Pediatr Urol. 2018;14:329. e1–7.
28. Figueroa V, Pippi-Salle JL, Braga LHP, et al. Comparative analysis of detorsion alone versus detorsion and tunica albuginea decompression (fasciotomy) with tunica vaginalis flap coverage in the surgical management of prolonged testicular ischemia. J Urol. 2012;188:1417–22.
29. Kutikov A, Casale P, White MA, et al. Testicular compartment syndrome: a new approach to conceptualizing and managing testicular torsion. Urology. 2008;72:786–9.
30. Grimsby GM, Schlomer BJ, Menon VS, Ostrov L, Keays M, Sheth KR, et al. Prospective evaluation of predictors of testis atrophy after surgery for testis torsion in children. Urology. 2018;116:150 5.
31. Lala S, Price N, Upadhyay V. Re-presentations and recurrent events following initial management of the acute paediatric scrotum. ANZ J Surg. 2019;89:e117–21.
32. Arap MA, et al. Late hormonal levels, semen parameters and presence of antisperm antibodies in patients treated for testicular torsion. J Androl. 2007;28:528–32.
33. Bush NC, Bagrodia A. Initial results for combined orchiectomy and prosthesis exchange for unsalvageable testicular torsion in adolescents: description of intravaginal prosthesis placement at orchiectomy. J Urol. 2012;188:1424–8.
34. Peycelon M, Rossignol G, Muller CO, Carricaburu E, Philippe-Chomette P, Paye-Jaouen A, et al. Testicular prostheses in children: is earlier better? J Pediatr Urol. 2016;12:e1-6.
35. Mneimneh WS, Nazeer T, Jennings TA. Torsion of the gonad in the pediatric population: Spectrum of histologic findings with focus on aspects specific to neonates and infants. Pediatr Develop Pathol 2013, 16:74-9.
36. Monteilh C, Calixte R, Burjonrappa S. Controversies in the management of neonatal testicular torsion: a meta-analysis. J Pediatr Surg. 2019;54:815–9.
37. Das S, Singer A. Controversies of perinatal torsion of the spermatic cord: a review, survey and recommendations. J Urol. 1990;143:231–3.
38. Abdelhalim A, Chamberlin JD, McAleer IM. A survey of the current practice patterns of contralateral testis fixation in unilateral testicular conditions. Urology. 2018;116:156–60.
39. Kim JS, Shin YS. Clinical features of acute scrotum in childhood and adolescence, based on 17 years experience in primary care clinic. Am J Emerg Med. 2018;36:1300–20.
40. Lev M, Ramon J, Mor Y, Jacobson JM, Soudack M. Sonographic appearances of torsion of the apêndix testis and apêndix epididymis in children. J Clin Ultrasound. 2015;43:485–9.
41. Park SJ, Kim HL, Yi BH. Sonography of intrascrotal appendage torsion: varying echogenicity of the torsed appendage according to the time from onset. J Ultrasound Med. 2011;30:1391–6.
42. Gagliardi L, Bertacca C, Centenari C, Merusi I, Parolo E, et al. Orchiepididymitis in a boy with Covid-19. Pediatr Infect Dis J. 2020;39:e201–2.
43. Pillai SB, Besner GE. Pediatric testicular problems. Pediatr Clin North Am. 1998;45:813–30.
44. Adorisio OA, Marchetti P, de Peppo F, Silveri M. Ultrasound in the acute scrotum: the truth and the false. BMJ Case Rep. 2013;bcr2013009011.

45. Bhatt S, Ahmad M, Batra P, Tandon A, Roy S, Mandal S. Neonatal adrenal hemorrhage presenting as "acute scrotum"—looking beyond the obvious: a sonographic insight. J Ultrasound. 2017;20:253–9.
46. Gupta A, Puri A. Neonatal perforation peritonitis masquerading as acute scrotum: significance of a preoperative abdominal X-ray. Pediatr Emerg Care. 2012;28:1254–5.
47. Gunez M, Kaya C, Koca O, Keles MO, Karaman MI. Acute scrotum in Henoch-Schonlein purpura: fact or fiction? Turk J Pediatr. 2012;54:194–7.
48. Verim L, Cebeci F, Remzi Erdem M, Somay A. Henoch-Schonlein purpura without systemic involvement beginning with acute scrotum and mimicking torsion of testis. Arch Ital Urol Androl. 2013;85:50–2.
49. Messina M, Fusi G, Ferrara F, Bindi E, Pellegrino C, Molinaro F, Angotti R. A rare cause of acute scrotum in a child: torsion of an epididymal cyst. Case report and review of the literature. Pediatr Med Chir 2019;21:41. https://doi.org/10.4081/pmc.2019.210.

# Chapter 23
# Common Acquired Diseases of the Scrotum

Clécio Piçarro and Daniel Xavier Lima

## 23.1  Inguinal Hernia

Inguinal hernia is a common disease that affects 0.8–4.4% of the general pediatric population. It is more frequent in boys than girls (5:1), and the right side is more involved. The incidence is higher in premature. The incarceration of the inguinal hernia in children is 6–18%, but it increases to 30% when considering infants (less than 1 year of age) [1].

The incidence of inguinal hernia in males is as high as 27% of adult population, and only 3% on women [2]. There is association of family history. Other conditions of higher incidence in adults are pulmonary obstructive pneumopathy, smoking, situations with high intra-abdominal pressure, collagen disease and abnormal connective tissue homeostasis.

The pathophysiology of the inguinal hernia, in the vast majority of cases (95%), is related to the persistence of the *processus vaginalis*. This type of inguinal hernia is known as indirect hernia.

On the other hand, the pathophysiology of the adult could also be related to the *processus vaginalis*, but more often is because an acquired weakness of the posterior wall of the inguinal region. In adults the types of inguinal hernia could be direct, indirect and femoral.

The clinical presentation is similar in childhood and adulthood, with a groin bulging related to increase of the intra-abdominal pressure. Sometimes, the patient could complain of local pain. The majority of cases this bulging occurs only in the

C. Piçarro (✉) · D. X. Lima
Department of Surgery, Faculty of Medicine, Federal University of Minas Gerais, Belo Horizonte, Brazil

C. Piçarro
Division of Pediatric Surgery, Hospital das Clínicas, Federal University of Minas Gerais, Belo Horizonte, Brazil



M. A. B. Fahmy (ed.), *Normal and Abnormal Scrotum*,
https://doi.org/10.1007/978-3-030-83305-3_23

groin, but it could extend to the scrotum. Although, in children, the pathophysiology is related to a congenital problem, the presentation is almost always acquired.

Physical examination is easier in adults due to better cooperation. In children the herniation may not occur during the examination, despite a good Valsalva maneuver. In the suspicion of inguinoscrotal herniation, beyond the scrotal bulging, invariably there must have an inguinal bulge associated. The herniation could spontaneously reduce when the abdominal pressure ceases, or be easily manually reduced, if there is no incarceration of the hernia content (Fig. 23.1).

The diagnosis of the inguinal hernia is eminently clinical. A baby with a consistent history of a groin bulging, even without seen the herniation during the examination, could be diagnostic, and all of these children needs to be referred to the surgeon. In some doubtful cases, a groin ultrasonography may be necessary.

The differential diagnosis of inguinal hernia are hydroceles and testicular tumors.

The management of a not incarcerated inguinal or inguinoscrotal is the prompt surgical correction, electively. The surgical access could be either through an open incision or laparoscopically. In children the open surgical treatment consists in the proximal closing of hernia sac, after dissecting it from the spermatic cord (Fig. 23.2). In adults, depending on the type of the hernia, there are different types of surgical correction, such use of mesh to reinforce the weakness of the posterior inguinal wall, in the direct inguinal hernia.

When the content of the hernia cannot be reduced manually, this constitutes an incarcerated hernia. It causes severe groin pain, and in some can causes could secondary intestinal obstruction (Fig. 23.3). If it takes much time to be corrected, it may have ischemia in the hernia content, especially in the bowel loop, or in testis, because the compression of the spermatic cord. The surgical operation is an urgency.

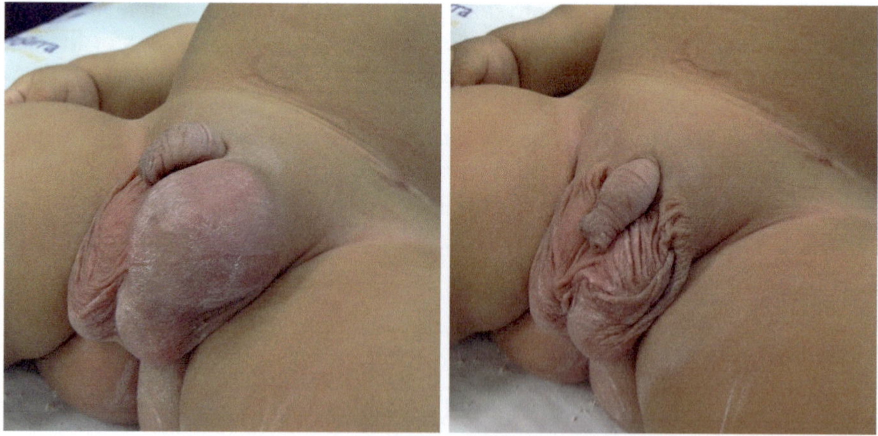

**Fig. 23.1** Children with left inguinoscrotal hernia, before (**a**) and after (**b**) reduction

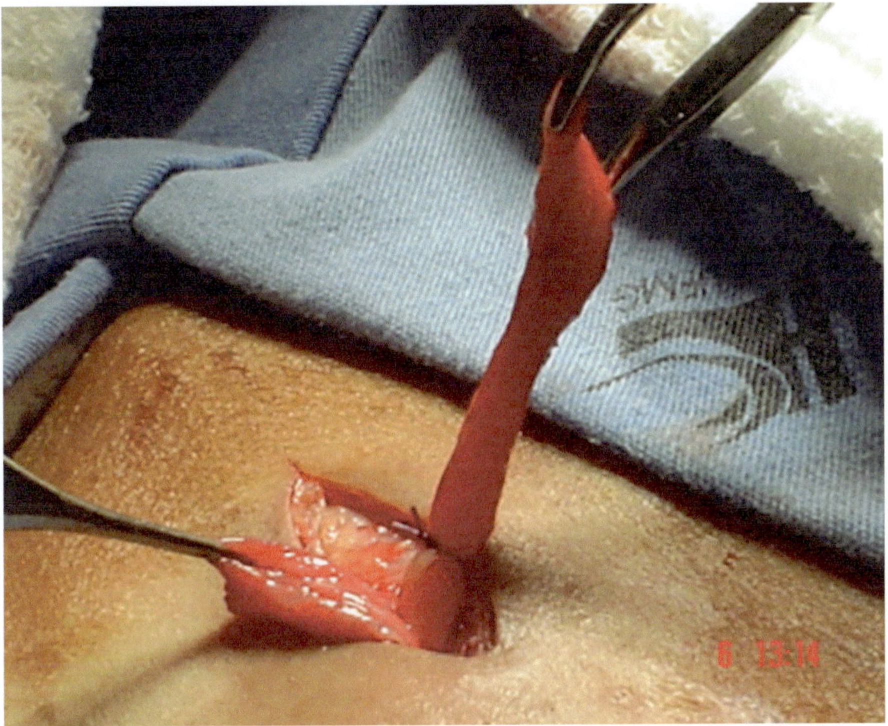

**Fig. 23.2** Surgical correction of an inguinal hernia in a child, with high ligation of the hernia sac, after dissection of the spermatic cord

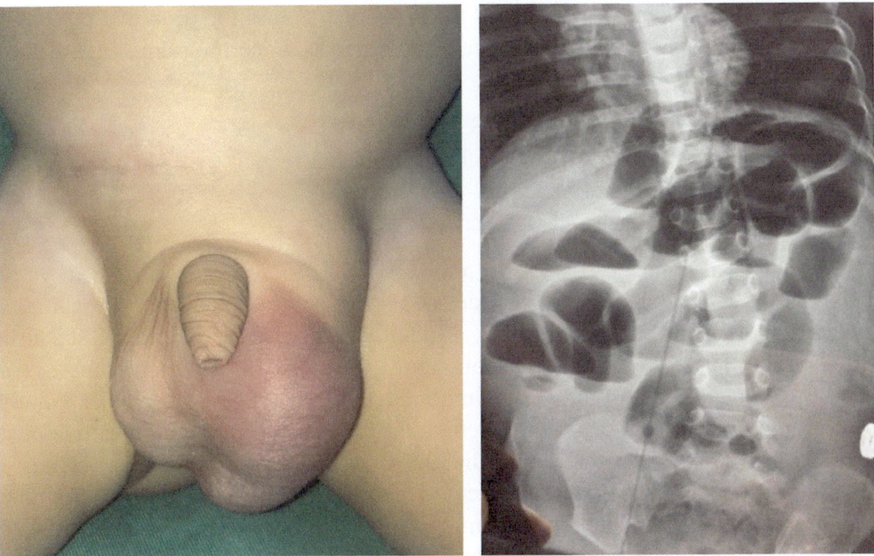

**Fig. 23.3** Boy with incarcerated inguinoscrotal hernia, with consequent bowel obstruction

## 23.2   Varicocele

Varicocele is a varicosity of the pampiniform plexus within the upper scrotum. It is very frequent in adults—if affects 15% of the male population, but it could appear since adolescence. It is much more common on the left side (80–90%). Approximately 40% of the infertility in male is related to varicocele, which is the main cause of infertility in male. The late consequences of varicocele in the adolescent are not well established, but it commonly leads to testicular atrophy [3].

The etiology of the varicosity of the distal testicular vein is related to the lack of the testicular vein valves, and some anatomical purposes, such as the angle entry of left testicular vein on the left renal vein, and compression of the proximal renal vein by the aorta and superior mesentery vein—the nutcracker phenomenon. Moreover, it causes a higher testis temperature and increases local venous pressure, which can result in testicular hypoxia.

In the anamnesis of the adult man or adolescent, in addition to the visual alteration in the scrotum, there may be pain complaint. In adults, the varicocele can be found on the assessment infertility. Physical examination shows the characteristic vein enlargement at the upper scrotum, which resemble a "bag of worms" (Fig. 23.4). On palpation it can sometimes be painful. The patient should be examined in prone and orthostatic position and using Valsalva maneuver. The sizes of the testicles have to be checked, to rule out testicular ipsilateral atrophy.

It is important to perform ultrasonography (US) (Fig. 23.5), not only to confirm the clinical suspicion, but also to verify the inversion of the testicular venous flow, and to measure its speed—a peak flow greater than 38 cm/s is related to a worst prognosis [4]. It is helpful also to check the testicular volume of both sides. With a more detailed US, it is possible (and desirable) to look for the nutcracker phenomenon in the left renal vein, as well the flow inversion in the proximal portion of the left gonadal vein. In adults and in late adolescence, a spermogram is mandatory.

The varicocele is graded from 0 to III, as follow:

  0. Subclinical, only seen by the US.
  I. Mild varicosity, just palpable with the Valsalva maneuver.
 II. Moderates veins dilations, easily palpable.
III. Severe veins dilations, easily seen by ectoscopy.

The treatment of the varicocele in adults is easier to define. A man with varicocele, symptomatic or not, with a decreased spermatozoid count needs treatment. The decision in adolescents is more difficult because some long-term scientific doubts, especially when the sexual immaturity is not completed, and the sperm count is not available. A boy with pain complaint and decreased testicular volume (discrepancy of more 15–20% on the contralateral side), is candidate for treatment. The ideal treatment is another doubt. In adults and adolescents, without nutcracker phenomenon, the surgical treatment could be performed through a low inguinal incision, just above the upper scrotum [4–6]. By this approach, a specific vein identification and ligation is done, with the aid of a microscope. Another alternative

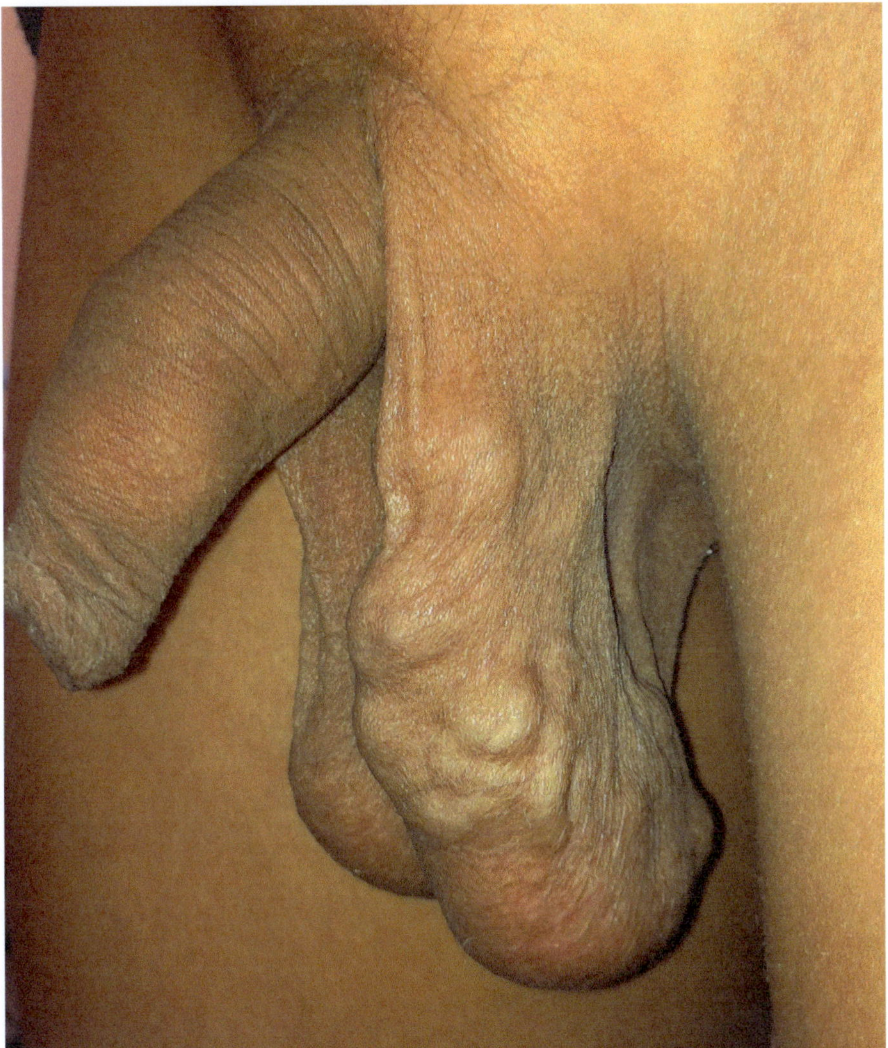

**Fig. 23.4** Left varicocele. It resembles a "bag of worm"

is the Palomo technique, that consists in a high retroperitoneal ligature of the testicle pedicle (vein, artery and lymphatics), close to kidney, that is accessed laparoscopically. There are several pro and cons in between these approaches. In patients with identification of the nutcracker phenomenon, and with indication of treatment, is another scientific doubt. Some authors demonstrated that the use routine surgical techniques have a higher rate of recurrency, and they suggest some more conservative management, and they consider the endovascular sclerotherapy of the distal testicular vein. On the other hand, some authors demonstrated that there

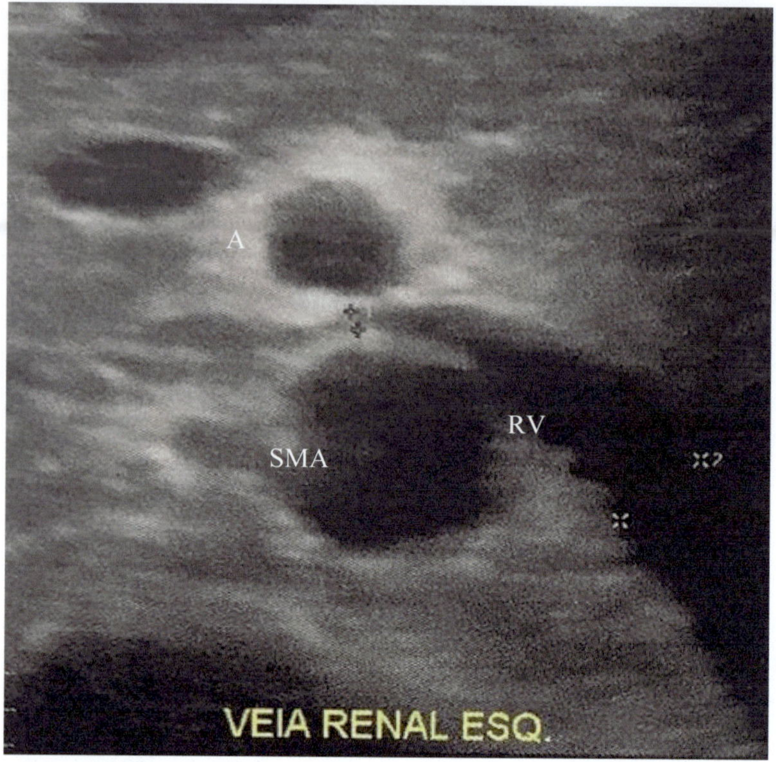


**Fig. 23.5** US showing the compression of the proximal renal vein (RV) by the aorta (A) and the superior mesenteric artery (SMA)—nutcracker phenomenon

is no difference in the long term with the usual surgical treatment (specific vein ligation and Palomo) [3–6].

## 23.3　Acute Idiopathic Scrotal Edema

It was first described by Qvist in 1956, and it is characterized by self-limited scrotal edema without any kind of affection of the testis or other types of intravaginal disease, like inguinoscrotal hernia. It causes no sequalae and could be recurrent. It is uncommon but it could be more frequent than reported in the literature. The etiology is uncertain, and could be related to insect bite, allergy, trauma, parasitic infection or cellulitis [7] (Chap. 21).

Clinically there a scrotal edema with erythema, that could be unilateral or bilateral, but without tenderness or systemic findings (Fig. 23.6). It may affect younger children and adolescents. There must have a careful palpation of the testis,

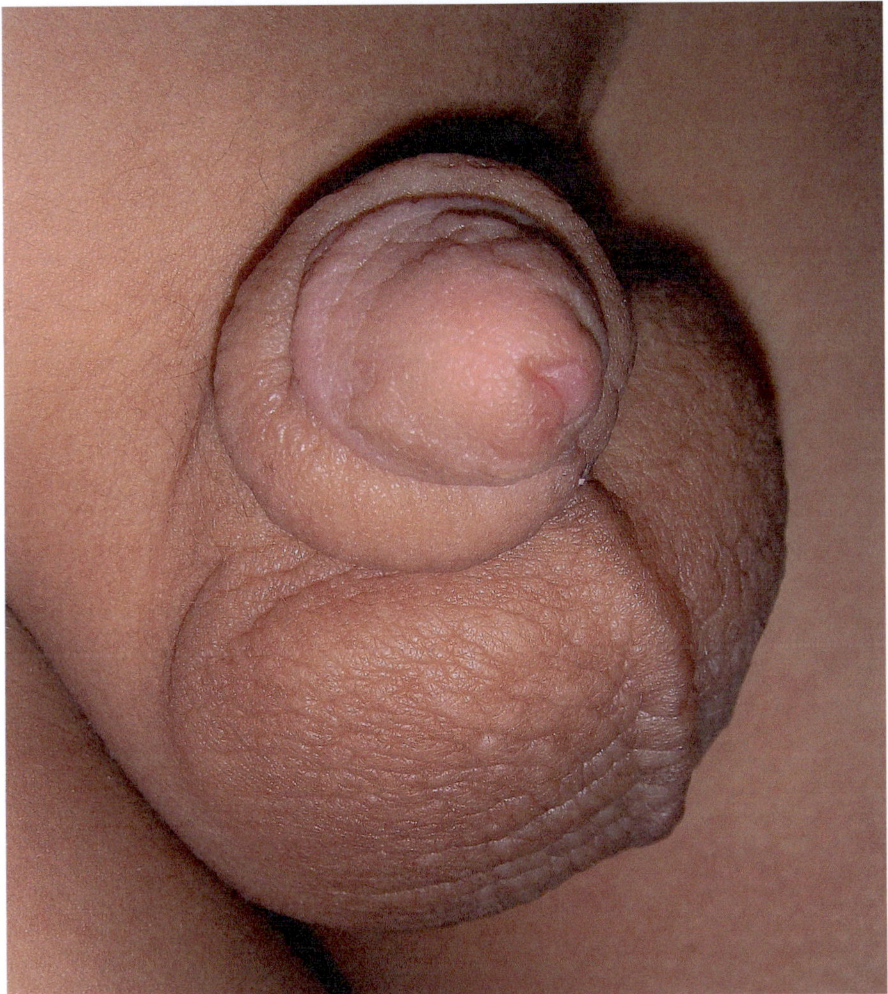

**Fig. 23.6** Boy with right acute idiopathic oedema

that is also nontender. It must be confirmed by scrotal ultrasonography, to rule out others causes of acute scrotum, like orchiepidimytis, testicular torsion or torsion of the testicular appendix.

The differential diagnosis includes others causes of acute scrotum, tumors and vasculitis.

The treatment is conservative, and the use of anti-inflammatories and antibiotics must be considered. These boys should be follow-upped because the chance of recurrence.

## 23.4   Genital Lymphedema

Lymphedema is a chronic swelling of tissues related to inadequate lymphatic function. This edema results in inflammation of the tissues, and later deposition of adipose tissue and fibrosis, and consequent local enlargement. It could be primary —anomalous lymphatics, or secondary—related to trauma to lymphatic nodes, malignancy and infection (filariasis). The vast majority of cases (90%) are secondary, and caused by filarial infestation, especially in the lower extremities.

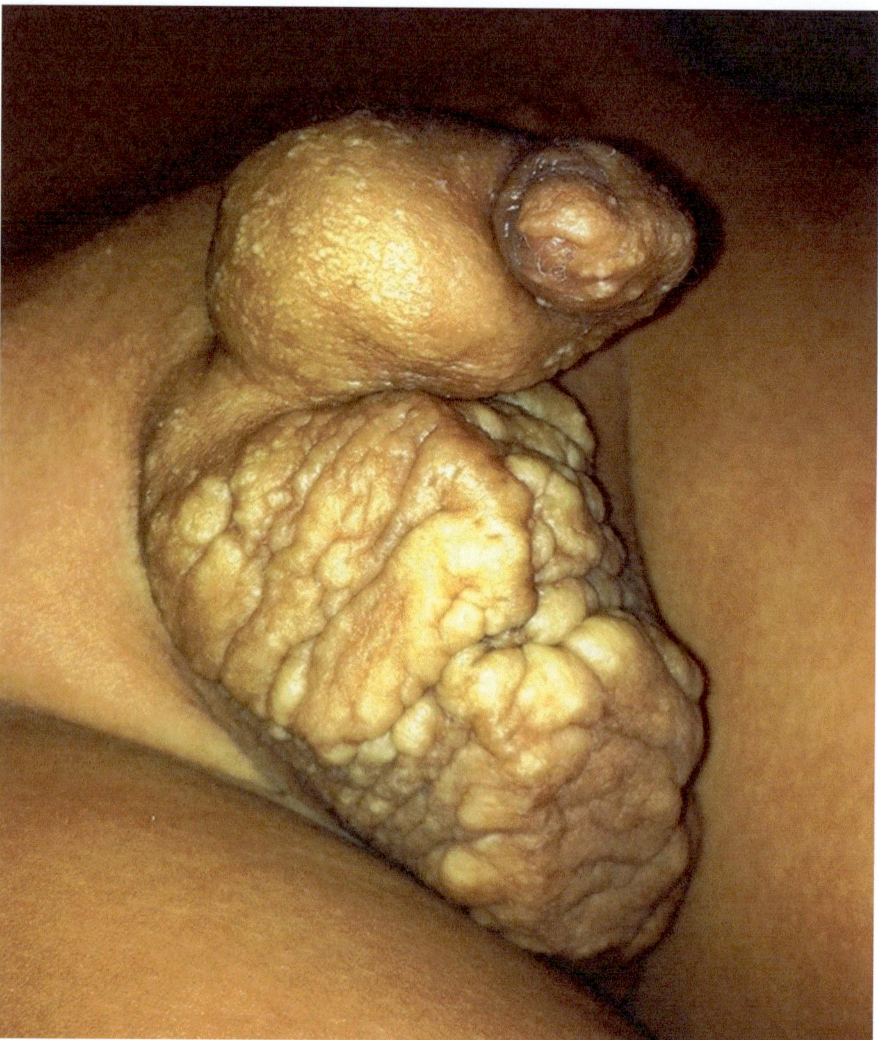

**Fig. 23.7**  Boy with genital lymphedema

Lymphedema of the male genitalia are uncommon, that can affect children and adults, and can cause profound functional and psychological distress. Some non-infection granulomatous disease are described as the cause of genital lymphedema in children, such as Chron's disease [8, 9].

The diagnosis is made by the history and physical examination, and sometimes with complementary images, especially magnetic resonance. The characteristic finding is the enlargement of the genitalia (Fig. 23.7), that could vary from affecting only the scrotum or the penis but could occur in both structures. It could have local cellulitis and lymphorrea. The correct diagnostic is imperative to provide the proper treatment. Others vascular anomalies should be considered.

The treatment of choice in the lower extremity lymphedema is compression. This can be difficult in the genitalia and cause discomfort. The focus of treatment is surgical correction. In children it could be postponed until the puberty. The enlarged subcutaneous tissue is resected with reconstruction of the genitalia, which needs to be previously well planned [8, 10].

## 23.5  Epididymal Cysts

Epididymal cyst may occur in adults and children, most commonly during adolescence, with incidence in children ranging from 5 to 20% [11]. In most cases they are benign lesions. The etiology is still not well defined. There are associations described with cryptorchidism, cystic fibrosis and von Hippel-Lindau disease. In adults there are confusions in terms of definition with spermatocele [11].

The diagnosis is based on scrotal pain or nodule, which can be confirmed by ultrasonography (US). It also could be found occasionally during scrotal US for other reasons or during surgical exploration. In adults, to differentiate from spermatocele, aspiration of the cysts would be necessary. The true epididymal cists only contain lymph.

Due to the benign behavior of these lesions, the initial management is conservative, with clinical and image (US) follow-up. Some authors recommend maintaining conservative management especially if the cyst is smaller than 10 mm [12]. The surgical excision is performed if there is no involution of the cyst during the follow-up, persistence of pain or anxiety from patient or their parents. In adults is describe treatment with sclerosing agents [11, 12].

## 23.6  Acquired Hydrocele

A hydrocele is characterized by a fluid-filled sac typically found in the scrotum, and less commonly in the external genitalia and pelvic regions Acquired hydrocele results from an imbalance of secretion and absorption within the tunica vaginalis. It is characteristically painless but can lead to physical and psychological complications and occasionally can be a cause of chronic scrotal pain in young adults [13].

Primary hydrocele results from a patent *processus vaginalis*, which leads to complications such as communicating hydrocele, inguinal hernia, or undescended testicle, and these will be discussed elsewhere. Acquired hydrocele can be communicating or noncommunicating. Communicating hydrocele occurs when a path exists between the peritoneal cavity and scrotum or the peritoneal cavity and inguinolabial region—a patent *processus vaginalis*. Hydrocele may be secondary to a dislocated testicle, testicular infarction, microlithiasis of testicle, lithiasis of tunica vaginalis, sarcoidosis of the testicle, retained foreign body, as well as sharp object injury [14]. Trauma and infection are common causes of the imbalance in lymphatic drainage, but it is most frequently idiopathic. Filarial hydrocele is a type of lymphatic filariasis prevalent in patients of developing countries and will be discussed in a specific part of this chapter.

Pelvic radiotherapy and surgery are potential causes of iatrogenic hydrocele, especially when there is disruption of the lymphatic system. Post-varicocelectomy hydrocele occurs as a complication in 3–33% of patients, because of damage to the lymphatics around the spermatic cord [15]. Hydroceles have also been reported as postoperative complications for inguinal herniorrhaphy, ventriculoperitoneal shunts, and renal transplants [16–18]. Although the post-herniorrhaphy hydrocele may resolve without further treatment, the surgeon should avoid radical dissection of the spermatic cord and carefully ligate lymphatics.

In addition to impairing self-esteem, hydrocele can lead to secondary complications, such as damage to spermatogenesis and delay in the diagnosis of testicular tumours, as it makes physical examination difficult. The reasons appointed for fertility impairment are the increased pressure on the blood supply on the testis from edema and a rise in intrascrotal temperature [19].

In children the diagnosis is easy clinically, and the main differential diagnosis is with inguino-scrotal hernia. In the history of hydrocele there is no complaint of inguinal bulging, only in the scrotum. And at the physical examination, also there only an isolated cystic lesion in the scrotum, with a normal inguinal region. In some doubt it could done a transillumination, that confirms the liquid content (Fig. 23.8). In some specific cases it could be necessary an ultrasonography (US) to discard an inguinal hernia.

In adults, hydroceles should be evaluated by US with duplex Doppler to properly rule out the possibility of an underlying testicular tumour. Patients should be placed in both supine and upright positions during examination as the hydrocele may reduce into the abdomen depending on the position of the patient [14]. Doppler US has a reported sensitivity to scrotal disease of 98% with 68% specificity. The colour image helps to differentiate benign from malignant lesions. Computed tomography (CT) scan with and without contrast and magnetic resonance imaging (MRI) of the scrotum or inguinal canal region provide additional information and increase diagnostic accuracy.

In children the management is conservative until the age of 2 years, with the exception of symptomatic (pain) or giant hydroceles. After this age, there is no

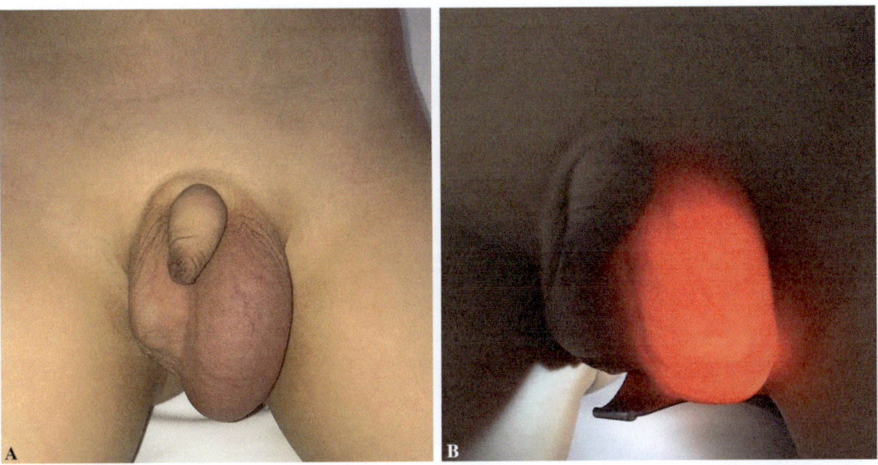

**Fig. 23.8  a** Boy with left hydrocele; **b** The transillumination confirms that cystic content

trend to spontaneous resolution, and the choice is the surgical treatment. The inguinal approach is performed, with high ligation of the *processus vaginalis*, after dissected apart of the inguinal cord (Fig. 23.9).

In adults, the most used non-invasive treatment options are aspiration and sclerotherapy, which are less expensive than hydrocelectomy. Aspiration alone has a high rate of recurrence [20]. Sclerotherapy has a place in the treatment of hydroceles in the adult population. However, there is little literature relating to children. Hydrocelectomy is also more invasive and subjected to complications, when compared to the percutaneous treatment, but presents a higher success rate. Postoperative complications include scrotal oedema, hematoma, chronic pain, decreased fertility, persistent swelling, Fournier's gangrene, and infection.

The classical surgical approach in adults is the Jaboulay's procedure. In this technique, the testis is exposed through an incision in the scrotum, the tunica is opened and everted and most of the hydrocele sac is resected with electrocautery, leaving a cuff along the borders of the testicle. Bleeding is controlled by a running suture closing the free edges of the hydrocele sac and haemostasis is secured by the aid of electrocautery [21] (Fig. 23.10).

Minimally access hydrocelectomy is alternatively performed through fenestration of the tunica and pull–through technique to remove large hydrocele sacs through a small incision and with minimal dissection. Its proponents claim better operative result in relation to scrotal oedema and hardening and patient satisfaction when compared to conventional eversion-excision hydrocelectomies [22].

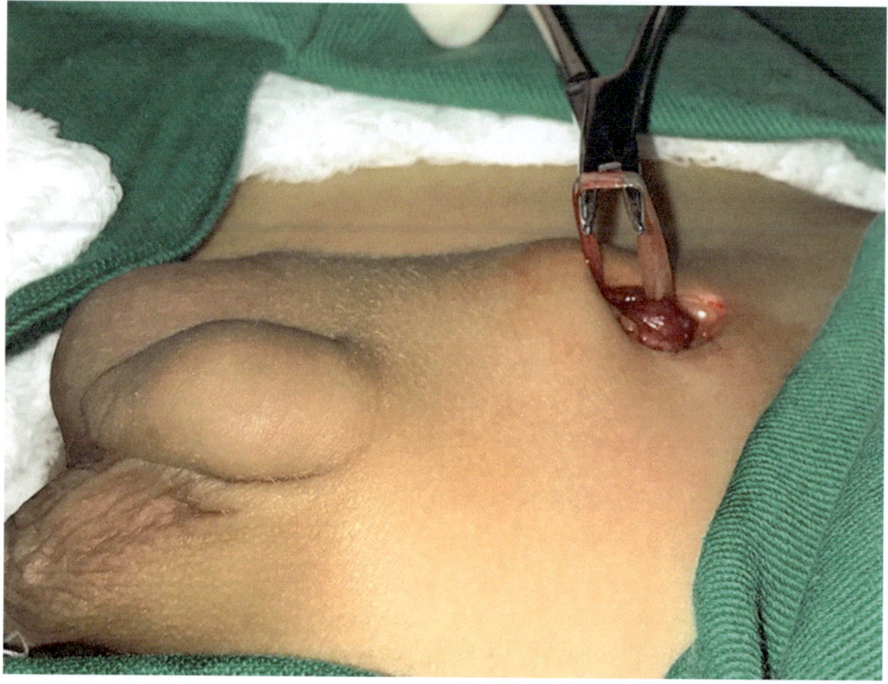

**Fig. 23.9** Correction of hydrocele in boy: inguinal approach with dissection of the *processus vaginalis* of the inguinal cord, to be high ligated

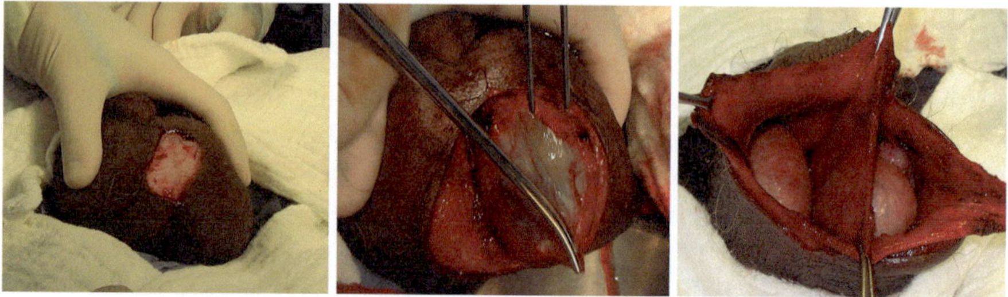

**Fig. 23.10** Jabulay's procedure for bilateral hydrocele

## 23.7 Hematocele

Another lesion that can simulate a neoplasm in the testis or paratesticular structures is the hematocele. Exceptionally, a true testicular neoplasia can indeed present clinically in the form of hematocele. It is commonly associated with a history of trauma to the scrotal region, when the diagnosis is simpler, as it has an acute onset and is accompanied by pain. However, in cases of severe blunt scrotal trauma, it can pose difficulty to the evaluation of a possible testicular rupture. Inasmuch as the degree of hematoma and swelling may not correlate with the severity of testicular injury, the presence of hematocele could impinge on a complete physical examination.

Moreover, hematocele may be idiopathic and of insidious onset, more commonly in elderly patients. In such cases, the most likely causes would be an asymptomatic trauma or infection or not initially noticed by patients. In another context, hematoceles may be secondary to coagulation disorders or vasculitis [23]. Characteristically, there is some difficulty in making an accurate diagnosis in the preoperative period, given that the form of clinical presentation is the same as that seen in cysts or testicular tumors [24]. Ultrasonography is an exam that can define the diagnosis, but in some cases it is inconclusive. In the setting of trauma, a normal or dubious ultrasound study should not delay surgical exploration when physical examination findings suggest testicular rupture. It is safer to establish the correct diagnosis in the operating room.

Magnetic resonance imaging, as it presents greater diagnostic sensitivity, can be indicated to demonstrate the presence of hematic content [25]. Chronic idiopathic hematoceles can present as firm and painless masses, often with fibrosis and calcification, which results in greater difficulty in differentiating them from tumors. For this reason, in many situations it is not possible to avoid surgical exploration, treating the case as a tumor until proven otherwise. Radical orchidectomy is indicated in uncertain settings [24].

The presence of fibrous wall and significant volume difficults the differential diagnosis with tumour lesions in the preoperative period [26].


## 23.8  Pyocele

Pyocele of the scrotum is a rare clinical entity poorly described in the literature. Also known as infected hydrocele, it is considered a urologic emergency that must be identified and treated swiftly to avoid testicular damage or Fournier's gangrene. It consists of purulent collections inside the potential space between the visceral and parietal tunica vaginalis surrounding the testicle and can appear as a complication after the treatment of the hydrocele by aspiration, after trauma, secondary to suppurative epididymo-orchitis or even as a manifestation of peritoneal meconium. The patients usually present with subacute onset of pain and swelling, fever, right hemiscrotal redness, and discomfort which may simulate other disease [27].

Laboratory testing may reveal leukocytosis. The diagnosis is suspected clinically, but usually only established by ultrasound. Characteristically, pyoceles show internal echoes with the fluid collection, because of cellular debris. Besides that, there might be loculations, septae, and fluid-fluid or air-fluid levels in the tunica vaginalis. On the other hand, a hydrocele will appear as a simple fluid region. The suggestion of a pyocele or a hematocele comes from internal echoes in the fluid collection [28].

The most worrying complication of a scrotal pyocele is the Fournier's gangrene, which will be discussed ahead. Computed tomography is recommended in such settings to delineate the extent of the disease and to define surgical resection. Pyocele treatment requires the use of broad-spectrum antibiotics and surgical drainage. Most of the cases reported previously are secondary to *E. coli* or *Staphylococcus* species. Broad-spectrum antibiotics are recommended until a specific organism is isolated and coverage can be reduced. There are two cases of pyocele in the literature in which surgical intervention was contraindicated due to clinical comorbidities and patients were treated only with antibiotics. Another case report described successful percutaneous drainage of pyocele, but those are not considered as standard treatments [29]. Unfortunately, many patients require orchiectomy, given that surgical drainage with preservation of the testis can be challenging [30].

## 23.9  Scrotal Abscess

Epididymitis is the most frequent cause of scrotal abscess. On the other hand, in the paediatric population, recurrent epididymitis is usually associated with anatomical abnormalities of the urinary tract. Wolffian duct caudal obstruction or abnormal insertion into the posterior urethra, for example, are predisposing factors for epididymitis [31]. They may be solitary or multiple, unilateral/bilateral, recurrent, and often secondary to urethra-ejaculatory reflux.

Other potential causes are neglected testicular torsion, spread of intra-abdominal abscess via patent *processus vaginalis*, idiopathic, and hematogenous route of systemic infection [32]. Acute necrotizing pancreatitis may also involve the scrotum through the retroperitoneal space. This leads to oedema of the scrotum and corresponding inguinal region, the so-called pancreatic hydrocele, but eventually this can lead to a scrotal abscess [33]. Although being rare, primary squamous cell carcinoma of the scrotum should be ruled out in cases of elderly men if a scrotal abscess shows suspicious features such as sudden increase in size, irregular consistency and associated inguinal lymphadenopathy and if wound fails to heal timely [34].

In cases of scrotal abscess associated with imprisoned ipsilateral hernia, appendicitis associated with Amyand's hernia (presence of the appendix in the inguinal hernia) must be suspected. The presence of normal appendix in the hernia sac is a rare condition, with an incidence of about 1% (Fig. 23.11). Much rarer is the case of an appendix complicated by acute appendicitis (AA) and peri appendicular abscess, with an incidence between 0.08 and 0.13%, but an accurate incidence cannot be estimated because few cases have been reported in the literature [35].

The diagnosis of a scrotal abscess is usually made by anamnesis and physical examination. The scrotum is generally oedematous and erythematous, sometimes with scrotal fluctuance. If the origin of the abscess is epididymitis, the affected epididymis presents tenderness, and the scrotal wall may be fixed to the underlying

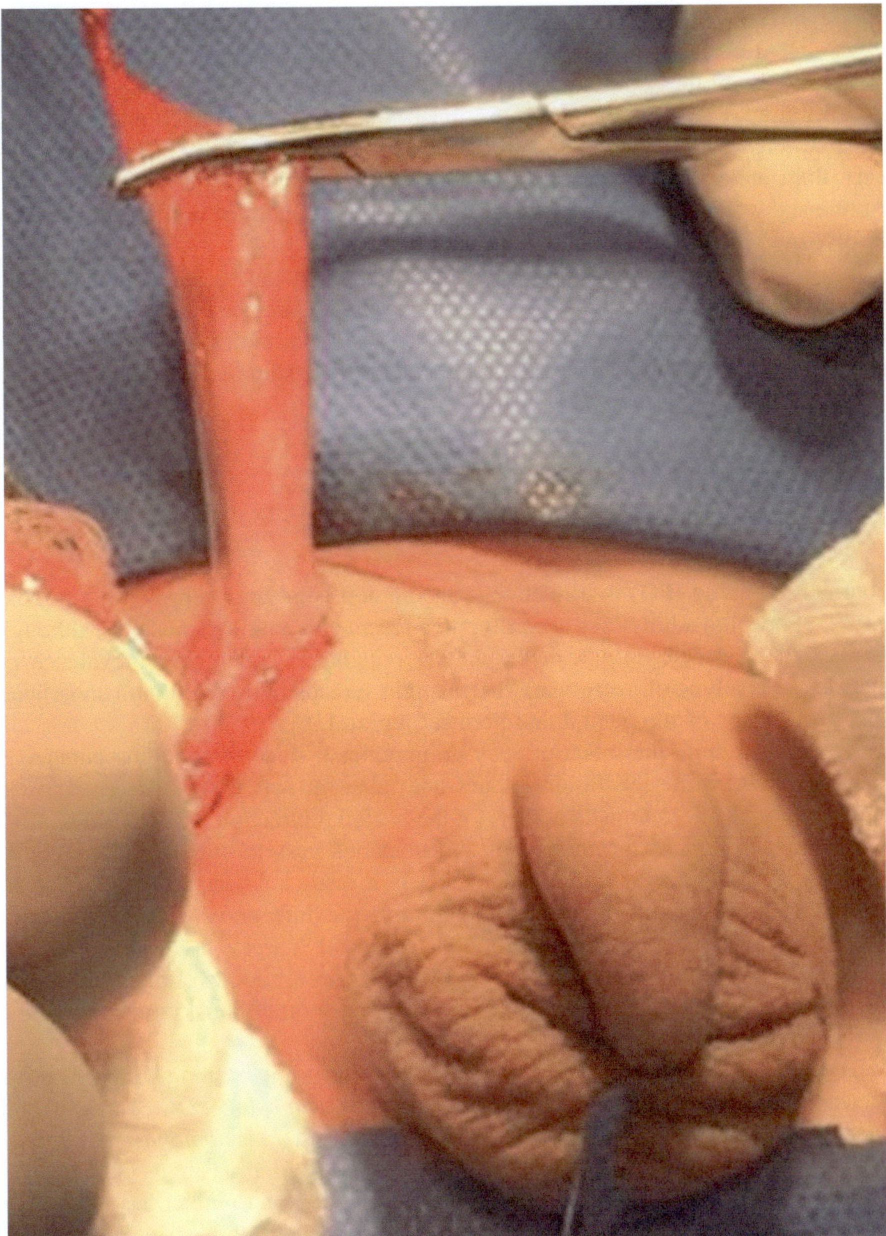

**Fig. 23.11** Boy with Amyand's inguinal hernia. Note the cecal appendix inside the hernia sac

epididymis. Scrotal ultrasound is useful in the diagnosis and can define the involvement of the abscess to the scrotal wall, epididymis, and/or testis.

Regardless of the aetiology, scrotal abscess requires surgical drainage, as occurs in other sites of abscess. The scrotum must be opened and drained and the cavity must be left with a drain. Broad-spectrum antibiotics to cover skin and genitourinary flora are used. Postoperative antibiotic therapy should be tailored to urine culture and wound culture sensitivities and should be continued until the infection is resolved.

Incomplete drainage or debridement of devitalized tissue may lead to persistence/extension of the abscess. It is crucial to recognize the origin of the infection to prevent recurrence. A dreadful possible complication is the Fournier gangrene, which can spread to abdominal and perineal skin and is potentially fatal. This issue will be discussed ahead.

## 23.10  Fournier Gangrene

Fournier gangrene (FG) is a relatively uncommon condition, representing a mere 0.02% of hospital admissions according to a recent epidemiological study, although its incidence is increasing with the ageing population and higher prevalence of diabetes. It is a type of necrotizing fasciitis that spreads quickly through superficial and deep planes of the genital and perineal region [36].

In the beginning, the infection may go unnoticed, since there are no cutaneous manifestations, while the fascial planes and adjacent soft tissues present intense inflammation. The synergistic activity of the bacterial infection leads to obliterative endarteritis, the micro thrombosis of subcutaneous vessels, ultimately leading to gangrene of the surrounding tissue, which is a result of bacterial production of various endotoxins and enzymes. In addition, the infectious and inflammatory process spreads to the dartos fascia, Colle's fascia and Scarpa's fascia, which allows for the involvement of the abdominal wall. It requires a high level of suspicion for the clinician to diagnose in a timely manner, because often the skin may not show any signs of disease [37].

The microorganisms involved are aerobic and anaerobic bacteria. Gram-positive bacteria, such as group A *Streptococci* and *Staphylococcus aureus*, and Gram-negative bacteria, such as *Escherichia coli* and *Pseudomonas aeruginosa* from several sources, including intestine, urinary tract or dermis are usually present. Some fungal infections have also been reported. In addition to infections from these regions, trauma and surgical manipulation of the genital and perineal area may trigger FG.

The disease is much more common among men, with a 10 to 1 ratio. Men in their 50's and 80's are the most affected worldwide [38]. The main risk factors are diabetes mellitus, malignancy, alcoholism, and immunosuppression. It can occur in children and usually is related to immunodeficiency status.

The most common form of presentation is the pain to genital or perineal area. With the progression of the inflammatory response, patients may experience fever, urinary retention, nausea, vomiting and malaise. On physical examination, there is a disproportion between related pain and skin findings, which can be minimal. The patient may have progressive oedema, hyperaemia, skin discoloration and a strong, putrid smell from the genital area (Fig. 23.12). Characteristically, there is a crepitus due to the air in the inner layers [39].

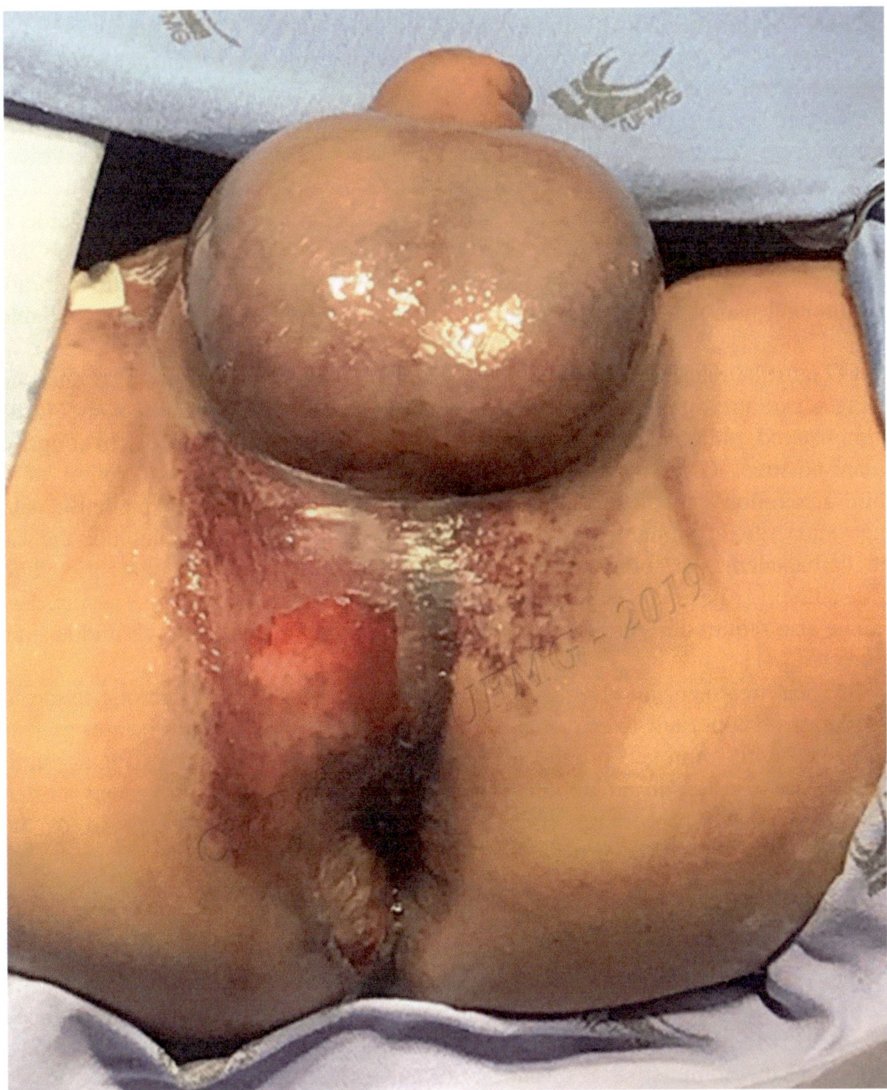

**Fig. 23.12** Fournier gangrene

For a proper evaluation of FG, it is necessary a combination of blood tests and imaging. A complete blood count will usually show elevated white blood count with a left shift. There are often also electrolyte abnormalities such as hyponatremia and metabolic acidosis, as well as any concurrent renal failure. Blood cultures and lactate can help to evaluate for associated bacteremia and sepsis. Arterial blood gas may be obtained to assess for acid/base status. Bacterial cultures are required to guide antibiotic treatment.

Ultrasonography (US) can be useful to identify the subcutaneous air in the underlying soft tissue. It can also assess the extent of the edema by measuring the thickness of the affected soft tissue. Computed tomography (CT) is more specific in this scenario, being the preferred method to better assess the extent of the disease. The main findings include fascial thickening, subcutaneous air, and fluid collections, such as an abscess. Most men and women will have genital and perineal involvement. However, women will almost always have vulvar or labial involvement, while men are more likely to have scrotal involvement than penis involvement. As magnetic resonance imaging (MRI) has become more readily available, it is increasingly used as a problem-solving resource when US or CT findings are equivocal or suboptimal to make a definitive diagnosis. Overall, the authors do not recommend use of MRI for clinically suspected FG when CT is readily available [40].

FG must be managed with both surgical interventions and medical resuscitation, being a true urological emergency. Empiric broad-spectrum antibiotics should be administered while culture is performed. A triple therapy is indicated, covering for Gram-positive, Gram-negative and anaerobic organisms. The association of a third-generation cephalosporin or aminoglycoside, in addition to penicillin and metronidazole, is commonly employed. Current antibiotic regimens include the use of carbapenems or piperacillin-tazobactam. Besides antibiotic therapy, fluid resuscitation is necessary, as patients may present with hypotension. Vasopressors can be also required in refractory situations. Electrolyte disturbances should also be corrected [41].

Surgical treatment involves extensive and radical resection of necrotic tissue. It is extremely important to perform it quickly in the course of the disease, as it is correlated with improved prognosis. Debridement is performed centrifugally until the subcutaneous tissue can no longer be easily separated from the skin, which often requires repeated procedures (Fig. 23.13). After controlling the spread of the infection, patients will need to undergo reconstructive surgery of the affected area. This will require a joint effort by different specialists, such as plastic surgeons, proctologists, and urologists. Colostomy deviation is sometimes necessary, especially when the infectious process originated in the anorectal area and later involved the anal sphincter. Hyperbaric oxygen has been shown to be useful for treatment, although it remains a controversial complementary treatment option. It is postulated that the hyperbaric environment results in improved tissue oxygenation, thus improving the administration of antibiotics and wound healing [42].

Vacuum Assisted Closure (VAC) is a method employed to accelerate the healing of surgical wounds and complicated wounds that fail primary healing. The open

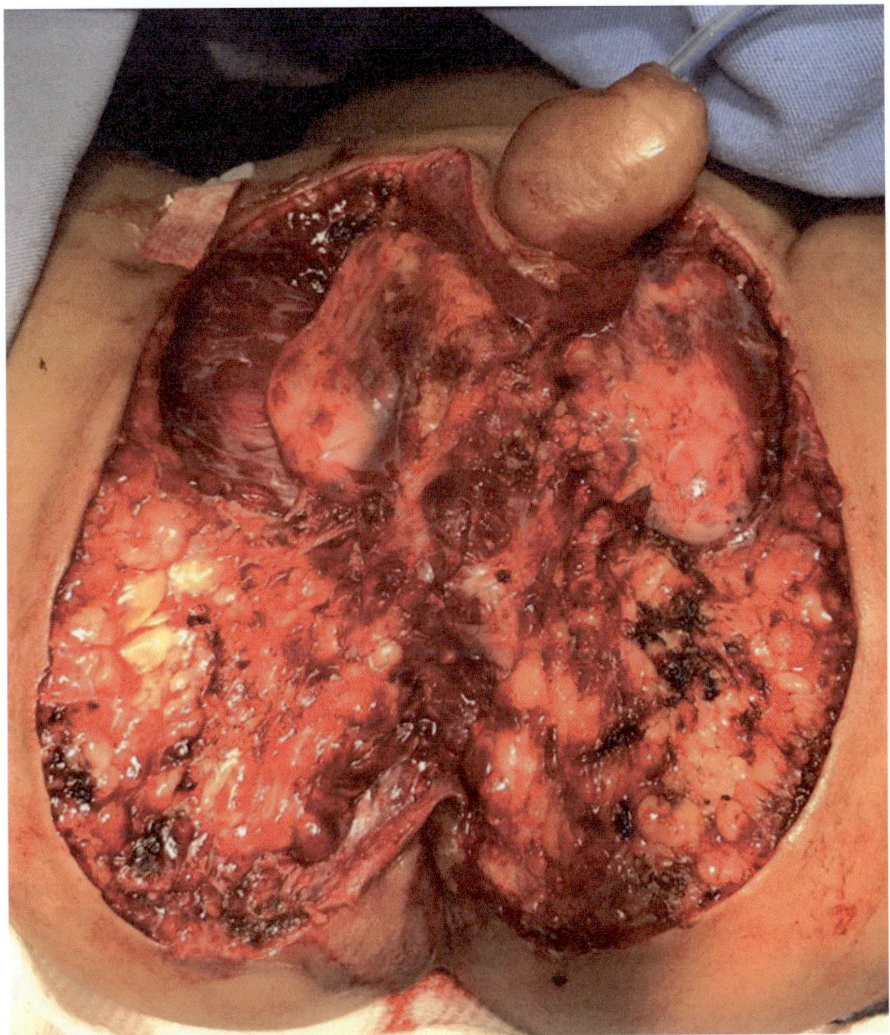

**Fig. 23.13**   Aggressive debridement of necrotic tissues

wound is exposed to negative pressure, which is thought to reduce oedema of the tissues, increase blood flow, and thereby promote healing and debridement. There is some evidence that suggests VAC is advantageous over conventional wound treatment in certain patients, reducing hospitalization, patient morbidity and allowed early reconstructive surgery [43].

Despite the advancements made in understanding the aetiology and the pathophysiology of FG, mortality rates remain high. Complications are quite common, both in the short term as well as the long term, including acute renal failure, acute respiratory distress syndrome, heart failure, sepsis, faecal incontinence and urinary tract infections. Psychological issues are also prevalent, given the devastating effect the disease may have.

# References


1. Esposito C, Escolino M, Turrà F, Roberti A, Cerulo M, Farina A, Caiazzo S, Cortese G, Servillo G, Settimi A. Current concepts in the management of inguinal hernia and hydrocele in pediatric patients in laparoscopic era. Semin Pediatr Surg. 2016;25(4):232–40.
2. Kingsnorth A, LeBlanc K. Hernias: inguinal and incisional. Lancet. 2003;362(9395):1561–71.
3. Evers JL, Collins JA. Assessment of efficacy of varicocele repair for male subfertility: a systematic review. Lancet. 2003;361(9372):1849–52.
4. Khasnavis S, Kogan BA. Natural history of testicular size in boys with varicoceles. J Pediatr Urol. 2015;11(3):148.e1–5.
5. Bong GW, Koo HP. The adolescent varicocele: to treat or not to treat. Urol Clin N Am. 2004;31(3):509–15.
6. Locke JA, Noparast M, Afshar K. Treatment of varicocele in children and adolescents: a systematic review and meta-analysis of randomized controlled trials. J Pediatr Urol. 2017;13(5):437–45.
7. Klin B, Lotan G, Efrati Y, Zlotkevich L, Strauss S. Acute idiopathic scrotal edema in children-revisited. J Pediatr Surg. 2002;37(8):1200–2.
8. Schook CC, Kulungowski AM, Greene AK, Fishman SJ. Male genital lymphedema: clinical features and management in 25 pediatric patients. J Pediatr Surg. 2014;49(11):1647–51.
9. Dederichs F, Iesalnieks I, Sladek M, Tzivinikos C, Hansen R, Muñoz C, Pavli P, Cavicchi M, Abitbol V, Rahier JF, VavrickaS, Katsanos K, Domènech E, ECCO-CONFER investigators. Genital granulomatosis in male and female patients with Crohn'sdisease: clinical presentation and treatment outcomes. J Crohns Colitis. 2018;12(2):197–203.
10. Lim KH, Speare R, Thomas G, Graves P. Surgical treatment of genital manifestations of lymphatic filariasis: a systematic review. World J Surg. 2015;39(12):2885–99.
11. Erikci V, Hoşgör M, Aksoy N, Okur Ö, Yildiz M, Dursun A, Demircan Y, Örnek Y, Genişol İ. Management of epididymal cysts in childhood. J Pediatr Surg. 2013;48(10):2153–6.
12. Niedzielski J, Miodek M, Krakós M. Epididymal cysts in childhood—conservative or surgical approach? Pol Przegl Chir. 2012;84(8):406–10.
13. Rottenstreich M, Glick Y, Gofrit ON. Chronic scrotal pain in young adults. BMC Res Notes. 2017;10(1):241.
14. Dagur G, Gandhi J, Suh Y, et al. Classifying hydroceles of the pelvis and groin: an overview of etiology, secondary complications, evaluation, and management. Curr Urol. 2017;10(1):1–14.
15. Salama N, Blgozah S. Immediate development of post-varicocelectomy hydrocele: a case report and review of the literature. J Med Case Rep. 2014;8:70.
16. Gulino G, Antonucci M, Palermo G, et al. Urological complications following inguinal hernioplasty. Arch Ital Urol Androl. 2012;84(3):105–10.
17. Ozveren MF, Kazez A, Cetin H, Ziyal IM. Migration of the abdominal catheter of a ventriculoperitoneal shunt into the scrotum—case report. Neurol Med Chir (Tokyo). 1999;39(4):313–5.
18. Beiko DT, Watterson JD, Cook AJ, Denstedt JD. Group A streptococcal hydrocele infection and sepsis in a renal transplant recipient. Can J Urol. 2003;10(1):1768–9.

19. Dandapat MC, Padhi NC, Patra AP. Effect of hydrocele on testis and spermatogenesis. Br J Surg. 1990;77(11):1293–4.
20. Shakiba B, Heidari K, Jamali A, Afshar K. Aspiration and sclerotherapy versus hydroco-electomy for treatinghydrocoeles. Cochrane Database Syst Rev. 2014;(11):CD009735.
21. Rioja J, Sánchez-Margallo FM, Usón J, Rioja LA. Adult hydrocele and spermatocele. BJU Int. 2011;107(11):1852–64.
22. Saber A. Minimally access versus conventional hydrocelectomy: a randomized trial. Int Braz J Urol. 2015;41(4):750–6.
23. McKenney MG, Fietsam R Jr, Glover JL, Villalba M. Spermatic cord hematoma: case report and literature review. Am Surg. 1996;62(9):768–9.
24. Barale M, Oderda M, Faletti R, et al. The strange case of a hematocele mistaken for a neoplastic scrotal mass. Can Urol Assoc J. 2015;9(3–4):E217–9.
25. Alvarez-Alvarez C, Farina-Perez LA, Barros CR. Idiopathic chronic hematocele of the vaginal sac. Int Braz J Urol. 2005;31(6):555–7.
26. Okubo N, Kobayashi M, Kusakabe T, Kamai T. A case of a hematocele of the spermatic cord mimicking epididymal tumor.Urol Case Rep. 2020;33:101318.
27. Slavis SA, Kollin J, Miller JB. Pyocele of scrotum: consequence of spontaneous rupture of testicular abscess. Urology. 1989;33(4):313–6.
28. Ragheb D, Higgins JL Jr. Ultrasonography of the scrotum: technique, anatomy, and pathologic entities. J Ultrasound Med. 2002;21(2):171–85.
29. Oberlin DT, Cheng EY. Management of pediatric pyocele using percutaneous imaging-guided aspiration. Int J Surg Case Rep. 2015;16:119–21.
30. Bruner DI, Ventura EL, Devlin JJ. Scrotal pyocele: uncommon urologic emergency. J Emerg Trauma Shock. 2012;5(2):206.
31. Desautel MG, Stock J, Hanna MK. Müllerian duct remnants: surgical management and fertility issues. J Urol. 1999;162(3 Pt 2):1008–14.
32. Kraft KH, Lambert SM, Snyder HM 3rd, Canning DA. Pyocele of the scrotum in the pediatric patient. J Pediatr Urol. 2012;8(5):504–8.
33. Sutalo N, Dragisic V, Miskovic J, Soljic M. Scrotal abscess as the first symptom of fatal necrotizing pancreatitis. Saudi Med J. 2019;40(11):1167–70.
34. Garg G, Sharma A, Aggarwal A, Sankhwar S. Squamous cell carcinoma of scrotum mimicking as scrotal abscess. BMJ CaseRep. 2018;2018:bcr2018226053.
35. Piedade C, Reis Alves J. Amyand's hernia in a 6-week-old infant: a delayed diagnosis. Case Rep Pediatr. 2013;2013:758171.
36. Singh A, Ahmed K, Aydin A, Khan MS, Dasgupta P. Fournier's gangrene. A clinical review. Arch Ital Urol Androl.2016;88(3):157–64.
37. Carroll PR, Cattolica EV, Turzan CW, McAninch JW. Necrotizing soft-tissue infections of the perineum and genitalia.Etiology and early reconstruction. West J Med. 1986;144(2):174–8.
38. Sorensen MD, Krieger JN. Fournier's gangrene: epidemiology and outcomes in the general US population. Urol Int. 2016;97(3):249–59.
39. Chernyadyev SA, Ufimtseva MA, Vishnevskaya IF, et al. Fournier's gangrene: literature review and clinical cases. Urol Int. 2018;101(1):91–7.
40. Ballard DH, Mazaheri P, Raptis CA, et al. Fournier gangrene in men and women: appearance on CT, ultrasound, and MRI and what the surgeon wants to know. Can Assoc Radiol J. 2020;71(1):30–9.
41. Mallikarjuna MN, Vijayakumar A, Patil VS, Shivswamy BS. Fournier's gangrene: current practices. ISRN Surg.2012;2012:942437.
42. Schneidewind L, Anheuser P, Schönburg S, Wagenlehner FME, Kranz J. Hyperbaric oxygenation in the treatment offournier's gangrene: A systematic review. Urol Int. 2021;105 (3-4):247–256.
43. Assenza M, Cozza V, Sacco E, et al. VAC (Vacuum Assisted Closure) treatment in Fournier's gangrene: personal experience and literature review. Clin Ter. 2011;162(1):e1–5.

# Chapter 24
# Neoplastic Lesions of Scrotum

Michal Yaela Schechter, Erik Van Laecke, and Anne-Françoise Spinoit

## Abbreviations

| | |
|---|---|
| AFP | Alpha-fetoprotein |
| BEP | Bleomycin, etoposide, and cisplatin |
| β-hCG | Beta-human chorionic gonadotropin |
| CT | Computed tomography |
| CXR | Chest X-ray |
| DES | Diethylstilbestrol |
| EP | Etoposide and cisplatin |
| FSH | Follicle-stimulating hormone |
| GCNIS | Germ cell neoplasia in situ |
| GCT | Germ cell tumor |
| IGCCCG | International germ cell cancer collaborative group |
| IGCNU | Intratubular germ cell neoplasia of unclassified type |
| LDH | Lactate dehydrogenase |
| LH | Luteinizing hormone |
| MRI | Magnetic resonance imaging |
| NSGCT | Non-seminomatous germ cell tumor |
| RPLND | Retroperitoneal lymph node dissection |
| RR | Relative risk |
| SCST | Sex cord-stromal tumor |
| TIP | Paclitaxel, ifosfamide, and cisplatin |
| TNMS | Tumor-node-metastasis-serum tumor marker |
| TTAGS | Testicular tumor of adrenogenital syndrome |

Michal Y. Schechter is fully funded by the Gianni Eggermont fund for advancement of research in Pediatric Urology.

M. Y. Schechter · E. Van Laecke · A.-F. Spinoit (✉)
Department of Urology, ERN eUROGEN Accredited Centre, Ghent University Hospital, Ghent, Belgium


M. A. B. Fahmy (ed.), *Normal and Abnormal Scrotum*,
https://doi.org/10.1007/978-3-030-83305-3_24

| US | Ultrasound |
| USPSTF | U.S. Preventive Services Task Force |
| VIP | Vinblastine, ifosfamide, and cisplatin |
| WHO | World Health Organization |

## 24.1 Introduction to Scrotal Neoplasms

Proper recognition and management of scrotal neoplasms necessitates an adequate knowledge of the contents of the scrotum and its functions, as discussed in the earlier book chapters. Some points to recall in this chapter include the scrotum as the site of spermatogenesis and therefore as a vital component of the male reproductive system. The testicular interstitial cells of Leydig produce androgens, in particular testosterone, which is another key scrotal function.

Some anatomical points particularly relevant to neoplasms of the scrotum include the the scrotal lymphatic and innervation systems. The scrotal lymphatic system drains to the ipsilateral nodes without crossing the septum. In contrast to the scrotal walls which drain into the nearby superficial inguinal nodes, the testis and epididymis are embryologically retroperitoneal organs, so their lymphatics drain into the lumbar and para-aortic nodes along the lumbar vertebrae. This difference in drainage pathway is relevant for testicular neoplasm cases, as it affects their potential for local versus regional dissemination. Scrotal wall innervation is controlled by the genitofemoral, ilioinguinal, pudendal, and posterior femoral cutaneous nerves. Some afferent and efferent nerves have been observed to cross over to the contralateral pelvic plexus, which may help explain how some pathologic processes in one testis can also affect the function of the other testis.

The scrota and its contents are complex and as such can present in various diseased states. This chapter highlights many of the neoplastic lesions found in scrotum and discusses the background, diagnosis, and management of testicular cancer, an umbrella term used to describe all scrotal neoplasms.

### 24.1.1  Incidence

Testicular cancer has a double incidence peak: It can present as a pediatric testicular neoplasia, causing 2–4% of childhood cancers.[1] Testicular cancer is also the most common neoplasm found in men ages 15- to 40-years-old. Overall, testicular neoplasms account for 1–2% of all neoplasms in males.[2] Assessment of recent trends in testicular cancer incidence and estimations of future rates has projected a continuing increase in worldwide incidence of cancer cases in the coming years.

Although population aging had been expected to reduce prevalence, increasing risk factors for testicular cancer indicate an expected increase in future testicular cancer development.

The table below is an outline of the testicular tumor subtypes with the highest incidence, stratified by age: While reviewing this table, it is important to remember that although testicular cancer has the greatest incidence rates at ages 30–34 years old, there are two incidence peaks: the first in the pediatric population, and the second in the 3rd and 4th decades of life. The discerning urologist should also keep in mind that after pure seminoma, mixed GCTs are the second most common testicular cancer subtype in adults.

| Age (years old) | Tumor subtype |
| --- | --- |
| 0–<11 | Prepubertal-type yolk sac tumor |
| ≥ 11–<35 | Embryonal carcinoma |
| ≥ 35–<74 | Seminoma[a] |
| ≥ 75+ | Lymphoma |

[a]It should be noted that although spermatocytic tumors occur most commonly in men ≥ 50 years old, regardless of patient age the incidence of spermatocytic tumors is always less than that of seminomatous tumors

## 24.1.2  Risk Factors

Well-established risk factors for testicular neoplasms include cryptorchidism or a personal or family history of testicular cancer. Males with undescended testes have a relative risk (RR) of 4.0–5.7 of a testicular cancer diagnosis, which falls to 2.0 to 3.0 in patients who undergo a protective orchiopexy prior to reaching 12 years of age. An orchiectomy may be performed in healthy males between 12 and 50 years old, as studies have shown that risk of mortality from testicular malignancy is higher than the risk of anesthetic or postoperative mortality in that age bracket. Recommendations regarding a contralateral, normally descended testis in a patient with cryptorchidism are conflicting, with some sources reporting a slightly increased risk of a testicular tumor as compared to the normal male population[3] and others suggesting no increased risk in the contralateral testis.

Personal or family history of testicular cancer has been shown to substantially increase risk of a testicular germ cell tumor (GCT) , with a personal history leading to a RR of 12. However, the 15-year cumulative incidence in this patient population is 2%.[4] Infertility has also been associated with a higher incidence of testicular cancer development. Current theories suggest a common etiology for infertility and testicular cancer, possibly due to poor germ cell quality. In addition, some studies have indicated an increased risk in patients born with hypospadias.

Additional risks for testicular neoplasms include genetic and environmental components. Chemical pollutants lead to disruption of endocrine activity, helping explain predictions of increasing testicular cancer incidence. Endocrine-disrupting chemicals associated with development of testicular cancer include those with estrogenic effects and may impair normal cell differentiation in perinatal and peripubertal germ stem cells, opening the possibility of considering the GCT type as an estrogen-dependent cancer. Exposure to synthetic estrogen diethylstilbestrol (DES) in utero and possibly exposure to exogenous estrogen therapy in the transgender population have been associated with increased risk for testicle cancer.

Testicular microlithiasis is a condition involving intratubular calcifications and is typically discovered incidentally on imaging. It is visualized on ultrasound (US) as multiple small echogenic foci disseminated across the testicular parenchyma. Up to 44% of microlithiasis patients have been diagnosed with testicular cancer,[5] however a cause-and-effect relationship has as of yet not been proven. This association has led to disagreement on the best approach for patients with testicular microlithiasis. Recent recommendations suggest follow-up for this patient population in cases of either a solid mass or of risk factors in the patient history (including maldescent testis, orchiopexy, testicular atrophy, or personal or family history of GCT), with an emphasis on an individualized approach for each patient.

## 24.2  Diagnosis

### 24.2.1  Presentation

The most common presentation of scrotal neoplasms involves a painless scrotal mass or swelling. Acute testicular pain is present in less than one-third of cases, and may be explained by intratumor hemorrhage or infarction caused by tumor growth. Patients may also report a sense of scrotal heaviness or achiness, as well as a history of scrotal trauma. Up to 20% of patients present with complaints related to metastatic spread.[6] A minority of patients also experience gynecomastia.

The clinical evaluation of a suspected scrotal neoplasm should begin with a history and physical exam. In addition to obtaining a clinical description of the mass, the patient should also be asked about any personal history of cryptorchidism, orchiopexy, inguinal hernia repair, or trauma, as well as any personal or family history of testicular cancer in first-degree relatives. Symptoms of metastatic disease may involve systemic symptoms, cough, shortness of breath, and back, abdominal, or flank pain.

A thorough physical examination should be performed by gently holding each testis and rolling it between the fingers to palpate the mass. It is critical to examine both testes, as 0.6% of patients with a testicular neoplasm also have a contralateral testis tumor.[7] Examination signs indicating metastasis should be evaluated, in particular palpation of the supraclavicular lymph nodes for lymphadenopathy and the abdomen for any masses. A breast exam should be performed as well, evaluating for signs of gynecomastia.

## 24.2.2 Differential Diagnosis

An important concept regarding scrotal neoplasms is that until proven otherwise, a hard intratesticular mass should be regarded as cancerous. However, some of the more important differential diagnoses under consideration during evaluation of a scrotal mass evaluation include epididymo-orchitis and hydrocele. These diseases are mistakenly diagnosed in up to one-third of testicular cancer cases, causing a missed earlier cancer diagnosis. Epididymitis and hydrocele have an increased prevalence of diagnosis in the three months prior to testicular cancer diagnosis. This may indicate hydrocele as a common misdiagnosis in testicular cancer cases or as a condition associated with cancer, and epididymitis as a possible complication of testicular cancer.

An US can be used to help further narrow down the differential diagnosis. Testicular cancer may be accompanied by a hydrocele, hindering the ability for a more thorough clinical evaluation. Therefore, an US is especially warranted in cases with an uncertain diagnosis of hydrocele.

Although epididymo-orchitis may be unilateral or bilateral while neoplastic scrotal lesions are usually unilateral, cases of epididymitis may exhibit a similar US appearance to testicular lymphoma and leukemia with a heterogenous echotexture on imaging. Therefore, patients with suspected epididymitis should be reevaluated with a follow-up US after resolution of infection to rule out a scrotal neoplasm.

## 24.2.3 Diagnostic Workup

Since a solid testicular mass is considered testicular cancer until proven otherwise, the initial classification of a scrotal mass as intra or extratesticular is important as malignant extratesticular masses are uncommon (3%).[8] US imaging is the primary imaging modality for identification of scrotal mass location and should be viewed as an extension of the physical examination. An US can also be used to help better determine the size and specific anatomical location of the mass. When combined with a clinical exam, a bilateral testicular US provides a nearly 100% sensitivity for testicular cancer diagnosis.[9] Imaging of the contralateral scrotum is also vital, as its assessment can not only help ensure that it is not pathologic but may also aid in the assessment of the scrotum under evaluation.

Testicular cancer on US typically appears as a hypoechoic, solid, and heterogenous lesion, with imaging differences present in the various cancer subtypes. When US findings are vague, magnetic resonance imaging (MRI) can be used as an adjunctive diagnostic tool and help check the mass. Nonpalpable or incidentally detected masses on US that measure <2 cm may be managed by serial examinations and a repeat US in 6–8 weeks, testis-sparing surgery, or orchiectomy.

Concerning clinical and US findings should prompt further workup with serum tumor markers, including lactate dehydrogenase (LDH), alpha-fetoprotein (AFP), and beta-human chorionic gonadotropin (β-hCG), along with a basic chemistry panel. These serum tumor markers are nonspecific, with AFP and LDH overexpression found in various other disorders and higher β-hCG levels present in other cancer types. However, LDH elevations are linked to an increased tumor burden in GCTs (LDH-1 is expressed on chromosome 12p). While AFP is never elevated in pure seminomas and pure choriocarcinomas, higher levels can be found in yolk sac, embryonal, and teratoma GCTs. β-hCG is produced by GCT syncytiotrophoblasts and is often overexpressed in choriocarcinomas and sometimes in seminomas.

Patients with a suspected sex cord-stromal tumor (SCST) should be evaluated for hormonal markers in addition to the serum tumor markers. These hormonal markers include testosterone, luteinizing hormone (LH), and follicle-stimulating hormone (FSH). If tumor markers are not detected or if patients have signs of feminization, serum levels of estrogen, estradiol, progesterone, and cortisol are also evaluated. Patients with normal serum tumor marker levels and inconclusive physical exam and US findings should have repeat imaging in 6–8 weeks for evaluation of testicular cancer.

Definitive diagnosis is achieved via histological analysis. A suspected tumor during workup is an indication for a radical transinguinal orchiectomy, providing tissue for the histological diagnosis (in addition to a therapeutic treatment) . Trans-scrotal biopsy is not conducted due to the possibility of local dissemination, as there is an increased risk of local recurrence with performance of biopsy as opposed to orchiectomy.

Suspicious findings are also an indication for cross-sectional imaging to evaluate retroperitoneal spread to the lymph nodes (the most frequent site of tumor spread) or distant metastases. This imaging includes a chest X-ray (CXR) and abdomino-pelvic computed tomography (CT) imaging. If the histological report indicates a nonseminomatous tumor, a CT chest should also be performed. If a seminomatous tumor is found, a CT chest should only be performed if the CXR or abdominopelvic CT is abnormal. The chest and abdominopelvic CT are used together for the purposes of staging. A bone scan or brain MRI is suitable when clinically indicated.

## 24.3 Classification and Staging

### 24.3.1 Tumor Classification

Classification of a testicular tumor type is based on its histological analysis. Together with staging, tumor classification is used to develop an appropriate treatment plan. While there are several diverse types of testicular tumors, 95% are classified as GCTs, with the majority of testicular tumors in men $\leq 50$ years of age classified as malignant GCTs.[10] Recent changes to the World Health Organization (WHO) classification of testicular cancer have led to an updated characterization based on histology as well as pathogenesis. These changes include the term germ cell neoplasia in situ (GCNIS) as a new label for the precursor lesion to GCTs, replacing the previous term of intratubular germ cell neoplasia of unclassified type (IGCNU). Spermatocytic tumor was placed in the non-GCNIS derived group, reflected by its name change from spermatocytic seminoma. Another adjustment is the distinction of GCNIS derived tumors from non-GCNIS derived tumors as generally representing postpubertal and prepubertal tumors, respectively. Specifically, yolk sac tumors and teratomas were divided into prepubertal- and postpubertal-types. There is growing data that testicular prepubertal and postpubertal tumors differ in clinical features and prognosis.

The following list provides an overview of the WHO testicular cancer classification, with a more detailed account from the 2016 WHO report found in Fig. 24.1:

## WHO classification of tumours of the testis

| | |
|---|---|
| **Germ cell tumours derived from germ cell neoplasia in situ** | |
| *Non-invasive germ cell neoplasia* | |
| Germ cell neoplasia in situ | 9064/2 |
| Specific forms of intratubular germ cell neoplasia | |
| *Tumours of a single histological type (pure forms)* | |
| Seminoma | 9061/3 |
| Seminoma with syncytiotrophoblast cells | |
| *Non-seminomatous germ cell tumours* | |
| Embryonal carcinoma | 9070/3 |
| Yolk sac tumour, postpubertal-type | 9071/3 |
| Trophoblastic tumours | |
| Choriocarcinoma | 9100/3 |
| Non-choriocarcinomatous trophoblastic tumours | |
| Placental site trophoblastic tumour | 9104/1 |
| Epithelioid trophoblastic tumour | 9105/3 |
| Cystic trophoblastic tumour | |
| Teratoma, postpubertal-type | 9080/3 |
| Teratoma with somatic-type malignancy | 9084/3 |
| *Non-seminomatous germ cell tumours of more than one histological type* | |
| Mixed germ cell tumours | 9085/3 |
| *Germ cell tumours of unknown type* | |
| Regressed germ cell tumours | 9080/1 |
| **Germ cell tumours unrelated to germ cell neoplasia in situ** | |
| Spermatocytic tumour | 9063/3 |
| Teratoma, prepubertal-type | 9084/0 |
| Dermoid cyst | |
| Epidermoid cyst | |
| Well-differentiated neuroendocrine tumour (monodermal teratoma) | 8240/3 |
| Mixed teratoma and yolk sac tumour, prepubertal-type | 9085/3 |
| Yolk sac tumour, prepubertal-type | 9071/3 |
| **Sex cord–stromal tumours** | |
| *Pure tumours* | |
| Leydig cell tumour | 8650/1 |
| Malignant Leydig cell tumour | 8650/3 |
| Sertoli cell tumour | 8640/1 |
| Malignant Sertoli cell tumour | 8640/3 |
| Large cell calcifying Sertoli cell tumour | 8642/1 |
| Intratubular large cell hyalinizing Sertoli cell neoplasia | 8643/1* |
| Granulosa cell tumour | |
| Adult granulosa cell tumour | 8620/1 |
| Juvenile granulosa cell tumour | 8622/1* |
| Tumours in the fibroma–thecoma group | 8600/0 |
| *Mixed and unclassified sex cord–stromal tumours* | |
| Mixed sex cord–stromal tumour | 8592/1 |
| Unclassified sex cord–stromal tumour | 8591/1 |
| **Tumour containing both germ cell and sex cord–stromal elements** | |
| Gonadoblastoma | 9073/1 |
| **Miscellaneous tumours of the testis** | |
| Ovarian epithelial-type tumours | |
| Serous cystadenoma | 8441/0 |
| Serous tumour of borderline malignancy | 8442/1 |
| Serous cystadenocarcinoma | 8441/3 |
| Mucinous cystadenoma | 8470/0 |
| Mucinous borderline tumour | 8472/1 |
| Mucinous cystadenocarcinoma | 8470/3 |
| Endometrioid adenocarcinoma | 8380/3 |
| Clear cell adenocarcinoma | 8310/3 |
| Brenner tumour | 9000/0 |
| Juvenile xanthogranuloma | |
| Haemangioma | 9120/0 |
| **Haematolymphoid tumours** | |
| Diffuse large B-cell lymphoma | 9680/3 |
| Follicular lymphoma, NOS | 9690/3 |
| Extranodal NK/T-cell lymphoma, nasal-type | 9719/3 |
| Plasmacytoma | 9734/3 |
| Myeloid sarcoma | 9930/3 |
| Rosai–Dorfman disease | |
| **Tumours of collecting duct and rete testis** | |
| Adenoma | 8140/0 |
| Adenocarcinoma | 8140/3 |

The morphology codes are from the International Classification of Diseases for Oncology (ICD-O) {917A}. Behaviour is coded /0 for benign tumours; /1 for unspecified, borderline, or uncertain behaviour; /2 for carcinoma in situ and grade III intraepithelial neoplasia; and /3 for malignant tumours. The classification is modified from the previous WHO classification (756A), taking into account changes in our understanding of these lesions.
*New code approved by the IARC/WHO Committee for ICD-O.

**Fig. 24.1** WHO classification image[12]

GCTs derived from GCNIS.
GCTs unrelated to GCNIS.
Sex cord-stromal tumors (SCSTs).
Miscellaneous tumors of the testis.
Hemato-lymphoid tumors.
Tumors of collecting duct and rete testis.[11]

### 24.3.2 Tumor Staging

Proper clinical staging, in conjunction with histological assessment and tumor type classification, is key for the determination of management of testicular cancer patients. Staging is based on imaging results of the anatomical extent of disease and tumor marker levels and consists of tumor–node–metastasis-serum tumor marker (TNMS) staging. The T relates to tumor characteristics, N to presence of spread to lymph nodes, and M to presence of metastasis. The additional value of S is based on post-orchiectomy tumor markers including LDH, AFP, and β-hCG. For patients receiving chemotherapy, these values should be assessed prior to its initiation.

The TNMS classification is then translated to prognostic groups of levels 0, I, II, and III, with further subdivisions. Stage 0 is for patients with GCNIS, stage I patients have a tumor limited to the testis area, Stage II patients have regional spread to the lymph nodes, and stage III patients have distant metastases.

Patients with metastatic testicular cancer may be further classified into an International Germ Cell Cancer Collaborative Group (IGCCCG) risk group. This classification uses histology, location of primary tumor and metastases, and pre-chemotherapy tumor markers levels to categorize patients into different prognoses: good, intermediate, or poor risk. 5-year survival rates published by the IGCCCG are 91% for good-risk, 79% for intermediate-risk, and 48% for poor-risk.[13] Admittedly this data is from over two decades ago, and current statistics from more recently treated patients indicate some increased survival rates since publication of the IGCCCG statistics.

## 24.4 Treatment

Each case of testicular cancer should be overseen by a multidisciplinary team that includes the patient and his preferences in the discussion. The treatment plan must be determined in a shared decision-making process, as different treatment options often have comparable outcomes but also have variable side effects and toxicities, mandating the patient's role in treatment selection.

Treatment guidelines in this section will focus on GCTs, with treatment beyond orchiectomy for SCSTs and other testicular tumors outlined in their respective sections further on in this chapter.

## 24.4.1 *Treatment Modalities*

The primary treatment for a testicular mass with suspected cancer is radical inguinal orchiectomy, with spermatic cord division at the internal inguinal ring to prevent a potential malignant spread to the retroperitoneal lymph nodes. Adjuvant post-orchiectomy therapies include RPLND, radiation therapy, and chemotherapy. Patients with residual disease after the treatment course may be further treated with salvage chemotherapy, consisting of paclitaxel, ifosfamide, and cisplatin (TIP), or vinblastine, ifosfamide, and cisplatin (VIP).

Prior to treatment, all patients undergoing an orchiectomy should be educated on the risks of infertility and the option of sperm cryopreservation prior to treatment. A pre-treatment fertility assessment may be considered, as at time of diagnosis nearly one-quarter of testicular cancer patients are azoospermic and nearly half are oligozoospermic. Patients should also be counseled on the risk of decreased androgen levels and the possibility of testosterone replacement therapy. Finally, patients must be informed regarding the option of testicular prosthesis for aesthetic appearance.

Testis-sparing surgery, or partial orchiectomy, may be desired for preservation of fertility and hormonal function. Currently there is limited data on the reliability of testicular enucleation as a cure for testicular cancer. As it carries a higher risk of local recurrence, it is not recommended in cases of suspected testicular malignancy with a normal contralateral testis. Testis-sparing surgery through an inguinal incision may be considered for patients with masses <2 cm in the following cases: inconclusive physical exam or US findings and negative tumor markers, solitary testis, or bilateral synchronous tumors. If testis-sparing surgery is performed, an intraoperative frozen section must also be completed for histological analysis. Complications following enucleation include testicular atrophy and patients should be counseled on this possibility along with the option of testosterone replacement therapy.

RPLND is a complex surgery which involves removal of retroperitoneal lymph nodes while attempting to preserve the nearby organs, vessels, and ejaculatory nerves to the greatest extent possible. This procedure should only be performed as a treatment, and not simply as a tool to better determine the disease stage. Recent nerve-sparing approaches to RPLND have reduced risk of retrograde ejaculation caused by nerve damage during the surgery, with more than 90% of patients maintaining anterograde ejaculation. The preservation of ejaculation via these nerve-sparing surgical techniques can also help conserve fertility. RPLND is rarely performed in children, mainly due to a much higher complication rate including postoperative bowel obstruction and wound infection in the pediatric population. Chemotherapy and radiation therapy are associated with an increased risk of cardiovascular disease and secondary non-germ cell neoplasms in testicular cancer survivors. Therefore, survivors should be followed by a primary care provider to be monitored for modifiable cardiovascular disease risk factors and receive appropriate cancer screenings.

### *24.4.2   GCNIS*

As GCNIS has a high risk of progression to a GCT, treatment options for GCNIS include close surveillance with ultrasonography, orchiectomy, or radiotherapy, and are often dependent on patient values. Surveillance may be considered in patients who prioritize maintaining their fertility and androgen production. Patients who prioritize cancer risk reduction should be offered orchiectomy or radiation. Orchiectomy removes the risk of testicular cancer. Low-dose radiation has very low rates of GCNIS on follow-up biopsy, although it is important to keep in mind that radioactive scatter to the other testis (which can be minimized via scrotal shielding) can cause decreased fertility or require testosterone replacement therapy. Chemotherapy has not been shown to be an effective treatment in GCNIS.

### *24.4.3   Stage I GCTs*

Once radical inguinal orchiectomy is performed for testicular cancer, management options are dependent on staging of the disease. Patients with stage I seminoma fall into two categories: those at high risk for relapse who have 2 risk factors (tumor size >4 cm and rete testis invasion), and those at lower risk with 0–1 risk factor. Patients with both risk factors have a 32% chance of relapse, while patients without both risk factors have a 6% risk of relapse.[14] Current recommendations are for the patients at high risk to receive adjuvant chemotherapy treatment with carboplatin, while patients at low risk should be monitored long-term with serial CT scans. Low risk patients who do not want to be surveillanced may be offered primary retroperitoneal and ipsilateral pelvic radiotherapy, a treatment which has a 1% risk of relapse but can cause long-term sequelae such as secondary cancers.[15] In addition, although the rate of relapse is low, it is still higher than the relapse risk in patients treated with chemotherapy for stage II seminoma.

Patients with a stage I nonseminomatous germ cell tumor (NSGCT) may be further classified into NSGCT stage IA or IB. 80–90% of men with NSGCT stage IA are completely cured after orchiectomy and are therefore typically followed with surveillance.[16] Patients who do not want to be surveillanced and want to have a decreased risk of relapse or those who are not good candidates for surveillance should be offered either RPLND or chemotherapy with BEP as an effective supplement to the orchiectomy. As there is a much higher risk of relapse for stage IB NSGCTs (~50%) as compared to stage IA, patients should be offered surveillance, RPLND, or BEP chemotherapy post-orchiectomy, with the final treatment modality determined via shared decision-making.[17]

### 24.4.4  Metastatic Disease: Stages IIA/B GCTs

Standard treatment for patients with stage IIA seminoma is radiotherapy, with an approximately 100% recurrence-free survival rate.[18] However, chemotherapy with bleomycin, etoposide, and cisplatin (BEP) or with etoposide and cisplatin (EP) has been shown to be equally effective. Stage IIB seminoma patients should be offered treatment with BEP or EP, as chemotherapy has a decreased relapse rate and fewer long-term side effects than in comparison to radiotherapy and is therefore recommended. Seminomas stage IIC or higher are treated with primary chemotherapy, applying the same standards used in NSGCTs.

Although RPLND is typically reserved for non-seminomatous tumors rather than for seminomas, initial research on its implementation as a primary treatment for testicular seminomas in stages I and II has shown high surgical cure rates comparable to chemotherapy or radiotherapy, while also bypassing any toxicities associated with adjuvant chemotherapy, radiotherapy, or multiple high-dose radiation CTs in younger men.

Overall, Stage II A/B NSGCTs with normal serum tumor markers may be treated by either chemotherapy or RPLND with comparable oncological outcomes. Stage IIA treatment with either chemotherapy or RPLND has a good prognosis. However, chemotherapy in stage IIB is the preferred initial treatment modality, as if the tumor is found to include any non-postpubertal teratoma GCT it will necessitate chemotherapy due to a higher risk of relapse with only RPLND. Additionally, any stage IIA/B NSGCT without elevated serum markers necessitates histological rule out of embryonal carcinoma via RPLND or biopsy.

NSGCTs in stages IIA/B with elevated tumor markers are classified in the good or intermediate IGCCCG prognosis groups and are treated with BEP, as high-relapse rates have been noted after primary RPLND. Salvage resection is recommended for residual lesions following chemotherapy.

### 24.4.5  Metastatic Disease: Stages IIC and III GCTs

Management in advanced GCTs does not differ much between seminomatous and nonseminomastous tumors and is more dependent on the IGCCCG risk stratification. Treatment in the good-risk group is BEP or EP, intermediate-risk is BEP, and poor-risk is BEP.

Nonseminomatous tumors in the good-risk group have shown inferior treatment results with EP as compared to BEP. However, this is not true for seminomatous tumors. Therefore, patients with NSGCTs in the good-risk group should only be administered EP when they have contraindications to bleomycin. Patients with seminomatous tumors in the intermediate-risk group who have bleomycin contraindications may be offered cisplatin, etoposide, and ifosfamide (PEI).

Reassessing serum tumor marker levels after the first cycle of chemotherapy is mandatory. Recent clinical research has demonstrated that a more aggressive treatment may be indicated for patients with poor-risk NSGCTs who do not have a decrease in tumor markers following the first BEP treatment. Dose-intensified chemotherapy has been shown to improve progression free survival but not overall survival rates. Therefore, patients in this category may be switched to dose-dense chemotherapy if their serum tumor markers are not sufficiently decreased after their first BEP treatment.

### 24.4.6 Postpubertal Versus Prepubertal

The new WHO classification further categorizes teratomas and yolk sac tumors into prepubertal- and postpubertal-types. This is largely due to the more aggressive behavior present in the postpubertal types, impacting their management.

Prepubertal teratomas do not metastasize. Therefore, orchiectomy, and in the case of small tumors a partial orchiectomy, is the only indicated treatment. Similarly, epidermoid cysts are treated with testis-sparing surgery. Post-treatment, prepubertal teratomas do not require further follow-up for radiographic assessment for recurrence. This sharply contrasts with postpubertal teratomas, which are more malignant and have lower survival rates. These tumors require the typical management in adult patients with NSGCTs. Metastases are resistant to chemotherapy and radiotherapy, leaving surgical removal as the only available option. It should also be noted that teratoma with somatic type malignancy can further worsen the prognosis in the event of its metastatic spread.

Correspondingly, prepubertal-type yolk sac tumors display more benign behavior than their postpubertal-type counterparts. Following tumor resection, patients are simply surveillanced, with chemotherapy only performed in the event of tumor recurrence. RPLND is no longer performed for prepubertal yolk sac tumors as it does not address the usual route of hematological spread in children and because the complication rate of RPLND in children is much greater than in adults. Postpubertal yolk sac tumors require the typical management in adult patients with NSGCTs.

### 24.4.7 COVID-19

At the time of this chapter publication, the coronavirus disease 2019 (COVID-19) global pandemic continues to affect hospital systems, leading to decreased available resources and delays in urological cancer treatment. Regarding testicular cancer, current recommendations are in agreement that it should be immediately treated as indicated and without delay.

## 24.5 Germ Cell Tumors Derived from GCNIS

This classification includes GCNIS and seminoma, along with NSGCTs such as embryonal carcinoma, postpubertal-type yolk sac tumor, trophoblastic tumor (especially choriocarcinoma), postpubertal type teratoma, teratoma with somatic-type malignancy, and mixed GCT. Regressed GCTs are also included in this category. GCNIS derived tumors form a homogenous group with comparable epidemiologic backgrounds, despite some differences in morphology and behavior. Their pathogenesis is typically due to testicular dysgenesis, which can be characterized by weakened spermatogenesis and immature Sertoli cells. Most of these GCTs also have an extra copy of the short arm of chromosome 12 in the form of an isochromosome 12p. Additionally, all GCTs originating from GCNIS can present with elevated β-hCG tumor marker levels.

GCNIS derived tumors are more typically found in the adult population and exhibit a tendency for invasion and spread to the contralateral testis in up to 8% of affected patients.[19] It should be noted that while NSGCTs often present in their pure form in children, adult NSGCTs are more likely to appear as mixed GCTs and contain two or more different histological GCT components.

### 24.5.1 Germ Cell Neoplasia in Situ

GCNIS is found in the seminiferous tubules of about 0.4–0.8% of healthy men, and microscopically appears as atypical germ cells with narrowed seminiferous tubules.[20] Within 7 years, up to 90% of GCNIS evolves into malignant GCTs and infiltrates the seminiferous tubule wall.[21]

As testicular cancer survivors have an increased risk for cancer development in the contralateral testis, there is some geographical disagreement over contralateral testis management in patients with GCTs. American urologists are less keen to biopsy the contralateral testis, as GCTs are only bilateral in 3% of cases and are not difficult to cure.[22] However, urologists in Europe are more inclined to biopsy due to the high probability of GCNIS becoming invasive.

### 24.5.2 Seminoma

Pure seminomas make up nearly 50% of all testicular GCTs, and rarely invade paratesticular tissue.[23]These tumors typically occur in adults and rarely in adolescents, with an age of presentation 10 years older than in other GCTs. Seminomas are comprised of large cells with clear cytoplasm and central nuclei with prominent nucleoli, often forming lobules composed of several cells separated by fibrinous septae. The majority of these tumors show lymphoid infiltration, with some developing noncaseating granulomas. Macroscopically, they appear as a homogenous well-circumscribed mass with no large hemorrhagic or necrotic areas. Increased tumor marker levels are rare in seminoma cases, although approximately 15% of seminomas exhibit β-hCG overexpression.[24]

Overall, prognosis for seminomas is highly favorable, with a survival rate of >95% after treatment.[25] The main indications for an unfavorable prognosis in seminoma cases include a tumor diameter >4 cm and invasion of the rete testis, with risk of tumor relapse found to be proportional to size of tumor diameter.

Treatment for seminomas is often different than for non-seminomas. Additionally, seminomas have a far more favorable prognosis than do NSGCTs. It is therefore important to carefully distinguish between these two tumor types for the development of an appropriate management plan. Aside from histological analysis, MR imaging can be used to help distinguish seminomatous tumors from their nonseminomatous counterparts. Seminomatous GCTs present on MRI as homogenously T2 hypointense and T1 isointense masses, along with internal T2 hypointense bands (which are more enhanced than the tumor). Unlike seminomas, non-seminomatous GCTs appear as T1 and T2 heterogeneous masses on MRI. Sometimes they can also present with a T2 hypointense fibrous pseudocapsule. Additionally, high AFP levels in a suspected pure seminoma indicates that the tumor is actually a mixed GCT containing nonseminomatous components, as AFP is never elevated in pure seminomas.

### 24.5.3 Embryonal Carcinoma

Embryonal carcinoma is a highly aggressive tumor composed of immature primitive cells with early hematogenous spread. Its growth patterns are varied and can be solid, glandular, tubular, or papillary. Microscopically, the undifferentiated polymorphous tumor cells have scant cytoplasm and overlapping nuclei, with abundant mitotes. Macroscopically, the tumor appears with focal areas of hemorrhage and necrosis. AFP or β-hCG may be elevated. Embryonal carcinomas often extend into the extratesticular space, distorting the testicle contour in 25% of cases.[26] At presentation, 40% of patients have spread to the regional retroperitoneal lymph nodes and 20% have distant metastases.[27] Although embryonal carcinoma is extremely aggressive, it can be cured with chemotherapy treatments (Fig. 24.2).

### 24.5.4 Yolk Sac Tumor: Postpubertal-Type

The pure form of yolk sac tumor nearly always occurs in children, but in rare instances can present in its postpubertal-type form, which is differentiated from the prepubertal type due to the postpubertal type's more malignant nature, despite no apparent differences in morphology. On a macroscopic level, yolk sac tumors have

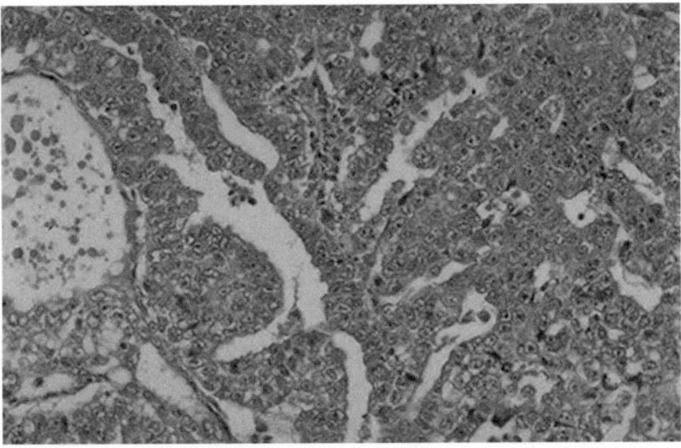

**Fig. 24.2** Embryonal carcinoma, microscopic appearance. The author

a grayish nodular surface with areas of hemorrhage and necrosis. Histologically, these tumors can exhibit a wide diversity of cell patterns that rarely present as a single pattern, often appearing with a microcystic (reticular) or solid pattern, and sometimes with papillary, myxoid, or hepatoid patterns, in addition to the cytoplasmic inclusions of hyaline bodies. Characteristic Schiller-Duval bodies containing glomerulus-like perivascular structures are not frequently encountered.

In adult patients, misdiagnosis of a postpubertal yolk sac tumor with another NSGCT is not important as therapy is the same. However, as yolk sac tumor can appear with a solid pattern with cells of clear cytoplasm, they can be mistaken for seminoma and care should be taken to determine whether rule out of yolk sac tumor is appropriate. Although AFP markers are typically positive in yolk sac tumors, diagnosis should be based on histological characteristics and not on AFP levels.

### 24.5.5 Choriocarcinoma (Trophoblastic Tumor)

Choriocarcinoma embodies a classic example of trophoblastic tumors and represents the testicular cancer subtype with the highest mortality. In its pure form, it is the least frequently occurring GCT (0.3%).[28] Morphologically, choriocarcinomas appear as small tumors with hemorrhagic nodules comprised of a mix of cytotrophoblastic clear cells and syncytiotrophoblastic giant cells, the latter of which can directly invade local blood vessels. β-hCG levels are characteristically elevated and 10% of patient present with gynecomastia.[29]

Choriocarcinoma is a highly malignant tumor with a predilection for early invasion of the vasculature and spread via hematogenous routes, particularly to the lungs, brain, or gastrointestinal tract. At presentation, it typically appears as a metastasis and not as a testicular tumor. Patients with high levels of β-hCG should have brain imaging in addition to their basic workup to detect possible brain metastases.

### 24.5.6 Teratoma: Postpubertal-Type and with Somatic-Type Malignancy

All teratoma types are composed of immature and mature fetal tissue derived from the three germinal layers ectoderm, mesoderm, and endoderm. Its lesions appear as cysts, fibroses, calcifications, and cartilage. Elevations in AFP levels may or may not be present. These tumors are classified by histological and prognostic differences into three subtypes: prepubertal-type, postpubertal-type, and with somatic-type malignancy.

In its pure form, postpubertal-type teratoma is less common than the prepubertal type and is defined by the presence of GCNIS tissue under microscopy, accompanied by disordered tissue organization and cytological atypia with mitosis. The postpubertal-type is more malignant than the prepubertal-type and can develop retroperitoneal metastases that are histologically comparable to testicular teratomas in up to 37% of cases.[30] The existence of GCNIS in these tumors is considered to be responsible for the high rate of retroperitoneal metastases present at time of diagnosis. GCNIS may also be the cause behind the development of adjoining types of testicular tumors in postpubertal-type teratomas, which would explain their frequent manifestation in mixed GCTs and their low prevalence in their pure forms. It should be noted that teratomas can present in adult patients without GCNIS on histology, in which case they are diagnosed as prepubertal-type teratomas.

Teratomas with somatic-type malignancy are defined by a significant histological overgrowth of carcinomatous or sarcomatous components in teratomas. If the somatic-type malignancy does not metastasize, the overall teratoma prognosis generally remains unaffected. However, if the malignancy spreads beyond the testis, the prognosis becomes quite poor.

### 24.5.7 Mixed Germ Cell Tumor

Mixed GCTs are classified as NSGCT tumors with two or more histological germ cell types. This classification constitutes 30–54% of all GCTs[31] and about 70% of all NSGCTs.[32] Age of presentation is variable and follows the predominant tumor type. The most frequent component present is embryonal carcinoma (80%).[33]

Prognosis is largely based on the most invasive tumor type and its percentage, as invasion of lymph or blood vessels is the most accurate predictor of metastases or relapse. A large embryonal carcinoma component present in a mixed GCT carries a more negative prognosis, as does a choriocarcinoma component of greater than 5% of the tumor.

A seminomatous component is not uncommonly found in mixed GCT cases. As discussed earlier, it is critical for appropriate treatment purposes to rule out non-seminomatous components in seminomatous tumors by extensive sampling.

## 24.5.8  *Regressed Germ Cell Tumor*

Regressed GCTs, also known as burned-out GCTs, represent tumors with a high metabolism that have outgrown their blood supply and regressed. These masses are typically only discovered during a search in the testes for a primary source of already discovered retroperitoneal GCTs. The testicular primary tumor is thought to "burn out" after it metastasizes, so that only its retroperitoneal metastases are left behind. A small testicular scar or calcification is an indicator of a burned-out GCT, which might be detected by US, biopsy, or surgical exploration in some cases. Often, the parenchyma surrounding the regressed GCT is atrophic and can also contain GCNIS.

## 24.6  GCTs not Derived from GCNIS

The classification of non-GCNIS derived GCTs is a less homogenous group than that of GCNIS derived GCTs, but tumors in this group are brought together due to their lack of the following qualities: GCNIS derivation, 12p chromosome amplification, and testicular dysgenesis. Included in this classification are spermatocytic tumors, prepubertal-type teratomas, prepubertal-type yolk sac tumors, and prepubertal-type mixed teratoma and yolk sac tumors. Non-GCNIS derived tumors are more often found in the pediatric population as compared to their GCNIS derived counterparts. Additionally, they are also more inert and less likely to metastasize.

## 24.6.1  *Spermatocytic Tumor*

Spermatocytic tumor, originating from spermatogonia, represents a highly curable non-GCNIS derived subtype. Although spermatocytic tumors typically have an older age of presentation than GCNIS derived GCTs, they are included in the same classification as prepubertal teratomas and yolk sac tumors due to the shared characteristics described above.

This rare tumor has a rather specific macroscopic appearance, presenting as a large, well-delineated grayish-white tumor with a soft consistency, without hemorrhagic or necrotic areas. It contains three cell types: small cells resembling lymphocytes, medium sized cells, and giant cells with a high mitotic index. Serum tumor markers in spermatocytic tumors are negative.

Pure spermatocytic tumors nearly exclusively appear in the testicle and exhibit benign behavior in the majority of cases. Therefore, these tumors do not require therapy post-orchiectomy. Metastasizing spermatocytic tumors are incredibly rare and are resistant to chemotherapy treatment.

Previously termed spermatocyctic seminoma, this tumor can be easily misdiagnosed due to its rarity and sometimes similar microscopic appearance to other testicular tumors. It should be noted that spermatocytic tumors have a similar appearance to seminomatous tumors on imaging as hypoechoic heterogenous lesions and are therefore difficult to distinguish apart from each other.

### 24.6.2 Teratoma: Prepubertal-Type

Prepubertal-type teratomas account for up to 20% of pediatric GCTs and are most common in children under 2 years of age. [34]Teratomas have both a different histogenesis and prognosis in pediatric patients in comparison to postpubertal patients. Although they present with a similar cystic macroscopic appearance also found in postpubertal-type teratomas, prepubertal teratomas show a very different microscopic appearance with an organoid distribution, resembling normal anatomical arrangement. They do not exhibit atypical cytology, high mitotic index, or most importantly presence of GCNIS. Prepubertal-type teratomas also have a normal serum AFP.

Additionally, in contrast to the postpubertal-type teratoma, the prepubertal-type is considered universally benign in children and does not metastasize. Therefore, although teratomas prior to puberty are not associated with GCNIS and have an excellent prognosis, postpubertal teratomas are considered malignant and therefore a diagnosis of postpubertal-type should be under consideration in older children and pubertal patients.

Incorporated into the prepubertal-type teratoma classification are more specialized forms including epidermoid cyst, dermoid cyst, and carcinoid tumor. Epidermoid cysts consisting of lamellar keratin are the most common of these specialized forms, accounting for 1% of all intrascrotal tumors.[35] These tumors may arise at any age but are classified as prepubertal teratomas even when presenting in adults, as they are considered benign. Epidermoid cysts are easily visualized on testicular ultrasonography as well-defined, encapsulated lesions with a characteristic "onion skin" appearance consisting of alternating concentric rings of hypo and hyperechogenicity, the latter representing the keratinized deposits.

### 24.6.3 Yolk Sac Tumor: Prepubertal-Type

Although pure prepubertal-type yolk sac tumors are rare in adults, they are the most common testicular tumor in children, comprising 70%[36] of all prepubertal GCTs, and with a median age of presentation at 19 months. The macro- and microscopic appearances of yolk sac tumors are identical in children and adults, with both populations exhibiting increased AFP levels. However, its age-based prognosis is what differentiates yolk sac tumors into prepubertal- and postpubertal-types, with resultant differences in management due to the more benign nature of the prepubertal-type. At diagnosis, 85% of prepubertal yolk sac tumors present as stage I, while the same is true for only 35% of postpubertal yolk sac tumors.[37] Overall, prognosis in children with yolk sac tumors is much better than in their adult counterparts.

## 24.7 Non-Germ Cell Tumors: Sex Cord-Stromal Tumors

This testicular tumor classification of sex cord-stromal tumors includes Leydig cell tumors, Sertoli cell tumors, and granulosa cell tumors, as well as other miscellaneous lesions. Also included in this category are gonadoblastomas, which are tumors containing elements of both GCTs and SCSTs. SCSTs are usually benign and are more frequent in the pediatric population, accounting for over 30% of all testicular tumors, while in adults they only make up 3–6% of testicular cancers (which is likely related to the high prevalence of GCTs in the adult population).[38]

About 10% of SCSTs are metastatic, typically in affected adults.[39] Metastatic behavior can be difficult to predict, as even SCSTs with bland histological features have shown the ability to seemingly metastasize without warning signs. Additionally, since confirmatory evidence of malignancy requires the presence of metastasis, prognosis based on the tumor's histological aspects can be helpful but should also be treated with caution. However, metastatic tumors have been shown to demonstrate a similar set of features including large size ($\geq 5$ cm), nuclear atypia, high mitotic index, necrosis and hemorrhage, infiltration of margins with extension into paratesticular tissue, and vascular invasion.

As mentioned earlier in this chapter, US is an important and helpful tool for distinguishing testicular cancer from more benign causes of a scrotal mass, such as hydrocele. Since US findings for GCTs and SCSTs may be similar, histological assessment should be used to differentiate between these two classifications. However, MRI has recently been shown as a superior imaging method to US with greater sensitivity for SCSTs, especially for Leydig cell tumors. It should be noted that testicular SCSTs do not have elevated tumor markers such as LDH, AFP, or β-hCG, and instead may show increased LH, FSH, or testosterone levels.

### 24.7.1 Leydig Cell Tumor

Leydig cell tumors are the most common type of SCST and can present in any age group. Presentation involves the bilateral testes in 3% of cases.[40] Macroscopically, Leydig cell tumors appear as a yellowish-brown homogenous mass, encapsulated within a thin fibrous capsule. Histologically, these tumors present with a wide variety of patterns, including solid, nodular, spindle-shaped, and trabeculae, leading to a wider differential diagnosis. Reinke crystals are characteristic for diagnosis but are only detectable in about 40% of cases.[41]

The differential diagnosis for Leydig cell tumor includes Leydig cell hyperplasia, malakoplakia, and testicular tumor of adrenogenital syndrome (TTAGS). Leydig cell tumors must be distinguished from Leydig cell hyperplasia particular in patients with testicular atrophy, cryptorchidism, or Klinefelter syndrome, as they commonly exhibit hyperplasia of their Leydig cells. Such cases are histologically differentiated from Leydig cell tumors by the microscopic appearance of a nodular and multifocal hyperplastic pattern, as well as atrophic seminiferous tubules entrapped among the hyperplastic nodules, a feature which rules out a cancerous diagnosis. Of note, less than 25% of Leydig cell tumors have associated Leydig cell hyperplasia.[42]

Though it is an extremely rare condition, malakoplakia of the testis should also be considered in the differential for Leydig cell tumor. Its classic macroscopic yellow nodular appearance appears similarly to a testicular tumor. Microscopically, malakoplakia contains large histiocytes with eosinophilic granular cytoplasm and may be mistaken for a Leydig cell tumor. These macrophages contain pathognomonic basophilic inclusions called Michaelis-Gutmann bodies, which are diagnostic of malakoplakia. Parenthetically, although testicular malakoplakia is a benign condition, it is usually treated by orchiectomy to exclude malignancy more definitively (Figs. 24.3 and 24.4).

Finally, the differential diagnosis for a Leydig cell tumor also includes TTAGS, which is another rare benign neoplasm that typically presents in the bilateral testes. Similarly to Leydig cell hyperplasia, it may be diagnosed histologically by visualization of entrapped tubules among the proliferating tumor cells. TTAGS spontaneously regresses with steroid therapy, making it an important diagnosis to rule out in suspected cases of Leydig cell tumor and potentially avoid an unnecessary orchiectomy.

Leydig cell tumors can be functioning or non-functioning, with androgen overproduction from functioning tumors causing precocious puberty, gynecomastia, decreased libido, and infertility. Clinical symptoms are dependent on the

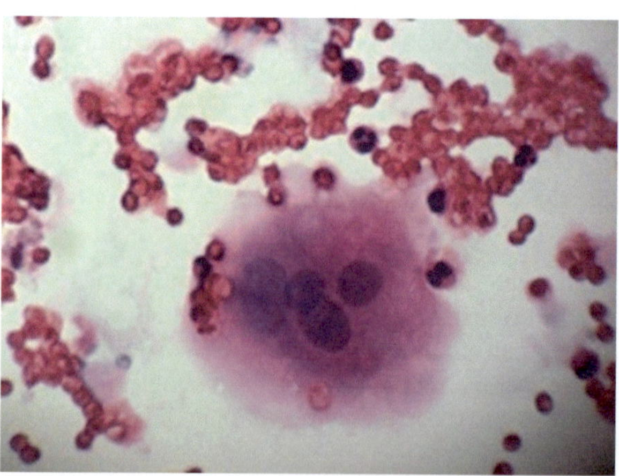

**Fig. 24.3** Malakoplakia, microscopic appearance with Michaelis-Gutmann bodies. From the author M A Fahmy

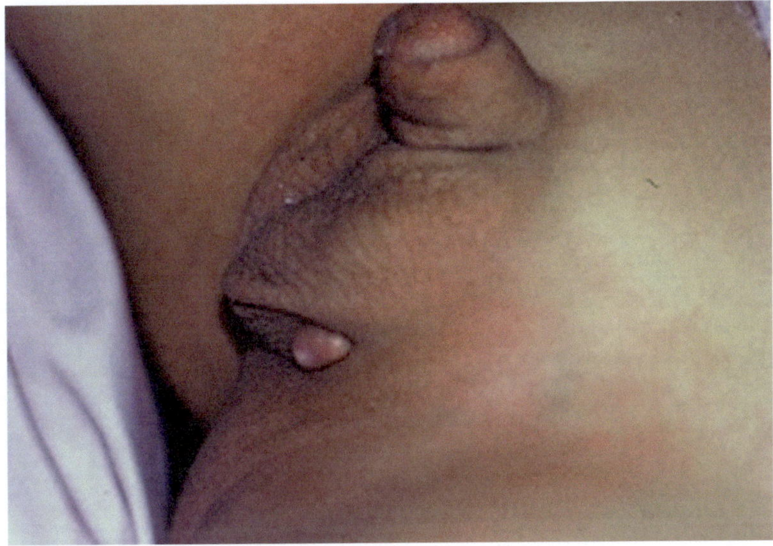

**Fig. 24.4**  Malakoplakia chronic granuloma. From the author M A Fahmy

produced hormone type, which is usually testosterone in the prepubertal population and estrogen in the postpubertal population. Leydig cell tumors are responsible for 10% of all precocious puberty cases in children.[43] Close to 30% of affected adults have gynecomastia or decreased libido.[44] Infertility in patients with these tumors is understood as a secondary manifestation of their abnormally high androgen secretion levels.

About 10% of Leydig cell tumors display malignant behavior,[45] with 20% of malignant tumors already metastasized by the time of diagnosis.[46] The most important indicator of malignancy in these tumors is the lesion size, as tumors with a diameter $\geq 5$ cm are nearly always malignant. As Leydig cell tumors are resistant to chemotherapy, the only therapeutic options beyond orchiectomy are RPLND and radiotherapy. The survival rate is low, with the average adult patient not surviving more than 5 years after diagnosis. As malignancy in prepubertal patients with Leydig cell tumors is rare and metastasis does not occur, children may be appropriately treated with only orchiectomy.

### 24.7.2  Sertoli Cell Tumor

Sertoli cell tumors represent about 1% of testicular tumors and can present in any age group.[47] Morphologically, they usually appear as grayish-yellow encapsulated masses. Like Leydig cell tumors, they possess a large heterogeneity of morphological presentations. Most commonly, the cells form a tubular growth pattern with a marked stromal hyalinization.

Special care should be taken to avoid mistaking Sertoli cell nodules for Sertoli cell tumors. Sertoli cell nodules consist of small hypoplastic zones comprised of prepubertal tubules lined by immature Sertoli cells and are a common finding especially in cryptorchid testes. Sertoli cell tumors can also be confused with the tubular variant of seminoma, so the surrounding tubules should be carefully checked for the presence of GCNIS.

Sertoli cell tumors are generally clinically silent, but occasionally patients may present with gynecomastia. About 12% of these tumors display malignant behavior, usually in adult patients.[48] The only treatment option remains orchiectomy and RPLND, as chemotherapy and radiotherapy have not shown to affect Sertoli cell tumors.

### 24.7.3 Granulosa Cell Tumor

Granulosa cell tumors are divided into an adult type and a juvenile type. The adult type can cause gynecomastia in 25% of affected patients and is malignant in 10% of cases.[48] While the adult type is very rare, the juvenile-type granulosa cell tumor is the most common testicular tumor in the perinatal period. The juvenile type is usually encountered prior to 6 months of age and may be diagnosed by prenatal ultrasound. There is an association with cryptorchidism in cases of ambiguous genitalia. Macroscopically, it often appears as a lobulated yellowish masse, often with a cystic component. The characteristic microscopic presentation consists of cysts lined by granulosa-like cells, intermixed with solid tubular structures.

Juvenile-type granulosa cell tumors may be mistaken for prepubertal-type yolk sac tumors, as they both may appear in the first few months after birth and have similar sized cysts on histology. Although yolk sac tumors are associated with high AFP levels, it is considered normal for children less than 6 months old to have elevated AFP levels. Juvenile granulosa cell tumors may be differentiated via a more repetitive morphology, as well as a lack of immunohistochemical AFP expression. A mistaken diagnosis can have severe consequences, as the juvenile-type granulosa cell tumor is completely benign with no reported cases of recurrence or metastases. It therefore may be cured with a simple testis-sparing surgical enucleation rather than an orchiectomy which would be indicated in a yolk sac tumor.

### 24.7.4 Gonadoblastoma

Gonadoblastomas are rare tumors consisting of both germ cells and sex cord-stromal cells. This tumor is unusual in patients younger than 12 years of age, with the great majority of its diagnoses occurring within the first few decades of life. Typical presentation involves the virilization of a phenotypic female upon reaching puberty. Gonadoblastomas arise most commonly in phenotypic females with DSD and rudimentary gonads with a 46-X,Y karyotype. Bilateral testes involvement is not uncommon.

Macroscopically, a gonadoblastoma appears as a yellowish multinodular tumor, with the nodules consisting of two main cell types: large cells representing germ cells, and small cells representing immature Sertoli and granulosa cells. It should be noted that this tumor is visible only with microscopy in a quarter of cases. If this testicular neoplasm is not removed, it can either regress and completely involute or it can progress into a germ cell tumor, most often a pure seminoma. If the germ cells overgrow the gonadal stromal cells, therapy follows the protocol for the specific GCT type of the cells.

## 24.8 Non-Germ Cell Tumors: Miscallaneous

### 24.8.1 Hemato-Lymphoid Tumors

Included in this classification are diffuse large B-cell lymphomas and plasmacytomas. Testicular plasmacytomas are monoclonal proliferations of plasma cells and are extremely rare, with the latest tally counting fewer than 100 reported cases in total.

Although lymphoma makes up a small percentage of all testicular tumors, it is the most common malignant testicular neoplasm in older men. It is also the most frequent neoplasm found in the bilateral testes. Testicular lymphoma rarely presents as a primary malignancy and is often secondary to non-Hodgkin lymphoma B-cell tumors.

Diffuse large B-cell lymphoma of the testis typically affects the entire organ, with replacement of the testicular parenchyma with a nodular and yellow-pink mass, occasionally with areas of hemorrhage and necrosis. The diffuse interstitial infiltration frequently spreads beyond the parenchyma to destroy the epididymis and invade the vasculature. Diffuse large B-cell lymphomas are highly aggressive tumors. Standard therapy is complex, involving orchiectomy with adjuvant chemotherapy and/or radiotherapy. Testicular lymphoma has a poor prognosis with a median survival time of 5 years, largely due to a high risk of relapse after therapy particularly to the central nervous system and contralateral testis. Testicular plasmacytomas exhibit a similar histological pattern, unfortunately with an even more dismal prognosis.

Although the affected patient age for testicular lymphoma is typically over 60 years of age, children may sometimes present with this cancer as well. While the histology is similar, the immunohistochemistry is different. In particular, pediatric testicular lymphomas do not exhibit Bcl2 overexpression or increased p53 expression. Additionally, affected children have an excellent prognosis unlike their adult counterparts.

## 24.8.2  Tumors of Collecting Duct and Rete Testis

This class of tumors is quite rare, with two reported types: adenoma (benign) and adenocarcinoma (malignant). The mortality rate for adenocarcinomas with local spread is more than 50%,[50] with an overall median survival of 1 year.

## 24.8.3  Metastases

Metastases to the testicles typically have different origins in children and adults. Pediatric patients tend to have metastases from leukemias, neuroblastomas, and rhabdomyosarcomas. Testicular metastases in adult patients are rare and are most commonly due to solid primary neoplasms including prostate, lung, and melanoma.

Lymphoma and leukemia are the most common metastatic malignancies in the pediatric testicle, accounting for up to 5% of all pediatric testicular tumors and most of tumors with bilateral presentation.[51] Morphologically, leukemias and lymphomas are difficult to distinguish from each other. Testicular leukemia incidence in children is 10–30%, with the testes acting as the second most common site of extramedullary relapse (after the central nervous system) in acute myelogenous or lymphoblastic leukemia.[52] Treatment does not usually necessitate an orchiectomy, with local control completed through low-dose radiotherapy in the bilateral testes. Since recurrences are found in such a high percentage of cases, previous recommendations have advised testicular biopsies for diagnosis confirmation in boys presenting with a history of leukemia and a painless testicular mass. However, early diagnosis has not been shown to improve what is a generally poor prognosis for these cases due to their associated diseases and is therefore no longer recommended.

## 24.8.4  Scrotal Skin Neoplasms

Primary malignant melanoma of the scrotum is a rare condition. Treatment entails wide local excision which achieves effective local control but does not prevent regional recurrence. As patients who show positive lymph nodes generally die of the melanoma despite surgery and chemotherapy, current recommendations advocate for wide local excision together with prophylactic modified inguinal lymphadenopathy.

As most cutaneous malignant melanomas arise from preexisting nevi, a long-standing scrotal skin lesion with haphazard shape, color and surface characteristics warrants immediate biopsy. Otherwise, a nevus that remains uniform in color, size and surface texture over time should be managed with regular self-examinations and follow-up appointments.

Squamous and basal cell carcinoma may also affect the scrotal skin. Risk factors include industrial exposure, poor hygiene, and chronic irritation. Survival rates are lower in patients with greater cancer progression at the initial diagnosis. Scrotal skin neoplasms may also be metastatic in nature and act as the initial presenting sign of an underlying primary malignancy. The discerning urologist should have a high index of suspicion for both primary and metastatic cancer when evaluating scrotal skin lesions.

## 24.9  Paratesticular Neoplasms

The range of scrotal structures surrounding the testicle can give rise to several varieties of paratesticular neoplasms. These masses are usually found to be benign, although in rare cases malignancy may be present. Benign neoplasms include lipomas, leiomyomas, and adenomatoid tumors. Malignant neoplasms are very rare and include liposarcomas, leiomyosarcomas, and rhabdomyosarcomas. Another form of paratesticular neoplasm is mesothelioma, which can be benign or malignant.

As US of paratesticular neoplasms usually demonstrates a solid mass but cannot differentiate well between benign and malignant tumors, any solid extratesticular mass found on imaging should be biopsied and evaluated.

### 24.9.1  Lipoma, Leiomyoma, and Adenomatoid Tumor

Lipomas are the most common extratesticular non-malignant neoplasm, accounting for about 90% of tumors in this category.[53] Leiomyomas are the second most common neoplasm in this category, usually arising in the epididymis. Treatment for lipomas and leiomyomas just involves their excision, as they do not exhibit recurrence. Adenomatoid tumors also have a predilection for the epididymis and appear on microscopy as tumors comprised of epithelial-like cells containing vacuoles and fibrous stroma. Adenomatoid tumors are managed by surgical excision as well.

### 24.9.2  Liposarcoma, Leiomyosarcoma, and Rhabdomyosarcoma

In adults, liposarcoma is the most frequent paratesticular sarcoma subtype, presenting as a slowly enlarging paratesticular mass. Spermatic cord liposarcomas in the inguinal canal may be mistaken for a hernia. Therefore, CT or MRI can be used to better define a liposarcoma, which appears on imaging as a well-defined mass composed of fat. Despite performance of radical orchiectomy with high ligation of the spermatic cord, liposarcomas are characterized by a high local recurrence rate, rarely with retroperitoneal spread.

Leiomyosarcoma is the second most frequent sarcoma subtype in the paratesticular region. Histological analysis of these tumors is important for determination of prognosis, as paratesticular leiomyosarcomas with low-grade behavior are typically indolent while lesions with high-grade behavior are more aggressive. Interestingly, epididymal leiomyosarcomas are mostly low-grade while leiomyosarcomas in the spermatic cord are more likely to be categorized as high-grade. Leiomyosarcomas have a high recurrence rate with metastases in the retroperitoneal lymph nodes as well as in the lung.

Rhabdomyosarcoma is a pediatric malignancy with a bimodal distribution, mostly affecting 3–4-month-old infants and teenagers. It has a variety of histological subtypes, most commonly the embryonal subtype representing 97% of all paratesticular rhabdomyosarcomas.[54] Rhabdomyosarcoma has nonspecific findings on MRI and cannot be distinguished from other extratesticular neoplasms via imaging. Of note, β-hCG may be produced from rhabdomyosarcoma cells in addition to its main production from syncytiotrophoblasts, so patients with rhabdomyosarcoma may present with elevated β-hCG. It exhibits highly aggressive behavior particularly in affected teenagers, and overall has a retroperitoneal spread incidence rate of 30–40%.[55] Pediatric patients with paratesticular rhabdomyosarcoma have a good 3-year survival rate of 80%.[56]

Sarcomas are initially treated with an orchiectomy with high ligation. It should be noted that patients with sarcomas other than liposarcomas who present with a negative metastatic evaluation after orchiectomy should still undergo a RPLND. Metastases in any sarcoma should be treated with chemotherapy.

### 24.9.3 Mesothelioma

Paratesticular mesothelioma originates from the tunica vaginalis and can present in patients of any age. Mesotheliomas can be benign or malignant, which are differentiated based on histology and behavior. The malignant version of the tumor is considered rare and may be associated with asbestos exposure. Despite orchiectomy treatment, prognosis is often poor.

## 24.10    Rare Scrotal Neoplasms

There are several rare neoplasms that may arise in the scrotum. They are described throughout this chapter, with some subtypes specifically outlined in this section. Evaluation of scrotal swellings should always include rare neoplasms in the differential diagnosis.

Scrotal angiolipomas are very rare neoplasms composed of mature adipose tissue and abnormal vasculature that are usually discovered during physical examination. Angiolipomas are benign lesions with an excellent prognosis that are completely cured via surgical resection.

Scrotal schwannoma is another rare and benign tumor, with fewer than ten recorded cases. Schwannomas are derived from Schwan cells and are typically asymptomatic until they present as painless scrotal swellings due to mass effect. There is no preferred imaging modality for diagnosis, and schwannomas do not exhibit pathognomonic findings on imaging. However, US may be helpful for localization of the lesion, which generally appears as a hypoechoic well-circumscribed mass. Definitive diagnosis is only achieved with histopathological analysis, so surgical resection is the standard approach for both diagnostic and therapeutic purposes, followed by long term follow-up.

Solitary fibrous tumors are an extremely rare neoplasm when presenting in the testicular or paratesticular tissue. Only five such cases have been reported up to date. Differential diagnosis in suspected paratesticular solitary fibrous tumors includes angiomyolipomas, leiomyomas, fibrosarcomas, and gastrointestinal stromal tumors. These tumors are often benign but have some chance of malignancy. Treatment entails surgical resection and long term follow-up, with a definitive diagnosis performed via immunohistochemistry (in particular with nuclear expression of STAT6). Histologically malignant features are associated with a worse prognosis.

Chondroid syringoma of the scrotum is another extremely rare neoplasm, with only eight reported cases in the literature. It is a benign tumor originating from epithelial and mesenchymal cells, most commonly occurring in the head and neck regions. Surgical resection must be performed as with every suspected scrotal neoplasm for treatment and evaluation of its histological features. Accurate diagnosis is dependent on excisional biopsy. Since a few cases of malignant chondroid syringoma have been reported, it is particularly important for affected patients to have regular follow-up and be examined for recurrence.

## 24.11    Fertility

As testicular cancer often appears in males prior to and especially during their prime reproductive years, fertility is a critical issue for many affected patients. Even prior to treatment, the presence of testicular cancer itself reduces sperm quality and quantity, more so than in men with other cancers. Additionally, the hypothalamic-pituitary–gonadal axis in testicular cancer can be dysfunctional, with affected patients more likely to have increased FSH and LH levels with low testosterone levels, a pattern typically associated with subfertile men. Studies have suggested that among GCTs, impact on fertility is more pronounced in the non-seminomatous subtype as compared to the seminomatous subtype.

Treatment with chemotherapy and radiation can have a negative effect on fertility potential, with alkylating agents having the potential for a more serious and permanent effect on spermatogenesis than platinum-based drugs. Negatively affected spermatogenesis is usually regained 1–4 years post-chemotherapy. Damage from radiotherapy is dose dependent, although the use of gonadal shielding during the radiation can reduce the impact. It should be noted that both chemotherapy and radiation therapy have teratogenic properties. Therefore, contraception should be implemented during treatment and continued for 6 months after its completion.

The only currently established option for preservation of fertility in postpubertal men remains sperm cryopreservation, preferably performed prior to initiation of treatment. The sperm can be collected through ejaculation or surgical retrieval, and if needed may be used with assisted reproductive technologies. Fertility preservation methods in prepubertal boys are still experimental but have shown potential for future use of spermatogonial stem cells either for in vitro spermatogenesis or autotransplantation.

Physicians treating testicular cancer patients should provide counseling on the potential impact on fertility along with the option of sperm banking, in particular when planning treatments that may cause permanent infertility. Such a discussion is crucial, as infertility is a potential long-term complication of testicular cancer and can cause a large amount of anxiety and fear in patients who desire to father children. Sperm cryopreservation has also been shown to invigorate young patients undergoing treatment and provide encouragement to them.

Patients should also be advised regarding the health effects in children born to fathers with testicular cancer. Although offspring of men with testicular cancer have a significantly 30% increased risk of congenital malformations, this risk is not further increased for children conceived after chemotherapy or radiotherapy and is therefore unlikely to be due to treatment.[57] This may help reassure patients concerned about the effects of cancer treatment on any of their future children.

## 24.12 Psychosexual Effects

In addition to handling the physical and emotional burden experienced by patients with malignancy, men with testicular cancer struggle also struggle in the sexual realm. The psychological impact of testicular cancer can be worsened by societal notions of masculinity and expectations to father children. These detrimental effects on quality of life often continue after treatment is over and must be addressed by healthcare providers both during and after treatment in the course of the adjustment period back to normal life.

Conditions affecting testicular cancer patients and survivors include fatigue, anxiety, depression, stress, and poor body image, negatively affecting their quality of life. Among younger adult patients, anxiety is more common than depression. Men treated with orechiectomy have reported a more minimal impact on their quality of life than those who also underwent chemotherapy or radiotherapy, in particular patients who suffered from chemotherapy-related side effects including gonadal dysfunction.

Low testosterone levels are not uncommon in testicular cancer, in particular in patients who have received both chemotherapy and radiotherapy. Although patients with normal and abnormal testosterone levels have similar rates of conception (as opposed to a decreased rate in patients with elevated FSH), low testosterone levels are associated with decreased quality of life in the sexual, physical, and social realms. Low testosterone has also been shown to increase cardiac risk factors such as body mass index and blood pressure. Therefore, screening for hormonal dysfunction and testosterone replacement therapy should be regularly performed for testicular cancer patients.

Additionally, testicular prosthesis should be offered for patients undergoing orchiectomy, irrespective of age. These implants are meant to improve self-image and mental health, and patient satisfaction with testicular prosthesis is typically high.

## 24.13 Preventative Measures

### 24.13.1 Disparities

Urologists should keep in mind that although multiple recent advances in treatment have significantly increased survival rates for testicular cancer, disparities in mortality outcomes and access to providers continue to exist. Although causcasian patients have the highest incidence of the disease, black patients are more likely to present at a later stage as compared to their white counterparts and are also nearly twice as likely to die from testicular cancer. Unlike GCTs, SCST's are more equally distributed in patients of different races.

### 24.13.2 Diagnostic Delay

Although testicular cancer is a well-known neoplasm in males, diagnostic delay is a common phenomenon. Contributions to delay in diagnosis may be due to both the patient and the physician. As testicular patients are often young, they may be more hesitant to consult a medical professional due to denial, limited access, or lack of information. Physicians have been found to frequently misdiagnose testicular cancer as a case of hydrocele or epididymitis, as well as focus on metastatic symptoms of the disease and miss the origination from the testis. This delay in diagnosis has serious consequences, including diminished response to treatment and decreased survival rates.

### *24.13.3  Prevention*

Various initiatives should be implemented to help minimize disparities and prevent diagnostic delays in testicular cancer. Improvement in physician and patient education may help achieve an earlier diagnosis and higher survival rates in patients. Healthcare providers, in particular primary care physicians, should be able to recognize signs and symptoms associated with testicular cancer and use their judgement regarding whether a referral is warranted. These signs and symptoms include a scrotal lump or swelling, particularly when combined with recurrent testicular pain. If testicular pain is linked to abdominal pain, groin pain, or raised inflammatory markers, these features also merit a referral. Additionally, as discussed earlier in this chapter, a diagnosis of hydrocele or epidiymo-orchitis should increase clinical suspicion for testicular cancer and prompt an ultrasound examination.

There is a lack of consensus on the subject of regular screenings for testicular cancer. The U.S. Preventive Services Task Force (USPSTF) has assigned it a grade D, recommending against testicular cancer screening in adolescent or adult males whether by the clinician or by the patient. The reasoning behind this statement includes the notion that testicular examination has minimal health benefits which are outweighed by potential harms such as false-positive results, anxiety, and harm from unnecessary tests and procedures. Additional points include a low incidence of testicular cancer and the highly favorable treatment outcomes. Other organizations have disagreed with the USPSTF's assessment to various extents. The American Cancer Society has attested that general agreement among physicians is to include a testicular exam in the general physical exam but does not comment regarding testicular self-examination by patients. The American Urological Association has included testicular self-examinations in its "Men's Health Checklist", a reference for patient care for healthcare providers, however the document also notes the USPSTF's recommendation against these screenings.

Advocates for testicular cancer screening have made their case by arguing that the benefits of testicular examination by clinicians and self-examination by patients outweigh any risks and provide the best care for the patient as an individual. Fear of malpractice due to the USPSTF recommendations has been cited as a deterrent for clinicians to improve patient care. Potential harms of testicular screening can be mitigated by better patient education and management of patient expectations, and early detection and treatment of testicular cancer can help increase the survival rate and give more years of life to patients. Additionally, this procedure has benefits other than cancer detection, as counseling male patients about testicular self-examination may help males feel more secure with their bodies and feel more comfortable seeking help from medical practitioners for health concerns. This is an especially important issue, as society generally discourages males from help-seeking behavior.

## Endnotes


1. Imaging.
2. Imaging.
3. Stephenson AJ, Gilligan TD. Neoplasms of the Testis. In: Wein B, Kavoussi L, Novick A, Partin A, Peters C, editors. Campbell-Walsh urology, 10th ed. Elsevier Saunders; 2012. p. 837–870.
4. Stephenson AJ, Gilligan TD. Neoplasms of the testis. In: Wein B, Kavoussi L, Novick A, Partin A, Peters C, editors. Campbell-Walsh urology, 10th ed. Elsevier Saunders; 2012. p. 837–870.
5. Imaging.
6. Stephenson AJ, Gilligan TD. Neoplasms of the testis. In: Wein B, Kavoussi L, Novick A, Partin A, Peters C, editors. Campbell-Walsh urology, 10th ed. Elsevier Saunders; 2012. p. 837–870.
7. Fosså SD, Chen J, Schonfeld SJ, McGlynn KA, McMaster ML, Gail MH, Travis LB. Risk of contralateral testicular cancer: a population-based study of 29,515 U.S. men. J Natl Cancer Inst. 2005 Jul 20;97(14):1056–66.
8. Imaging.
9. Imaging.
10. Stephenson AJ, Gilligan TD. Neoplasms of the testis. In: Wein B, Kavoussi L, Novick A, Partin A, Peters C, editors. Campbell-Walsh urology, 10th ed. Elsevier Saunders; 2012. p. 837–870.
11. Moch H, Cubilla AL, Humphrey PA, Reuter VE, Ulbright TM. The 2016 WHO classification of tumours of the urinary system and male genital organs-part a: renal, penile, and testicular tumours. Eur Urol. 2016 Jul;70(1):93–105.
12. Moch H, Cubilla AL, Humphrey PA, Reuter VE, Ulbright TM. The 2016 WHO classification of tumours of the urinary system and male genital organs-part a: renal, penile, and testicular tumours. Eur Urol. 2016 Jul;70(1):93–105.
13. International Germ Cell Consensus Classification: a prognostic factor-based staging system for metastatic germ cell cancers. International Germ Cell Cancer Collaborative Group. J Clin Oncol. 1997 Feb;15(2):594–603.
14. Laguna MP, Albers P, Algaba F, et al. EAU guidelines on testicular cancer. In: EAU Guidelines. 2020 Edition. EAU Guidelines Office; 2020. p. 1–60.
15. Tandstad T, Smaaland R, Solberg A, Bremnes RM, Langberg CW, Laurell A, Stierner UK, Ståhl O, Cavallin-Ståhl EK, Klepp OH, Dahl O, Cohn-Cedermark G. Management of seminomatous testicular cancer: a binational prospective population-based study from the Swedish norwegian testicular cancer study group. J Clin Oncol. 2011 Feb 20;29(6):719–25.

16. Stephenson A, Eggener SE, Bass EB, et al. Diagnosis and treatment of early stage testicular cancer: AUA guideline. J Urol. 2019;202:272.
17. Stephenson A, Eggener SE, Bass EB, et al. Diagnosis and treatment of early stage testicular cancer: AUA guideline. J Urol. 2019;202:272.
18. Schmidberger H, Bamberg M, Meisner C, Classen J, Winkler C, Hartmann M, Templin R, Wiegel T, Dornoff W, Ross D, Thiel HJ, Martini C, Haase W. Radiotherapy in stage IIA and IIB testicular seminoma with reduced portals: a prospective multicenter study. Int J Radiat Oncol Biol Phys. 1997 Sep 1;39 (2):321–6.
19. Imaging.
20. Mikuz G, Colecchia M. Tumors of the testis. In: Colecchia M, editor. Pathology of testicular and penile neoplasms. Springer; 2016. p. 97–158.
21. Mikuz G, Colecchia M. Tumors of the testis. In: Colecchia M, editor. Pathology of testicular and penile neoplasms. Springer; 2016. p. 97–158.
22. Mikuz G, Colecchia M. Tumors of the testis. In: Colecchia M, editor. Pathology of testicular and penile neoplasms. Springer; 2016. p. 97–158.
23. Imaging.
24. Gaddam SJ, Chesnut G. Testicle cancer. In: StatPearls. StatPearls Publishing; 2020.
25. Algaba F, Sesterhenn IA. Histological classification and pathology of testicular tumors. In: Laguna MP, Albers P, Bokemeyer C, Richie JP, editors. Cancer of the testis. Springer London; 2011. p. 3–26.
26. Imaging.
27. Mikuz G, Colecchia M. Tumors of the testis. In: Colecchia M, editor. Pathology of testicular and penile neoplasms. Springer; 2016. p. 97–158.
28. Nistal M, González-Peramato P. Germ cell tumors derived from germ cell Neoplasia In Situ. In: Nistal M, González-Peramato P, editors. Atlas of peculiar and common testicular and paratesticular tumors. Springer; 2020. p. 1–110.
29. Algaba F, Sesterhenn IA. Histological classification and pathology of testicular tumors. In: Laguna MP, Albers P, Bokemeyer C, Richie JP, editors. Cancer of the testis. Springer London; 2011. p. 3–26.
30. Nistal M, González-Peramato P. Germ cell tumors derived from germ cell Neoplasia In Situ. In: Nistal M, González-Peramato P, editors. Atlas of peculiar and common testicular and paratesticular tumors. Springer; 2020. p. 1–110.
31. Mikuz G, Colecchia M. Tumors of the testis. In: Colecchia M, editor. Pathology of testicular and penile neoplasms. Springer; 2016. p. 97–158.
32. Nistal M, González-Peramato P. Germ cell tumors Dderived from germ cell Neoplasia In Situ. In: Nistal M, González-Peramato P, editors. Atlas of Peculiar and Common Testicular and Paratesticular Tumors. Springer; 2020. p. 1–110.
33. Mikuz G, Colecchia M. Tumors of the testis. In: Colecchia M, editor. Pathology of testicular and penile neoplasms. Springer; 2016. p. 97–158.
34. Mikuz G, Colecchia M. Tumors of the testis. In: Colecchia M, editor. Pathology of testicular and penile neoplasms. Springer; 2016. p. 97–158.

35. Mikuz G, Colecchia M. Tumors of the testis. In: Colecchia M, editor. Pathology of testicular and penile neoplasms. Springer; 2016. p. 97–158.
36. Agarwal PK, Palmer JS. Testicular and paratesticular neoplasms in prepubertal males. J Urol. 2006 Sep;176(3):875–81.
37. Agarwal PK, Palmer JS. Testicular and paratesticular neoplasms in prepubertal males. J Urol. 2006 Sep;176(3):875–81.
38. Mikuz G, Colecchia M. Tumors of the testis. In: Colecchia M, editor. Pathology of testicular and penile neoplasms. Springer; 2016. p. 97–158.
39. Mikuz G, Colecchia M. Tumors of the testis. In: Colecchia M, editor. Pathology of testicular and penile neoplasms. Springer; 2016. p. 97–158.
40. Mikuz G, Colecchia M. Tumors of the testis. In: Colecchia M, editor. Pathology of testicular and penile neoplasms. Springer; 2016. p. 97–158.
41. Algaba F, Sesterhenn IA. Histological classification and pathology of testicular tumors. In: Laguna MP, Albers P, Bokemeyer C, Richie JP, editors. Cancer of the testis. Springer London; 2011. p. 3–26.
42. Nistal M, González-Peramato P. Sex Cord-Stromal Tumors. In: Nistal M, González-Peramato P, editors. Atlas of Peculiar and Common Testicular and Paratesticular Tumors. Springer; 2020. p. 145–220.
43. Nistal M, González-Peramato P. Sex Cord-Stromal Tumors. In: Nistal M, González-Peramato P, editors. Atlas of Peculiar and Common Testicular and Paratesticular Tumors. Springer; 2020. p. 145–220.
44. Algaba F, Sesterhenn IA. Histological Classification and Pathology of Testicular Tumors. In: Laguna MP, Albers P, Bokemeyer C, Richie JP, editors. Cancer of the testis. Springer London; 2011. p. 3–26.
45. Algaba F, Sesterhenn IA. Histological Classification and Pathology of Testicular Tumors. In: Laguna MP, Albers P, Bokemeyer C, Richie JP, editors. Cancer of the testis. Springer London; 2011. p. 3–26.
46. Mikuz G, Colecchia M. Tumors of the Testis. In: Colecchia M, editor. Pathology of testicular and penile neoplasms. Springer; 2016. p. 97–158.
47. Algaba F, Sesterhenn IA. Histological Classification and Pathology of Testicular Tumors. In: Laguna MP, Albers P, Bokemeyer C, Richie JP, editors. Cancer of the testis. Springer London; 2011. p. 3–26.
48. Mikuz G, Colecchia M. Tumors of the Testis. In: Colecchia M, editor. Pathology of testicular and penile neoplasms. Springer; 2016. p. 97–158.
49. Mikuz G, Colecchia M. Tumors of the Testis. In: Colecchia M, editor. Pathology of testicular and penile neoplasms. Springer; 2016. p. 97–158.
50. Albrecht W, Stein JP. Primary Non-Germ Cell Tumors of the Testis. In: Laguna MP, Albers P, Bokemeyer C, Richie JP, editors. Cancer of the testis. Springer London; 2011. p.329–334.
51. Agarwal PK, Palmer JS. Testicular and paratesticular neoplasms in prepubertal males. J Urol. 2006 Sep;176(3):875–81.
52. Agarwal PK, Palmer JS. Testicular and paratesticular neoplasms in prepubertal males. J Urol. 2006 Sep;176(3):875–81.

53. Franchi A, Santi R, Nesi G. Paratesticular Soft Tissue Neoplasms. In: Colecchia M, editor. Pathology of testicular and penile neoplasms. Springer; 2016. p. 191–202.
54. Agarwal PK, Palmer JS. Testicular and paratesticular neoplasms in prepubertal males. J Urol. 2006 Sep;176(3):875–81.
55. Agarwal PK, Palmer JS. Testicular and paratesticular neoplasms in prepubertal males. J Urol. 2006 Sep;176(3):875–81.
56. Agarwal PK, Palmer JS. Testicular and paratesticular neoplasms in prepubertal males. J Urol. 2006 Sep;176(3):875–81.
57. Al-Jebari Y, Glimelius I, Berglund Nord C, Cohn-Cedermark G, Ståhl O, Tandstad T, et al. Cancer therapy and risk of congenital malformations in children fathered by men treated for testicular germ-cell cancer: A nationwide register study. PLoS Med. 2019 Jun;16(6):e1–14.

## Suggested Further Reading

1. Acar C, Gurocak S, Sozen S. Current treatment of testicular sex cord-stromal tumors: critical review. Urology. 2009;73(6):1165–71.
2. Alexis O, Adeleye AO, Worsley AJ. Men's experiences of surviving testicular cancer: an integrated literature review. J Cancer Surviv. 2020;14(3):284–93.
3. Alrehaili M, Tashkandi E. Testicular mixed germ cell tumor combined with malignant transformation to chondrosarcoma: a very rare and aggressive disease. Am J Case Rep. 2020;21:e922933-1–e922933-5.
4. Alsunbul A, Alenezi M, Alsuhaibani S, AlAli H, Al-Zaid T, Alhathal N. Intra-scrotal extra-testicular schwannoma: a case report and literature review. Urol Case Rep. 2020;32:101205.
5. Aoun F, Slaoui A, Naoum E, Hassan T, Albisinni S, Azzo JM, et al. Testicular microlithiasis: systematic review and clinical guidelines. Prog Urol. 2019;29(10):465–73.
6. Capelouto CC, Clark PE, Ransil BJ, Loughlin KR. A review of scrotal violation in testicular cancer: is adjuvant local therapy necessary? J Urol. 1995;153(3 Pt 2):981–5.

# Chapter 25
# Scrotal Swelling and Cysts

Michal Yaela Schechter, Erik Van Laecke, and Anne-Françoise Spinoit

**Abbreviations**

| | |
|---|---|
| CEUS | Abdominal contrast-enhanced ultrasound |
| EMPD | Extramammary forms of Paget's Disease |
| MRI | Magnetic resonance imaging |
| US | Ultrasound |

## 25.1   Introduction

Cystic lesions are the most frequently encountered pathologies in the scrotum. This category includes paratesticular cysts, intratesticular cysts, and fluid collections. Of these, the paratesticular space represents the most common location for scrotal lesions. Scrotal cysts are typically asymptomatic and are either detected by (clinical) palpation (or self-examination) or as an incidental finding during ultrasound (US).

Unlike solid scrotal masses, once cystic scrotal masses are discovered, the most important component of the evaluation is not their location in relation to testis. Rather, it is whether they are pure cysts, as purely cystic cancers are extremely rare.[1] This determination may be achieved through clinical assessment combined with imaging, usually with grey-scale or color Doppler US. When US of the lesions

Michal Y. Schechter is fully funded by the Gianni Eggermont fund for advancement of research in Pediatric Urology.

M. Y. Schechter · E. Van Laecke · A.-F. Spinoit (✉)
Department of Urology, ERNeUROGEN Accredited Centre, Ghent University Hospital, Ghent, Belgium

is uncertain, an abdominal contrast-enhanced ultrasound (CEUS) or magnetic resonance imaging (MRI) can help locate and characterize the scrotal lesion.

In order for a scrotal lesion to be considered as an uncomplicated simple cyst, it must appear on imaging as a well-defined and relatively unattenuated rounded structure, with posterior acoustic enhancement and no wall thickening. A scrotal lesion that differs from this description is either a complicated cyst, pseudo cyst, or neoplasm.[2] This differentiation has practical implications for the urologist as pure cysts are considered benign and do not require surgical exploration (Figs. 25.1 and 25.2).

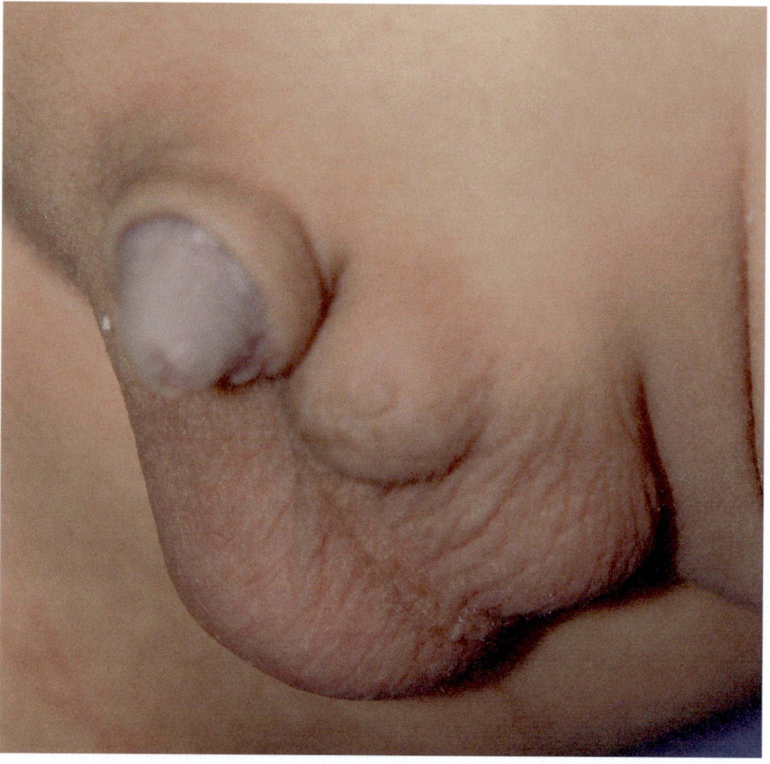

**Fig. 25.1** Scrotal cyst. From the author M A Fahmy

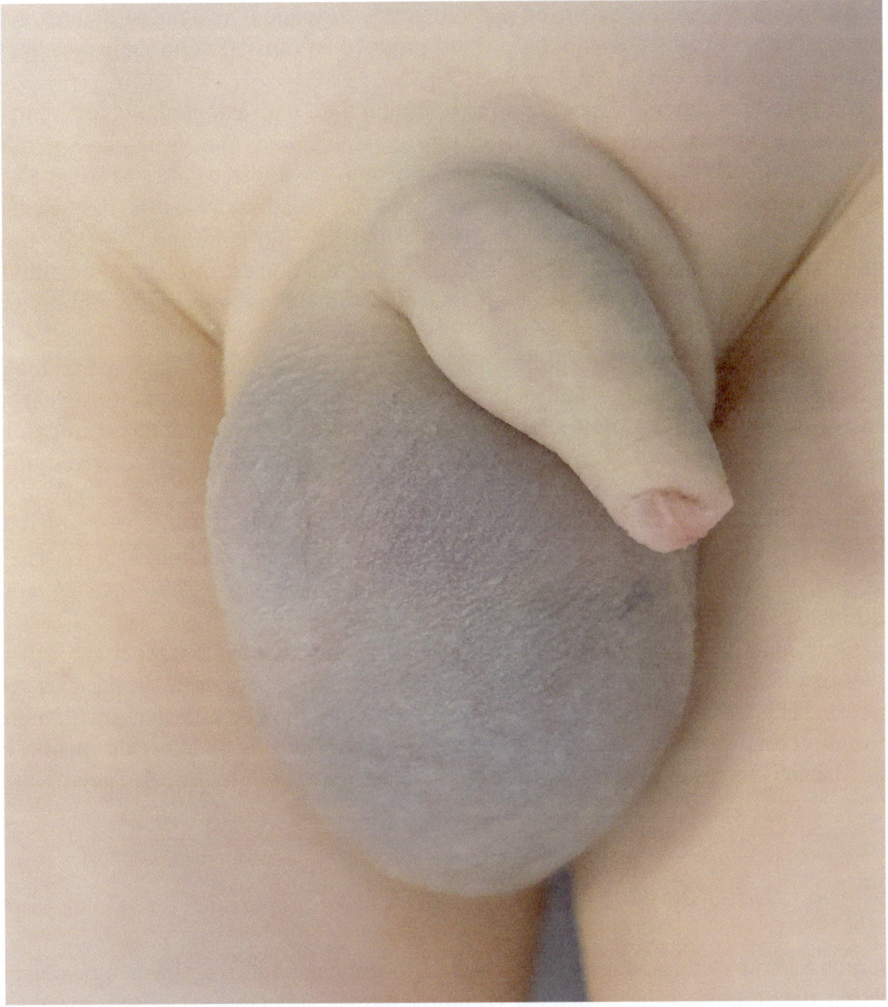

**Fig. 25.2** Scrotal cyst containing connective tissue. From the author Anne-Françoise Spinoit

## 25.2  Paratesticular Cysts

### 25.2.1  *Epididymis*

Epididymal cystic masses are the most common type of scrotal cysts and have been reported in 20–40% of asymptomatic patients undergoing an US examination.[3] Due to their small size and softness, they are usually not palpable during the clinical examination. Epididymal cysts may be categorized as congenital or acquired cysts.

Congenital cysts are formed from pathologically distended vestigial structures and are typically visualized as multiple cysts grouped in clusters, although they may also be large and solitary.[4]

Acquired epididymal cysts are more common than their congenial counterparts. Acquired cysts are further categorized into regular epididymal cysts and spermatoceles, with the former having a lymphatic origin while the latter are due to a tubular obstruction from an inflammatory process. Spermatoceles develop in the vaginal cavity and are mostly located in the head of the epididymis. While true epididymal cysts are usually single in number and are consist of clear serous fluid, spermatoceles may be multilocular and are full of proteinaceous fluid and spermatozoa.[5]

Finally, although regular epididymal cysts are more common than spermatoceles, postvasectomy patients are more likely to have spermatoceles than true cysts. Postvasectomy patients may also present with tubular ectasia of the epididymis several years after the procedure, with a vesicular dilation of the entire epididymis diagnosed on US.[6]

Both subtypes of regular epididymal cysts and spermatoceles are completely benign and appear on US as well-defined, homogenous, hypoechoic lesions. They are indistinguishable on US, which does not carry practical significance as their differentiation is not clinically relevant.[7]

Occasionally, very large epididymal cysts (whether true cysts or spermatoceles) may be difficult to distinguish from hydroceles on US if septations in the cyst are present. This differentiation is important as hydroceles may be associated with more serious scrotal pathologies, as will be discussed later in this chapter. Confusion is alleviated by remembering that while cysts displace the testis, a hydrocele envelops it.[8]

### 25.2.2 Appendiceal Cysts

Scrotal anatomy varies among individuals, and some patients may have appendages within the scrotum. The two most common scrotal appendages are the appendix testis (a remnant of the Mullerian duct) at the superior head of the testis and the appendix epididymis (a remnant of the Mesonephron) at the head of the epididymis.[9] The appendix testis and epididymis are usually noticeable on imaging in the presence of paratesticular fluid and present with an echogenic or cystic appearance on US. The appendices themselves are clinically insignificant; however, they may undergo torsion and cause severe pain in the affected patient.[10]

In the case of an appendiceal torsion, a classic physical examination finding is the "blue dot sign," which refers to the small, firm nodule on the upper pole of the testis that is palpable and presents as a bluish discoloration through the overlying skin. US imaging is useful for exclusion of more common causes of severe testicular pain, in particular testicular torsion and acute epididymo-orchitis. A Doppler US with absent internal appendiceal blood flow combined with increased periappendiceal peripheral flow is extremely suggestive of appendiceal torsion.[11]

### 25.2.3  Spermatic Cord

Spermatic cord cysts are congenital or acquired during adulthood, with the congenital type only becoming apparent during adulthood.[12] They are formed secondary to incomplete obliteration of the peritoneal vaginal duct or residual coelomic epithelium or may occur due to a chronic hydrocele.

Cysts of the spermatic cord are typically slow growing and asymptomatic. On clinical examination, the cyst may be palpated as a variably sized, tense, elastic mass along the course of the spermatic cord. It is easily diagnosed on US as either a typical unilocular simple cyst or as a slightly complicated multilocular cyst. Care should be taken to avoid confusing this benign lesion with a hydrocele or inguinal hernia, the latter of which may be known as a pseudocyst of the spermatic cord. If multiloculated, spermatic cord cysts should also be distinguished from cystadenomas of Mullerian origin.[13]

### 25.2.4  Tunica Albuginea

Tunica albuginea cysts are very rare, benign lesions. They typically manifest as small palpable masses within the tunica albuginea along the upper anterior or lateral aspect of the testicle and may present as single or multiple cysts. Although tunica albuginea cysts are usually small, they may become large and compress the adjacent testicular parenchyma, simulating an intratesticular mass. Diagnosis via US is straight forward as long as the lesion is a simple cyst. Less commonly, cysts of the tunica albuginea are complex and present with internal echoes, raising concern for a neoplasm. In the case of equivocal US findings and diagnostic doubt, a contrast-enhanced MRI can help localize and better define the lesion.[14]

### 25.2.5  Extramammary Scrotal Paget's Disease

Scrotal extramammary forms of Paget's Disease (EMPD) are rare lesions composed of an intra-epidermal adenocarcinoma that may progress to epidermis invasion and metastasis. Primary scrotal EMPD is more common than secondary. On clinical examination, its typical presentation is a single, well-delineated, chronic plaque which may be squamous, keratotic, or erosive and exhibits show centrifugal spread. Affected patients frequently describe a burning sensation or intense pruritus. Scrotal EMPD is often misdiagnosed and treated with antifungals and topical steroids. As this lesion is resistant to these treatments, if these treatments fail the discerning urologist should suspect scrotal EMPD and order a skin biopsy to prevent further diagnostic delay.[15]

First-line treatment is surgical excision, allowing for a more comprehensive histological analysis and confirmation of scrotal EMPD. It also enables screening for invasive Paget's Disease or associated neoplasia. Secondary scrotal EMPD often involves a nearby organ, in particular the prostate, or in some cases an underlying cutaneous adnexal tumor. Metastatic EMPD therapy consists of chemotherapy. Prognosis is good for primary forms that are non-invasive in terms of mortality, but morbidity assessment is dependent on the presence of chronic pruritis, pain, oozing, and recurrent lesions. Patients should be monitored long-term due to risk of relapse or metastasis.[16]

## 25.3 Intratesticular Cysts

Previously considered a rare finding, testicular cysts are now recognized as more commonplace due to the more frequent use of scrotal US in recent years. They are usually solitary but may be multiple, and are generally small in size (a few mm to cm).[17]

Intratesticular cysts may be further classified as simple, complex, dermoid, epidermoid, or neoplastic. Another type of intratesticular cystic lesion is cystic dysplasia of the rete testis, which much be differentiated from tubular ectasia of the rete testis.

### 25.3.1 Simple Testicular Cysts

If simple in nature, cysts are considered to be benign and do not require any treatment. Simple intratesticular cysts may develop anywhere within the testis but are often visualized near the mediastinum testis.[18]

### 25.3.2 Complex Testicular Cysts

If any imaging characteristics suggestive of a complex cyst are present, such as non-cystic content, septa, or vegetations, it must be evaluated for a potential neoplasm. In cases of complex cysts that display mobility of the echoic material when the patient moves, the cyst is always considered benign. However, if the cyst is fixed in place, rule out of a neoplasm is required. Follow-up of complex testicular cysts often shows reduction in complexity and size or disappearance, revealing their benign nature.[19]

### 25.3.3  Dermoid and Epidermoid Testicular Cysts

Included in the typically benign germ cell prepubertal-type teratoma category are the dermoid and epidermoid cyst subtypes. Dermoid cysts are far less common than their epidermoid counterparts and do not have malignant potential. They appear on US imaging as a hypoechoic mass, at times containing low-level echoes with tiny echogenic foci due to desquamated keratin crystals. Absence of internal vascularity is present on Doppler.[20]

Epidermoid cysts have an uncertain pathogenesis. Current suggestions include their origination as a result of monodermal teratoma development or squamous metaplasia of surface mesothelium. Visualization on US is varied but epidermoid cysts often present with a classic "Onion Skin" appearance of alternating concentric rings of hypo- and hyper-echogenicity representing the layers of lamellar keratin.[21] Although this presentation is characteristic, it is not pathognomonic.

In cases with uncertain US findings for suspected epidermoid cysts, color Doppler or CEUS may be used for further evaluation. They may also present on MRI with alternating low and high signal intensity areas on T1- and T2-weighted images, in addition to a "Target Sign" pattern on T1-weighted images due to the hyperintense central area of the lesion.[22] Once an epidermoid cyst is suspected on imaging, teratomas and other tumors must be ruled out via partial orchiectomy with intraoperative pathological analysis (Fig. 25.3).[23]

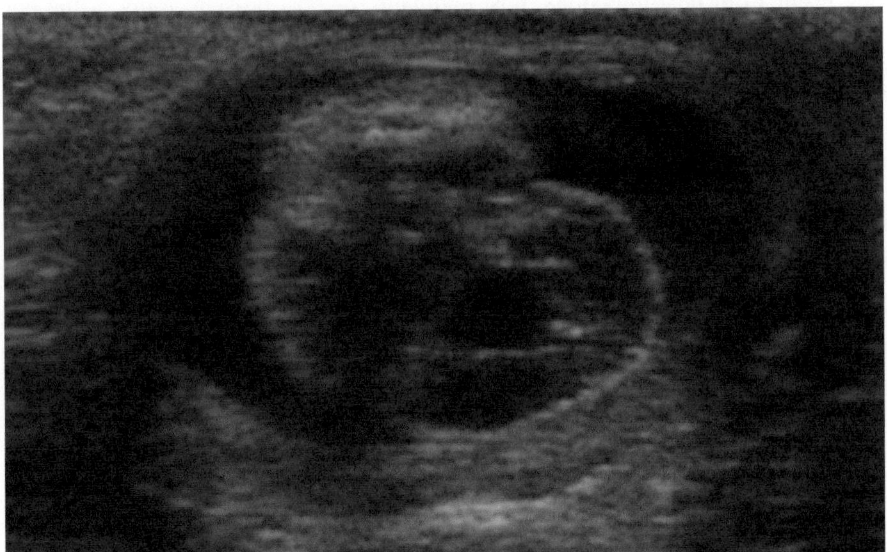

**Fig. 25.3** Dermoid cyst on US. Note it has replaced all normal testicular tissue. On pathology report, no normal testicular tissue could be found. Printed with permission from the author Anne-Françoise Spinoit

### 25.3.4  Cystic Testicular Tumors

Purely cystic testicular malignancies are extremely rare.[24] However, the presence of cystic component in testicular neoplasms is uncommon, and when present is most often found in the form of a cystic teratoma.[25] Therefore, any cyst that does not fulfill all of the previously mentioned imaging criteria for classification of a simple cyst must be considered malignant until its benign nature is confirmed.

Careful inspection of the cyst for vascular solid components is performed via imaging. As solid materials often lack vascularization on color Doppler, absence of blood flow on Doppler imaging does not have sufficient sensitivity to rule out vegetations. Instead, CEUS and MRI imaging may solve diagnostic doubts related to the solid component of the cyst. Virtually all tumors with cystic components display intralesional vascularization following microbubble contrast injection on CEUS[26] and enhance after gadolinium injection on MRI.[27]

### 25.3.5  Tubular Ectasia of the Rete Testis

The rete testis is formed at the confluence of the seminiferous tubules within the mediastinum testis that eventually drains into the epididymal head. Dilation of the rete testis is a benign and common condition, mostly affecting patients over 50 years of age. Presentation is bilateral in about one-third of cases.[28] The etiology may result from post-infectious, post-traumatic, or post-prostatectomy at the epididymal obstruction. Possible contributing factors for rete testis ectasia include epididymitis, testicular biopsy, and vasectomy. It is also often associated with epididymal abnormalities such as spermatoceles or dilated efferent ducts. Although this dilation is a benign condition, ectasia of the rete testis may cause oligospermia and azoospermia and consequent infertility.[29]

Ectasia of the rete testis appears on US as branching hypoechoic cystic figures in the mediastinum. It is important to accurately diagnose this condition on pre-operative imaging as it may easily be confused with a hypoechoic mass and, therefore, cause an unnecessary biopsy for rule out of testicular cancer.[30] Differential diagnosis includes cystic dysplasia of the rete testis, which is usually seen in the pediatric population and is associated with ipsilateral urogenital lesions,[31] and varicocele which is easily diagnosed on Doppler US. The age of the patient at presentation, clinical features, and appearance on US allow for pre-operative diagnosis of tubular ectasia of the rete testis.

## 25.4   Scrotal Fluid Collections

### 25.4.1   *Varicoceles*

Varicoceles occur when the venous valves of the pampiniform plexus become ineffective. The resulting impairment in plexus drainage leads to its dilation and hyperthermia, causing a progressive decline in testicular function. Varicoceles may be diagnosed via characteristic clinical findings such as scrotal fullness with Valsalva in a standing position or a "bag of worms" mass that shrinks in the recumbent position.[32]

Varicoceles do not require confirmation with US, although there is some disagreement among urologists as to whether the diagnosis must be confirmed by Doppler US. Nevertheless, if the clinical exam findings are equivocal or if an obese body habitus prevents proper examination, it is agreed that Doppler imaging should be used to support the diagnosis via the demonstration of reversal of venous blood flow with Valsalva or spermatic vein diameter measurement of $\geq 3$ mm.[33]

Venography had the highest sensitivity for varicocele diagnosis and is therefore often used as a gold standard by researchers. However, it is not typically used in general clinical practice as venography is both invasive and time consuming. Current recommendations discourage routine use of US for identification of non-palpable varicoceles as their repair does not demonstrate clinical benefit.[34]

Testicular varicoceles are commonly associated with infertility and their correction can help improve the sperm count. The clinician should recall that over 80% of varicocele cases are not associated with infertility, but up to 40% of men with primary infertility and up to 81% of men with secondary infertility have diagnosed varicoceles.[35]

Varicoceles may be intratesticular as well, in which case they are usually idiopathic but can also be secondary to renal vein obstruction. They are bilateral in about one-quarter of cases and are more prevalent on the left side.[36] Ultrasound findings are similar to those of extra testicular varicoceles.

### 25.4.2   *Hydroceles*

The parietal and visceral layers of the tunica vaginalis normally have a minimal amount of fluid between them. The presence of a more abundant fluid collection is called a hydrocele. Hydroceles are the most common cause of painless scrotal swelling and can present either as congenital lesions due to a patent processus vaginalis or can present in their adult form. An acute presentation in adults may be associated with underlying scrotal pathology, including inflammation, trauma, torsion, or testicular tumors.[37]

This diagnosis is confirmed by an US exam, where the hydrocele is visualized as anechoic fluid collections around the anterolateral testis.[38] If the lesion is chronic, wall thickening and septations may also be present.

Large hydroceles can exert pressure on testicular parenchyma, causing impaired blood flow and mimicking testicular torsion. These cases mandate fluid aspiration to restore normal testicular blood circulation. It should be noted that a hydrocele may be the presenting symptom of malignant mesothelioma of the tunica vaginalis, which is a rare but highly aggressive testicular cancer. It is often missed on imaging, leading to a delayed diagnosis with higher recurrence and mortality rates. Color Doppler can be helpful for a more accurate preoperative diagnosis of mesothelioma.[39]

### 25.4.3    Hematoceles and Hematomas

Hydroceles caused by trauma contain an accumulation of blood within the tunica vaginalis and are known as hematoceles. Post-traumatic testicular hematomal collections may present as intratesticular hematomas, extratesticular hematomas in the epididymis and scrotal wall, or as hematoceles.

US appearance of these blood collections varies with time. Acute hematomas on US appear more hyperechoic and may have a diffusely heterogenous mixture, but as these hematomas become chronic and resolve, they decrease in their echogenicity and size and become more complex with cystic components. On Doppler, intratesticular hematomas appear as focal areas of avascularity. If an acute hematoma is suspected but imaging is negative, repeat imaging should be performed within 12–24 hours after the initial US evaluation, as the initial echotexture of a hematoma may be indistinguishable from the surrounding parenchyma.[40]

As the testicular parenchyma underlies the tunica albuginea, an injury to one structure very often means an injury to the other as well. However, a heterogeneous intratesticular lesion may appear in cases of intratesticular hematomas without testicular rupture. These cases require imaging, in particular a CEUS, to better assess if surgical exploration for testicular rupture is warranted.[41]

Finally, about 10–15% of testicular tumors first manifest and are incidentally discovered after scrotal trauma.[42] This is likely because testicular tumors are the most common solid malignancy in 15–35-year-old males, and the highest incidence of traumatic injury is in that age group. Testicular tumors often appear similarly to hematomas, and in cases of trauma it can be difficult to differentiate between lesions. Therefore, cases with abnormal intratesticular US readings without immediate surgical intervention should be followed up with a repeat US to rule out malignancy, as over time scrotal hematomas are expected to shrink and scrotal masses are expected to grow. If US findings are equivocal, MRI may be used for a more conclusive diagnosis.[43]

### 25.4.4  Pyoceles and Abscesses

Pyoceles occur when the mesothelial lining of the tunica vaginalis is breached as a complication of trauma, surgery, or epididymo-orchitis, allowing for an infectious process to ensue. Patients typically appear with a painful scrotum along with US findings of a septate or complex heterogenous collection of fluid. A pyocele organized as an abscess always lacks vascularity on Doppler US, sometimes with peripheral hyperemia. In a minority of cases, the particulate matter within the lesion creates gas bubbles in the abscess cavity which appear as focal hyperechoic spots with posterior shadowing on US. Most patients are completely cured with a treatment of antibiotics. However, in cases with an abscess complicated by a perineal necrotizing infection requires emergency surgery and debridement.[44]

### 25.4.5  Inguinoscrotal Hernias

Inguinoscrotal hernias typically consist of bowel or omentum that passes into the scrotal cavity via an incompletely obliterated processus vaginalis. While this condition is more commonly in preterm neonates, it may also present in adults. As clinical examination is often insufficient for proper diagnosis, US is used for help with diagnosis and further characterization of the hernia.[45]

Bowel hernia appearance on US is dependent on bowel content. Imaging showing specular reflection within fluid indicates bowel containing fluid, while bowels containing air or solid stool appear with a bright echotexture. US also allows for visualization of peristalsis within the bowel hernia, thus firmly establishing the diagnosis. Omental hernias can be visualized on US as paratesticular masses with diffuse echotextures due to their fat content.[46]

**Endnotes**


1. Imaging article.
2. Martin B. Cystic structures of the scrotal contents. In: Atlas of scrotal ultrasound. Springer Berlin Heidelberg; 1992. p. 175–95.
3. Valentino M, Bertolotto M, Ruggirello M, Pavlica P, Barozzi L, Rossi C. Cystic lesions and scrotal fluid collections in adults: Ultrasound findings. J Ultrasound. 2011 Dec;14(4):208–15.
4. Martin B. Cystic structures of the scrotal contents. In: Atlas of scrotal ultrasound. Springer Berlin Heidelberg; 1992. p. 175–95.
5. Imaging article.
6. Valentino M, Bertolotto M, Ruggirello M, Pavlica P, Barozzi L, Rossi C. Cystic lesions and scrotal fluid collections in adults: Ultrasound findings. J Ultrasound. 2011 Dec;14(4):208–15.

7. Imaging article.
8. Valentino M, Barozzi L, Pavlica P, Rossi C. Imaging scrotal lumps in adults-2: cysts and fluid collections. In: Bertolotto M, Trombetta C, editors. Scrotal pathology. Springer Berlin Heidelberg; 2011. p. 179–89.
9. Imaging article.
10. Valentino M, Bertolotto M, Ruggirello M, Pavlica P, Barozzi L, Rossi C. Cystic lesions and scrotal fluid collections in adults: Ultrasound findings. J Ultrasound. 2011 Dec;14(4):208–15.
11. Imaging article.
12. Martin B. Cystic structures of the scrotal contents. In: Atlas of sucrotal Ultrasound. Springer Berlin Heidelberg; 1992. p. 175–95.
13. Valentino M, Barozzi L, Pavlica P, Rossi C. Imaging scrotal lumps in adults-2: cysts and fluid collections. In: Bertolotto M, Trombetta C, editors. Scrotal pathology. Springer Berlin Heidelberg; 2011. p. 179–89.
14. Valentino M, Bertolotto M, Ruggirello M, Pavlica P, Barozzi L, Rossi C. Cystic lesions and scrotal fluid collections in adults: Ultrasound findings. J Ultrasound. 2011 Dec;14(4):208–15.
15. Dauendorffer JN, Herms F, Baroudjian B, Basset-Seguin N, Cavelier-Balloy B, Fouéré S, Bagot M, Lebbé C. Penoscrotal Paget's disease. Ann Dermatol Venereol. 2021 Jan 15:S0151-9638(20)31,154–6.
16. Dauendorffer JN, Herms F, Baroudjian B, Basset-Seguin N, Cavelier-Balloy B, Fouéré S, Bagot M, Lebbé C. Penoscrotal Paget's disease. Ann Dermatol Venereol. 2021 Jan 15:S0151-9638(20)31,154–6.
17. Martin B. Cystic structures of the scrotal contents. In: Atlas of Scrotal Ultrasound. Springer Berlin Heidelberg; 1992. p. 175–95.
18. Bertolotto M, Valentino M, Iannelli M, Neri F, Kaso G, Barozzi L, et al. The testicles: cystic lesions. In: Martino P, Galosi AB, editors. Atlas of ultrasonography in urology, andrology, and nephrology. Springer International Publishing; 2017. p. 471–82.
19. Bertolotto M, Valentino M, Iannelli M, Neri F, Kaso G, Barozzi L, et al. The testicles: cystic lesions. In: Martino P, Galosi AB, editors. Atlas of ultrasonography in urology, andrology, and nephrology. Springer International Publishing; 2017. p. 471–82.
20. Imaging article.
21. Imaging article.
22. Imaging article.
23. Bertolotto M, Valentino M, Iannelli M, Neri F, Kaso G, Barozzi L, et al. The testicles: cystic lesions. In: Martino P, Galosi AB, editors. Atlas of ultrasonography in urology, andrology, and nephrology. Springer International Publishing; 2017. p. 471–82.
24. Imaging article.

25. Valentino M, Bertolotto M, Ruggirello M, Pavlica P, Barozzi L, Rossi C. Cystic lesions and scrotal fluid collections in adults: ultrasound findings. J Ultrasound. 2011 Dec;14(4):208–15.

26. Bertolotto M, Valentino M, Iannelli M, Neri F, Kaso G, Barozzi L, et al. The testicles: cystic lesions. In: Martino P, Galosi AB, editors. Atlas of ultrasonography in urology, andrology, and nephrology. Springer International Publishing; 2017. p. 471–82.

27. Valentino M, Barozzi L, Pavlica P, Rossi C. Imaging scrotal lumps in adults-2: cysts and fluid collections. In: Bertolotto M, Trombetta C, editors. Scrotal pathology. Springer Berlin Heidelberg; 2011. p. 179–89.

28. Valentino M, Bertolotto M, Ruggirello M, Pavlica P, Barozzi L, Rossi C. Cystic lesions and scrotal fluid collections in adults: Ultrasound findings. J Ultrasound. 2011 Dec;14(4):208–15.

29. Valentino M, Bertolotto M, Ruggirello M, Pavlica P, Barozzi L, Rossi C. Cystic lesions and scrotal fluid collections in adults: Ultrasound findings. Journal of Ultrasound. 2011 Dec;14(4):208–15.

30. Imaging article.

31. Bertolotto M, Valentino M, Iannelli M, Neri F, Kaso G, Barozzi L, et al. The testicles: cystic lesions. In: Martino P, Galosi AB, editors. Atlas of ultrasonography in urology, andrology, and nephrology. Springer International Publishing; 2017. p. 471–82.

32. Imaging article.

33. Imaging article.

34. Imaging article.

35. Imaging article.

36. Bertolotto M, Valentino M, Iannelli M, Neri F, Kaso G, Barozzi L, et al. The testicles: cystic lesions. In: Martino P, Galosi AB, editors. Atlas of ultrasonography in urology, andrology, and nephrology. Springer International Publishing; 2017. p. 471–82.

37. Valentino M, Barozzi L, Pavlica P, Rossi C. Imaging scrotal lumps in adults-2: cysts and fluid collections. In: Bertolotto M, Trombetta C, editors. Scrotal pathology. Springer Berlin Heidelberg; 2011. p. 179–89.

38. Imaging article.

39. Valentino M, Barozzi L, Pavlica P, Rossi C. Imaging scrotal lumps in adults-2: cysts and fluid collections. In: Bertolotto M, Trombetta C, editors. Scrotal pathology. Springer Berlin Heidelberg; 2011. p. 179–89.

40. Imaging article.

41. Imaging article.

42. Imaging article.

43. Imaging article.

44. Valentino M, Barozzi L, Pavlica P, Rossi C. Imaging scrotal lumps in adults-2: cysts and fluid collections. In: Bertolotto M, Trombetta C, editors. Scrotal pathology. Springer Berlin Heidelberg; 2011. p. 179–89.
45. Valentino M, Barozzi L, Pavlica P, Rossi C. Imaging scrotal lumps in adults-2: cysts and fluid collections. In: Bertolotto M, Trombetta C, editors. Scrotal pathology. Springer Berlin Heidelberg; 2011. p. 179–89.
46. Imaging article.

# Chapter 26
# Dermatological Diseases Specific to Scrotum

Mohamed A. Baky Fahmy

**Abbreviations**

| | |
|---|---|
| AR | Androgen receptor |
| ER | Estrogen receptor |
| PD | Paget's disease |
| HPV | Human papillomavirus |
| LSC | lichen sclerosis |
| LP | lichen planus |
| BXO | Balanitis xerotica obliterans |

## 26.1 Special Characters of Scrotal Skin

The skin of the scrotum is thin and more deeply pigmented than the surrounding skin. It is closely adherent to the underlying dartos muscle, which gives it a rugose wrinkled appearance with contraction of the muscle (e.g. at rest in younger individuals, and in the cold at all ages). The scrotum has numerous pilosebaceous, eccrine and apocrine glands. Hair is sparse and coarse, this hair also covers the skin down to the anus and sweat and sebaceous glands are numerous [1].

The genital skin differs from skin of other body regions in different aspects:

- There is no subcutaneous fat tissue, no Scarp's fascia; instead there is the tunica dartos with smooth muscle cells.
- No tight attachment of the skin to underlying bone or cartilage.
- Little or minimal keratinizing epithelia.
- Reduced hair growth of the scrotal skin.
- Moist environment due to multitude of mucous secreting glands.

M. A. B. Fahmy (✉)
Al-Azhar University, Cairo, Egypt

- The dartos fascia is of paramount importance because it serves as a fixation point between layers whereas it provides elasticity and sliding properties to the scrotal skin.
- Notably, the male genital skin has to manage fast volume changes that occur during sexual activity and thermal regulation of the testes.
- Constant microbial contamination from cutaneous, genitourinary, and intestinal flora.
- AR expression differs between genital and nongenital skin with upregulation in genital fibroblasts. In general, it appears that sex steroid hormone expression is higher in stromal cells than in epithelial cells, implying higher responsiveness of fibroblasts to hormonal influences. Aside from receptor expression, the binding capacity and metabolism of sex steroid hormones differs between different skin regions. Testosterone binding capacity of the AR is higher in genital compared to nongenital skin cells from both sexes—independently of age—and testosterone degradation is up to 30 times faster in genital skin compared with nongenital skin [2].

These physiological tasks are addressed by several means:

(i)   Abundance of skin tissue on the scrotal sac.
(ii)  Presence of the dartos fascia and muscle in the scrotum.
(iii) A high amount of elastic fibers in the dermis.
      High skin elasticity and abundance of tissue are the prerequisite for tension-free acute wound healing with unapparent scars and optimal repair after injury. But the drawback is the tendency of the outer genitals to enormous swelling and edema after surgery, infection or trauma, due to its elasticity and intricate lymphatics, but the swelling of the genital tissue resolves as fast as it occurs in healthy subjects [3].

## 26.2   Specific Scrotal Dermatosis

**Inflammatory Dermatosis**

**Intertrigo**: Intertrigo is the name given to any dermatosis occurring in skin folds, genital skin is especially susceptible to secondary infection, e.g., with *Candida,* however *Candida* is a ready opportunist, so its presence may not always indicate primary infection as the cause of the genital inflammation. Bacteria have increasingly been implicated in the etiology of the disease, particularly *Staphylococcus aureus.* If the *Streptococcus pyogenes* is isolated; it has been suggested that the disease may be sexually transmitted possibly by penile–oral intercourse. Intertrigo usually affects the inguinal region with creeping to the scrotum; it is common in infants and incontinent patients. Males may harbour the organism (*Candida albicans*) in the inguinal or gluteal folds or in the scrotum and the penis. Factors predisposing to cutaneous candidiasis and other complications of intertrigo include immunosuppression, diabetes mellitus, and the administration of potent systemic antibiotics.

### Infectious Pustules (Scrotal Abscess)

One of the most common causes of genital pustules, especially with inflammation, is cutaneous candidiasis. Discrete, scattered pustules in hairy areas of the body generally are caused by *Staphylococcus aureus* and less frequently, *Streptococcus pyogenes*. In susceptible individuals, folliculitis may develop into a larger cutaneous abscess known as a carbuncle or a furuncle. Superficial infections usually respond well to topical antibiotics. Oral antibiotics should be used conservatively and cultures and sensitivities used to guide therapy as methicillin resistant strains of bacteria may be present, but fully developed walled-off abscesses may require incision and drainage.

**Secondary scrotal abscess**: As the scrotal wall is in direct communication with both the retroperitoneum and the peritoneal cavity; so it is not rare to have an extension and trickling of any fluid from these spaces into the scrotal wall (Figs. 26.1 and 26.2). Almost all faecal abscesses or enterocutaneous fistulas of the scrotum are due to incarcerated bowel loop in inguinal hernia.

Rarely, necrotic tissue and exudate may trickle to the scrotum from retroperitoneal extension of necrotic process. Several cases of scrotal abscesses complicating an acute necrotizing pancreatitis was reported [4]. Pneumoscrotum and faecal abscess of the scrotum are a rare presentation of retroperitoneal colonic perforation [5]. Many cases reported after duodenal and bowel perforation [6]. In neonates with

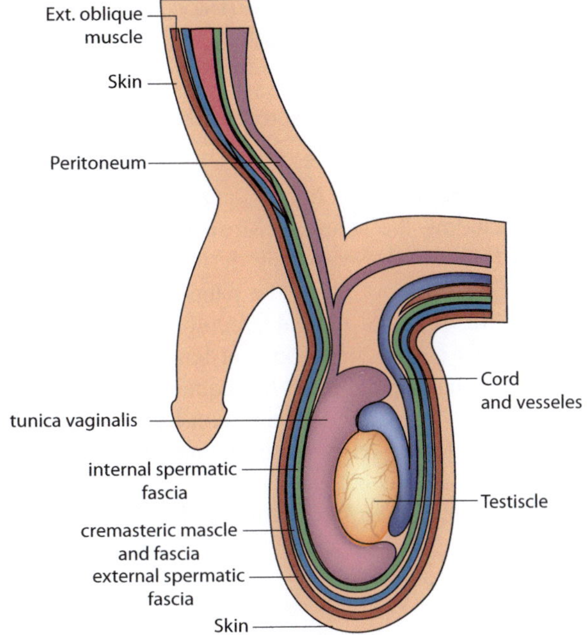


**Fig. 26.1** Peritoneal extension in the scrotal wall Needs refining

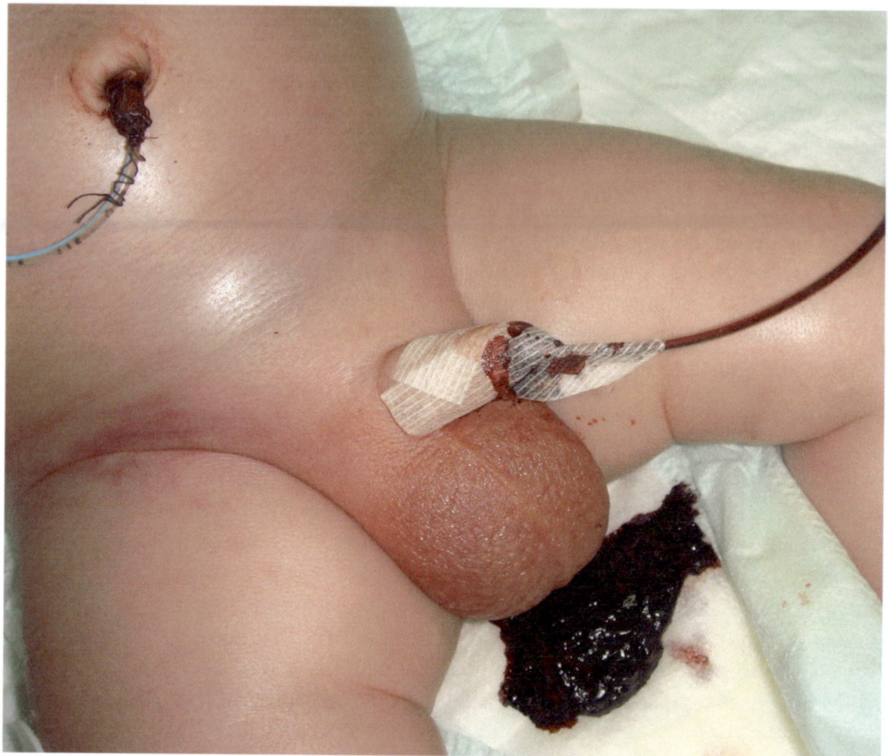

**Fig. 26.2** An infant with bleeding tendency; haematuria and bleeding per rectum are evident. The scrotum filled with blood trickling from an intraperitoneal haemorrhage

necrotizing enterocolitis, scrotal manifestation may indicating bowel perforation and faecal peritonitis (Fig. 26.3).

**Napkin dermatitis**: In infants, eczematous reactions are often seen in the napkin area, including the scrotum. Most of these cases represent a primary irritant dermatitis (Fig. 26.4). Seborrheic dermatitis and a psoriasiform napkin rash can also occur. Some but not all of the patients with the latter condition develop psoriasis late in life. Infantile gluteal granuloma (papuloerosive dermatitis of Jacquet and Sevestre) is a rare condition that has been described mainly in the newborn and infants in the napkin area. It frequently develops in a background of an irritant napkin rash [3]. A similar condition has been described in incontinent males with lesions developing on the scrotum and anogenital region (Fig. 26.5). The histology is mainly non-specific and includes superficial ulceration, focal necrosis and a prominent mixed inflammatory cell infiltrate with granulomata and numerous lymphocytes and plasma cells, haemorrhage and hemosiderin deposition may be detectable.

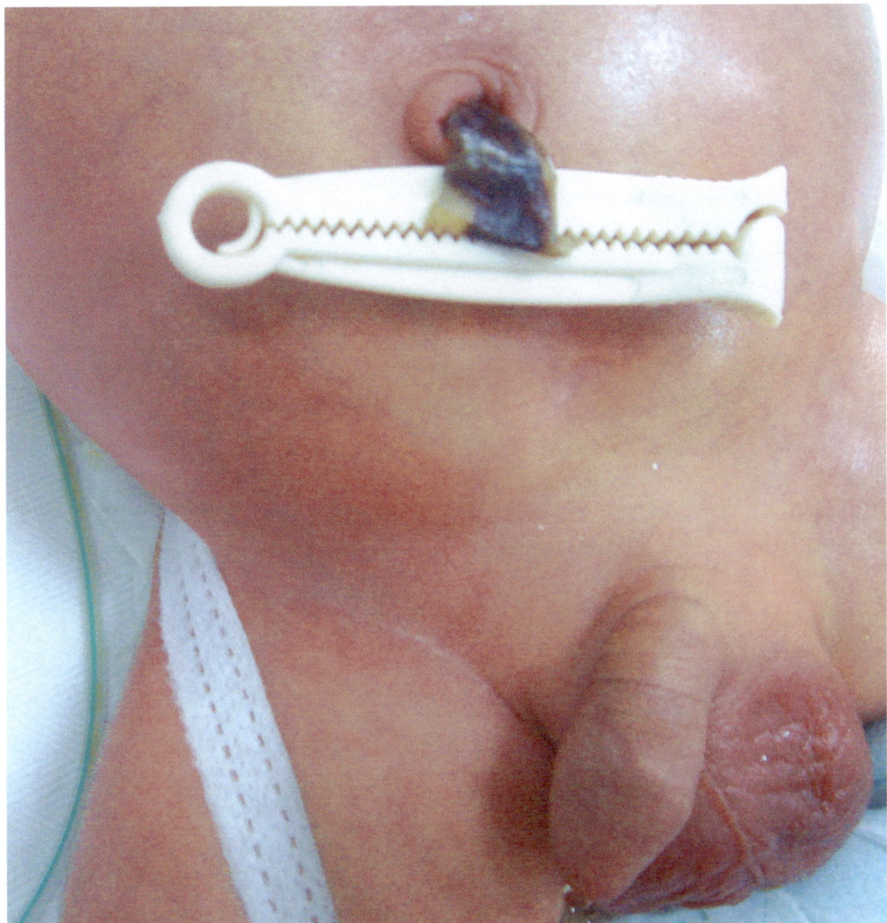

**Fig. 26.3** A neonate with NEC and bowel perforation with a secondary scrotal wall infection (Left)

Differential diagnosis: Crohn's disease and infective granulomatous conditions may have to be excluded.

**Granuloma Inguinale**: or donovanosis, this disease is also known as genital serpiginous ulceration. It is a genital ulcerative disease caused by the bacterium Klebsiella granulomatis (known as Calymmatobacterium granulomatis). The disease is endemic in some tropical and subtropical climates countries, in populations with low economic status, poor personal hygiene, active sexual activity and more often occurs at the age of 20–40 years with an equal ratio of men and women [7].

Clinically, the disease is commonly characterized by painless, slowly progressive ulcerative lesions on the genitalia or perineum without regional lymphadenopathy.

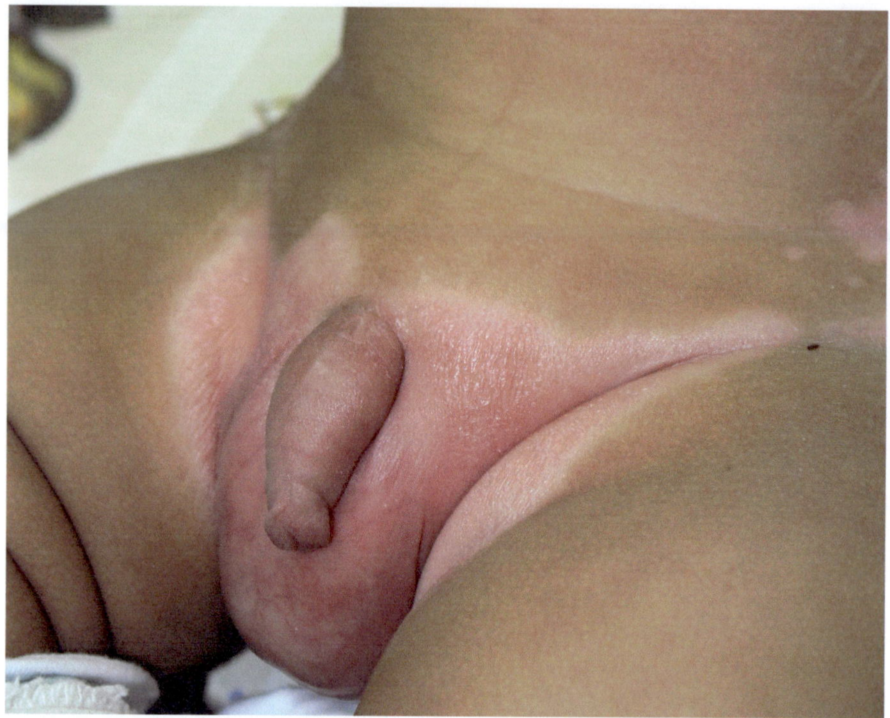

**Fig. 26.4** Extensive napkin dermatitis

The lesions are highly vascular and bleed easily on contact Extragenital lesions may occur but are rare and more common in newborns. In some countries this disease is often neglected, therefore it is misdiagnosed and inaccurately managed. The causative organisms are difficult to cluttered, and this has led to a debate about the definitive etiology [8].

Fournier's gangrene discussed in Chap. 23.

**Eczema**: Seborrheic dermatitis is the commonest form of eczema affecting anogenital skin, followed by irritant contact eczema, which is more common than many other inflammatory dermatosis. Allergic contact eczema is rare at genital sites and occurs more typically in a perianal distribution. Involvement of scrotal skin with atopic eczema is uncommon (Fig. 26.6).

**Seborrheic dermatitis** is commonly associated with an abnormal hypersensitivity to the normal commensal cutaneous yeast, *Pityrosporum ovale*. The groin, scrotum and penis not rarely involved, and it may be the sole site, leading to the patient presenting with pruritus ani or balanoposthitis. Some patients may also have a tendency to develop psoriasis on the scalp, the face, in the flexures and at anogenital sites, seborrheic dermatitis and psoriasis may be indistinguishable. Seborrheic

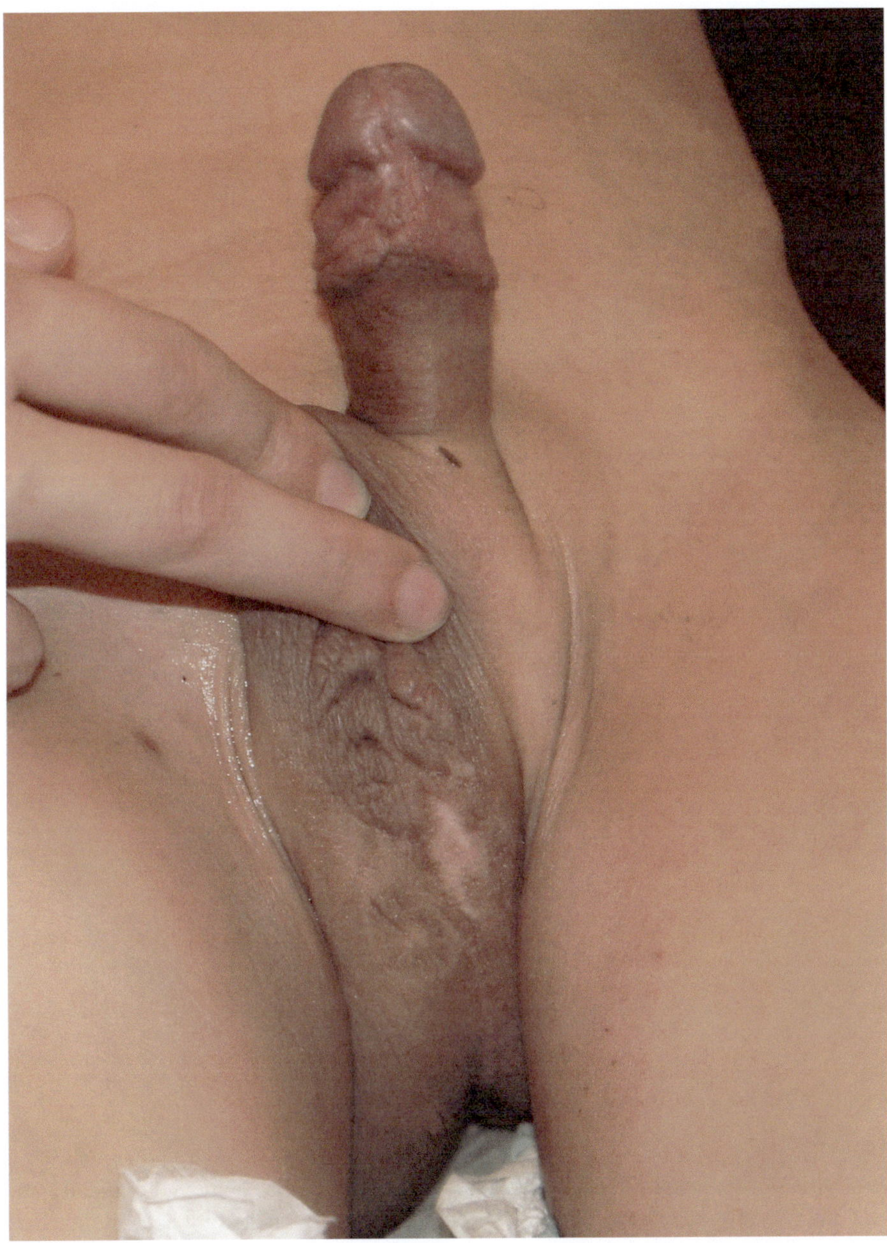

**Fig. 26.5** 7 years old boy with urinary incontinence secondary to spina bifida and a localised scrotal dermatitis

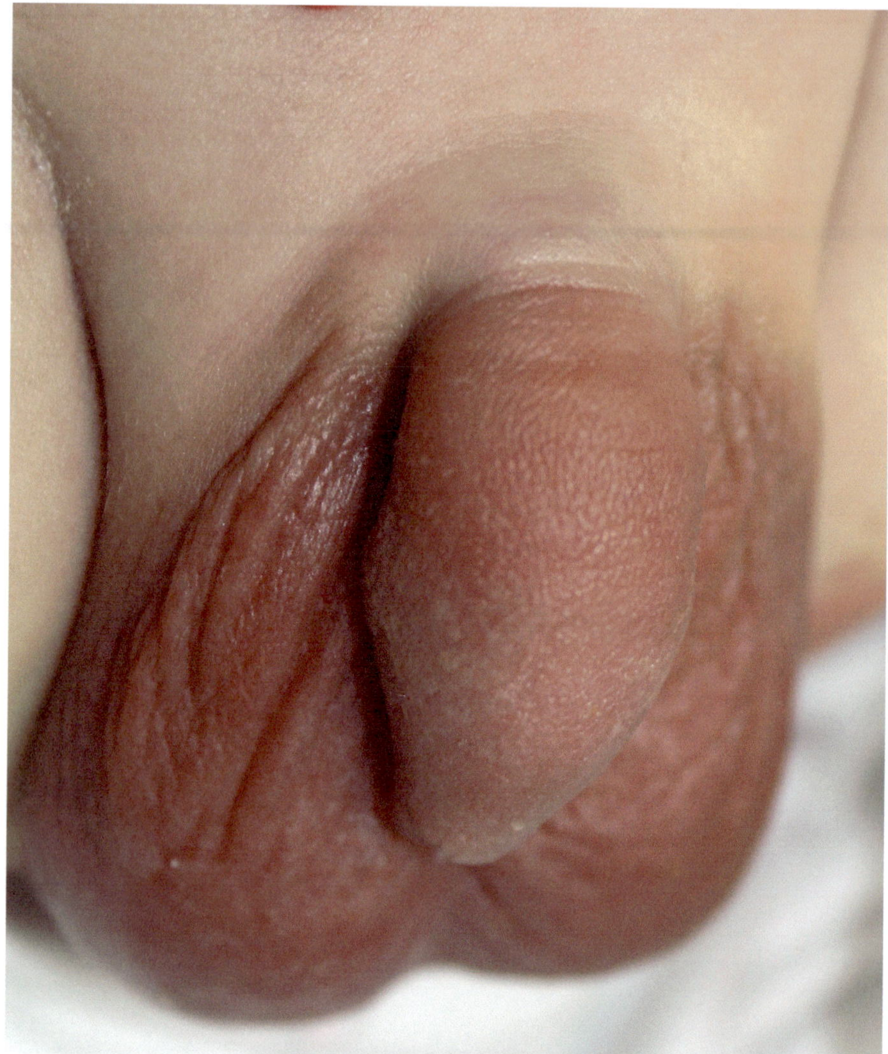

**Fig. 26.6** Allergic contact eczema of the scrotum in a neonate

dermatitis is very common after HIV infection. Diagnosis is achieved clinically and it is not usually necessary to do a biopsy. Histology is identical to seborrheic dermatitis occurring elsewhere.

**Condyloma acuminata**: It is one of the most common sexually transmitted diseases, caused by Human papillomavirus (HPV). Among various types, types 6 and 11 comprise 90% of the cases of the disease [9]. Its size and form can be various depending on each case. It is commonly presented as a huge pedunculated mass of the scrotum without any symptoms that appeared along months. Both the number and size of the masses are usually increase throughout a few months. The incidence of condyloma is reported to be around 5% among adults aged 20–40 years. The great majority are sexually transmitted. Men whose sexual partners have HPV-related cervical lesions have an increased (50–85%) incidence of penile condyloma. When genital condyloma occurs in children, sexual abuse should be suspected [9]. Condyloma is most often located on the corona of the glans, but also occurs on the scrotal skin and perineum. Condyloma is flat, delicately papillary, or warty and cauliflower-like. Histologically, it consists of a proliferation of squamous epithelium with an acanthotic and papillomatous architecture, showing orderly epithelial maturation (Fig. 26.7).

For both diagnostic and therapeutic purposes, excisional biopsy of the largest pedunculated mass is usually required. Small sessile masses could not be easily excised. Surgery usually performed for large lesions without major complications and the remnant lesions should be treated with topical 5-fluorouracil [10].

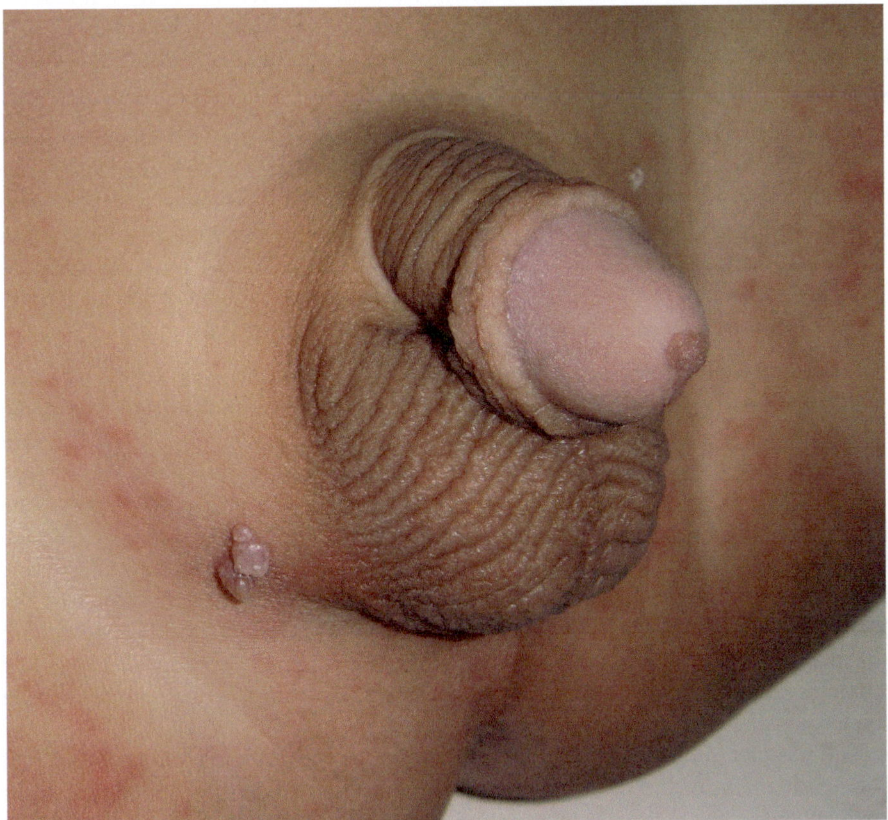

**Fig. 26.7** A small condyloma near to the scrotum in a 2 years circumcised child

**Giant condyloma**: is a rare scrotal exophytic tumor which reaches a very large size after many years of evolution, there has been much confusion in the correct classification of this lesion which has been confused with verrucous carcinoma. In giant condylomas, patients are older than those with condyloma acuminatum and younger than those with condylomatous (warty) carcinoma. Grossly, it presents as a cauliflower-like tumor showing a papillomatous growth with a sharp demarcation between the lesion and stroma on the cut surface. The deep border may affect lamina propria, dartos or corpus spongiosum. histologically, it may have an exo- and endophytic growth pattern with morphology identical to condyloma acuminatum.

**Verruciform xanthoma**: Verruciform xanthoma is a warty lesion characterized by acanthosis, hyperkeratosis, and parakeratosis, with long rete ridges associated with a neutrophilic infiltrate. A variable prominent xanthomatous infiltrate occupies the dermis between the rete ridges. This lesion is usually solitary and arises in the oral cavity, and only a few genital lesions have been described (scrotal, penile, and vulvar areas). Despite the architectural resemblance of verruciform xanthoma to other verruciform mucocutaneous lesions of the scrotum related to HPV infection, this lesion is most likely not an HPV-associated penile lesion. Mohsin et al. postulated that the xanthoma cells, which is the histologic hallmark of the lesion, are possibly derived from dermal dendritic cells [11].

**lichen planus (LP)**: LP is inflammatory, papulosquamous disorder affecting either or all of the skin, mucous membrane, hair, and nail. Isolated hypertrophic lesions on the scrotum are a rare phenomenon. Although very rarely, malignant transformation is possible. Majority of reported neoplasms have been histologically well differentiated squamous cell carcinomas. Potent local corticosteroid ointments are the mainstay of therapy for localized lesions of LP. In hypertrophic type, an intralesional injections of long acting steroid are usually effective [12].

**Scrotal Balanitis Xerotica Obliterans (BXO)**: also known as lichen sclerosis (LSC). In men it is the most common cause of acquired phimosis and affects the glans and the prepuce mainly. Typical symptoms are a thickening of the foreskin that impairs retraction. Whitish plaques can extend over the entire glans with affection of the urethral meatus followed by stenosis and voiding problems. The anogenital area is frequently affected forming an 8-shaped efflorescence around the perinium and the anal orifice with opaque plaques and papules. In chronic disease, these atrophic lesions can lead to a complete destruction of the scrotum. The patients' quality of life is severely reduced due to chronic pruritus, pain, and obstipation resulting from painful defecation and painful erection and hygienic problems. BXO is associated with squamous cell carcinoma formation in a variable percentage of men [13].

The posterior urethra and the rest of the external genitalia are generally spared. The involvement of the scrotum is not commonly known, but an extensive disease involvement of the entire anterior urethra along with scrotal skin, has been reported occasionally [14]. Scrotal involvement is usually secondary to urethral affection and urethrocutaneous fistulous formation [15]. Complications reported include phimosis, meatal stenosis, dense obliterative urethral strictures, urethral stone formation and the development of squamous cell carcinoma [16]. Other BXO associated diseases comprise autoimmune thyroiditis, vitiligo, or pernicious anemia. The etiology is not fully understood, an autoimmune origin with T- and B-cell-driven response to a yet unknown antigen is discussed, because dense T-lymphocytic infiltrates with concomitant vasculitis and extensive tissue destruction are found in the tissue sections. The glycoprotein extracellular matrix protein 1 (ECM 1) has been targeted as putative autoantigen because the symptoms of the autosomal recessive disorder lipoid proteinosis resemble acquired LSC with thickening and scarring of skin and mucosa [17].

**Angiokeratoma of scrotum**: also known as Angiokeratoma of Fordyce, it is the most common form of angiokeratoma affecting the scrotal skin. It is a distinctive vascular lesion of the scrotum, regarded as a variant distinct from systemic angiokeratoma corporis diffusum. Angiokeratomas are multiple, 1–4 mm in size, soft, and affect middle-aged to elderly patients.

Pathology: Histologic appearance of angiokeratomas includes marked dilatation of the papillary dermal vasculature with acanthosis and elongation of rete ridges forming a collarette circumferentially engulfing vascular lacunae. Thrombi may be present. There is moderate to marked hyperkeratosis and parakeratosis, dermal fibrosis, chronic inflammation, atrophy of the dartos muscle, and degeneration of the elastic tissue [18].

**Scrotal Fat Necrosis**: Fat necrosis of the scrotum usually occurs in obese children and adolescents. It is typically presents in prepubertal boys as a tender scrotal mass inferior and independent of the testis. The lesion can be unilateral but bilateral lesions are not rare. Usually there is no clear history of trauma, but a history of swimming in cold water frequently elicited. There is no associated urinary tract infection, fever, leukocytosis or constitutional symptomatology. Non expectation of the diagnosis frequently has led to scrotal exploration [19]. If the diagnosis is confirmed by ultrasound or clinically; a conservative measure will be sufficient to bring recovery in most cases. Conservative measures include rest, analgesics and avoidance of exposure to cold, which will result in complete resolution within one week. The exact etiology is not well known; but the injury from hypothermia is the result of liberation of lipases, vascular phenomenon or direct damage from the cold are a possible explanations. It has been suggested that the lesion develops when scrotal fat crystallizes following exposure to very low temperature. Some authors allude to chronic mechanical trauma, such as bicycle riding, as a possible cause of such scrotal masses [20].

Pathology: If surgical exploration done to elicit the diagnosis; a firm ill-defined, gray-yellow nodules in the lower portion the scrotal wall, are detectable. Such cases should be differentiated from other conditions such as testicular torsion and epididymo-orchitis (Chap. 23).

**Scrotal ganglioneuromas**: Ganglioneuromas are the most benign of the neuroblastic group of tumours, which include neuroblastoma and ganglioneuroblastoma. They consist of ganglion cells, Schwann cells and connective tissue. The most common locations are the posterior mediastinum and retroperitoneum. Few cases had been reported arising from the scrotum, it is presented as discrete scrotal masses and may cause diagnostic confusion with testicular tumours [21].

**Spindle Cell Nodule** (Inflammatory Myofibroblastic Tumor).

Scrotal myofibroblastic proliferation following trauma, with similar histology to nodular fasciitis, may mimic sarcoma. Clinicopathologic evaluation is mandatory in these cases to avoid misinterpretation (Chap. 25).

**Hidradenitis Suppurativa**: lesion results from obstruction of the drainage system of apocrine and eccrine glands by keratin plugs. Pilosebaceous units become distended, and infected with a variety of bacteria. It is an inflammatory process of apocrine and eccrine glands that are obstructed by follicular hyperkeratosis that extrudes keratin and eccrine and apocrine products and commensal bacteria into dermis then initiating the acute necrotizing and granulomatous reaction [22]. Histologically the lesions show a follicular hyperkeratosis, with apocrine and eccrine glands involvement by acute and chronic inflammation.

**Foreign body lipogranuloma**: This condition results from tissue reaction to the injection of foreign materials like wax, silicone or paraffin into the penoscrotal region. Nodules develop at the site of foreign material placement, sometimes causing marked deformity and it may raising concern for neoplasia. Histologically these nodules are consist of sclerotic fibroconnective tissue with numerous unlined cystic spaces of variable size, with an evidence of a granulomatous tissue reaction.

## 26.3   Scrotal Skin Involvement in Other Dermatosis

Various inflammatory autoimmune diseases (e.g., Behçet's syndrome or Crohn's disease with ulcerations, pyoderma gangraenosum, bullous skin diseases and sarcoidosis) may affect the scrotum.

**Scrotal Sarcoidosis**: Sarcoidosis is a multisystem granulomatous disease of unknown etiology that affects the skin in approximately 25% of patients. Cutaneous lesions manifest in 2 forms: specific and nonspecific. Noncaseating granulomas are considered specific. Nonspecific lesions include erythema nodosum, calcinosis cutis and nail clubbing. The most common sites of specific sarcoidosis lesions include the lips, neck, upper trunk, and extremities [23]. Few cases have reported with cutaneous sarcoidosis involving the genitalia; and rarely the scrotum is affected.

Although there have been reports of sarcoidosis involving the epididymis and testes, which presented as scrotal masses, cutaneous scrotal involvement with the skin as the primary site of involvement is very rare. Cutaneous sarcoidosis generally can precede any systemic involvement, it would be reasonable to consider skin biopsies in patients who present with atypical wart like lesions on the scrotum and penis to rule out sarcoidosis [24].

**Penoscrotal Paget's disease**: Paget's disease (PD) was originally described in mammary sites in 1874 by James Paget, before being described in the male genital region for the first time in 1889 by Crocker. It consists of an initially intra-epidermal adenocarcinoma associated with malignant proliferation of non-keratinocytic epithelial cells known as Paget cells. It can later invade the dermis (invasive PD) and become metastatic [25]. Extramammary PD (EMPD) is rarer and less frequently associated with underlying neoplasia than mammary PD (MPD), where it is found almost systematically. It accounts for only 6.5% of all cases of PD. Among EMPDs, the penoscrotal region forms (14%) and perianal forms (20%). In the 2018 WHO classification of cutaneous adnexal tumours, the EMPD is classed as a "site-specific appendageal tumour" along with MPD, papillary hidradenoma, fibroadenoma, phyllodes tumours and adenocarcinoma of mammary-like anogenital glands [26].

## 26.4 Scrotal Pigmentary Disorders

**Hypopigmentation**: By far the most common color change on the genitalia is the loss of pigment in the form of vitiligo. This pigment loss is quite remarkable in persons with dark complexions and may be overlooked entirely in fair-skinned people. Characteristically it is symmetric in distribution, but it may be seen as white patches on the glans penis. Asymmetric vitiligo is unusual but does occur, often in a dermatomal distribution [27]. Some vitiligo patients have autoimmune thyroid disorders or diabetes, but many have no systemic abnormalities (Fig. 26.8). Treatment should be directed to a dermatologist, but spontaneous repigmentation has been known to occur. Postinflammatory hypopigmentation may be seen after an episode of primary or secondary syphilis, any form of genital ulcer, a dermatophyte infection, or chronic dermatitis or intertrigo.

**Hyperpigmentation**

**Genital melanocytic nevi**: Genital pigmented lesions arise mainly on the vulva, although they may occur less often on the perineum, pubic region, and male genitalia (penis and scrotum). Friedman and Ackerman first described an atypical melanocytic nevus of genital type in a series of seven unusual vulvar nevi [28]. Giant congenital nevi have been defined variously as those larger than 20 cm in diameter, those greater in total area than 120 $cm^2$, or those that cannot be completely excised with primary suture closure in a single operative procedure (Fig. 26.9). This rare variant occur in less than 1 in 20,000 newborns but its impact is great because of considerable cosmetic disfigurement, psychosocial disruption,

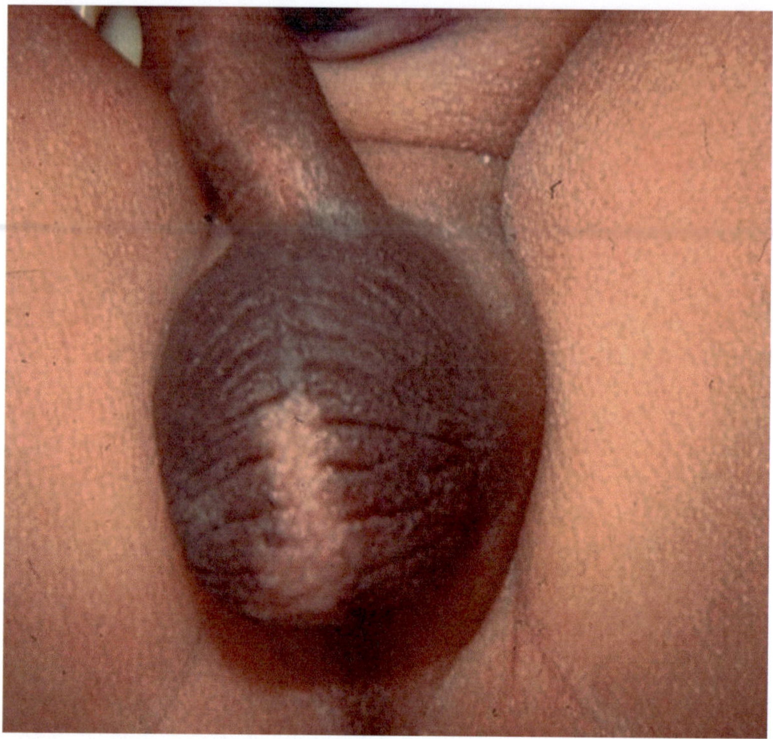

**Fig. 26.8** Congenital scrotal hypopigmentation

and the malignant potential of the lesion [29]. The mode of inheritance of giant pigmented nevi is probably multifactorial. At least 86% of nevi were pigmented and hairy. The lifetime risk of melanoma in patients with a giant congenital nevus is markedly increased and it is about 5% [30]. Very rarely a congenital melanocytic nevus presented as a large scrotal mass [31]. Biopsy remains the mainstay of diagnosis in cases of scrotal lesions along with the aid of immunohistochemistry.

A major challenge is to reconstruct the covering of the penile shaft or the scrotum, for which a large number of surgical techniques and procedures have been reported. The application of a split-thickness skin graft over the penile shaft promotes adequate skin coverage with minimal attenuation of penile sensation. Tissue expansion of the normal skin is another alternative option [32] (Fig. 26.10).

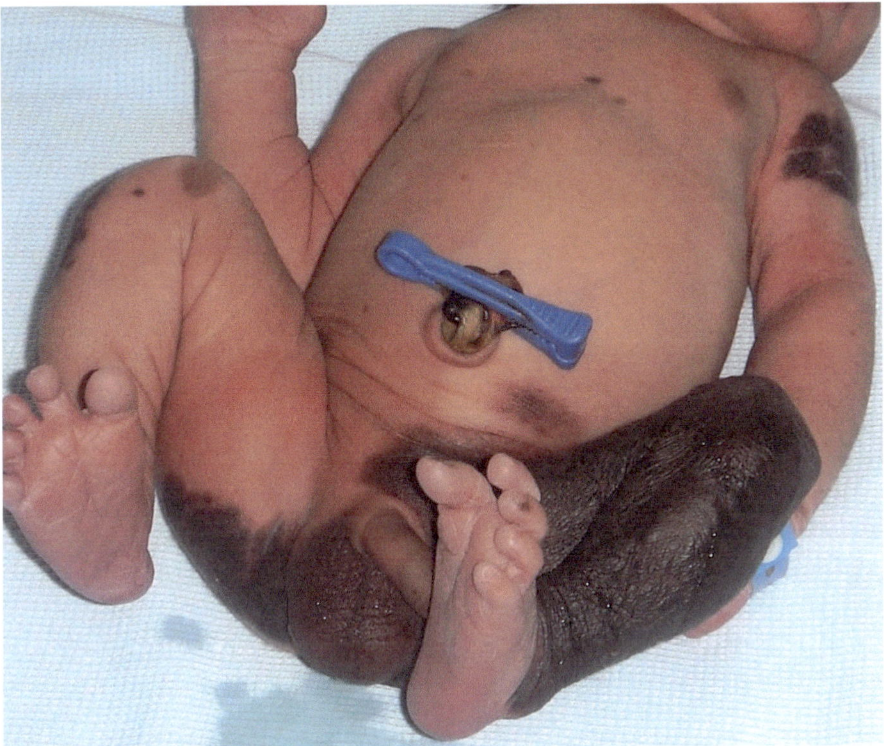

**Fig. 26.9** Giant melanocytic nevus affected the buttocks and the scrotum

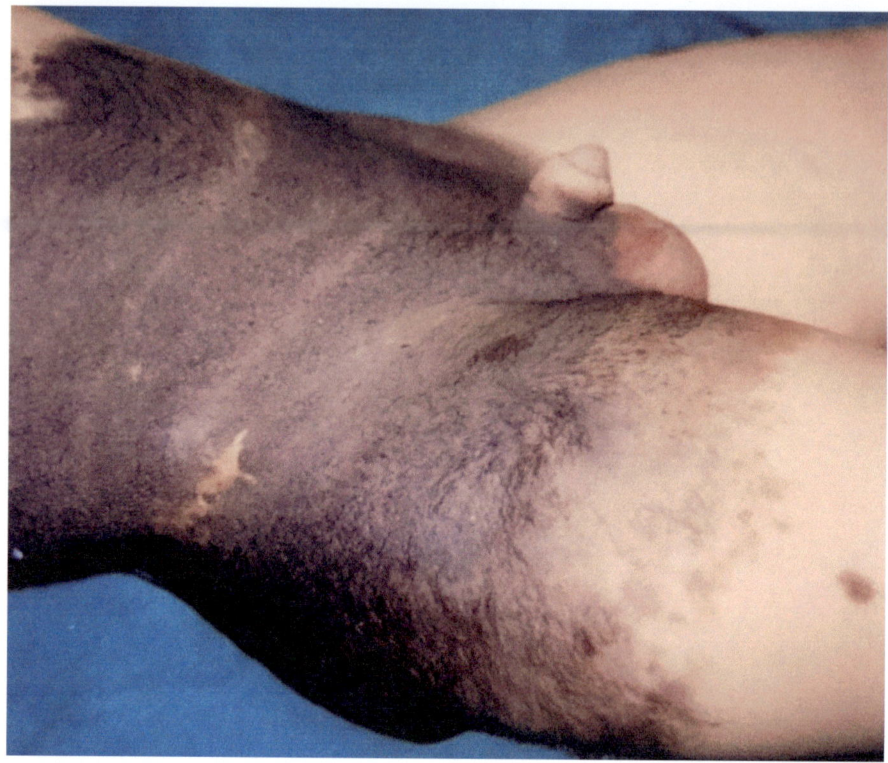

**Fig. 26.10** Giant melanocytic nevus involving most of the trunk, upper thigh and scrotum, managed by serial excision and tissue expansion

# References


1. Hewan-Lowe K, Moreland A, Finnerty DP. Penis and scrotum. In: Someren AE, editor. Urologic pathology with clinical and radiologic correlations. MacMillan Publishing Co.; 1989. p. 613.
2. Zouboulis CC, Chen WC, Thornton MJ, Qin K, Rosenfield R. Sexual hormones in human skin. Horm Metab Res. 2007;39:85–95.
3. Mirastschijski U. Genital scars. In: Téot L, Mustoe TA, Middelkoop E, Gauglitz GG, editors. Textbook on scar management. Cham: Springer; 2020. https://doi.org/10.1007/978-3-030-44766-3_47.
4. Mirhashemi S, Soori M, Faghih G, Peyvandi H, Shafagh O. Scrotal abscess: a rare presentation of complicated necrotizing pancreatitis. Arch Iran Med. 2017;20(2):0–0.
5. Bahadur A, Singh N, Kashmira M, Shukla A, Gupta V, Jain S. Fecal scrotal abscess secondary to spontaneous retroperitoneal perforation of ascending colon. Case Rep Med. 2021.
6. Aldohuky W, Mohammed AA. Scrotal abscess as a manifestation of posterior duodenal perforation; a very rare presentation. Urol Case Rep. 2019;27:101010.
7. Magalhaes BM, Veasey JV, Mayor SAS, Lellis RF. Donovanosis in a child victim of sexual abuse: response to doxycycline treatment. An Bras Dermatol. 2018;93(4):592–4.

8. Purwoko MIH, Devi M, Nugroho SA. Granuloma inguinale. Biosci Med J Biomed Transl Res. 2021;5(3):659–68.
9. Medeiros-Fonseca B, Mestre VF, Estêvão D, Sánchez DF, Cañete-Portillo S, Fernández-Nestosa MJ, Casaca F, et al. HPV16 induces penile intraepithelial neoplasia and squamous cell carcinoma in transgenic mice: first mouse model for HPV-related penile cancer. J Pathol. 2020;251(4):411–9.
10. Passos MRL. Infection with human papillomavirus (HPV). In: Atlas of sexually transmitted diseases. Cham: Springer; 2018. p. 239–319.
11. Mohsin SK, Lee MW, Amin MB, Stoler MH, Eyzaguirre E, Ma CK, Zarbo RJ. Cutaneous verruciform xanthoma: a report of five cases investigating the etiology and nature of xanthomatous cells. Am J Surg Pathol. 1998;22(4):479–87.
12. Surani A, Marfatia Y, Bavariya R. Multiple pruritic plaques on scrotum-what is your diagnosis? Indian J Sex Trans Dis AIDS. 2018; 39(2):141–2. https://doi.org/10.4103/ijstd.IJSTD_82_18.
13. Clouston D, Hall A, Lawrentschuk N. Penile lichen sclerosus (balanitis xerotica obliterans). BJU Int. 2011;108(Suppl 2):14–9.
14. Singh I, Ansari MS. Extensive balanitis xerotica obliterans (BXO) involving the anterior urethra and scrotum. Int Urol Nephrol. 2006;38(3):505–6. https://doi.org/10.1007/s11255-006-0100-8.
15. Kumar S, Nagappa B, Ganesamoniv R. Extensive balanitis xerotica obliterans of urethro-cutaneous fistula presenting as mass in scrotum. Urology. 2010;76(2):332–3.
16. Herschorn S, Colapinto V. Balanitis xerotica obliterans involving anterior urethra. Urology. 1979;14(6):592–6.
17. Saccucci M, Di Carlo G, Bossu M, Giovarruscio F, Salucci A, Polimeni A. Autoimmune diseases and their manifestations on oral cavity: diagnosis and clinical management. J Immunol Res. 2018;2018:6061825.
18. Hoekx L, Wyndaele J. Angiokeratoma: a cause of scrotal bleeding. Acta Urol Belg. 1998;66:27–8.
19. Hollander JB, Begun FP, Lee RD. Scrotal fat necrosis. J Urol. 1985;134(1):150–1. https://doi.org/10.1016/s0022-5347(17)47035-2.
20. Peterson LJ, Whitlock NW, Odom RB, Ramirez RE, Stutzman RE, Mcaninch JW. Bilateral fat necrosis of the scrotum. J Urol. 1976;116(6):825–6. https://doi.org/10.1016/s0022-5347(17)59033-3.
21. Thwalni A, Kumar R, Shergill I. Ganglioneuromas in the adult scrotum. J R Soc Med. 2005;98(6):295–295.
22. Maclennan GT, Cheng L. Penis and scrotum. In: Atlas of genitourinary pathology. London: Springer; 2010. https://doi.org/10.1007/978-1-84882-395-2_8.
23. Al Hajjaj SA, Rünger TM, Chung HJ. Flesh-colored papules on the scrotum. Cutis. 2019;104(3):E23–5.
24. McLaughlin SS, Linquist AM, Burnett JW. Cutaneous sarcoidosis of the scrotum: a rare manifestation of systemic disease. Acta Derm Venereol. 2002;82:216–7.
25. Kanitakis J. Mammary and extramammary Paget's disease. J Eur Acad Dermatol Venereol. 2007;21:581–90.
26. Elder DE, Massi D, Scolyer RA, Willemze R, editors. WHO classification of skin tumours, 4th ed. Lyon, France: IARC; 2018. p. 66–71. World Health Organization Classification of Tumours; vol. 11.
27. Taieb A, Picardo M. Vitiligo. N Engl J Med. 2009;360:2160–9.
28. Friedman RJ, Ackerman AB. Difficulties in the histologic diagnosis of melanocytic nevi on the vulvae of premenopausal women. In: Pathology of malignant melanoma. New York: Masson; 1981. p. 119.
29. Wyatt AJ, Hansen RC. Pediatric skin tumors. Pediatr Clin North Am. 2000;47(4):937–63.
30. Ruiz-Maldonado R, Tamayo L, Laterza AM, Durán C. Giant pigmented nevi: clinical, histopathologic, and therapeutic considerations. J Pediatr. 1992;120(6):906–11.

31. Elkiran YM, Abdelmaksoud MA, Abdelgawwad MS, Elsaadany NA, Elshafei AM. Giant scrotal swelling in association with a congenital giant melanocytic nevus: a case report. JPRAS Open. 2020;26:80–5.
32. Baky Fahmy MA, Mazy A. The feasibility of tissue expanders in reconstruction of giant congenital melanocytic nevi in children. Surg Innov. 2010;17(3):189–94. https://doi.org/10.1177/1553350610371627.

# Chapter 27
# Scrotal Imaging

Michal Yaela Schechter, Erik Van Laecke, and Anne-Françoise Spinoit

**Abbreviations**

| | |
|---|---|
| CT | Computed tomography |
| CEUS | Abdominal contrast-enhanced ultrasound |
| GCNIS | Germ cell neoplasia in situ |
| GCT | Germ cell tumor |
| MRI | Magnetic resonance imaging |
| NSGCT | Non-seminomatous germ cell tumor |
| SCST | Sex cord-stromal tumor |
| US | Ultrasound |

## 27.1  Introduction to Scrotal Imaging

The scrota contain complex anatomical, vascular, lymphatic, and innervation systems which aid its multiple functionalities including reproduction, thermoregulation, and endocrine hormone production. Clinical examination is critical for proper evaluation of the scrotum and may be aided by imaging, particularly when physical exam findings are equivocal.

Basic scrotal imaging involves the following modalities: Ultrasound (US), Doppler, Magnetic Resonance Imaging (MRI), and Computed Tomography (CT). Each technique is different in terms of the images it gathers, equipment required, and the conditions it may be used in.

US imaging, also called a sonogram, is one of the safest forms of medical imaging, and is quite cost-effective as well. It uses high-frequency sound waves

Michal Y. Schechter is fully funded by the Gianni Eggermont fund for advancement of research in Pediatric Urology.

M. Y. Schechter · E. Van Laecke · A.-F. Spinoit (✉)
Department of Urology, Ghent University Hospital, ERN eUROGEN Accredited Centre, Ghent, Belgium

which reflect off soft tissue to generate images of organs and other bodily structures. A subset of ultrasound imaging is known as doppler imaging, which uses sound waves to allow visualization of blood flow in arterial and venous vasculature.

CT imaging uses serial X-rays to produce 3D images of bones, organs, blood vessels, and other soft tissues within the body. While these scans were created to provide more detailed images than conventional X-rays, they also produce more radiation and are therefore limited in their use in children. However, the ongoing evolution of CT imaging has since created better imaging with limited radiation doses, and these improvements are expected to further develop in the future.

MRI scans are one of the highest quality imaging modalities available. These scans use a strong magnetic field along with radio waves to create 3D images of the body and realize differences in tissue that would not otherwise be seen with a CT scan. MRI is similar to CT in that they can both create cross-sectional imaging of the body but is different in that MRI does not use harmful radiation. MR imaging can also create higher quality images than CT, enabling it to better highlight differences in tissues. However, an MRI takes a considerably longer amount of time to scan than does a CT and is more expensive.[1]

Indications for imaging include scrotal abnormalities, pain, trauma, masses, infertility, and follow-up. As the scrota and its contents are relatively superficial, an ultrasound scan can produce quite detailed and accurate information and is therefore the primary imaging technique used for scrotal evaluation after initial clinical examination. Typical adults have a scrotal thickness of about 2–8 mm, with each testis measuring 3–5 cm in diameter and about 20 mL in volume.[2] Testicular volume evolves with pediatric growth curves, with a linear increase in volume related to pubertal physical growth and usually considered to be the first sign of the puberty.

Normal ultrasound findings show the testis as a structure with homogenous echogenicity containing a mildly coarse echotexture. The tunica vaginalis and albuginea appear as an echogenic outline of the testis, and the mediastinum testis is visualized as a linear echogenic invagination of the tunica albuginea. A minority of patients have an identifiable rete testis which can form a hypoechoic region near the mediastinum. The epididymis appears isoechoic or mildly hyperechoic relative to the testis. On doppler imaging, the testis and epididymis demonstrate a low-resistance arterial velocity. The appendix testis and appendix epididymis are not usually noticeable unless paratesticular fluid is present.

MRI is the imaging method of choice when US characterization of the lesion is insufficient. CT scans are performed less frequently than MRI and are mainly used for testicular neoplasm staging and treatment follow-up. MR Imaging of normal scrota demonstrates intermediate testicular signal intensity on T1-weighted images, with a low signal intensity of the tunica albuginea and a heterogenous and isointense epididiymis relative to the testis. On T2-weighted images, normal testes have high signal intensity with low signal intensity of the tunica albuginea, as well as a hypointense epididymis, making this the best MRI format for epididymal visualization and differentiation from the adjacent testis. Contrast-enhanced scrotal MRI

**Fig. 27.1** Normal scrotal US with mediastinum testis (arrow) visualized as a linear echogenic band[3]

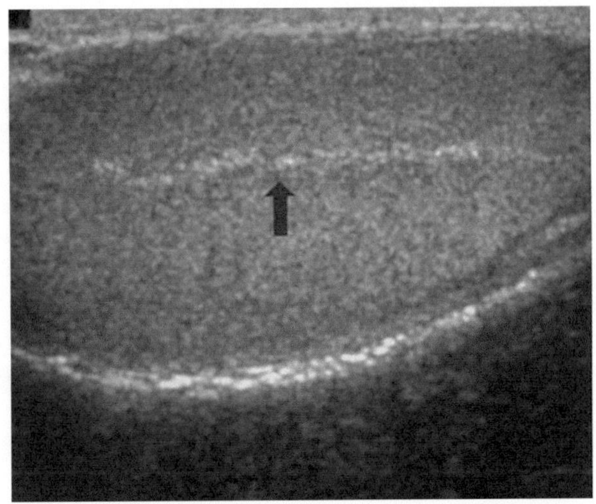

demonstrates homogenous testicular enhancement and can best show the rete testis radiating from the mediastinum testis to the tunical surface.

When imaging a scrotum it is critical to also assess the contralateral scrotum, both for ensuring that it is not pathologic and because the comparison between the scrotum may aid in evaluation of the scrotum in question (Figs. 27.1 and 27.2).

## 27.2 Acute Scrotum

Cases of acute scrotum include acute epididymitis/epididymo-orchitis, testicular torsion, appendiceal torsion, and trauma. The first step in evaluation of acute scrotum is performance of an US. Acute scrotum may also include Fournier gangrene.

**Infection**

Infection is the most common cause of an acute scrotum, and can include the epididymis (epididymitis), testis (orchitis), or if the infection spreads it can include both the epididymis and the testis (epididymo-orchitis).

Acute epididymitis typically appears on US as an enlarged hypo/hyperechoic epididymis along with heterogenous echogenicity secondary to diffuse testicular spread of the infection. While these findings are nonspecific, epididymo-orchitis is the most common disease with these combined findings on US. Cases may also exhibit indirect signs of inflammation such as scrotal wall thickening and reactive hydrocele.

The discerning urologist should keep in mind that a heterogenous testicular echotexture is not pathognomonic to epididymo-orchitis. Although neoplastic

**Fig. 27.2** Normal scrotal
T2-weighted MRI, with
hypointense epididymis
(arrowhead)[4]

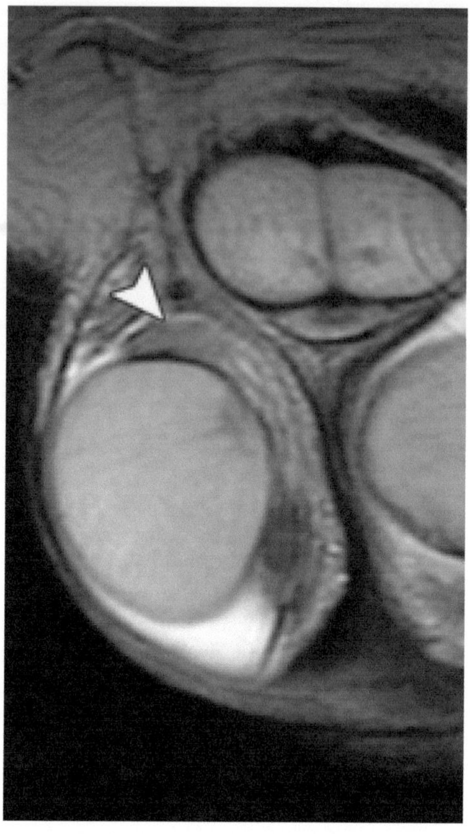

lesions are usually found in one testis while infection may be unilateral or bilateral, cases of testicular leukemia and lymphoma may have a similar appearance on US to epididymo-orchitis. As heterogeneous echogenicity does not always indicate scrotal infection, suspected cases should be monitored with a follow up US after their resolution to rule out neoplasms or infarctions.

The hallmark of doppler in epididymo-orchitis is increased blood flow, consistent with hyperemia of the epididymis, testis, or both. As grey-scale US findings can be within normal limits in cases of testicular infection and doppler has a nearly 100% sensitivity for scrotal inflammation detection, hyperemia in Doppler US can be used as a diagnostic tool in epididymo-orchitis cases.[5] Careful comparison with the contralateral asymptomatic testis is important to ensure that the doppler imaging is properly working to detect blood flow (Fig. 27.3).

## Testicular Torsion

Testicular torsion is considered a medical emergency of testicular ischemia, attributable to venous obstruction followed by arterial obstruction. The terminal nature

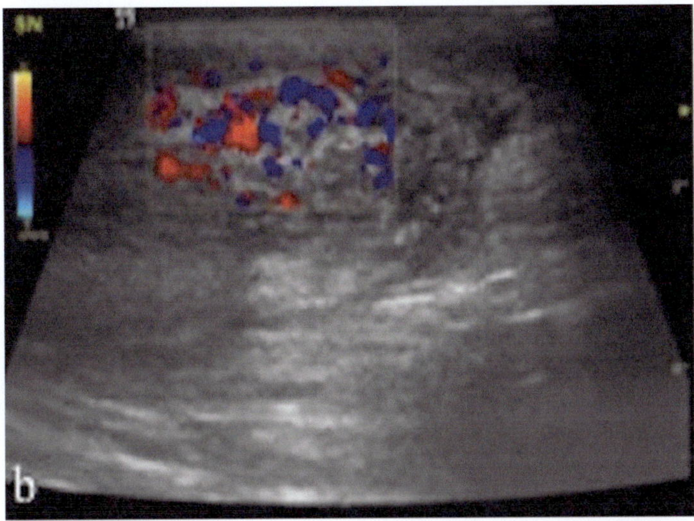



**Fig. 27.3** Acute epididymitis on doppler US, showing a heterogeneous echotexture with increased blood flow[6]

of testicular vascularization as outlined in the anatomy of scrotum chapter is critical for the development of torsion of the testis.

Two incidence peaks have been described, correlating with two different types of torsion: Extravaginal testicular torsion in neonates and intravaginal testicular torsion typically occurring in adolescents. Extravaginal torsion is caused when the tunica vaginalis is not affixed to the gubernaculum, increasing torsion risk of both the tunica vaginalis and the spermatic cord. Neonates with this condition typically present at birth with an already infarcted and necrotic testis. Intravaginal torsion occurs within the tunica vaginalis and often affects adolescents with bell-clapper deformity, a condition in which the tunica vaginalis attaches at a point higher than the posterolateral testis, allowing the spermatic cord to twist inside.

The diagnosis of testicular torsion is mostly clinical. If additional investigation is needed, an US should be performed urgently as the testicular salvage rate is dependent not only on the degree of torsion, but also on the duration of vascular congestion and ischemia. A 90–100% salvage rate with performance of detorsion exists within the first 6 hours after onset of symptoms, a 20–50% rate within 12–24 hours, and a 0–10% rate after 24 hours.[7]

Cases of suspected testicular torsion should be evaluated with a doppler study, the hallmark of which is an absence of intratesticular blood flow. This single criterion is 86% sensitive and 100% specific for a torsion diagnosis.[8] In some cases, paratesticular flow in epididymal collaterals also appears within hours of the onset of torsion. As with cases of testicular infection, careful comparison with the contralateral asymptomatic testis is important to ensure that the doppler imaging is properly working to detect blood flow.

The doppler component of the ultrasound is especially critical as grey-scale US findings are nonspecific for torsion and are often normal in the early phases of torsion. At 4–6 hours post onset of torsion, a common grey-scale US finding is testicular swelling and decreased echogenicity. Infarction can alter testicular echogenicity and is therefore used to help predict testicular viability. A case of late or missed torsion (24 hours post onset) is typically visible as an increasingly heterogenous testicular echotexture. Other US findings in torsion cases may include an enlarged hypoechoic epididymal head (secondary to torsion of the deferential artery which feeds the epididymis), an abnormally round or oval homogenous spermatic cord caudal to the point of torsion (secondary to twisting of the spermatic cord at the level of the superficial inguinal ring), and indirect signs of inflammation similarly found in testicular infection.[9]

Recently, near infrared spectroscopy has shown promising results in experimentation for testicular torsion diagnosis. It can provide a quicker diagnosis than a doppler and it measures the testicular $O_2$ saturation which can be more useful than the blood flow as measured by a doppler.[10] It remains to be seen whether this imaging modality will be widely implemented (Fig. 27.4).

## Trauma

Scrotal trauma can include testicular rupture, fracture, or hematomas. US is used in these cases to help inform which scrotal injuries warrant surgical intervention. Abdominal contrast-enhanced ultrasound (CEUS) is a form of US imaging that uses gas-filled microbubbles to better visualize abdominal and pelvic organs and blood vessels and can provide superior results to both grey-scale US and CT. It may be used as a rapid imaging modality in emergency cases that require more accurate identification of viable tissue to determine if surgical intervention is warranted.

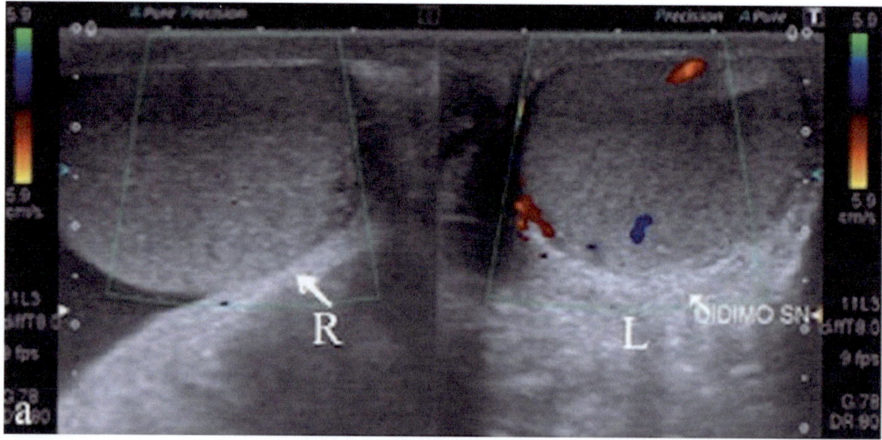

**Fig. 27.4** Testicular torsion on doppler US, showing absence of flow in the R testis as opposed to the L testis[11]

A testicular rupture is a surgical emergency that occurs when a tear in the tunica albuginea allows for extrusion of testicular contents. Exploratory surgery performed within 72 hours after the trauma can save up to 90% of ruptured testes. It should be noted that the tunica albuginea and the tunica vasculosa are situated right next to each other, so rupture of the tunica albuginea often also causes vascular loss to the testis due to the concurrent rupture of the tunica vasculosa. The main US findings include a heterogeneous testicular echotexture with irregular poorly defined borders due to hemorrhage and necrosis, contour abnormality due to testicular parenchyma extrusion, disruption of the tunica albuginea, and a large hematocele. The first two US findings of testicular heterogeneity with contour abnormality have a sensitivity of 100% and a specificity of 93.5%. Doppler US can demonstrate disruption of the normal blood flow of the tunica vasculosa (Fig. 27.5).[12]

Another scrotal surgical emergency is testicular fracture, which refers to a break in the normal testicular parenchyma that appears on US as a linear hypoechoic and vascular area within the testicular parenchyma. While it may be associated with a ruptured tunica albuginea and therefore become a case of testicular rupture, a fracture without rupture is contained within the testicular parenchyma. US doppler is critical in delineating the extent of viable tissue to determine salvageability and management. However, direct visualization of a fracture line is uncommon. When conventional ultrasound findings are equivocal, CEUS can both better define

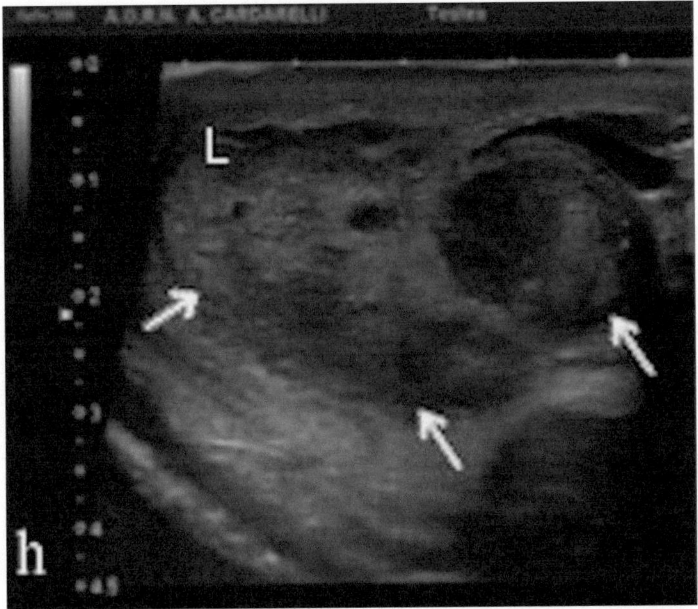

**Fig. 27.5** Testicular rupture on US, with heterogenous echotexture and contour abnormality (arrows)[13]

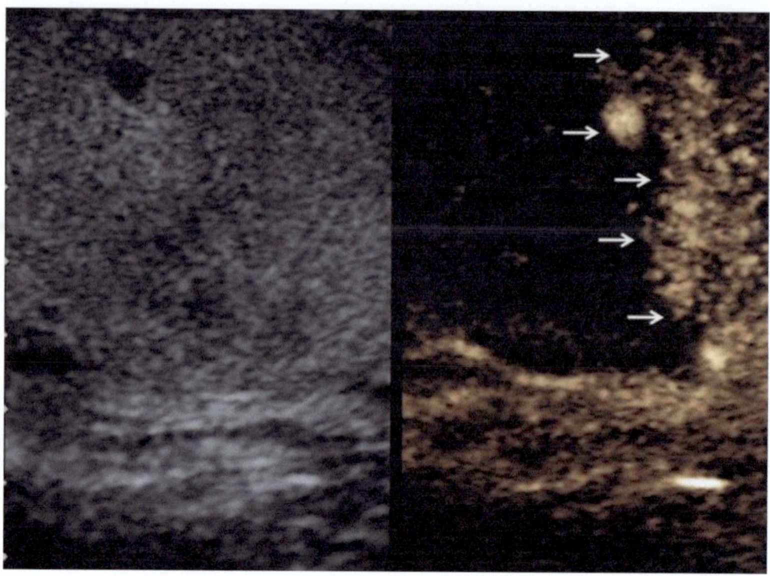

**Fig. 27.6** Testicular fracture on US (left) and CEUS (right), with a clear demarcation between vascularized and non-vascularized tissue (arrows)[15]

fracture lines and differentiate between enhancing viable vascularized tissue and nonenhancing nonvascularized tissue (Fig. 27.6).[14]

Post-traumatic testicular hematomas may present as intratesticular hematomas, extratesticular hematomas in the epididymis and scrotal wall, or as hematoceles (hematomas between the visceral and parietal layers of the tunica vaginalis). US appearance of hematomas varies with time. Acute hematomas on US appear more hyperechoic and may have a diffusely heterogenous mixture, but as these hematomas become chronic and resolve, they decrease in their echogenicity and size and become more complex with cystic components. On doppler, intratesticular hematomas appear as focal areas of avascularity (Fig. 27.7).[16]

There are a few caveats in the management of a suspected acute hematoma. If an acute hematoma is suspected but imaging is negative, repeat imaging should be performed within 12–24 hours after the initial US evaluation, as the initial echotexture of a hematoma may be indistinguishable from the surrounding parenchyma.

As mentioned earlier, the testicular parenchyma underlies the tunica albuginea and an injury to one structure very often means an injury to the other as well. However, a heterogeneous intratesticular lesion may appear in cases of intratesticular hematomas without testicular rupture. These cases require imaging, in particular a CEUS, to better assess if surgical exploration for testicular rupture is warranted.

Finally, about 10–15% of testicular tumors first manifest and are incidentally discovered after scrotal trauma.[18] This is likely because testicular tumors are the

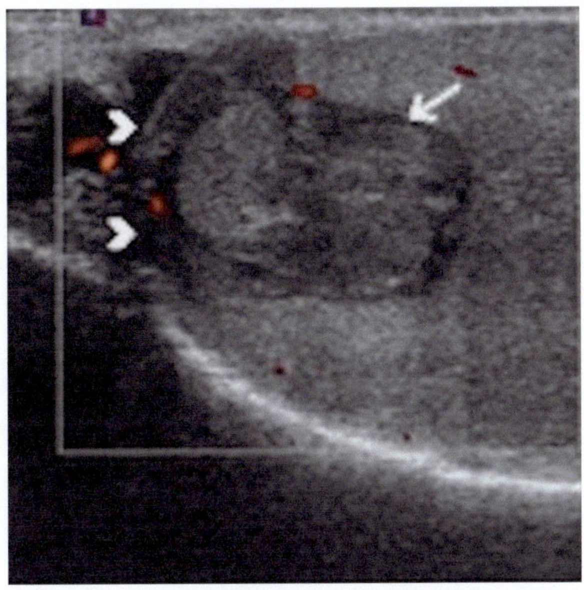

**Fig. 27.7** Intratesticular hematoma on doppler US, with an avascularized, hypoechoic, and heterogenous echotexture (arrows) with an intact tunica vaginalis (arrowheads)[17]

most common solid malignancy in 15–35-year-old males, and the highest incidence of traumatic injury is in that age group. Testicular tumors often appear similarly to hematomas, and in cases of trauma it can be difficult to differentiate between lesions. Therefore, cases with abnormal intratesticular US readings without immediate surgical intervention should be followed up with a repeat US to rule out malignancy, as over time scrotal hematomas are expected to shrink and scrotal masses are expected to grow. If US findings are equivocal, MRI may be used for a more conclusive diagnosis.

## Appendiceal Torsion

US evaluation of torsion of the appendix testis or appendix epididymis is useful in terms of excluding testicular torsion and acute epididymo-orchitis. A classic physical examination finding in cases of appendiceal torsion is the "blue dot sign", referring to a small firm nodule palpable on the upper pole of the testis presenting as a bluish discoloration through the overlying skin. US typically shows a hypo or hyperechoic mass in comparison to the echotexture of the adjacent testis or epididymis, and these findings are often associated with a reactive hydrocele and scrotal skin thickening. Color doppler with no internal blood flow and increased peri-appendiceal peripheral flow is highly suggestive of appendiceal torsion (Fig. 27.8).[19]

## Fournier Gangrene

Fournier gangrene is a fulminant necrotizing fasciitis caused by mixed aerobic and anaerobic bacteria that frequently extends to the perineal, perianal, and lower abdominal wall regions. This condition typically presents in adults with high

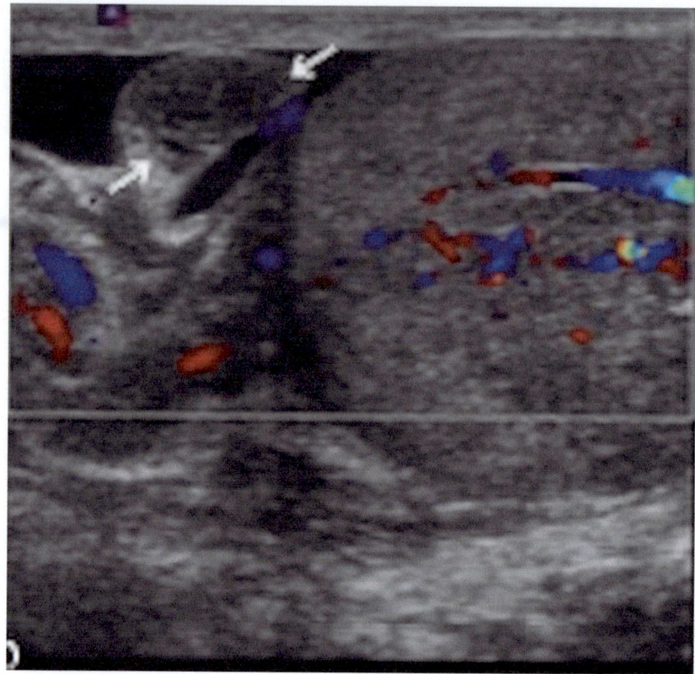

**Fig. 27.8** Appendiceal torsion on doppler US, with an enlarged and avascularized mass (arrows)[20]

comorbidities such as diabetes, obesity, and alcoholism. As rapid progression of tissue necrosis can lead to multiorgan failure and a mortality rate of up to 75%,[21] this condition constitutes a urologic emergency necessitating prompt diagnosis and initiation of surgical debridement and antibiotics. Fournier gangrene is a clinical diagnosis and treatment should not be delayed for imaging confirmation unless exam findings are ambiguous. Characteristic crepitus can present at physical exam in 19–64% of patients.[22]

Imaging techniques include US and CT in determining the location and cause of scrotal gas when clinical signs cannot produce a definitive diagnosis. CT is the preferred modality of imaging and demonstrates soft tissue thickening, fat stranding, and subcutaneous emphysema dissecting the fascial layers. Although US is not considered first-line imaging in suspected cases, it can still help with early disease recognition in emergency department settings. The hallmark of Fournier gangrene on US is multiple hyperechoic and hyperreflective foci with posterior acoustic dirty shadowing relating to the underlying subcutaneous gases within the scrotal wall. Other US findings include scrotal wall swelling and thickening, with doppler showing increased blood flow in the affected area (Fig. 27.9).

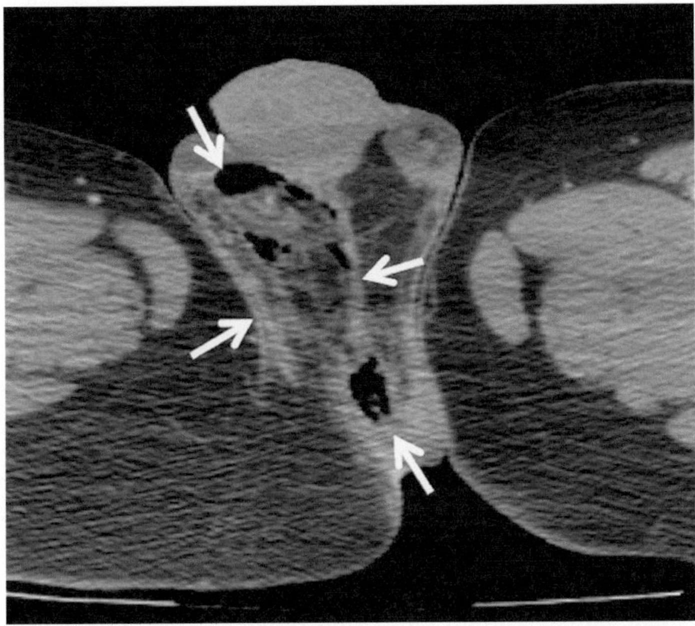

**Fig. 27.9** Fournier gangrene on CT, with inflammation and gaseous changes in the scrotal wall (arrows)[23]

## 27.3   Scrotal Masses

The initial classification of a scrotal mass as intratesticular or extratesticular is important because intratesticular masses are considered cancerous until proven otherwise, while extratesticular masses are rarely malignant (3%).[24] US is the primary imaging modality used to assess the location of scrotal masses, with the possibility of vascularity assessment through use of doppler. When US findings are indeterminate, MR imaging can act as an adjunctive diagnostic tool and help localize the lesion as well as evaluate for local tumor extension and regional spread. CT imaging is used to assess the presence of metastases and determine tumor resectability. CT also plays a pivotal role in tumor surveillance and evaluation of response to treatment.

Extratesticular cysts appear similarly to intratesticular cysts on US and doppler. The differentiation of intra and extratesticular cysts does not have clinical significance, and purely cystic cancers are extremely rare.

## 27.3.1 Extratesticular Masses

The variety of scrotal structures surrounding the testicle can give rise to several types of extratesticular masses. Malignant neoplasms are rare and can include rhabdomyosarcomas, leiomyosarcomas, and liposarcomas. The more commonly found benign neoplasms are lipomas, adenomatoid tumors, and leiomyomas. Extratesticular cysts include epididymal cystic masses and hydroceles. Another form of an extratesticular benign mass is an inguinal hernia.

### Rhabdomyosarcoma, Leiomyosarcoma, and Liposarcoma

Rhabdomyosarcoma is a pediatric malignancy which has nonspecific findings on MRI. It typically presents as an encapsulated gray-white mass with focal areas of hemorrhage and cystic degeneration and cannot be well-differentiated from other malignant or benign extratesticular neoplasms. Leiomyosarcoma appears on US and CT as a heterogenous enhancing mass and can be evaluated for tumor spread with MRI. Due to its fat content, liposarcoma has nonspecific hyperechoic findings on US but CT and MRI can be used to better determine its presence and show well-defined macroscopic fat masses (Fig. 27.10).

### Lipoma, Adenomatoid Tumor, and Leiomyoma

Lipomas are the most common extratesticular non-malignant neoplasm. They appear on US as well-defined homogenous hyperechoic masses and are absent of blood flow on doppler. Adenomatoid tumors are visualized on US as well-defined hypoechoic masses with variable doppler flow. Leiomyomas are rare and present on US as solid iscoechoic lesions with shadowing at transition zones.[26]

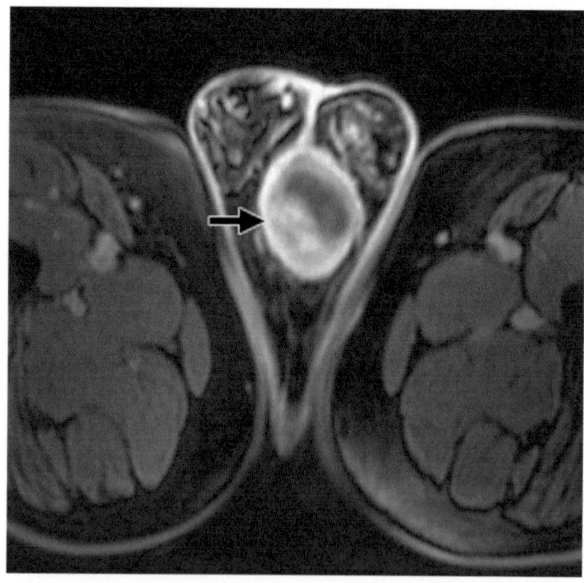

**Fig. 27.10** Liposarcoma of the spermatic cord on T1-weighted MRI, showing as an enhanced scrotal mass (arrow)[25]

## Epididymal Cystic Masses

Epididymal masses can be further categorized into a single epididymal cyst or a spermatocele, which is a cystic dilation of the tubular efferent ductules in the head of the epididymis. Single epididymal cysts are made up of clear serous fluid, while spermatoceles can be multilocular and contain proteinaceous fluid and spermatozoa. It should be noted that all cysts lack internal vascularity on doppler. These two subtypes appear as well-defined, homogeneous, hypoechoic lesions with posterior acoustic enhancement on US. Although imaging cannot be used to accurately distinguish one from another, this does not present a challenge as these conditions usually do not have clinical relevance.

## Hydrocele

Hydroceles are the most common cause of painless scrotal swelling and can present either as congenital lesions due to a patent processus vaginalis or in their adult form which may be associated with underlying scrotal pathology. This diagnosis is confirmed by an US exam where they are visualized as anechoic fluid collections around the anterolateral testis (Fig. 27.11).

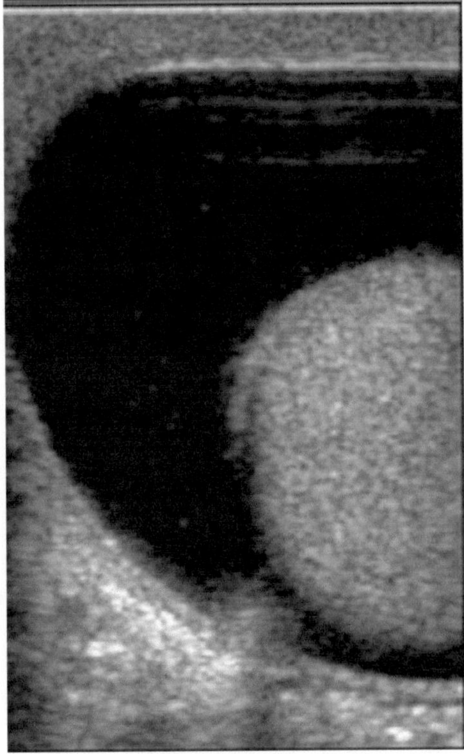

**Fig. 27.11** Hydrocele on US, showing as a peritesticular fluid collection[27]

**Inguinal Hernia**

Inguinal hernias typically consist of bowel or omentum. Bowel hernia appearance is dependent on bowel content. US imaging showing specular reflection within fluid indicates bowel containing fluid, while bowels containing air or solid stool appear with a bright echotexture. US also allows for visualization of peristalsis within the bowel hernia, thus establishing the diagnosis. Omental hernias can be visualized on US as paratesticular masses with diffuse echotextures due to their fat content.[28]

## 27.3.2  Intratesicular Masses

Intratesticular scrotal masses include testicular neoplasms and cysts. Testicular cancer is the most common neoplasm found in men aged 15–40 years old. It accounts for 1–2% of all neoplasms in males. Testicular cancer can also present in the pediatric population, in particular during the neonatal period and puberty, accounting for 2–4% of childhood cancers.[30]

Testicular tumors may arise from germ cells, sex cord-stroma, or lymph, and are classified based on their origins. 90–95% of testicular tumors are germ cell tumors (GCTs), which are further categorized based on the most recent 2016 WHO classification system regarding their derivation status from germ cell neoplasia in situ (GCNIS). The classification system of testicular tumors is critical as it guides their treatment and determines the prognosis. It includes testicular GCTs derived from GCNIS, testicular GCTs not derived from GCNIS, non-germ cell testicular tumors: sex cord-stromal tumors, and hemato-lymphoid tumors. It should be noted that GCNIS tumors have a tendency for invasion and have been found in the contralateral testis in up to 8% of patients with GCNIS.[32] Overall, GCNIS tumors are more typically found in the adult population as opposed to the pediatric population, and vice-versa for non-GCNIS tumors which are more common in children. There is growing evidence that testicular prepubertal tumors and postpubertal tumors differ both in terms of clinical features and prognosis.

Intratesticular cysts include cysts of the tunica albuginea, tubular ectasia of the rete testis, and testicular cysts. Another type of testicular mass includes testicular microlithiasis.

When combined with a clinical examination, US has been shown to have a nearly 100% sensitivity in diagnosis of testicular cancer.[33] Doppler can show hypervascularity in the majority of cases involving malignant tumors, but an absence of blood flow cannot be used for exclusion of malignancy as it is more difficult to demonstrate increased vascularity in small tumors. Although MRI does not have a clear diagnostic benefit in testicular cancer as compared to US, it is helpful in cases where US findings are equivocal. MRI can help differentiate seminomatous GCTs from their nonseminomatous counterparts by demonstrating seminomatous GCTs as homogenously T2 hypo- and T1 isointense masses along with internal T2 hypointense bands which enhance more than the tumor.

Non-seminomatous GCTs present with T1 and T2 heterogeneous appearance on MRI and may be associated with a T2 hypointense fibrous pseudocapsule.

## Testicular GCTs Derived from GCNIS

This classification includes pure seminoma along with non-seminomatous (NSGCT) tumors such as embryonal carcinoma, choriocarcinoma, postpubertal type teratoma, and regressed GCTs. While NSGCTs are typically found in pure form in the pediatric population, adult NSGCTs often present as mixed GCTs and contain two or more different histological GCT components. Mixed GCTs appear on US as ill-defined masses with a heterogenous echotexture and possible echogenic foci.

## Seminoma

Pure seminomas make up about 50% of all testicular GCTs. Sonographically, seminomas appear as homogenous hypoechoic solid lesions and rarely invade paratesticular tissues. If multilobulated, they show increased blood flow on doppler along their echogenic fibrinous septae (Fig. 27.12).

## Embryonal Carcinoma

Embryonal carcinoma is an aggressive tumor which extends into the extratesticular space and distorts the contour of the testis in about 25% of cases.[35] US imaging typically shows ill-defined predominantly hypoechoic lesions with widespread necrosis, hemorrhage, and fibrosis (Fig. 27.13).

## Choriocarcinoma

Choriocarcinoma is a highly malignant tumor composed of both cytotrophoblasts and syncytiotrophoblasts and represents the form of testicular cancer with the highest mortality. It has a propensity for early vascular invasion leading to hematogenous dissemination, particularly to the lungs. On US, choriocarcinoma appears as a solitary mass or multifocal ill-defined heterogenous masses with mixed

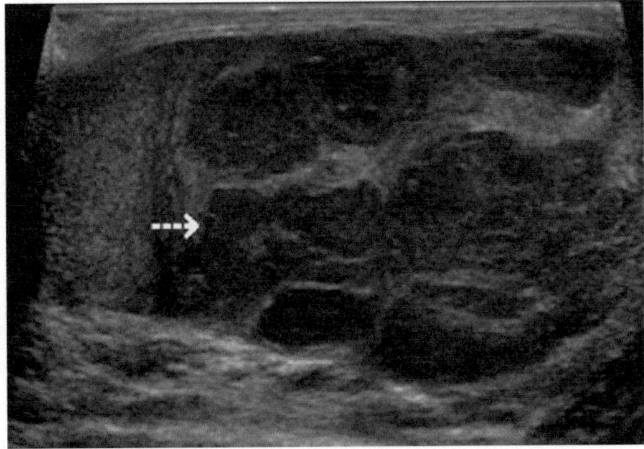

**Fig. 27.12** Pure seminoma on US, with multilobulated hypoechoic masses separated by fibrinous septae (dotted arrow)[34]

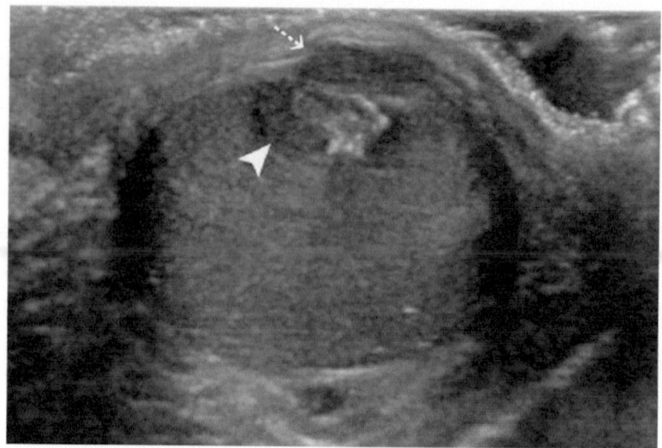

**Fig. 27.13** Embryonal carcinoma on US, showing extension into the extratesticular space (dotted arrow)[36]

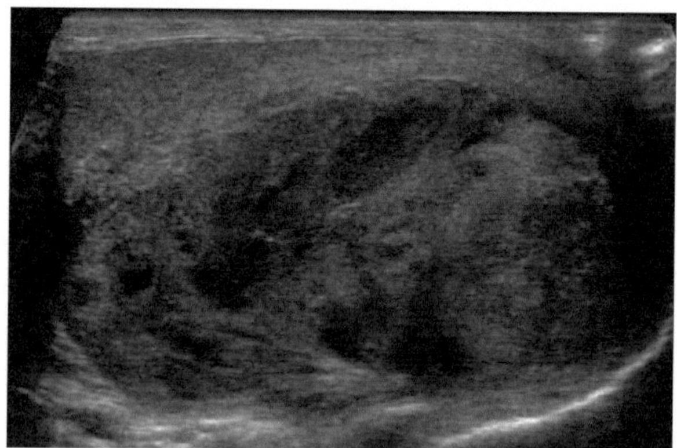

**Fig. 27.14** Choriocarcinoma on US, showing an ill-defined heterogenous solid mass with necrosis[37]

cystic and solid components due to hemorrhagic necrosis in the center of the tumor (Fig. 27.14).

## Postpubertal-Type Teratoma

Postpubertal type teratoma is more common than the prepubertal type, and unlike the prepubertal type it is often malignant. Teratomas are composed of fetal tissue derived from all three germ cell layers (ectoderm, mesoderm, and endoderm) and present sonographically as large complex heterogenous masses with focal echogenic lesions. These lesions can represent cysts, fibrosis, calcifications, immature bone, and cartilage (Fig. 27.15).

## Burned-Out GCTs

Burned-out GCTs represent tumors with a high metabolism, resulting in outgrowth of their blood supply and tumor regression. Appearance on US varies from a hypoechoic mass to small echogenic foci. These masses are typically discovered while searching for a primary source of retroperitoneal GCTs. The testicular

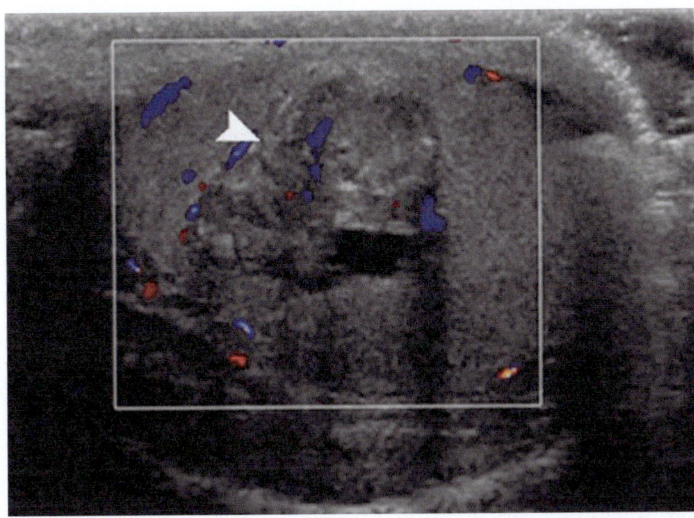

**Fig. 27.15** Postpubertal teratoma on doppler US, as a complex heterogeneous mass with calcifications and cystic lesions (arrowhead)[38]

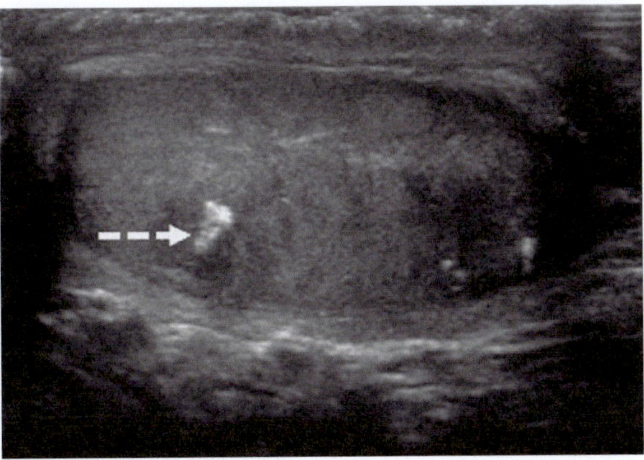

**Fig. 27.16** Burned out GCT on US, showing as a small focal intratesticular calcification (dotted arrow)[39]

primary tumor is thought to metastasize and then "burn out", leaving its retroperitoneal metastases behind with only a small testicular scar or calcification to mark its origination. Therefore, the discovery of an irregular scar should prompt consideration for GCT regression (Fig. 27.16).

## Testicular GCTs Not Derived from GCNIS

This category includes spermatocytic tumors, prepubertal-type teratomas (epidermoid cyst and dermoid), and prepubertal-type yolk sac tumors. Non-GCNIS GCT's are more inert and less likely to metastasize than their GCNIS counterparts and are more often found in the pediatric population.

## Spermatocytic Tumor

Spermatocytic tumors represent a highly curable non-GCNIS subtype. They present on US as well-defined hypoechoic heterogenous masses containing cystic spaces due to hemorrhagic changes with necrosis. Linear calcification may be visualized at the tumor periphery. Spermatocytic tumors, previously termed spermatocyctic seminomas, are difficult to distinguish from seminomatous lesions based on imaging alone (Fig. 27.17).

## Prepubertal-Type Teratoma

In contrast to the postpubertal-type teratoma, the prepubertal-type is typically benign and does not metastasize. Included in this category are the epidermoid cyst and dermoid subtypes. Epidermoid cysts contain lamellar keratin and are visualized as encapsulated round to oval lesions on imaging. Sonographically, they appear with a characteristic "onion skin" appearance of alternating concentric rings of hypo and hyperechogenicity. Epidermoid cysts may also present on MRI with alternating low and high signal intensity areas on T1- and T2-weighted images, in addition to a "target sign" pattern on T1-weighted images due to the hyperintense central area of the lesion (Fig. 27.18).

Dermoid testicular cysts are much less common than epidermoid cysts and do not have malignant potential. They are visualized on US as a hypoechoic mass,

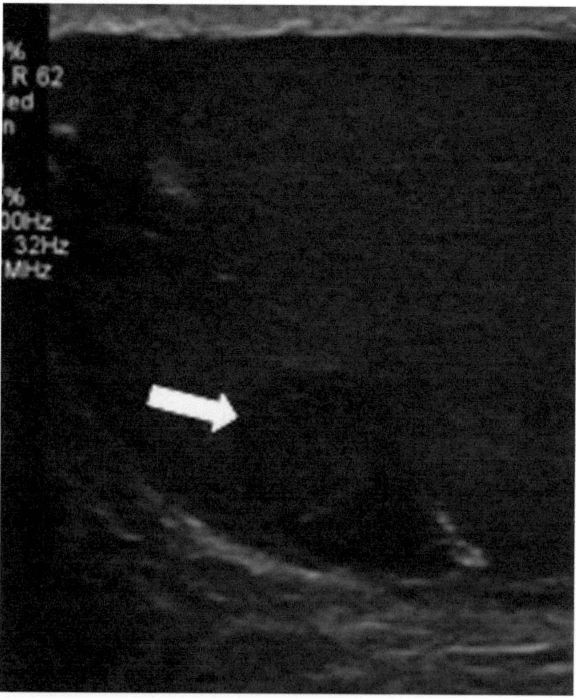

**Fig. 27.17** Spermatocytic tumor on US, demonstrating a well-defined hypoechoic heterogenous lesion (arrow)[40]

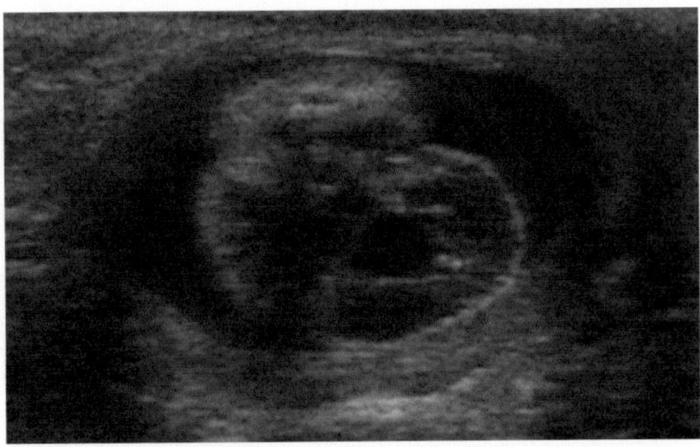

**Fig. 27.18** Epidermoid cyst on US, showing an "onion skin" appearance. The author

possibly containing low-level echoes with tiny echogenic foci due to desquamated keratin crystals. Doppler imaging shows lack of internal vascularity.

## Prepubertal-Type Yolk Sac Tumor

Prepubertal-type yolk sac tumors account for up to 80% of prepubertal malignant testicular tumors.[41] US imaging shows a heterogenous appearance with varying proportions of cystic change and echogenic foci secondary to hemorrhage or necrosis. The prepubertal type is similar to the rarer postpubertal type, although the prepubertal type is a much more malignant subtype.

## Non-Germ Cell Testicular Tumors: Sex Cord-Stromal Tumors

This testicular tumor classification includes sex cord-stromal tumors (SCSTs) including Leydig cell tumors and Sertoli cell tumors, and rarer subtypes such as granulosa cell tumors and other miscellaneous lesions.

## Leydig and Sertoli Cell Tumor

As the most common type of SCST, Leydig cell tumors are commonly benign and can occur in any age group. As they appear on US as small hypoechoic masses and show increased blood flow on doppler, it is difficult to properly differentiate these tumors from seminomas based on US alone. Recently, MRI has been shown as superior to US in Leydig cell tumors diagnosis with a high sensitivity and specificity. Leydig cell tumor MRI demonstrates well-defined margins with a significant T2 hypointense signal and rapid and marked wash-in, which is then followed by a slow and late wash-out. Conversely, seminoma on MRI appears as a tumor with ill-defined margins and a mild T2 hypointensity, along with a weak, progressive wash-in without a wash-out. Additionally, Leydig cell tumor tumors may show a T2 hyperintense central scar on MR imaging with a capsular high T2 signal intensity (Fig. 27.19).

Sertoli cell tumors typically only present in patients less than 40 years old, with a minority of cases involving metastasis. US reveals increased echogenicity, with a dense collagenous matrix causing a multicystic "spoke wheel" pattern. MR imaging

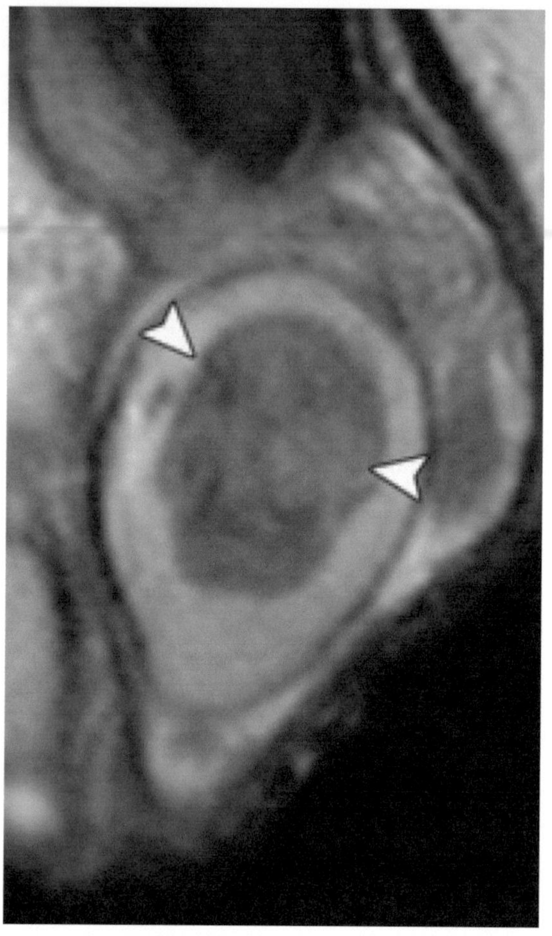

**Fig. 27.19** Leydig cell tumor on T2-weighted MRI, appearing as a hypointense intratesticular mass (arrowheads)[42]

demonstrates a homogenous mass with intermediate T1 signal intensity lesions, hyperintense T2-weighted images, and rim enhancement.

## Hemato-Lymphoid Tumor

Although lymphoma is a rare testicular tumor, it is the most common malignant testicular neoplasm in elderly men and is often secondary to non-Hodgkin lymphoma B-cell tumors. It is the most frequent bilateral testes neoplasm. Testicular lymphoma presents on grey-scale US as diffuse or focal hypoechoic lesions with increased vascularity on doppler. Some studies have described sonographic images of lymphoma as alternating hypo and hyperechoic striated bands radiating peripherally from the mediastinum testis.[43]

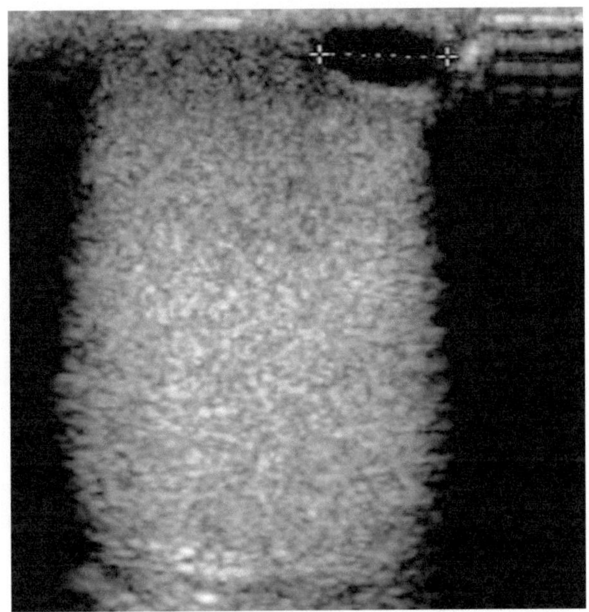

**Fig. 27.20** Cyst of the tunica albuginea on US, appearing as a well-defined anechoic space[44]

## Intratesticular Cysts

Intratesticular cysts include tubular ectasia of the rete testis and and testicular cysts. These intratesticular cysts appear on US as typical cysts with well-defined anechoic structures. Tubular ectasia of the rete testes is a benign condition visualized on US as branching hypoechoic cystic figures in the mediastinum testis. It is important to accurately diagnose this condition on US as it can easily be confused with a hypoechoic mass and therefore cause an unnecessary biopsy (Fig. 27.20).

## Testicular Microlithiasis

Testicular microlithiasis is an infrequently encountered condition involving intratubular calcifications. It is typically discovered incidentally on US and is visualized as echogenic foci 2–3 mm in size disseminated across the testicular parenchyma without acoustic shadowing. While some testicular microcalcification is considered normal, testicular microlithiasis is defined as the presence >5 foci per transducer field per testis. This condition has been associated with multiple urological conditions, most importantly testicular cancer which has been found in up to 44% of microlithiasis patients.[45] A cause-and-effect relationship between any of these associations has yet to be proven.

The association between microlithiasis and testicular neoplasms has produced much disagreement on how to best manage the uncertain status of microlithiasis as a precursor to carcinoma. Potential approaches including serial clinical examinations, US, tumor marker screenings, or immediate biopsy. The most recent recommendations are against follow up of isolated microlithiasis in the absence of a

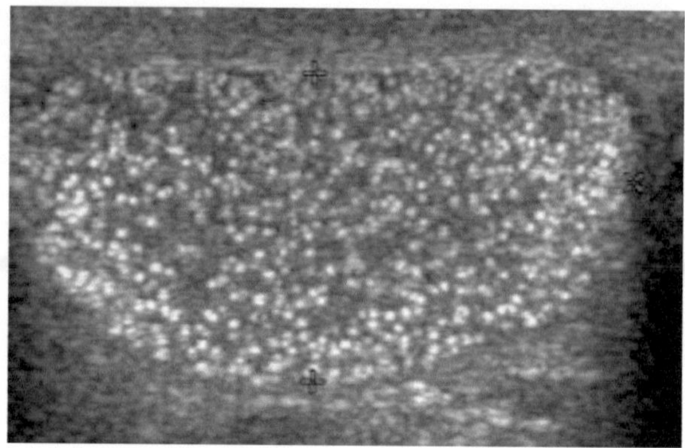

**Fig. 27.21** Testicular microlithiasis on US, visualized as multiple disseminated echogenic foci with no acoustic shadowing[47]

solid mass or risk factors in the patient's history including maldescent, orchidopexy, testicular atrophy, or personal or family history of GCT. Some sanction annual serial US exams for microlithiasis patients up to age 55 years with risk factors and no solid mass (Fig. 27.21).[46]

## 27.4 Infertility

Infertility is estimated to affect about 7% of the male population. The etiology of infertility can be challenging to identify, and half of all infertile men remain without a diagnosed etiology. Due to its ability to accurately present intrascrotal contents, ultrasonography is widely used as the primary imaging modality for assessment of male infertility and can assess for presence of varicocele, cryptorchidism, and testicular hypotrophy. US can also provide details on a number of conditions which are associated to varying degrees with male infertility, such as epididymitis, epididymal cysts, spermatoceles, testicular GCT's, and testicular microlithiasis. It should be noted that it is not uncommon for small testicular masses to incidentally be discovered during a workup of male infertility. These masses generally do not demonstrate substantial growth and may be safely observed with follow-up.[48]

**Varicocele**

Varicoceles occur when the venous valves of the pampiniform plexus become ineffective. The resulting impairment in plexus drainage leads to its dilation and hyperthermia, causing a progressive decline in testicular function. As discussed in the anatomy of scrotum chapter, testicular venous drainage consists of a complex anastomotic and varying system which must be taken into consideration in cases of suspected varicocele. The variation in venous drainage on the left and right sides is clinically relevant for the pathogenesis of varicocele.

Testicular varicoceles are commonly associated with infertility and their correction can help improve the sperm count. The clinician should recall that over 80%

of varicocele cases are not associated with infertility, but up to 40% of men with primary infertility and up to 81% of men with secondary infertility have diagnosed varicoceles.[49]

Varicoceles may be diagnosed via characteristic clinical findings such as scrotal fullness with Valsalva or a "bag of worms" mass that shrinks in the recumbent position and do not require confirmation with grey-scale US, although there is some contention as to whether the diagnosis should be confirmed by doppler. Nevertheless, if the clinical exam findings are equivocal or if an obese body habitus prevents proper examination, it is agreed that doppler imaging can support the diagnosis by demonstrating reversal of venous blood flow with Valsalva or spermatic vein diameter measurement of $\geq 3$ mm.[50] Current practice discourages routine use of US for identification of nonpalpable varicoceles as their repair does not demonstrate clinical benefit.

Venography had the highest sensitivity for varicocele diagnosis and is therefore often used as a gold standard for researchers. However, it is not typically used in general clinical practice as it is both invasive and time consuming (Fig. 27.22).

**Cryptorchidism**

Cryptorchidism is a congenital disorder involving an undescended testicle and is the most common malformation in newborn males. This irregular positioning of the testes can cause increased risk of infertility as well as testicular cancer, with decreased risk of these disorders in cases of early orchiopexy. On US, cryptorchid testes appear as hypotrophic, inhomogenous, and hypoechoic figures. Although US is the main form of imaging used in cryptorchidism, meta-analyses have reported sonography as an unreliable resource for localization of nonpalpable testes and rule out of intraabdominal testes, with a weak sensitivity and specificity especially in comparison to diagnostic and therapeutic laparoscopy (which has nearly 100% sensitivity and specificity). Imaging is therefore not routinely used to evaluate

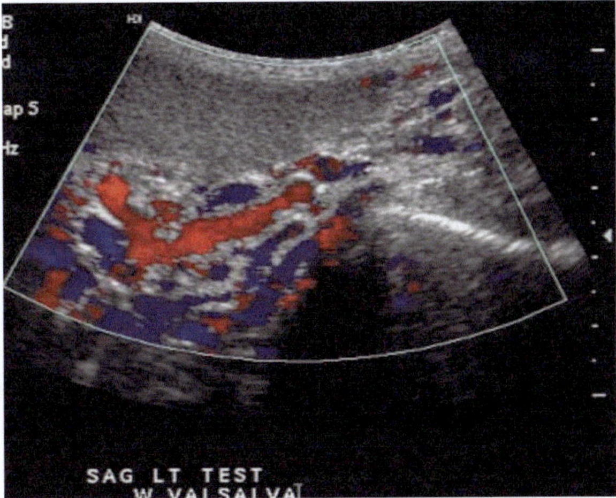


**Fig. 27.22** Varicocele on doppler US, demonstrating significant refluxing vascular flow with Valsalva[51]

differential diagnoses or for preoperative planning prior to orchiopexy, except in cases with obese patients in whom testes palpation is difficult or when searching for Mullerian structures in cases of suspected DSD.

## Testicular Hypotrophy

Testicular volume is positively correlated to total sperm count, sperm motility, normal sperm morphology, and testosterone levels. Testicular hypotrophy is defined as a testicular volume less than 12 ml. US has greater precision in measurement of testicular volume than does Prader's orchidometer.

## Endnotes


1. Brant W. Diagnostic imaging methods. In: Klein J, Brant W, Helms C, Vinson E, editors. Fundamentals of diagnostic radiology, 5th ed. Lippincott Williams & Wilkins; 2012, p. 9–16.
2. Sakamoto H, Saito K, Oohta M, Inoue K, Ogawa Y, Yoshida H. Testicular volume measurement: comparison of ultrasonography, orchidometry, and water displacement. Urology. 2007 Jan;69(1):152–7.
3. Dogra VS, Gottlieb RH, Oka M, Rubens DJ. Sonography of the scrotum. Radiology. 2003 Apr;227(1):18–36.
4. Cassidy FH, Ishioka KM, McMahon CJ, Chu P, Sakamoto K, Lee KS, et al. MR imaging of scrotal tumors and pseudotumors. Radiographics. 2010 May;30 (3):665–83.
5. Sweet DE, Feldman MK, Remer EM. Imaging of the acute scrotum: keys to a rapid diagnosis of acute scrotal disorders. Abdom Radiol (NY). 2020 Jul;45 (7):2063–81.
6. Di Serafino M, Acampora C, Iacobellis F, Schillirò ML, Borzelli A, Barbuto L, et al. Ultrasound of scrotal and penile emergency: how, why and when. J Ultrasound. 2020 Jul 11.
7. Ringdahl E, Teague L. Testicular torsion. Am Fam Physician. 2006 Nov 15;74 (10):1739–43.
8. Dogra VS, Gottlieb RH, Oka M, Rubens DJ. Sonography of the scrotum. Radiology. 2003 Apr;227(1):18–36.
9. Dogra VS, Gottlieb RH, Oka M, Rubens DJ. Sonography of the scrotum. Radiology. 2003 Apr;227(1):18–36.
10. Aydogdu O, Burgu B, Gocun PU, Ozden E, Yaman O, Soygur T, et al. Near infrared spectroscopy to diagnose experimental testicular torsion: comparison with Doppler ultrasound and immunohistochemical correlation of tissue oxygenation and viability. J Urol. 2012 Feb;187(2):744–50.
11. Di Serafino M, Acampora C, Iacobellis F, Schillirò ML, Borzelli A, Barbuto L, et al. Ultrasound of scrotal and penile emergency: how, why and when. J Ultrasound. 2020 Jul 11.
12. Sweet DE, Feldman MK, Remer EM. Imaging of the acute scrotum: keys to a rapid diagnosis of acute scrotal disorders. Abdom Radiol (NY). 2020 Jul;45 (7):2063–81.

13. Di Serafino M, Acampora C, Iacobellis F, Schillirò ML, Borzelli A, Barbuto L, et al. Ultrasound of scrotal and penile emergency: how, why and when. J Ultrasound. 2020 Jul 11.

14. Sweet DE, Feldman MK, Remer EM. Imaging of the acute scrotum: keys to a rapid diagnosis of acute scrotal disorders. Abdom Radiol (NY). 2020 Jul;45 (7):2063–81.

15. Hedayati V, Sellars ME, Sharma DM, Sidhu PS. Contrast-enhanced ultrasound in testicular trauma: role in directing exploration, debridement and organ salvage. Br J Radiol. 2012 Mar;85(1011):e65–68.

16. Di Serafino M, Acampora C, Iacobellis F, Schillirò ML, Borzelli A, Barbuto L, et al. Ultrasound of scrotal and penile emergency: how, why and when. J Ultrasound. 2020 Jul 11.

17. Di Serafino M, Acampora C, Iacobellis F, Schillirò ML, Borzelli A, Barbuto L, et al. Ultrasound of scrotal and penile emergency: how, why and when. J Ultrasound. 2020 Jul 11.

18. Sweet DE, Feldman MK, Remer EM. Imaging of the acute scrotum: keys to a rapid diagnosis of acute scrotal disorders. Abdom Radiol (NY). 2020 Jul;45 (7):2063–81.

19. Dogra VS, Gottlieb RH, Oka M, Rubens DJ. Sonography of the scrotum. Radiology. 2003 Apr;227(1):18–36.

20. Di Serafino M, Acampora C, Iacobellis F, Schillirò ML, Borzelli A, Barbuto L, et al. Ultrasound of scrotal and penile emergency: how, why and when. J Ultrasound. 2020 Jul 11.

21. Dogra VS, Gottlieb RH, Oka M, Rubens DJ. Sonography of the scrotum. Radiology. 2003 Apr;227(1):18–36.

22. Sweet DE, Feldman MK, Remer EM. Imaging of the acute scrotum: keys to a rapid diagnosis of acute scrotal disorders. Abdom Radiol (NY). 2020 Jul;45 (7):2063–81.

23. Sweet DE, Feldman MK, Remer EM. Imaging of the acute scrotum: keys to a rapid diagnosis of acute scrotal disorders. Abdom Radiol (NY). 2020 Jul;45 (7):2063–81.

24. Sharbidre KG, Lockhart ME. Imaging of scrotal masses. Abdom Radiol (NY). 2020 Jul;45(7):2087–108.

25. Parker RA, Menias CO, Quazi R, Hara AK, Verma S, Shaaban A, et al. Mr imaging of the penis and scrotum. Radiographics. 2015 Aug;35(4):1033–50.

26. Sharbidre KG, Lockhart ME. Imaging of scrotal masses. Abdom Radiol (NY). 2020 Jul;45(7):2087–108.

27. Ragheb D, Higgins JL. Ultrasonography of the scrotum: technique, anatomy, and pathologic entities. J Ultrasound Med. 2002 Feb;21(2):171–85.

28. Ragheb D, Higgins JL. Ultrasonography of the scrotum: technique, anatomy, and pathologic entities. J Ultrasound Med. 2002 Feb;21(2):171–85.

29. Park JS, Kim J, Elghiaty A, Ham WS. Recent global trends in testicular cancer incidence and mortality. Medicine (Baltimore). 2018 Sep;97(37):e12390.

30. Sangüesa C, Veiga D, Llavador M, Serrano A. Testicular tumours in children: an approach to diagnosis and management with pathologic correlation. Insights Imaging. 2020 May 27;11(1):74.

31. Dogra VS, Gottlieb RH, Oka M, Rubens DJ. Sonography of the scrotum. Radiology. 2003 Apr;227(1):18–36.

32. Sharbidre KG, Lockhart ME. Imaging of scrotal masses. Abdom Radiol (NY). 2020 Jul;45(7):2087–108.

33. Kreydin EI, Barrisford GW, Feldman AS, Preston MA. Testicular cancer: what the radiologist needs to know. AJR Am J Roentgenol. 2013 Jun;200(6):1215–25.

34. Sharbidre KG, Lockhart ME. Imaging of scrotal masses. Abdom Radiol (NY). 2020 Jul;45(7):2087–108.

35. Sharbidre KG, Lockhart ME. Imaging of scrotal masses. Abdom Radiol (NY). 2020 Jul;45(7):2087–108.

36. Sharbidre KG, Lockhart ME. Imaging of scrotal masses. Abdom Radiol (NY). 2020 Jul;45(7):2087–108.

37. Sharbidre KG, Lockhart ME. Imaging of scrotal masses. Abdom Radiol (NY). 2020 Jul;45(7):2087–108.

38. Sharbidre KG, Lockhart ME. Imaging of scrotal masses. Abdom Radiol (NY). 2020 Jul;45(7):2087–108.

39. Sharbidre KG, Lockhart ME. Imaging of scrotal masses. Abdom Radiol (NY). 2020 Jul;45(7):2087–108.

40. Sharbidre KG, Lockhart ME. Imaging of scrotal masses. Abdom Radiol (NY). 2020 Jul;45(7):2087–108.

41. Sharbidre KG, Lockhart ME. Imaging of scrotal masses. Abdom Radiol (NY). 2020 Jul;45(7):2087–108.

42. Cassidy FH, Ishioka KM, McMahon CJ, Chu P, Sakamoto K, Lee KS, et al. MR imaging of scrotal tumors and pseudotumors. Radiographics. 2010 May;30 (3):665–83.

43. Dogra VS, Gottlieb RH, Oka M, Rubens DJ. Sonography of the scrotum. Radiology. 2003 Apr;227(1):18–36.

44. Ragheb D, Higgins JL. Ultrasonography of the scrotum: technique, anatomy, and pathologic entities. J Ultrasound Med. 2002 Feb;21(2):171–85.

45. Ragheb D, Higgins JL. Ultrasonography of the scrotum: technique, anatomy, and pathologic entities. J Ultrasound Med. 2002 Feb;21(2):171–85.

46. Balawender K, Orkisz S, Wisz P. Testicular microlithiasis: what urologists should know. A review of the current literature. Cent European J Urol. 2018;71 (3):310–4.

47. Ragheb D, Higgins JL. Ultrasonography of the scrotum: technique, anatomy, and pathologic entities. J Ultrasound Med. 2002 Feb;21(2):171–85.

48. Bieniek JM, Juvet T, Margolis M, Grober ED, Lo KC, Jarvi KA. Prevalence and management of incidental small testicular masses discovered on ultrasonographic evaluation of male infertility. J Urol. 2018 Feb;199(2):481–6.

49. Schlegel PN, Sigman M, Collura B, De Jonge CJ, Eisenberg ML, Lamb DJ, et al. Diagnosis and treatment of infertility in men: AUA/ASRM guideline part I. J Urol. 2021 Jan;205(1):36–43.
50. Sabanegh A, Agarwal A. Anatomy of the Lower Urinary Tract and Male Genitalia. In: Wein B, Kavoussi L, Novick A, Partin A, Peters C, editors. Campbell-Walsh urology, 10th ed. Elsevier Saunders; 2012, p. 628–31.
51. Ragheb D, Higgins JL. Ultrasonography of the scrotum: technique, anatomy, and pathologic entities. J Ultrasound Med. 2002 Feb;21(2):171–85.
52. Tasian GE, Copp HL, Baskin LS. Diagnostic imaging in cryptorchidism: utility, indications, and effectiveness. J Pediatr Surg. 2011 Dec;46(12):2406–13.

## Suggested Further Reading

1. Fulgham P, Bishoff JT. Urinary tract imaging: basic principles. In: Wein B, Kavoussi L, Novick A, Partin A, Peters C, editors. Campbell-Walsh urology, 10th ed. Elsevier Saunders; 2012, p. 122–124.
2. Garcia RA, Sajjad H. Anatomy, abdomen and pelvis, scrotum. In: StatPearls. StatPearls Publishing; 2020.
3. Wibmer AG, Vargas HA. Imaging of testicular and scrotal masses: the essentials. In: Hodler J, Kubik-Huch RA, von Schulthess GK, editors. Diseases of the Abdomen and Pelvis 2018–2021. Springer International Publishing; 2018. p. 257–64.
4. Stephenson A, Eggener SE, Bass EB, Chelnick DM, Daneshmand S, Feldman D, et al. Diagnosis and treatment XE "treatment" of early stage testicular cancer: AUA guideline. J Urol. 2019;202(2):272–81.
5. Aoun F, Slaoui A, Naoum E, Hassan T, Albisinni S, Azzo JM, et al. Testicular XE "testicular" microlithiasis: systematic review and clinical guidelines. Prog Urol. 2019;29(10):465–73.
6. Jungwirth A, Giwercman A, Tournaye H, Diemer T, Kopa Z, Dohle G, et al. European association of urology guidelines on male infertility XE "infertility": the 2012 update. Eur Urol. 2012;62(2):324–32.

# Chapter 28
# Scrotoplasty

Mohamed A. Baky Fahmy

**Abbreviations**

| | |
|---|---|
| VRAM | Vertical Rectus Abdominis Myocutaneous Flap |
| CSA | Congenital Scrotal Agenesis |
| FTSGs | Full Thickness Skin Grafts |
| STSGs | Split Thickness Skin Grafts |

**Definition:** Scrotoplasty, also known as oscheoplasty, is reconstructive surgery to repair or create a scrotum. Scrotoplasty term is commonly used to indicates the surgical procedure used to replace partially or completely a damaged scrotum, but sometimes the procedures used to reconstruct the penoscrotal junction, penoscrotal fusion and webbed penis repairs are called inaccurately as scrotoplasty. Also a scrotal lifting procedure, scrotum tightening, or scrotum reduction surgeries that involve removing the excess scrotal skin to improve the appearance and comfort of the scrotum sometimes also termed as scrotoplasty.

Partial scrotal loss is seldom a problem, and primary closure of the scrotal defect with the remaining scrotal skin can usually be accomplished due to viscoelastic properties of the scrotum. Due to the special function and appearance of the scrotum, reconstructive options for total scrotal defect are always not satisfactory to achieve a native dynamic scrotum.

## 28.1   Common Causes of Scrotal Skin Loss

Genital skin loss in men may be caused by avulsion injuries, assaults, self-mutilation, burns, animal attacks, gangrene of the male genitalia and excision of scrotal skin in cases of neoplastic lesions, haemangiomas and lymphedema

M. A. B. Fahmy (⊠)
Al-Azhar University, Cairo, Egypt

  435
M. A. B. Fahmy (ed.), *Normal and Abnormal Scrotum*,
https://doi.org/10.1007/978-3-030-83305-3_28

repair. Scrotal construction may also be required for congenital anomalies and female to male intersex surgical intervention.

**1. Post traumatic penoscrotal avulsion injury**: the scrotum in 36% of the cases, and the penile shaft in 33% being popular sites for injury in multiply traumatised victims, penoscrotal defects caused by high-speed trauma are an important category of concern. Also, patients with combined skeletal injuries or those requiring respiratory care were prone to advanced wounds (Advanced wounds are a sub-category of surgically demanding wounds, which require surgical treatment, but the focus of treatment is tissue reconstruction) [1]. Scrotal firearm related injuries are a frequent occurrence, its incidence varies widely among countries and across demographic subgroups, and it is expected to be higher in war battles [1].

So common types of trauma associated with scrotal avulsion are:

- High-speed machines accidents
- Industrial accidents
- Traffic accidents
- Fall from height
- Firearm injuries
- Post circumcision trauma.

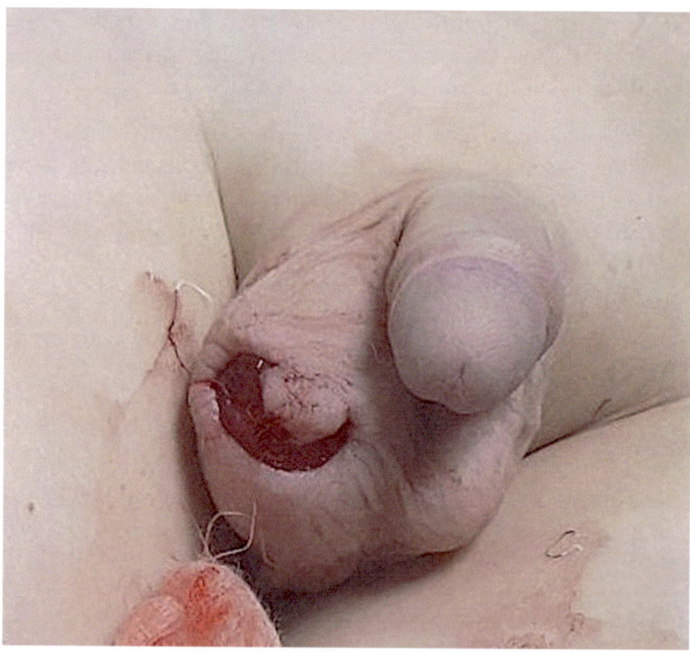

**Fig. 28.1** Small traumatic scrotal injury which could be repaired primarily

If the scrotal skin loss is less than 50%, it can often be closed immediately after patient resuscitation [2] (Fig. 28.1).

**2. Fournier gangrene** is a progressive necrotizing fasciitis of the genitalia and perineum, it is a common indication for scrotoplasty. Despite great advances in treatment, and pathophysiological understanding of necrotizing soft-tissue infections, Fournier gangrene remains a life-threatening urological emergency [3]. It can affects patients of any age and gender, it might be more prevalent in elder men even after a minor trauma to the genitalia, specially in immunocompromised patients such as patients with diabetes mellitus, obesity, HIV, substance abuse and cancer patients receiving chemotherapy [4]. In children Fournier gangrene may supervenes ischaemic gangrene after ritual circumcision; specially after the use of electro-cautery (Figs. 28.2 and 28.3). The polymicrobial flora may causes rapid extensive soft tissue necrosis and sepsis (Chap. 23).

**3. Scrotal neoplasm**: (Chap. 25) Scrotal wall excision is indicated in many primary or secondary scrotal neoplasms. Often defects from such resections are superficial and limited to skin and subcutaneous tissue. Primary closure if possible provides a good color match and potential scrotal function. Otherwise, a simple skin graft or

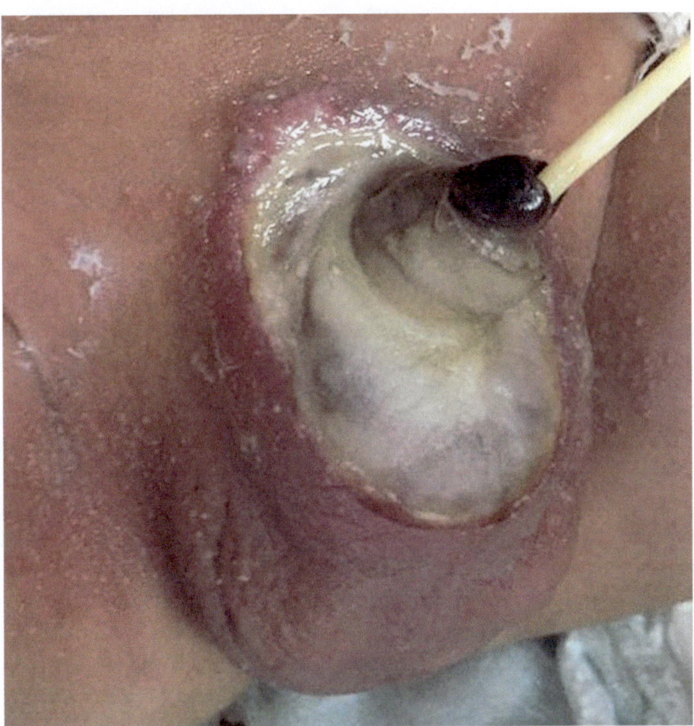

**Fig. 28.2** A child with penile gangrene and scrotal skin loss after monopolar diathermy injury during circumcision

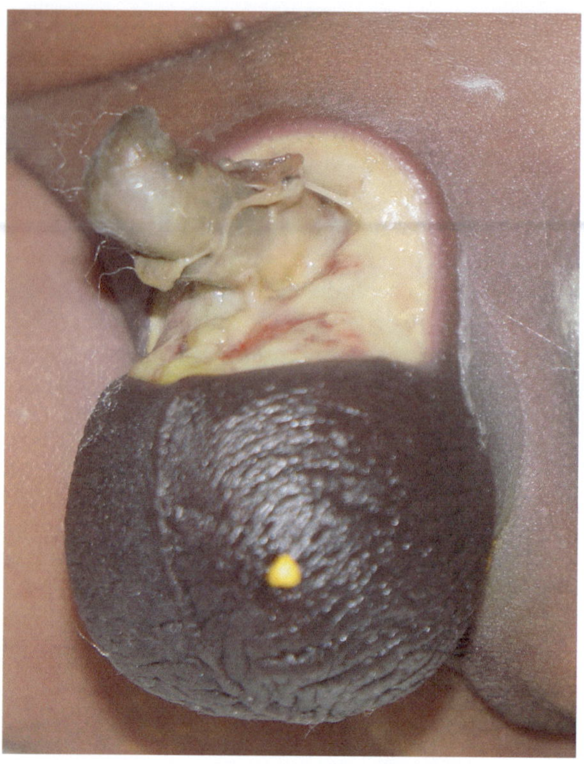

**Fig. 28.3** A neonate with Fournier gangrene involving the whole penis and upper scrotum after circumcision

local fasciocutaneous flap is often adequate to obtain wound healing, but fails to allow thermal regulation for the testes. In the case of advanced penile cancer, extended resection can still leave some residual viable scrotal tissue for wound closure without need of any other approaches. Pedicled anterolateral thigh flap without an irradiation injury can provide excellent coverage for this area. A local flap in case of irradiation has the disadvantage of using the irradiated tissue, which can increase wound complications and flap loss [5].

**4. Congenital anomalies**: Some transgender men, intersex, and non-binary people who were assigned female at birth may have an indication to create a neoscrotum, as part of their transition. In male to female (MTF) sex reassignment surgery the labia majora are dissected to form hollow cavities. Scrotoplasty achieved with the creation of a neoscrotum, which is typically constructed by fusing the labia majora to form a single sac. Also a number of skin flaps can be used to create the new scrotum [6]. Testicular prostheses need to be implanted in the neoscrotum with or without tissue expansion, testicular implants are used for enhanced cosmesis.

In cases of Congenital Scrotal Agenesis (CSA) and hypoplasia, which are the rarest scrotal anomaly, CSA is characterized by complete absence of scrotal rugae in the perineum between the penis and anus. It is commonly bilateral with an impalpable testicles, but rare cases of unilateral scrotal agenesis are sometimes recognizable (Chap. 11).

This anomaly may posses difficulty during orchidopexy or it may end with social anxiety around excessively small scrotal size when compared to peers, and where there may be concerns regarding the future sexual life. The management of congenitally absent and severely underdeveloped scrota has ranged from multiple procedures involving skin expanders and tissue flaps, such cases are usually presented early at childhood.

Scrotoplasty has become a common practice during insertion of penile prosthesis, for improving patient perception of penile length. Although scrotoplasty can improve patient satisfaction with inflatable penile prosthesis (IPP), but scrotoplasty can lead to increased patient morbidity, specially in diabetic patients [7].

**5. Scrotal lymphedema and vascular malformations**: Extensive lesions involving most of the scrotal tissue may deserve a substitutional scrotoplasty after primary excision (Chap. 21).

**6. Cock and ball torture injuries**: some practices like ball crusher, testicle cuff, and scrotal parachute, may carry a significant health risks, and can potentially be harmful to the male genitals as the circulation of blood can be easily cut off with a subsequent scrotal necrosis, which may be complicated by a sort of Fournier gangrene and scrotal loss [8].

**7. Reduction Scrotoplasty**: Excess scrotal skin, or scrotomegaly, is a poorly defined condition that can affect men of all ages and may indicate a sort of scrotoplastic surgery.

## 28.2  Timing of Reconstructive Options

The timing of scrotal reconstruction depends on the aetiology of defect. Traumatic and infectious defects require serial debridements until achieving a healthy local tissue wound bed. Scrotal specialized tissue and anal sphincters should be preserved as much as possible. Hence, reconstruction in those patients is frequently delayed and performed in a staged fashion.

In Fournier gangrene the guidelines are available for early, extensive and planned repeated debridement. The extensive debridement should be performed within the first 12 h [9]. Once necrotic tissue has been removed, the underlying infectious process should be treated systemically, and once the patient is recovering, options for definitive genital reconstruction should be planned. Oncologic defects are reconstructed after ensuring that the wound margins are free of tumor and preferentially immediately after resection. Immediate wound closure shortens the overall morbidity to the patient. Delayed reconstruction requires painful dressing changes and may cause progressive necrosis of irradiated wound [10].

On malignant cases with a tumor affecting the perineum and scrotum, radical resection of recurrent tumor after irradiation creates significant problems that require careful planning during resection and reconstruction. Preoperative planning must be communicated with the ablative team to optimize reconstruction and outcome [11].

For cases of CSA and other congenital scrotal defects the optimum time for surgery is early around the age of two years, and an associated undescended testicle could be fixed 4–6 months after completing scrotoplasty. A concomitant orchidopexy after accomplishment scrotoplasty was reported by Wright [12].

## 28.3 Modalities of Scrotoplasty

Various modalities of treatment advocated for scrotoplasty are skin grafting, flaps, temporary implantation of the exposed testes in the inguinal pouch and tissue expander.

### 28.3.1 Skin Grafts

Split-thickness skin grafting is the most commonly used reconstructive technique for the scrotal loss. The testicles should be brought to a dependent position (hanging between the thighs), without shortening by bluntly dissecting and freeing up the cords as much as possible before applying the graft [13]. The split-thickness skin graft of 0.012–0.016 inches thick is most often taken from the anterior or lateral thigh. When possible, healthy dartos tissue is maintained and used as a graft bed in order to allow for translocation of the scrotal skin over the deeper structures. In cases of scrotal lymphedema, it is essential to completely remove dartos fascia and graft directly to Buck's fascia or tunica albuginea in order to bypass the obstructed lymphatics. The testicles should be covered with the smallest possible amount of subcutaneous tissue to prevent over insulation and ensure low temperatures to maintain normal spermatogenesis [14].

Skin graft, works best on the proximal scrotum and penile shaft, as these areas have very thin epithelium and rich blood supply. Vacuum-assisted treatment is very helpful in such cases. Both full thickness skin grafts (FTSGs) and split thickness skin grafts (STSGs), which contain epidermis and a portion of dermis, have been successfully utilized on the penis and scrotum as well. STSGs are typically harvested at a depth of 0.012–0.018 inches, thinner grafts associated with improved graft take. STSGs are typically harvested from the anterolateral or medial thigh [12]. Compared to FTSGs, the advantages of STSGs include a thin graft that more closely resembles native penile skin, lack of hair follicles, improved graft take due to reduced metabolic requirements, and the ability to easily mesh and expand the graft to cover a larger recipient site [15].

## 28.3.2 Local Flap

Several loco-regional skin and fasciocutaneous flaps from thigh, perineum, abdominal wall and groin area have been described to reconstruct scrotum. These flaps represent an excellent tool in scrotal reconstruction. The range of local flaps used for scrotoplasty includes skin advancement using inguinal to upper thigh skin, local fasciocutaneous flaps, and musculocutaneous flaps. Simply a rotational fasciocutaneous thigh flaps can be brought together to cover the testicles.

The next step for a successful reconstruction in cases of Fournier gangrene is choosing a secondary refining reconstructive options by using the surrounding abdominal or thigh soft tissue. Anterolateral thigh flaps using the descending branch of the lateral circumflex femoris artery have been described, and show good results at a long term follow-up [16].

**Muscle flaps** like gracilis and rectus abdominis are well vascularized and have been used for scrotal reconstruction. A limitation of muscle flap includes hair bearing skin, sacrifice of functioning muscle, poor sensation and scarring on thighs. In cases with an existing laparotomy, a vertical rectus abdominis myocutaneous flap (VRAM) with skin from the supraumbilical area provides excellent soft tissue bulk to obliterate dead space to prevent abscess and hernia [17]. The vertical rather than the transverse skin island design because epigastric skin comfortably reaches the perineum without tension. Donor site fascial closure does not require a mesh because the intact anterior rectus sheath below the arcuate line can be simply reapproximated to the posterior sheath just above the arcuate line [10].

Gracilis myocutaneous flap is another option, although not ideal due to its small volume and its pedicle does not allow adequate reach into the pelvis and the sacrum. An additional flap such as pedicled omentum based on the right gastroepiploic vessel is necessary to fill the dead space induced after extensive resection in cases of neoplastic lesions [18]. All these flap reconstructive options have significant donor site morbidity and result in bulky coverage. These flaps provide a significant amount of subcutaneous tissue that is uncharacteristic of the native scrotum. Basically in cases of severe nercotizing fasciitis the muscle or omental flap is the best choice since the muscle is able to counter the infection in much better way. In cases of traumatic defects; temporary placing the testes in subcutaneous thigh pouch, and then a split skin graft or fasciocutaneous flap can be used.

**Preputial flap**: The most commonly cited technique for neoscrotum creation in cases of CSA was described by Wright [12] and Verga [19] in 1993 and 1996, respectively. Both created a preputial flap and then used the Beck-Ombrédanne technique to buttonhole the penile glans and shaft through a preputial dartos window to transpose the prepuce to the ventral base of the penile shaft as a neoscrotum. Wright [12] performed an immediate bilateral orchidopexy and although the long-term results appear acceptable. Benson et al. [20] reported their experience with an innovative surgical technique for creation of a neoscrotum in three children with CSA and a concomitant cryptorchidism. They created a neoscrotum using the foreskin. The prepuce was harvested on a pedicle of dartos and transposed over the perineal cleft to create a neoscrotal pouch. The flap was allowed to heal for 12–14 weeks, at which time the orchidopexy was performed with an acceptable aesthetic outcome [20]. In such cases of CSA any conservative modality applicable to ameliorate scrotal underdevelopment partially or completely will be useful either solely or before reconstructive surgery. Short term topical testosterone proved to be effective in a considerable percentage of cases of bilateral or unilateral scrotal hypoplasia; with a subsequent increase in scrotal surface area and number of rugae, it may substitutes the indication for surgical reconstruction [21]. Another technique utilized an inverted omega skin incision was made around the scrotal skin and base of the penis for management of cases with prepenile scrotum, where a scrotal flaps were prepared and these were brought beneath the penis. When complicated with hypospadias, scrotoplasty was performed as the third stage operation, following chordectomy and urethroplasty [22].

### 28.3.3 Tissue Expansion

Tissue expansion was first demonstrated in 1957 to increase the amount of local soft tissue coverage through prolonged mechanical creep [23]. This principle can be applied to patients who present for delayed or staged scrotoplasty. Goodman [24] first described a 2-tissue expander-based scrotal reconstruction for a traumatic injury in 1990. The use of tissue expanders for scrotal reconstruction has the advantages of excellent functional and cosmetic results with simple surgical technique provides reconstruction of native scrotal soft tissue without additional donor site morbidity. Tissue expanders have been used to reconstruct two-compartment scrotum provided that adjacent perineal or inguinal skin is uninvolved [25]. Scrotal sac reconstruction using tissue expansion usually entails a two-stage repair. The first stage consists of placing the tissue expander beneath the deep dartos fascia of the residual scrotal skin. The tissue expander is then gradually inflated to a volume large enough to accommodate both testes. The time required for tissue expansion sufficient for scrotal reconstruction varies and is dependent on the degree of tissue loss and pliability. During the second stage, the scrotal skin is moved posteriorly as expanded V–Y flaps, which allows the scrotum to hang in a more natural fashion. Testicular mobilization with orchiopexy is then performed [26].

Tissue expansion technique could be applied as a primary tool for scrotoplasty, or secondary in patients with contracted split thickness skin grafts or lost scrotal volume due to previous scrotal closure with testes stored in the inner thighs. Expansion results in soft tissue coverage of native scrotal skin with no additional donor site morbidity. This leads to improved aesthetics and functionality of the cremaster muscle which provides an ideal environment for spermatogenesis [2].

Hyaluronic acid gel scrotal injection can provide satisfactory improvement for enhancement of the scrotal volume to delay the placement of the definitive prosthesis until the child reaches adolescence, in cases of children with empty scrotum [27].

### 28.3.4  New Modalities

**Scrotum, penis and abdominal wall transplant**: A team from John Hopkins have reported the first total penis, scrotum and partial abdominal wall transplantation on a male who had sustained trauma from an improvised explosive device. Over 1 year after the transplant, the recipient has near-normal erectile and orgasmic function and reports substantial improvements in pleasure scores with normal sensation to the penile shaft and tip. He is also able to urinate standing. The team reported that testicular prostheses will be placed in the future [28].

Wu et al. [29] at 2007 developed a tissue engineered testicular prosthesis with high-density polyethylene and polyglycolic acid, after isolating the chondrocytes from swine cartilage, they were seeded onto scaffold and cultured for 2 weeks. Such modalities could be promising in the near future if it is extended to include scrotal tissue.

## 28.4  Complications and Outcome of Scrotoplasty

Primary repair of scrotal wound in inadequate circumstances, specially with ischaemic scrotal edges may end with skin necrosis and wound dehiscence (Fig. 28.4). Generally the long-term success with skin grafting for limited scrotal injury is excellent and only 20% of patients require significant revisions or reconstructions [30].

In sever injuries and wide grafting the complications of split skin grafting may have certain disadvantages like hair growth, contraction and distortion, lack of protection and less acceptable cosmetic results. Infertility may occur after total scrotal reconstruction. Skin graft impairs scrotal movement and has been reported to cause azoospermia in two of three cases after traumatic scrotal avulsion [31]. Also skin grafting procedure requires an additional donor site in patients that most likely have significant comorbidities including diabetes and obesity. Secondary contracture of meshed skin grafts results in loss of scrotal volume and high riding testicles [32]. High riding testicles and even ectopic testicular location at the root of

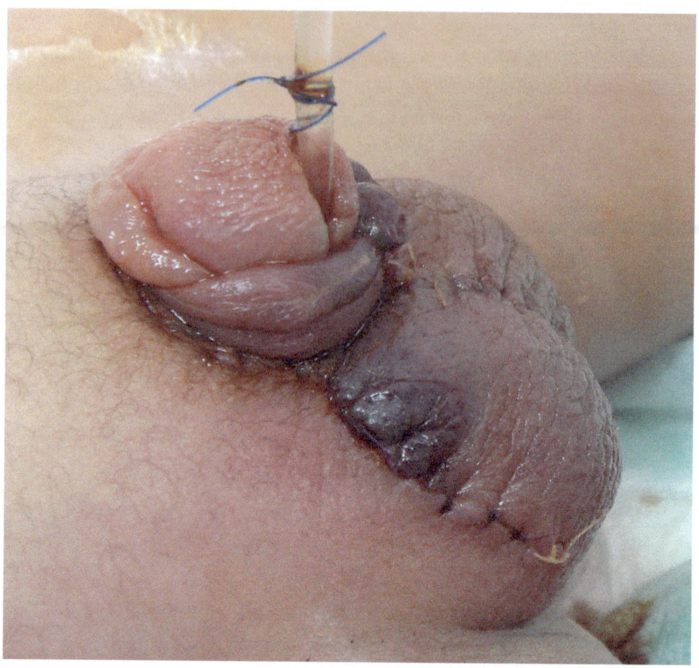

**Fig. 28.4** Scrotal skin necrosis after primary scrotal repair

**Fig. 28.5** A rare complication of testicular high riding at the distal penile shaft after improper scrotal grafting to cover a denuded penile shaft

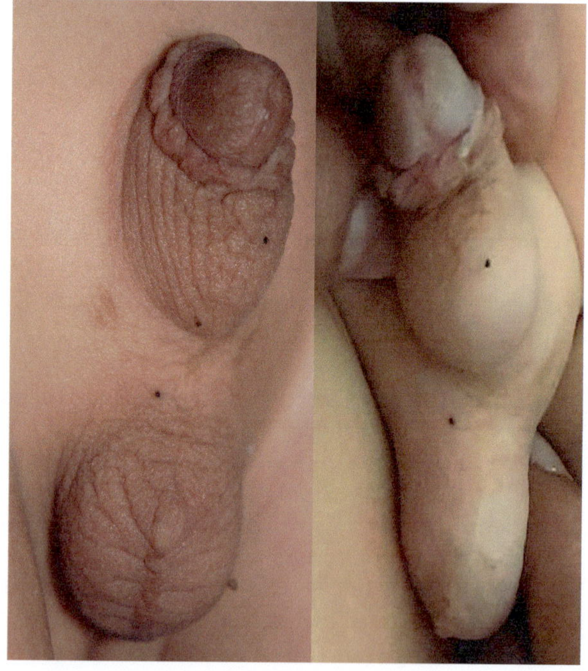

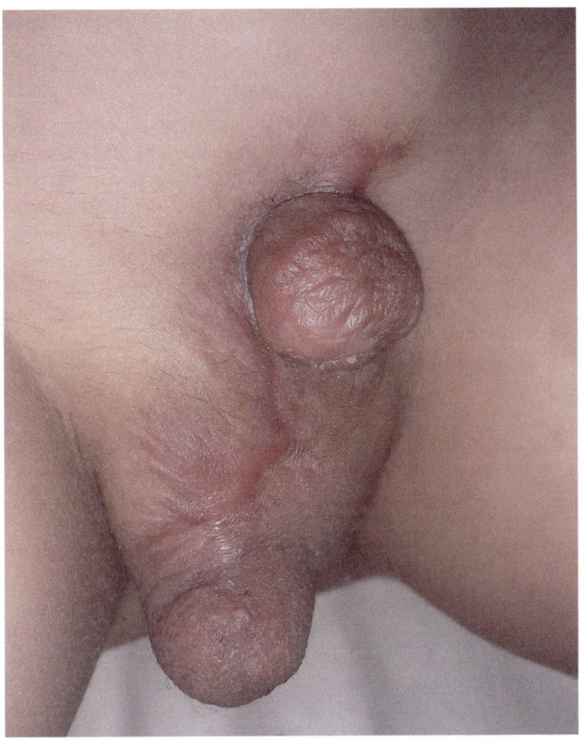

**Fig. 28.6** Non aesthetically reconstructed scrotum with a caudally placed neoscrotum and a wide penoscrotal distance

the penis may be encountered if the repair of scrotal layers not fully respected, specially in cases with combined penoscrotal skin loss (Fig. 28.5).

Bulky flap elevates testicular temperature and may impairs spermatogenesis, and debulking of such thick flap has been reported to improve sperm production by Wang [33]. Incorrect adjustment of the scrotal flaps without consideration of a normal penoscrotal angles, may end with a caudally positioned neoscrotum and a wide penoscrotal distance and results in a non aesthetic reconstructed scrotum with an unsightly outlook (Fig. 28.6). A tissue expander-based reconstruction can also have a higher incidence of infection risk or possible extrusion specially at the perineum.

# References


1. Kim MJ, Lee DH, Park DH, Lee IJ. Multivariate analysis of early surgical management factors affecting posttraumatic penoscrotal avulsion injury: a level I trauma center study. BMC Urol. 2021;21(1):1–8.
2. Kadouri Y, Zaoui Y, Sayegh HEL, Benslimane L, Nouini Y. Scrotal gunshot injury: a case report. Urol Case Rep. 2021;34:101437.

3. Masters FW, Robinson DW. The treatment of avulsions of the male genitalia. J Trauma Acute Care Surg. 1968;8:430–8.
4. Hagedorn JC, Wessells H. A contemporary update on Fournier's gangrene. Nat Rev Urol. 2017;14(4):205–14.
5. Yu P, Sanger JR, Matloub HS, Gosain A, Larson D. Anterolateral thigh fasciocutaneous island flaps in perineoscrotal reconstruction. Plast Reconstr Surg. 2002;109:610–6; discussion 617–8.
6. Shergill AK, Camacho A, Horowitz JM, Jha P, Ascher S, Berchmans E, Slama J, et al. Imaging of transgender patients: expected findings and complications of gender reassignment therapy. Abdom Radiol. 2019;44(8):2886–98.
7. Gupta NK, Sulaver R, Welliver C, Kottwitz M, Frederick L, Dynda D, Köhler TS. Scrotoplasty at time of penile implant is at high risk for dehiscence in diabetics. J Sex Med. 2019. https://doi.org/10.1016/j.jsxm.2019.02.001.
8. Langdridge D, Barker M. Safe, sane, and consensual: contemporary perspectives on sadomasochism. Palgrave Macmillan; 2008. p. 174. ISBN 978-0-230-51774-5. Archived from the original on 2013–06–20. Retrieved 2016–10–21.
9. Eckmann C. The importance of source control in the management of severe skin and soft tissue infections. Curr Opin Infect Dis. 2016;29:139–44.
10. Tran NV. Scrotal and perineal reconstruction. Semin Plast Surg. 2011;25(3):213. Thieme Medical Publishers.
11. Arnold PG, Lovich SF, Pairolero PC. Muscle flaps in irradiated wounds: an account of 100 consecutive cases. Plast Reconstr Surg. 1994;93(2):324–7; discussion 328–9.
12. Wright JE. Congenital absence of the scrotum: case report and description of an original technique of construction of a scrotum. J Pediatr Surg. 1993;28(2):264–6.
13. Black PC, Friedrich JB, Engrav LH, Wessells H. Meshed unexpanded split-thickness skin grafting for reconstruction of penile skin loss. J Urol. 2004;172:976–9.
14. McDougal WS. Scrotal reconstruction using thigh pedicle flaps. J Urol. 1983;129:757–9.
15. Cocci A, Cito G, Falcone M, Capece M, Di Maida F, et al. Subjective and objective results in surgical correction of adult acquired buried penis: a single-centre observational study. Arch Ital Urol Androl. 2019;91:25–9.
16. Gil T, Metanes I, Aman B, et al. The five-flap technique for the correction of post-circumcision peno-scrotal webbing. J Plast Reconstr Aesthet Surg. 2010;63:e325–6.
17. Sunesen KG, Buntzen S, Tei T, Lindegaard JC, Nørgaard M, Laurberg S. Perineal healing and survival after anal cancer salvage surgery: 10-year experience with primary perineal reconstruction using the vertical rectus abdominis myocutaneous (VRAM) flap. Ann Surg Oncol. 2009;16(1):68–77.
18. Shibata D, Hyland W, Busse P, et al. Immediate reconstruction of the perineal wound with gracilis muscle flaps following abdominoperineal resection and intraoperative radiation therapy for recurrent carcinoma of the rectum. Ann Surg Oncol. 1999;6(1):33–7.
19. Verga G, Avolio L. Agenesis of the scrotum: an extremely rare anomaly. J Urol. 1996;156(4):1467.
20. Benson M, Hanna MK. A novel technique to construct a neo-scrotum out of preputial skin for agenesis and underdeveloped scrotum. J Pediatr Urol. 2018. https://doi.org/10.1016/j.jpurol.2018.03.022.
21. Al Samahy O, Othman D, Gad D, Baky Fahmy MA. Efficacy of topical testosterone in management of scrotal hypoplasia and agenesis. J Pediatr Urol. 2021.
22. Mori Y, Yabumoto H, Shimada K, Ikoma F. Scrotoplasty for repair of prepenile scrotum Hinyokika kiyo. Acta Urologica Japonica. 1983;29(2):199–206.
23. Surg NC. The expansion of an area of skin by progressive distention of a subcutaneous balloon: use of the method for securing skin for subtotal reconstruction of the ear. Plast Reconstr Surg. 1957;19:124–30.
24. Goodman RC. Total reconstruction of a two-compartment scrotum by tissue expansion. Plast Reconstr Surg. 1990;85:805–7.

25. Still EF, Goodman RC. Total reconstruction of a two-compartment scrotum by tissue expansion. Plast Reconstr Surg. 1990;85:805–7.
26. Rapp DE, Cohn AB, Gottlieb LJ, Lyon MB, Bales GT. Use of tissue expansion for scrotal sac reconstruction after scrotal skin loss. Urology. 2005;65(6):1216–8.
27. Martín-Crespo Izquierdo R, Luque Pérez AL, Ramírez Velandia H, Luque Mialdea R. Escrotoplastia de relleno con acido hialurónico como alternativa mínimamente invasiva para aumentar el volumen escrotal hasta la pubertad [Hyaluronic acid scrotoplasty: minimally-invasive procedure to enhance the volume of scrotum until puberty]. Cir Pediatr. 2014;27(1):11–5. Spanish. PMID: 24783640.
28. Redett III RJ, Etra JW, Brandacher G, Burnett AL, Tuffaha SH, Sacks JM, Shores JT, et al. Total penis, scrotum, and lower abdominal wall transplantation. N Engl J Med. 2019;381(19):1876–8.
29. Wu Y. Experimental study on tissue engineered testicular prosthesis with internal support. Zhongguo Xiu Fu Chong Jian Wai Ke Za Zhi. 2007;21(11):1243–6.
30. Agarwal P. Scrotal reconstruction: our experience. J Surg Pakistan (Int). 2012;17(1):32–5.
31. Gencosmanoglu R, Bilkay U, Alper M, Gurler T, Cagdas A. Late results of split-grafted penoscrotal avulsion injuries. J Trauma Acute Care Surg. 1995;39(6):1201–3.
32. Thourani VH, Ingram WL, Feliciano DV. Factors affecting success of split-thickness skin grafts in the modern burn unit. J Trauma. 2003;54:562–8.
33. Wang D, Wei Z, Sun G, Luo Z. Thin-trimming of the scrotal reconstruction flap: long-term follow-up shows reversal of spermatogenesis arrest. J Plast Reconstr Aesthet Surg. 2009;62(11):e455–6.

# Index

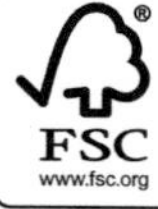